DBT® SKILLS TRAINING MANUAL

Also from Marsha M. Linehan

Books

Cognitive-Behavioral Treatment of Borderline Personality Disorder

DBT Skills Training Handouts and Worksheets, Second Edition

Dialectical Behavior Therapy with Suicidal Adolescents
Alec L. Miller, Jill H. Rathus, and Marsha M. Linehan

Mindfulness and Acceptance: Expanding the Cognitive-Behavioral Tradition
Edited by Steven C. Hayes, Victoria M. Follette, and Marsha M. Linehan

DVDs

Crisis Survival Skills, Part One: Distracting and Self-Soothing

Crisis Survival Skills, Part Two: Improving the Moment and Pros and Cons

From Suffering to Freedom: Practicing Reality Acceptance

Getting a New Client Connected to DBT (Complete Series)

Opposite Action: Changing Emotions You Want to Change

This One Moment: Skills for Everyday Mindfulness

Treating Borderline Personality Disorder: The Dialectical Approach

Understanding Borderline Personality: The Dialectical Approach

For more information and for DBT skills updates from the author,
see her websites:
www.linehaninstitute.org, http://blogs.uw.edu/brtc,
and *http://faculty.washington.edu/linehan/*

DBT® Skills Training Manual

SECOND EDITION

Marsha M. Linehan

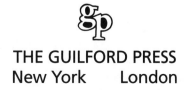

THE GUILFORD PRESS
New York   London

© 2015 Marsha M. Linehan

Published by The Guilford Press
A Division of Guilford Publications, Inc.
72 Spring Street, New York, NY 10012
www.guilford.com

Printed in the United States of America

This book is printed on acid-free paper.

Last digit is print number: 9   8   7   6   5   4   3   2   1

The author has checked with sources believed to be reliable in her efforts to provide information that is complete and generally in accord with the standards of practice that are accepted at the time of publication. However, in view of the possibility of human error or changes in behavioral, mental health, or medical sciences, neither the author, nor the editor and publisher, nor any other party who has been involved in the preparation or publication of this work warrants that the information contained herein is in every respect accurate or complete, and they are not responsible for any errors or omissions or the results obtained from the use of such information. Readers are encouraged to confirm the information contained in this book with other sources.

Library of Congress Cataloging-in-Publication Data

Linehan, Marsha, author.
    [Skills training manual for treating borderline personality disorder]
    DBT skills training manual / Marsha M. Linehan. — Second edition.
        p.   ;   cm.
    Dialectical behavior therapy skills training manual
    Preceded by: Skills training manual for treating borderline personality disorder / Marsha M. Linehan. c1993.
    Includes bibliographical references and index.
    ISBN 978-1-4625-1699-5 (paperback : alk. paper)
    1. Dialectical behavior therapy.   I. Title.   II. Title: Dialectical behavior therapy skills training manual.
    [DNLM: 1. Borderline Personality Disorder—therapy.   2. Behavior Therapy—methods.   3. Psychotherapeutic Processes.   4. Psychotherapy—methods.   5. Suicide—prevention & control.   WM 190.5.B5]
    RC489.D48
    616.89´142—dc23
                                                    2014026329

DBT is a registered trademark of Marsha M. Linehan.

When I teach my graduate students—who work with complex, difficult-to-treat individuals at high risk for suicide—I always remind them that they can choose whether to look out for themselves or to look out for their clients, but they cannot always do both. If they want to look out for themselves at a possible cost to their clients, I remind them that they are in the wrong profession.

I dedicate this book to all those who have found the courage to carry on this work at a possible cost to themselves.

I also dedicate it to my colleagues at the University of Washington Behavioral Research and Therapy Clinics: Elaine Franks, who has done everything possible to limit the costs to me; my students, who have kept me going when I wanted to stop; Katie Korslund, my second in command, who has given me such wise counsel; Melanie Harned, who has backed me up so many times in so many ways; and all those at the University of Washington Human Subjects Division, who have never even once impeded my often "out-of-the-box" research treating individuals at extremely high risk for suicide. Their willingness to allow such high-risk research when other universities likely would not sets an example for others—and made this book possible.

About the Author

Marsha M. Linehan, PhD, ABPP, is the developer of dialectical behavior therapy (DBT) and Professor of Psychology and of Psychiatry and Behavioral Sciences and Director of the Behavioral Research and Therapy Clinics at the University of Washington. Her primary research interest is in the development and evaluation of evidence-based treatments for populations with high suicide risk and multiple, severe mental disorders.

Dr. Linehan's contributions to suicide research and clinical psychology research have been recognized with numerous awards, including the Gold Medal Award for Life Achievement in the Application of Psychology from the American Psychological Foundation and the James McKeen Cattell Award from the Association for Psychological Science. In her honor, the American Association of Suicidology created the Marsha Linehan Award for Outstanding Research in the Treatment of Suicidal Behavior.

She is a Zen master and teaches mindfulness and contemplative practices via workshops and retreats for health care providers.

Preface

The original edition of this skills training manual was published in 1993. At that time, the only research conducted on Dialectical Behavior Therapy (DBT) was a 1991 clinical trial comparing DBT to treatment as usual for the treatment of chronically suicidal individuals meeting criteria for borderline personality disorder (BPD). Since then, an enormous amount of research has been conducted on "standard" DBT, which typically consists of DBT individual therapy, group skills training, telephone coaching, and a therapist consultation team. Research has also been conducted on stand-alone DBT skills training, and on the behavioral practices that together make up the DBT skills. The new skills in this edition are a product of my experience and research using the original skills; the wide-ranging research on emotions, emotion regulation, distress tolerance, and mindfulness, as well as new findings in the social sciences; and new treatment strategies developed within the cognitive-behavioral paradigm. The major changes in the revised skills package are described below.

Skills for Multiple Disorders and Nonclinical Populations

The original skills training manual was focused entirely on treating clients with high risk for suicide and BPD. This was primarily because the research on DBT, including DBT skills, had been conducted with clients meeting criteria for BPD and for high suicide risk. Since the first edition, however, a number of studies have been conducted focusing on skills training with different populations. For example, DBT skills training has been shown effective with eating disorders,[1, 2] treatment-resistant depression,[3, 4] and a variety of other disorders.[5] In

my colleagues' and my research, increases in use of skills mediates reductions in suicide attempts, nonsuicidal self-injury, difficulties regulating emotions, and interpersonal problems.[6] A subset of skills was also added to a treatment for problem drinkers and improved outcomes compared to a treatment without the skills.[7] A subset of DBT skills is taught in the evidence-based National Education Alliance for Borderline Personality Disorder's Family Connections program for family members of individuals with BPD. The entire set of core skills is taught in the friends and families skills groups at the University of Washington Behavioral Research and Therapy Clinics, which consist of individuals who want to learn skills for coping with and accepting individuals in their lives who are difficult. This could include friends or relatives with serious mental health problems, employees with problematic colleagues and/or managers, managers with problematic employees, and therapists treating very difficult client populations. Corporate consultants are looking at DBT skills as a way to improve corporate morale and productivity. New sets of specialized skills have been developed for specific disorders, including a module targeting emotion overcontrol,[8] middle path skills developed originally for parents and adolescents but appropriate for many populations,[9] skills for attention-deficit/hyperactivity disorder, and a set of skills specifically designed for individuals with addictions. DBT skills lesson plans are now being used in school systems to teach middle school and high school students,[10] are working their way into programs focused on resilience, and can be applied across work settings. DBT skills are widely taught in general mental health programs in community mental health, inpatient, acute care, forensic, and many other settings. In sum, there are substantial data and clinical experience suggesting that DBT skills are effective across a wide variety of both clinical and nonclinical populations and across settings.

Of course, it should not come as a surprise that DBT skills are widely applicable. I developed many of the skills by reading treatment manuals and treatment literature on evidence-based behavioral interventions. I then looked to see what therapists told patients to do for each problem, repackaged those instructions in skills handouts and worksheets, and wrote teaching notes for therapists. For example, for the skill "opposite action" (see Chapter 9) for fear, I repackaged exposure-based treatments for anxiety disorders in simpler language. I also applied the same principles of change across other disordered emotions. "Check the facts" is a core strategy in cognitive therapy interventions. DBT skills are what behavior therapists tell clients to do across many effective treatments. Some of the skills are entire treatment programs formulated as a series of steps. The new "nightmare protocol," an emotion regulation skill, is an example of this. The mindfulness skills are a product of my 18 years in Catholic schools, my training in contemplative prayer practices through the Shalem Institute's spiritual guidance program, and my 34 years as a Zen student and now as a Zen master. Other skills came from basic behavioral science and research in cognitive and social psychology. Some came from colleagues developing new DBT skills for new populations.

New Skills in This Edition

There are still four primary DBT skills training modules: mindfulness skills, interpersonal effectiveness skills, emotion regulation skills, and distress tolerance skills. Within these modules, I have added the following new skills.

1. In **mindfulness skills** (Chapter 7), I have added a section on teaching mindfulness from alternative perspectives, including a spiritual perspective.

2. In **interpersonal effectiveness skills** (Chapter 8), I have added two new sections. The first focuses on skills for finding and building relationships you want and ending relationships you don't want. The second focuses on balancing acceptance and change in interpersonal interactions. It closely duplicates the skills Alec Miller, Jill Rathus, and I developed for adolescent multifamily skills training, in which parents of adolescent clients also participate in skills training.[11]

3. The **emotion regulation skills** (Chapter 9) have been expanded greatly and also reorganized. The number of emotions described in detail has expanded from six to ten (adding disgust, envy, jealously, and guilt). A section on changing emotional responses adds two new skills: check the facts and problem solving. Also in that section, the opposite action skill has been extensively updated and expanded. Skills for reducing emotional vulnerability have been reorganized into a set of skills called the ABC PLEASE skills. In the section on accumulating positive emotions, I changed the Pleasant Events Schedule (now called the Pleasant Events List) to be appropriate for both adolescent and adult clients. I also added a values and priorities handout that lists a number of universal values and life priorities. Another new skill, cope ahead, focuses on practicing coping strategies in advance of difficult situations. Optional nightmare and sleep hygiene protocols are also included. Finally, a new section is added for recognizing extreme emotions ("Identify Your Personal Skills Breakdown Point"), including steps for using crisis survival skills to manage these emotions.

4. The **distress tolerance skills** (Chapter 10) now start with a new STOP skill—stop, take a step back, observe, and proceed mindfully—adapted from the skill developed by Francheska Perepletchikova, Seth Axelrod, and colleagues.[12] The crisis survival section now includes a new set of skills aimed at changing body chemistry to rapidly regulate extreme emotions (the new TIP skills). A new set of skills focused on reducing addictive behaviors has also been added: dialectical abstinence, clear mind, community reinforcement, burning bridges, building new ones, alternate rebellion, and adaptive denial.

5. Across modules I have also made a number of changes. Every module now starts with goals for that module along with a goals handout and a corresponding pros and cons worksheet. The worksheet is optional and can be used if the client is unwilling or ambivalent about practicing the skills in the module.

A mindfulness skill has been added to both the interpersonal module (mindfulness of others) and the distress tolerance module (mindfulness of current thoughts). Together with mindfulness of current emotion (emotion regulation), these additions are aimed at keeping the thread of mindfulness alive across time.

More Extensive Teaching Notes

Many people who have watched me teach DBT skills have commented that most of what I actually teach was not included in the first edition of this book. In this second edition, I have added much more information than was in the previous one. First, as much as possible I have included the research underpinnings for the skills included. Second, I have provided a very broad range of different teaching points that you can choose from in teaching, far more points than either you or I could possibly cover in a skills training class. The teaching notes may, at first, seem overwhelming. It is important to remember that this book is not to be read cover to cover at one sitting. Instead, teaching notes are organized by specific skills so that when teaching a specific skill you can find the notes just for that skill or set of skills. It will be important for you to read over the material for the skills you plan to teach and then highlight just those points that you wish to make when teaching. With practice over time, you will find that you expand your teaching to include different parts of the material. You will also find that some parts of the material fit some of your clients and other parts fit other clients. The material is meant to be used flexibly. With experience, you will no doubt start adding your own teaching points.

More Clinical Examples

A larger number of clinical examples are also included in this second edition. Examples are essential for good teaching. However, you should feel free to modify the examples provided and to substitute new ones to meet the needs of your clients. In fact, this is the major difference in teaching skills for various populations; one set of examples may be needed for clients with high emotion dysregulation and impulse control difficulties, another for those with emotion overcontrol, and another for substance-dependent clients. Differences in culture, ethnicity, nationality, socioeconomic status, and age may each necessitate different sets of examples. In my experience, it is the examples but not the skills that need to be changed across populations.

More Interactive Handouts and Optional Handouts

Many of the handouts have been modified to allow greater interaction during skills training sessions. Most have check boxes so participants can check items of importance to them or skills they are willing to practice in the coming weeks. Each module also now includes a number of optional handouts.

These have the same number as the core handout with which they are associated plus a letter (e.g., 1a, 1b). These optional handouts can be given out and taught to participants, given out but not formally taught, used by the skills trainer to teach but not given out, or simply ignored if not viewed as useful. My experience is that these optional handouts are extremely useful for some groups and individuals but not for others.

Improved Worksheets

By popular demand, homework sheets have been relabeled worksheets. Also, on each handout the corresponding worksheets are listed, and on each worksheet the corresponding handouts are listed.

There are now multiple alternative worksheets associated with many of the handouts. The increase in worksheets is due to a number of factors. First, it became clear over the years that a worksheet that works very well for one person may not be good for another person. As a result, I have developed a range of worksheets for each handout. For most skills sections, there is one set of worksheets that covers the skills in the entire section. This is for clients who are unlikely to complete much homework practice and can help those who have already completed skills training and are now working on maintaining their practice of skills.

Second, different clients like different types of practice. There are clients who want to check off what homework they have done, clients who prefer to describe their homework and rate its effectiveness, and those who like to write diaries describing what they have done and how it affected them. I have found it most effective to let clients choose worksheets to fill out from a set.

Multiple Teaching Schedules Outlined

The 1993 edition of the skills manual included the specific skills and worksheets that were used in the first randomized clinical trial of DBT. At that time, DBT had not spread very far, and there were not many examples of how to choose skills for situations in which some but not all of the skills could be taught, nor were skills developed at that time for special populations such as adolescents or individuals with addictions, eating disorders, and so forth. Given the many new skills in this edition, it is not possible to teach all the skills in a 24-week skills group, even when the skills are repeated for a second 24 weeks, as in a 1-year DBT treatment program. This edition includes a number of schedules for teaching skills, including schedules for 1-year, 6-month, and briefer skills training in acute care units and nontraditional settings. Schedules for particular populations (such as adolescents and substance abusers) are also provided. As often as possible, the teaching schedules are based on clinical trials that showed that the specific skills schedule was effective. With this in mind, there are now several sets of core DBT skills that are outlined in the appendices to Part I. My general strategy in teaching skills is to give participants all the DBT handouts and worksheets. I then follow a teaching schedule I determine based on the population, the number of weeks of treatment, and current research. Along the way, I tell participants that if we have time I will teach them other skills—if they talk me into it.

A Word about Terms

There are many terms for a person who teaches and coaches behavioral skills: therapist, psychotherapist, individual therapist, marital therapist, family therapist, milieu therapist, group therapist, group leader, counselor, case manager, skills trainer, behavioral coach, skills coach, crisis worker, mental health worker, mental health care provider, and so on. In this manual, the term "therapist" refers to a person who is providing psychotherapy or other mental health services. In standard DBT, this would be the person's individual therapist. The terms "skills trainer," "skills leader," "skills co-leader," and "leader" refer to individuals who are providing skills training either individually or in a group. In standard DBT, this refers to the group skills leaders. On occasion I use the term "provider" as a general reference to any person providing health care services.

References

1. Telch, C. F., Agras, W. S., Linehan, M. M. (2001). Dialectical behavior therapy for binge eating disorder. *Journal of Consulting and Clinical Psychology, 69*(6), 1061–1065.

2. Safer, D. L., & Jo, B. (2010). Outcome from a randomized controlled trial of group therapy for binge eating disorder: Comparing dialectical behavior therapy adapted for binge eating to an active comparison group therapy. *Behavior Therapy, 41*(1), 106–120.

3. Lynch, T. R., Morse, J. Q., Mendelson, T., & Robins, C. J. (2003). Dialectical behavior therapy for depressed older adults: A randomized pilot study. *American Journal of Geriatric Psychiatry, 11*(1), 33–45.

4. Harley, R., Sprich, S., Safren, S., Jacobo, M., & Fava, M. (2008). Adaptation of dialectical behavior therapy skills training group for treatment-resistant depression. *Journal of Nervous and Mental Disease, 196*(2), 136–143.

5. Soler, J., Pascual, J. C., Tiana, T., Cebria, A., Barrachina, J., Campins, M. J., & Pérez, V. (2009). Dialectical behaviour therapy skills training compared to standard group therapy in borderline personality disorder: A 3-month randomised controlled clinical trial. *Behaviour Research and Therapy, 47*, 353–358.

6. Neacsiu, A. D., Rizvi, S. L., & Linehan, M. M. (2010). Dialectical behavior therapy skills use as a mediator and outcome of treatment for borderline personality disorder. *Behaviour Research and Therapy, 48*(9), 832–8.

7. Whiteside, U. (2011). *A brief personalized feedback intervention integrating a motivational interviewing therapeutic style and dialectical behavior therapy skills for depressed or anxious heavy drinking young adults.* Unpublished doctoral dissertation, University of Washington.

8. Lynch, T. R. (in press). *Radically open DBT: Treating the overcontrolled client.* New York: Guilford Press.

9. Miller, A. L., Rathus, J. H., & Linehan, M. M. (2007). *Dialectical behavior therapy with suicidal adolescents.* New York: Guilford Press.

10. Mazza, J. J., Dexter-Mazza, E. T., Murphy, H. E., Miller, A. L., & Rathus, J. L. (in press). *Dialectical behavior therapy in schools.* New York: Guilford Press.

11. Miller, A. L., Rathus, J. H., Linehan, M. M., Wetzler, S., & Leigh, E. (1997). Dialectical behavior therapy adapted for suicidal adolescents. *Journal of Psychiatric Practice, 3*(2), 78–86.

12. Perepletchikova, F., Axelrod, S., Kaufman, J., Rounsaville, B. J., Douglas-Palumberi, H., & Miller, A. (2011). Adapting dialectical behavior therapy for children: Towards a new research agenda for paediatric suicidal and non-suicidal self-injurious behaviors. *Child and Adolescent Mental Health, 16*, 116–121.

Acknowledgments

There is truly something magical about being a university professor. Students arrive excited but often with threadbare knowledge, and before you know it they have not only climbed on your shoulders but have built a ladder from there reaching to the sky. I have been enormously privileged to have had many such students and postdoctoral fellows in my research clinic while I wrote this book. They have read countless versions of the skills presented here and tried out new skills, correcting, improving, and throwing them out as they went. They have radically accepted canceled meetings and frantic requests to find missing references, rearrange entire reference lists, and find research I knew I had read but could not locate to save my soul. They have helped me early in the day, at night, and when I called on weekends. They have stayed by my side even though my door said: "Do Not Disturb: Please Do Not Ignore This Message!" Although I am sure that I have missed some names here (please let me know for the next printing), I want especially to thank the following students and former students, now colleagues: Milton Brown, Linda Dimeff, Safia Jackson, Alissa Jerud, Anita Lungu, Ashley Maliken, Lyndsey Moran, Andrada Neacsiu, Shireen Rizvi, Cory Secrist, Adrianne Stevens, Stephanie Thompson, Chelsey Wilks, and Brianna Woods; and fellows and former fellows, now colleagues: Alex Chapman, Eunice Chen, Melanie Harned, Erin Miga, Marivi Navarro, and Nick Salman. Many others have jumped in when asked: colleagues Seth Axelrod, Kate Comtois and her entire DBT team, Sona Dimidjian, Anthony Dubose, Thomas Lynch, Helen McGowan, and Suzanne Witterholt. When I had something controversial to say, I sent it to the DBT strategic planning executive group (also known as the Linehan Institute Research Advisory Board) for approval: Martin Bohus, Alan Fruzzetti, André Ivanoff, Kathryn Korslund, and Shelley McMain.

No one with multiple jobs and never-ending demands on their time can get much done without strong administrative help. I could not have gotten this book done without the help of Elaine Franks, my fabulous administrative assistant. She canceled phone calls and meetings, said no before I could say yes, called me at all hours—morning, noon, and night—to see what I was doing and how I was progressing, and sent me repeated copies of things I had lost. Thao Truong, our office and financial manager, made sure that the whole place did not fall apart while everyone was waiting on me to finish tasks well beyond deadline.

Much of what is in this manual I learned from the many clients who participated in skills training groups that I have conducted over the years. I am grateful to all those who put up with the many versions that did not work or were not useful, and to those among them who gave enough feedback for me to make needed revisions in the skills being taught.

I want to thank Copyeditor Marie Sprayberry, Editorial Project Manager Anna Brackett, Senior Editor Barbara Watkins, Executive Editor Kitty Moore, and the staff at The Guilford Press. In getting this manual out in a timely fashion, they each had occasion to practice all the distress tolerance skills in this book. Their concern for the manuscript and for this form of treatment was evident at every step. Last, but certainly not least, I want to thank my family: Nate and Geraldine, who supported me at every step, and Catalina, who brought enough joy to keep us all going.

Contents

PART I

An Introduction to DBT Skills Training

PART II

Teaching Notes for DBT Skills Modules

Chapter 7   Mindfulness Skills   151

Chapter 8   Interpersonal Effectiveness Skills   231

Chapter 9   Emotion Regulation Skills   318

Chapter 10 Distress Tolerance Skills

List of Online Handouts and Worksheets

Purchasers can download and print the handouts and worksheets at *www.guilford.com/skills-training-manual*.

General Skills: Orientation and Analyzing Behavior

General Handouts

Orientation Handouts

General Handout 1: Goals of Skills Training
General Handout 1a: Options for Solving Any Problem
General Handout 2: Overview—Introduction to Skills Training
General Handout 3: Guidelines for Skills Training
General Handout 4: Skills Training Assumptions
General Handout 5: Biosocial Theory

Handouts for Analyzing Behavior

General Handout 6: Overview—Analyzing Behavior
General Handout 7: Chain Analysis
General Handout 7a: Chain Analysis, Step by Step
General Handout 8: Missing-Links Analysis

General Worksheets

Orientation Worksheet

General Worksheet 1: Pros and Cons of Using Skills

Worksheets for Analyzing Behavior

General Worksheet 2: Chain Analysis of Problem Behavior
General Worksheet 2a: Example—Chain Analysis of Problem Behavior
General Worksheet 3: Missing-Links Analysis

Mindfulness Skills

Mindfulness Handouts

Handouts for Goals and Definitions

Mindfulness Handout 1: Goals of Mindfulness Practice

Mindfulness Handout 1a: Mindfulness Definitions

Handouts for Core Mindfulness Skills

Mindfulness Handout 2: Overview—Core Mindfulness Skills

Mindfulness Handout 3: Wise Mind—States of Mind

Mindfulness Handout 3a: Ideas for Practicing Wise Mind

Mindfulness Handout 4: Taking Hold of Your Mind—"What" Skills

Mindfulness Handout 4a: Ideas for Practicing Observing

Mindfulness Handout 4b: Ideas for Practicing Describing

Mindfulness Handout 4c: Ideas for Practicing Participating

Mindfulness Handout 5: Taking Hold of Your Mind—"How" Skills

Mindfulness Handout 5a: Ideas for Practicing Nonjudgmentalness

Mindfulness Handout 5b: Ideas for Practicing One-Mindfulness

Mindfulness Handout 5c: Ideas for Practicing Effectiveness

Handouts for Other Perspectives on Mindfulness Skills

Mindfulness Handout 6: Overview—Other Perspectives on Mindfulness

Mindfulness Handout 7: Goals of Mindfulness Practice—A Spiritual Perspective

Mindfulness Handout 7a: Wise Mind from a Spiritual Perspective

Mindfulness Handout 8: Practicing Loving Kindness to Increase Love and Compassion

Mindfulness Handout 9: Skillful Means—Balancing Doing Mind and Being Mind

Mindfulness Handout 9a: Ideas for Practicing Balancing Doing Mind and Being Mind

Mindfulness Handout 10: Walking the Middle Path—Finding the Synthesis between Opposites

Mindfulness Worksheets

Worksheets for Core Mindfulness Skills

Mindfulness Worksheet 1: Pros and Cons of Practicing Mindfulness

Mindfulness Worksheet 2: Mindfulness Core Skills Practice

Mindfulness Worksheet 2a: Mindfulness Core Skills Practice

Mindfulness Worksheet 2b: Mindfulness Core Skills Practice

Mindfulness Worksheet 2c: Mindfulness Core Skills Calendar

Mindfulness Worksheet 3: Wise Mind Practice

Mindfulness Worksheet 4: Mindfulness "What" Skills—Observing, Describing, Participating

Mindfulness Worksheet 4a: Observing, Describing, Participating Checklist

Mindfulness Worksheet 4b: Observing, Describing, Participating Calendar

Mindfulness Worksheet 5: Mindfulness "How" Skills—Nonjudgmentalness,
   One-Mindfulness, Effectiveness
Mindfulness Worksheet 5a: Nonjudgmentalness, One-Mindfulness, Effectiveness Checklist
Mindfulness Worksheet 5b: Nonjudgmentalness, One-Mindfulness, Effectiveness Calendar
Mindfulness Worksheet 5c: Nonjudgmentalness Calendar

Worksheets for Other Perspectives on Mindfulness Skills

Mindfulness Worksheet 6: Loving Kindness
Mindfulness Worksheet 7: Balancing Being Mind with Doing Mind
Mindfulness Worksheet 7a: Mindfulness of Being and Doing Calendar
Mindfulness Worksheet 8: Mindfulness of Pleasant Events Calendar
Mindfulness Worksheet 9: Mindfulness of Unpleasant Events Calendar
Mindfulness Worksheet 10: Walking the Middle Path to Wise Mind
Mindfulness Worksheet 10a: Analyzing Yourself on the Middle Path
Mindfulness Worksheet 10b: Walking the Middle Path Calendar

Interpersonal Effectiveness Skills

Interpersonal Effectiveness Handouts

Handouts for Goals and Factors That Interfere

Interpersonal Effectiveness Handout 1: Goals of Interpersonal Effectiveness
Interpersonal Effectiveness Handout 2: Factors in the Way of Interpersonal Effectiveness
Interpersonal Effectiveness Handout 2a: Myths in the Way of Interpersonal Effectiveness

Handouts for Obtaining Objectives Skillfully

Interpersonal Effectiveness Handout 3: Overview—Obtaining Objectives Skillfully
Interpersonal Effectiveness Handout 4: Clarifying Goals in Interpersonal Situations
Interpersonal Effectiveness Handout 5: Guidelines for Objectives Effectiveness—
   Getting What You Want (DEAR MAN)
Interpersonal Effectiveness Handout 5a: Applying DEAR MAN Skills to a Difficult
   Current Interaction
Interpersonal Effectiveness Handout 6: Guidelines for Relationship Effectiveness—
   Keeping the Relationship (GIVE)
Interpersonal Effectiveness Handout 6a: Expanding the V in GIVE—Levels of Validation
Interpersonal Effectiveness Handout 7: Guidelines for Self-Respect Effectiveness—
   Keeping Respect for Yourself (FAST)
Interpersonal Effectiveness Handout 8: Evaluating Options for Whether or How Intensely
   to Ask for Something or Say No
Interpersonal Effectiveness Handout 9: Troubleshooting—When What You Are Doing
   Isn't Working

Handouts for Building Relationships and Ending Destructive Ones

Interpersonal Effectiveness Handout 10: Overview—Building Relationships
   and Ending Destructive Ones
Interpersonal Effectiveness Handout 11: Finding and Getting People to Like You

Interpersonal Effectiveness Worksheets

Worksheets for Walking the Middle Path

Interpersonal Effectiveness Worksheet 11: Practicing Dialectics
Interpersonal Effectiveness Worksheet 11a: Dialectics Checklist
Interpersonal Effectiveness Worksheet 11b: Noticing When You're Not Dialectical
Interpersonal Effectiveness Worksheet 12: Validating Others
Interpersonal Effectiveness Worksheet 13: Self-Validation and Self-Respect
Interpersonal Effectiveness Worksheet 14: Changing Behavior with Reinforcement
Interpersonal Effectiveness Worksheet 15: Changing Behavior by Extinguishing or Punishing It

Emotion Regulation Skills

Emotion Regulation Handouts

Emotion Regulation Handout 1: Goals of Emotion Regulation

Handouts for Understanding and Naming Emotions

Emotion Regulation Handout 2: Overview—Understanding and Naming Emotions
Emotion Regulation Handout 3: What Emotions Do for You
Emotion Regulation Handout 4: What Makes It Hard to Regulate Your Emotions
Emotion Regulation Handout 4a: Myths about Emotions
Emotion Regulation Handout 5: Model for Describing Emotions
Emotion Regulation Handout 6: Ways to Describe Emotions

Handouts for Changing Emotional Responses

Emotion Regulation Handout 7: Overview—Changing Emotional Responses
Emotion Regulation Handout 8: Check the Facts
Emotion Regulation Handout 8a: Examples of Emotions That Fit the Facts
Emotion Regulation Handout 9: Opposite Action and Problem Solving—Deciding Which to Use
Emotion Regulation Handout 10: Opposite Action
Emotion Regulation Handout 11: Figuring Out Opposite Actions
Emotion Regulation Handout 12: Problem Solving
Emotion Regulation Handout 13: Reviewing Opposite Action and Problem Solving

Handouts for Reducing Vulnerability to Emotion Mind

Emotion Regulation Handout 14: Overview—Reducing Vulnerability to Emotion Mind: Building a Live Worth Living
Emotion Regulation Handout 15: Accumulating Positive Emotions—Short Term
Emotion Regulation Handout 16: Pleasant Events List
Emotion Regulation Handout 17: Accumulating Positive Emotions—Long Term
Emotion Regulation Handout 18: Values and Priorities List
Emotion Regulation Handout 19: Build Mastery and Cope Ahead
Emotion Regulation Handout 20: Taking Care of Your Mind by Taking Care of Your Body
Emotion Regulation Handout 20a: Nightmare Protocol, Step by Step—When Nightmares Keep You from Sleeping
Emotion Regulation Handout 20b: Sleep Hygiene Protocol

Distress Tolerance Skills

Distress Tolerance Handouts

Distress Tolerance Handout 1: Goals of Distress Tolerance

Handouts for Crisis Survival Skills

Distress Tolerance Handout 2: Overview—Crisis Survival Skills

Distress Tolerance Handout 3: When to Use Crisis Survival Skills

Distress Tolerance Handout 4: STOP Skill

Distress Tolerance Handout 5: Pros and Cons

Distress Tolerance Handout 6: TIP Skills—Changing Your Body Chemistry

Distress Tolerance Handout 6a: Using Cold Water, Step by Step

Distress Tolerance Handout 6b: Paired Muscle Relaxation, Step by Step

Distress Tolerance Handout 6c: Effective Rethinking and Paired Relaxation, Step by Step

Distress Tolerance Handout 7: Distracting

Distress Tolerance Handout 8: Self-Soothing

Distress Tolerance Handout 8a: Body Scan Meditation Step by Step

Distress Tolerance Handout 9: Improving the Moment

Distress Tolerance Handout 9a: Sensory Awareness, Step by Step

Handouts for Reality Acceptance Skills

Distress Tolerance Handout 10: Overview—Reality Acceptance Skills

Distress Tolerance Handout 11: Radical Acceptance

Distress Tolerance Handout 11a: Radical Acceptance—Factors That Interfere

Distress Tolerance Handout 11b: Practicing Radical Acceptance Step by Step

Distress Tolerance Handout 12: Turning the Mind

Distress Tolerance Handout 13: Willingness

Distress Tolerance Handout 14: Half-Smiling and Willing Hands

Distress Tolerance Handout 14a: Practicing Half-Smiling and Willing Hands

Distress Tolerance Handout 15: Mindfulness of Current Thoughts

Distress Tolerance Handout 15a: Practicing Mindfulness of Thoughts

Handouts for Skills When the Crisis Is Addiction

Distress Tolerance Handout 16: Overview—When the Crisis Is Addiction

Distress Tolerance Handout 16a: Common Addictions

Distress Tolerance Handout 17: Dialectical Abstinence

Distress Tolerance Handout 17a: Planning for Dialectical Abstinence

Distress Tolerance Handout 18: Clear Mind

Distress Tolerance Handout 18a: Behavior Patterns Characteristic of Addict Mind and of Clean Mind

Distress Tolerance Handout 19: Community Reinforcement

Distress Tolerance Handout 20: Burning Bridges and Building New Ones

Distress Tolerance Handout 21: Alternate Rebellion and Adaptive Denial

Distress Tolerance Worksheets

Worksheets for Crisis Survival Skills

Distress Tolerance Worksheet 1: Crisis Survival Skills

Distress Tolerance Worksheet 1a: Crisis Survival Skills

Distress Tolerance Worksheet 1b: Crisis Survival Skills

Distress Tolerance Worksheet 2: Practicing the STOP Skill

Distress Tolerance Worksheet 2a: Practicing the STOP Skill

Distress Tolerance Worksheet 3: Pros and Cons of Acting on Crisis Urges

Distress Tolerance Worksheet 3a: Pros and Cons of Acting on Crisis Urges

Distress Tolerance Worksheet 4: Changing Body Chemistry with TIP Skills

Distress Tolerance Worksheet 4a: Paired Muscle Relaxation

Distress Tolerance Worksheet 4b: Effective Rethinking and Paired Relaxation

Distress Tolerance Worksheet 5: Distracting with Wise Mind ACCEPTS

Distress Tolerance Worksheet 5a: Distracting with Wise Mind ACCEPTS

Distress Tolerance Worksheet 5b: Distracting with Wise Mind ACCEPTS

Distress Tolerance Worksheet 6: Self-Soothing

Distress Tolerance Worksheet 6a: Self-Soothing

Distress Tolerance Worksheet 6b: Self-Soothing

Distress Tolerance Worksheet 6c: Body Scan Meditation, Step by Step

Distress Tolerance Worksheet 7: IMPROVE the Moment

Distress Tolerance Worksheet 7a: IMPROVE the Moment

Distress Tolerance Worksheet 7b: IMPROVE the Moment

Worksheets for Reality Acceptance Skills

Distress Tolerance Worksheet 8: Reality Acceptance Skills

Distress Tolerance Worksheet 8a: Reality Acceptance Skills

Distress Tolerance Worksheet 8b: Reality Acceptance Skills

Distress Tolerance Worksheet 9: Radical Acceptance

Distress Tolerance Worksheet 9a: Practicing Radical Acceptance

Distress Tolerance Worksheet 10: Turning the Mind, Willingness, Willfulness

Distress Tolerance Worksheet 11: Half-Smiling and Willing Hands

Distress Tolerance Worksheet 11a: Practicing Half-Smiling and Willing Hands

Distress Tolerance Worksheet 12: Mindfulness of Current Thoughts

Distress Tolerance Worksheet 12a: Practicing Mindfulness of Thoughts

Worksheets for Skills When the Crisis Is Addiction

Distress Tolerance Worksheet 13: Skills When the Crisis Is Addiction

Distress Tolerance Worksheet 14: Planning for Dialectical Abstinence

Distress Tolerance Worksheet 15: From Clean Mind to Clear Mind

Distress Tolerance Worksheet 16: Reinforcing Nonaddictive Behaviors

Distress Tolerance Worksheet 17: Burning Bridges and Building New Ones

Distress Tolerance Worksheet 18: Practicing Alternate Rebellion and Adaptive Denial

PART I

An Introduction to DBT Skills Training

Chapter 1

Rationale for Dialectical Behavior Therapy Skills Training

What Is DBT?

The behavioral skills training described in this manual is based on a model of treatment called Dialectical Behavior Therapy (DBT). DBT is a broad-based cognitive-behavioral treatment originally developed for chronically suicidal individuals diagnosed with borderline personality disorder (BPD). Consisting of a combination of individual psychotherapy, group skills training, telephone coaching, and a therapist consultation team, DBT was the first psychotherapy shown through controlled trials to be effective with BPD.[1] Since then, multiple clinical trials have been conducted demonstrating the effectiveness of DBT not only for BPD, but also for a wide range of other disorders and problems, including both undercontrol and overcontrol of emotions and associated cognitive and behavioral patterns. Furthermore, an increasing number of studies (summarized later in this chapter) suggest that skills training alone is a promising intervention for a variety of populations, such as persons with drinking problems, families of suicidal individuals, victims of domestic abuse, and others.

DBT, including DBT skills training, is based on a dialectical and biosocial theory of psychological disorder that emphasizes the role of difficulties in regulating emotions, both under and over control, and behavior. Emotion dysregulation has been linked to a variety of mental health problems[2] stemming from patterns of instability in emotion regulation, impulse control, interpersonal relationships, and self-image. DBT skills are aimed directly at these dysfunctional patterns. The overall goal of DBT skills training is to help individuals change behavioral, emotional, thinking, and interpersonal patterns associated with problems in living. Therefore, understanding the treatment philosophy and theoretical underpinnings of DBT as a whole is critical for effective use of this manual. Such understanding is also important because it determines therapists' attitude toward treatment and their clients. This attitude, in turn, is an important component of therapists' relationships with their clients, which are often central to effective treatment and can be particularly important with suicidal and severely dysregulated individuals.

A Look Ahead

This manual is organized into two main parts. Part I (Chapters 1–5) orients readers to DBT and to DBT skills training in particular. Part II (Chapters 6–10) contains the detailed instructions for teaching the specific skills. The client handouts and worksheets for all of the skills modules can be found at a special website for this manual (*www.guilford.com/skills-training-manual*). They can be printed out for distribution to clients, and modified as necessary to fit a particular setting. A separate, printed volume of handouts and worksheets, ideal for client use, which has its own website where clients can print their own forms, is also available for purchase.

In the rest of this chapter, I describe the dialectical world view underpinning the treatment, and the assumptions inherent in such a view. The biosocial model of severe emotion dysregulation (including BPD) and its development are then described, as well as how variations on the model apply to difficulties in emotion regulation in general. As noted above, the DBT skills presented in this manual are specifically designed to address emotion dysregulation and its maladaptive consequences. Chapter 1 concludes with a brief overview of the research on standard DBT (individual psychotherapy, phone coaching, consultation team, and skills training), as well as the research on DBT skills training minus the individual therapy component. In Chapters 2–5, I discuss practical aspects of skills training: planning skills training, including ideas for different skills curricula based on client population and the setting (Chapter 2); structuring session format and starting skills training (Chapter 3); DBT skills training treatment targets and procedures (Chapter 4); and applying other DBT strategies and procedures to behavioral skills training (Chapter 5). Together, these chapters set the stage for deciding how to conduct skills training in a particular clinic or practice. A set of Appendices to Part I consists of 11 different curricula for skills training programs.

In Part II, Chapter 6 begins the formal skills training component of DBT. It covers how to introduce clients to DBT skills training and orient them to its goals. Guidelines on how to teach specific skills then follow, grouped into four skills modules: Mindfulness Skills (Chapter 7), Interpersonal Effectiveness Skills (Chapter 8), Emotion Regulation Skills (Chapter 9), and Distress Tolerance Skills (Chapter 10).

Every skill has corresponding client handouts with instructions for practicing that skill. Every handout has at least one (usually more than one) associated worksheet for clients to record their practice of the skills. Again, all of these client handouts and worksheets can be found at the special Guilford website for this manual (see above for the URL), as well as in the separate volume. Descriptions of handouts and related worksheets are given in boxes at the start of each main section within the skill modules' teaching notes (Chapters 6–10).

I should note here that all skills training in our clinical trials was conducted in groups, although we do conduct individual skills training in my clinic. Many of the treatment guidelines in this manual assume that skills training is being conducted in groups, mainly because it is easier to adapt group skills training techniques for individual clients than vice versa. (The issue of group vs. individual skills training is discussed at some length in the next chapter.)

This manual is a companion to my more complete text on DBT, *Cognitive-Behavioral Treatment of Borderline Personality Disorder*.[3] Although DBT skills are effective for disorders other than BPD, the principles underlying the treatment are still important and are discussed fully there. Because I refer to that book often throughout this manual, from

here on I simply call it "the main DBT text." The scientific underpinnings and references for many of my statements and positions are fully documented in Chapters 1–3 of that text; thus I do not review or cite them here again.

The Dialectical World View and Basic Assumptions

As its name suggests, DBT is based on a dialectical world view. "Dialectics" as applied to behavior therapy has two meanings: that of the fundamental nature of reality, and that of persuasive dialogue and relationship. As a world view or philosophical position, dialectics forms the basis of DBT. Alternatively, as dialogue and relationship, dialectics refers to the treatment approach or strategies used by the therapist to effect change. These strategies are described in full in Chapter 7 of the main DBT text and are summarized in Chapter 5 of this manual.

Dialectical perspectives on the nature of reality and human behavior share three primary characteristics. First, much as dynamic systems perspectives do, dialectics stresses the fundamental interrelatedness or wholeness of reality. This means that a dialectical approach views analyses of individual parts of a system as of limited value unless the analysis clearly relates the parts to the whole. Thus dialectics directs our attention to the individual parts of a system (i.e., one specific behavior), as well as to the interrelatedness of the part to other parts (e.g., other behaviors, the environmental context) and to the larger wholes (e.g., the culture, the state of the world at the time). With respect to skills training, a therapist must take into account first the interrelatedness of skills deficits. Learning one new set of skills is extremely difficult without learning other related skills simultaneously—a task that is even more difficult. A dialectical view is also compatible with both contextual and feminist views of psychopathology. Learning behavioral skills is particularly hard when a person's immediate environment or larger culture do not support such learning. Thus the individual must learn not only self-regulation skills and skills for influencing his or her environment, but also when to regulate them.

Second, reality is not seen as static, but as made up of internal opposing forces (thesis and antithesis) out of whose synthesis evolves a new set of opposing forces. A very important dialectical idea is that all propositions contain within them their own oppositions. As Goldberg put it, "I assume that truth is paradoxical, that each article of wisdom contains within it its own contradictions, that *truths stand side by side*" (pp. 295–296, emphasis in original).[4] Dialectics, in this sense, is compatible with psychodynamic conflict models of psychopathology. Dichotomous and extreme thinking, behavior, and emotions are viewed as dialectical failures. The individual is stuck in polarities, unable to move to syntheses. With respect to behavioral skills training, three specific polarities can make progress extremely difficult. The therapist must pay attention to each polarity and assist each client in moving toward a workable synthesis.

The first of these polarities is the dialectic between the need for clients to accept themselves as they are in the moment and the need for them to change. This particular dialectic is the most fundamental tension in any psychotherapy, and the therapist must negotiate it skillfully if change is to occur.

The second is the tension between clients' getting what they need to become more competent, and losing what they need if they become more competent. I once had a client in skills training who every week reported doing none of the behavioral homework assignments and insisted that the treatment was not working. When after 6 months I suggested that maybe this wasn't the treatment for her, she reported that she had been trying the new skills all along and they *had* helped. However, she had not let me know about it because she was afraid that if she showed any improvement, I would dismiss her from skills training.

A third very important polarity has to do with clients' maintaining personal integrity and validating their own views of their difficulties versus learning new skills that will help them emerge from their suffering. If clients get better by learning new skills, they validate their view that the problem all along was that they did not have sufficient skills to help themselves. They have not been trying to manipulate people, as others have accused them of doing. They are not motivated to hurt others, and they do not lack positive motivation. But the clients' learning new skills may also seem to validate others' opinions in other ways: It may appear to prove that others were right all along (and the client was wrong), or that the client was the problem (not the environment). Dialectics not only focuses the client's attention on these polarities, but also suggests ways out of them. (Ways out are discussed in Chapter 7 of the main DBT text.)

The third characteristic of dialectics is an assumption, following from the two characteristics above, that the fundamental nature of reality is change and process rather than content or structure. The most important implication here is that both the individual and the environment are undergoing continuous transition. Thus therapy does not focus on maintaining a stable, consistent environment, but rather aims to help the client become comfortable with change. An example of this is that we discourage people from sitting in exactly the same seats in a skills training group for the whole time they are in the group. Within skills training, therapists must keep aware not only of how their clients are changing, but also of how they themselves and the treatment they are applying are changing over time.

Biosocial Theory: How Emotion Dysregulation Develops*

As noted earlier, DBT was originally developed for individuals who were highly suicidal, and secondarily for individuals who met criteria for BPD. Effective treatment, however, requires a coherent theory. My first task, therefore, was to develop a theory that would let me understand the act of suicide, as well as BPD. I had three criteria for my theory: It had to (1) guide treatment implementation, (2) engender compassion, and (3) fit the research data. The biosocial theory I developed was based on the premise that both suicide and BPD are, at their core, disorders of emotion dysregulation. Suicidal behavior is a response to unbearable emotional suffering. BPD is a severe mental disorder resulting from serious dysregulation of the affective system. Individuals with BPD show a characteristic pattern of instability in affect regulation, impulse control, interpersonal relationship, and self-image.

---

*The ideas discussed in this section on the biosocial theory in general (and the DBT model of emotions in particular) are not only drawn from the main DBT text, but also based on the following: Neacsiu, A. D., Bohus, M., & Linehan, M. M. (2014). Dialectical behavior therapy: An intervention for emotion dysregulation. In J. J. Gross (Ed.), *Handbook of emotion regulation* (2nd ed., pp. 491–507). New York: Guilford Press; and Crowell, S. E., Beauchaine, T. P., & Linehan, M. M. (2009). A biosocial developmental model of borderline personality: Elaborating and extending Linehan's theory. *Psychological Bulletin, 135*(3), 495–510. Neacsiu et al. discuss emotion dysregulation as central to BPD and mental disorder, and Crowell et al. present an elaboration and extension of my original biosocial theory.

Emotion dysregulation has also been related to a variety of other mental health problems. Substance use disorders, eating disorders, and many other destructive behavioral patterns often function as escapes from unbearable emotions. Theorists have proposed that major depressive disorder should be conceptualized as an emotion dysregulation disorder, based partly on a deficit in up-regulating and maintaining positive emotions.[5] Similarly, literature reviews have demonstrated that anxiety disorders, schizophrenia, and even bipolar disorders are directly linked to emotion dysregulation.[6,7]

The DBT Model of Emotions

To understand emotion dysregulation, we have to first understand what emotions actually are. Proposing any definition of the construct "emotion," however, is fraught with difficulty, and there is rarely agreement even among emotion researchers on any one concrete definition. That being said, teaching clients about emotions and emotion regulation requires some attempt at a description of emotions, if not an exact definition. DBT in general, and DBT skills in particular, are based on the view that emotions are brief, involuntary, full-system, patterned responses to internal and external stimuli.[8] Similar to others' views, DBT emphasizes the importance of the evolutionary adaptive value of emotions in understanding them.[9] Although emotional responses are systemic responses, they can be viewed as consisting of the following interacting subsystems: (1) emotional vulnerability to cues; (2) internal and/ or external events that, when attended to, serve as emotional cues (e.g., prompting events); (3) appraisal and interpretations of the cues; (4) response tendencies, including neurochemical and physiological responses, experiential responses, and action urges; (5) nonverbal and verbal expressive responses and actions; and (6) aftereffects of the initial emotional "firing," including secondary emotions. It is useful to consider the patterned actions associated with emotional responses to be part and parcel of the emotional responses rather than consequences of the emotions. By combining all these elements into one interactional system, DBT emphasizes that modifying any component of the emotional system is likely to change the functioning of the entire system. In short, if one wants to change one's own emotions, including emotional actions, it can be done by modifying any part of the system.

Emotion Dysregulation

Emotion dysregulation is the inability, even when one's best efforts are applied, to change or regulate emotional cues, experiences, actions, verbal responses, and/or nonverbal expressions under normative conditions. Pervasive emotion dysregulation is seen when the inability to regulate emotions occurs across a wide range of emotions, adaptation problems, and situational contexts. Pervasive emotion dysregulation is due to vulnerability to high emotionality, together with an inability to regulate intense emotion-linked responses. Characteristics of emotion dysregulation include an excess of painful emotional experiences; an inability to regulate intense arousal; problems turning attention away from emotional cues; cognitive distortions and failures in information processing; insufficient control of impulsive behaviors related to strong positive and negative affect; difficulties organizing and coordinating activities to achieve non-mood-dependent goals during emotional arousal; and a tendency to "freeze" or dissociate under very high stress. It can also present as emotion overcontrol and suppression, which leads to pervasive negative affect, low positive affect, an inability to up-regulate emotions, and difficulty with affective communication. Systemic dysregulation is produced by emotional vulnerability and by maladaptive and inadequate emotion modulation strategies. Emotional vulnerability is defined by these characteristics: (1) very high negative affectivity as a baseline, (2) sensitivity to emotional stimuli, (3) intense response to emotional stimuli, and (4) slow return to emotional baseline once emotional arousal has occurred.

Emotion Regulation

Emotion regulation, in contrast, is the ability to (1) inhibit impulsive and inappropriate behavior related to strong negative or positive emotions; (2) organize oneself for coordinated action in the service of an external goal (i.e., act in a way that is not mood-dependent when necessary); (3) self-soothe any physiological arousal that the strong emotion has induced; and (4) refocus attention in the presence of strong emotion. Emotion regulation can be automatic as well as consciously controlled. In DBT, the focus is first on increasing conscious control, and second on eliciting sufficient practice to overlearn skills such that they ultimately become automatic.

Biological Vulnerabilities (the "Bio" in the Biosocial Theory)[10]*

Dispositions to negative affectivity, high sensitivity to emotion cues, and impulsivity are biologically based precursors to emotion dysregulation. The biological influences include heredity, intrauterine factors, childhood or adulthood physical insults affecting the brain, and the effects of early learning experiences on both brain development and brain functioning. A dysfunction in any part of the extremely complex human emotion regulation system can provide the biological basis for initial emotional vulnerability and subsequent difficulties in emotion modulation. Thus the biological disposition may be different in different people.

Two dimensions of infant temperament, effortful control and negative affectivity, are particularly relevant here. Effortful control, which contributes to both emotional and behavioral regulation, is a general term for a number of self-regulation behaviors (including inhibiting dominant responses to engage in less dominant responses, planning, and detecting errors in behavior). Children at risk for pervasive emotion dysregulation and behavioral dyscontrol are likely to be low on effortful control and high on negative affectivity, which is characterized by discomfort, frustration, shyness, sadness, and inability to be soothed.

The Caregiving Environment (the "Social" in the Biosocial Theory)

The contributions of the social environment, particularly the family, include (1) a tendency to invalidate emotions and an inability to model appropriate expressions of emotion; (2) an interaction style that reinforces emotional arousal; and (3) a poor fit between the child's temperament and the caregivers' parenting style. This final point is emphasized here because it highlights the biology × environment transactions that shape both child and caregiver behaviors. In theory, a child with low biological vulnerability may be at risk for BPD and/or high emo-

tion dysregulation if there is an extreme discrepancy between child and caregiver characteristics, or if the family's resources are extremely taxed (e.g., by a family member's alcoholism or a sibling with cancer). Such situations have the potential to perpetuate invalidation, because the demands of the child often exceed the ability of the environment to meet those demands.

The converse is also likely: A biologically vulnerable child may be resilient in a well-matched environment where strong family supports are in place. Such differential outcomes led me to propose three primary types of families that increase risk for BPD: the disorganized family (e.g., one that is pervasively neglectful or maltreating); the perfect family (e.g., one where expressing negative emotions is taboo), and the normal family (one characterized primarily by poorness of fit). Importantly, caregiver characteristics are not necessarily fixed or preexisting. Rather, the caregiver is also a product of complex biological, social, and psychological transactions, including evocative effects of the child on parenting style.

The Role of the Invalidating Environment

The role of invalidation in the development of emotion dysregulation makes a lot of sense, once you realize that a primary function of emotions in humans (as well as other mammals) is to serve as a rapid communication system. Invalidation of emotions sends the message that the communication was not received. When the message is important, the sender understandably escalates the communication by escalating the emotion. When the receiver does not "get" the communication or disbelieves it, he or she understandably increases efforts to stop the communication, usually by some means of invalidation. And so it goes, around and around, escalating on both sides until one side backs down. It is often the receiver who finally stops and listens or gives in to the demands of the highly emotional sender. Ergo, escalation has been reinforced. When this continues intermittently, the pattern of escalated emotion dysregulation is cemented.

Such an environment is particularly damaging for a child who begins life with high emotional vulnerability. The emotionally vulnerable and reactive individual elicits invalidation from an environment that might have otherwise been supportive. A defining characteristic of an invalidating environment is the

*The "Biological Vulnerabilities (the "Bio" in the Biosocial Theory)" section is adapted from Crowell, S. E., Beauchaine, T. P., & Linehan, M. M. (2009). A biosocial developmental model of borderline personality: Elaborating and extending Linehan's theory. *Psychological Bulletin, 135*(3), 495–510. Copyright 2009 by the American Psychological Association. Adapted by permission.

tendency to respond erratically and inappropriately to private experience (e.g., beliefs, thoughts, feelings, sensations), and in particular to be insensitive to private experience that does not have public accompaniments. Invalidating environments also tend to respond in an extreme fashion (i.e., to over- or underreact) to private experiences that do have public accompaniments. Phenomenological, physiological, and cognitive components of emotions are prototypic private experiences that lead to invalidation in these settings. To clarify the invalidating environment's contribution to emotionally dysregulated behavioral patterns, let us contrast it to environments that foster more adaptive emotion regulation skills.

In the optimal family, public validation of private experience is given frequently. For example, when a child says, "I'm thirsty," parents give him or her a drink (rather than saying, "No, you're not. You just had a drink"). When a child cries, parents soothe the child or attempt to find out what is wrong (rather than saying, "Stop being a crybaby!"). When a child expresses anger or frustration, family members take it seriously (rather than dismissing it as unimportant). When the child says, "I did my best," the parent agrees (rather than saying, "No, you didn't"). And so on. In the optimal family, the child's preferences (e.g., for color of room, activities, or clothes) are taken into account; the child's beliefs and thoughts are elicited and responded to seriously; and the child's emotions are viewed as important communications. Successful communication of private experience in such a family is followed by changes in other family members' behavior. These changes increase the probability that the child's needs will be met and decrease the probability of negative consequences. Parental responding that is attuned and is not aversive results in children who are better able to discriminate their own and others' emotions.

By contrast, an invalidating family is problematic because the people in it respond to the communication of preferences, thoughts, and emotions with nonattuned responses—specifically, with either nonresponsiveness or extreme consequences. This leads to an intensification of the differences between an emotionally vulnerable child's private experience and the experience the social environment actually supports and responds to. Persistent discrepancies between a child's private experience and what others in the environment describe as the child's experience provide the fundamental learning environment necessary for many of the behavioral problems associated with emotion dysregulation.

In addition to early failures to respond optimally, an invalidating environment more generally emphasizes controlling emotional expressiveness, especially the expression of negative affect. Painful experiences are often trivialized and attributed to negative traits, such as lack of motivation, lack of discipline, and failure to adopt a positive attitude. Strong positive emotions and associated preferences may be attributed to other negative traits, such as lack of judgment and reflection or impulsivity. Other characteristics of the invalidating environment include restricting the demands a child may make upon the environment, discriminating against the child on the basis of gender or other arbitrary characteristics, and using punishment (from criticism up to physical and sexual abuse) to control behavior.

The invalidating environment contributes to emotion dysregulation by failing to teach the child to label and modulate arousal, to tolerate distress, or to trust his or her own emotional responses as valid interpretations of events. It also actively teaches the child to invalidate his or her own experiences by making it necessary for the child to scan the environment for cues about how to act and feel. By oversimplifying the ease of solving life's problems, it fails to teach the child how to set realistic goals. Moreover, by punishing the expression of negative emotion and erratically reinforcing emotional communication only after escalation by the child, the family shapes an emotional expression style that vacillates between extreme inhibition and extreme disinhibition. In other words, the family's usual response to emotion cuts off the communicative function of ordinary emotions.

Emotional invalidation, particularly of negative emotions, is an interaction style characteristic of societies that put a premium on individualism, including individual self-control and individual achievement. Thus, it is quite characteristic of Western culture in general. A certain amount of invalidation is, of course, necessary in raising a child and teaching self-control. Not all communications of emotions, preferences, or beliefs can be responded to in a positive fashion. The child who is highly emotional and who has difficulty controlling emotional behaviors will elicit from the environment (especially parents, but also friends and teachers) the greatest efforts to control the emotionality from the outside. Invalidation can be quite effective at temporarily inhibiting emotional expression. Invalidating environments, however, have different effects on different children. The emotion control strategies used in invalidating families may have little negative impact on children who are physiologically well equipped to regulate their emotions, or may even be useful to some such children. However, such strategies are hypothesized to have a devastating impact on emotionally vulnerable children.

This transactional view of the development of pervasive emotion dysregulation generally should not be used to diminish the importance of trauma in the etiology of BPD and emotion dysregulation. Researchers have estimated that up to 60–75% of individuals with BPD have histories of childhood trauma,[11, 12] and many continue to experience further trauma during adulthood.[13, 14] In one study, researchers found that 90% of inpatients with BPD reported some experience of adult verbal, emotional, physical, and/or sexual abuse, and that these rates of adult abuse were significantly higher than those reported by comparison participants with Axis II disorders other than BPD.[14] It is unclear, however, whether the trauma in and of itself facilitates the development of BPD and of high emotion dysregulation patterns, or whether the trauma and the development of the disorder both result from the extant familial dysfunction and invalidation. In other words, the occurrence of victimization and emotion regulation problems may arise from the same set of developmental circumstances.

Development of Emotion Dysregulation: Summary

Emotion dysregulation in general, as well as the dysregulation encountered in BPD specifically, is an outcome of biological disposition, environmental context, and the transaction between the two during development. The biosocial developmental model proposes the following: (1) The development of extreme emotional lability is based on characteristics of the child (e.g., baseline emotional sensitivity, impulsivity), in transaction with a social context that shapes and maintains the lability; (2) reciprocal reinforcing transactions between biological vulnerabilities and environmental risk factors increase emotion dysregulation and behavioral dyscontrol, which contribute to negative cognitive and social outcomes; (3) a constellation of identifiable features and maladaptive coping strategies develops over time; and (4) these traits and behaviors may exacerbate risk for pervasive emotion dysregulation across development, due to evocative effects on interpersonal relationships and social functioning, and via

interference with healthy emotional development. This model is illustrated in Figure 1.1.

The Consequences of Emotion Dysregulation

Maccoby has argued that the inhibition of action is the basis for the organization of all behavior.[15] The development of self-regulatory repertoires (as in effortful control, described above), especially the ability to inhibit and control affect, is one of the most important aspects of a child's development. The ability to regulate the experience and expression of emotion is crucial, because its absence leads to the disruption of behavior, especially goal-directed behavior and other prosocial behavior. Alternatively, strong emotion reorganizes or redirects behavior, preparing the individual for actions that compete with the nonemotionally or less emotionally driven behavioral repertoire.

The behavioral characteristics of individuals meeting criteria for a wide range of emotional disorders, can be conceptualized as the effects of emotion dysregulation and maladaptive emotion regulation strategies. Impulsive behavior, and especially self-injurious and suicidal behaviors, can be thought of as maladaptive but highly effective emotion regulation strategies. For example, overdosing usually leads to long periods of sleep, which in turn reduce susceptibility to emotion dysregulation. Although the mechanism by which self-mutilation exerts affect-regulating properties is not clear, it is very common for individuals engaging in such behavior to report substantial relief from anxiety and other intense negative emotional states following such acts. Suicidal behavior is also very effective in eliciting helping behaviors from the environment, which may be effective in avoiding or changing situations that elicit emotional pain. For example, suicidal behavior is generally the most effective way for a nonpsychotic individual to be admitted to an inpatient psychiatric unit. Suicide ideation, suicide planning, and imagining dying from suicide, when accompanied with a belief that pain will end with death, can bring an intense sense of relief. Finally, planning suicide, imagining suicide, and engaging in a self-injurious act (and its aftereffects if it becomes public) can reduce painful emotions by providing a compelling distraction.

The inability to regulate emotional arousal also interferes with the development and maintenance

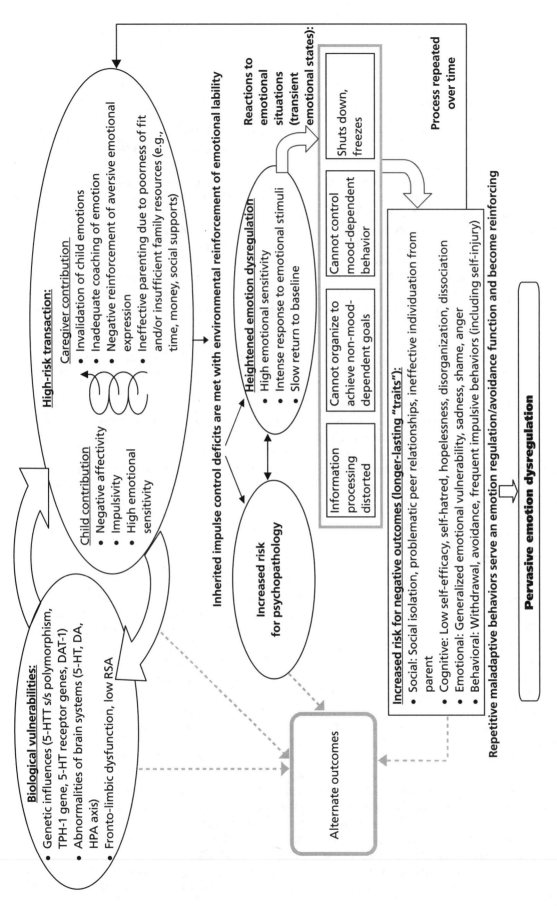

FIGURE 1.1. Illustration of the biosocial developmental model of BPD. 5-HT, serotonin; 5-HTT, serotonin transporter; TPH-1, tryptophan hydroxylase 1; DA, dopamine; DAT-1, dopamine transporter 1; HPA, hypothalamic–pituitary–adrenocortical; RSA, respiratory sinus arrhythmia. Adapted from Crowell, S. E., Beauchaine, T. P., & Lenzenweger, M. F. (2008). The development of borderline personality and self-injurious behavior. In T. P. Beauchaine & S. Hinshaw (Eds.), *Child psychopathology* (p. 528). Hoboken, NJ: Wiley. Copyright 2008 by John Wiley & Sons, Inc. Adapted by permission.

of a sense of self. Generally, one's sense of self is formed by observations of oneself and of others' reactions to one's actions. Emotional consistency and predictability, across time and similar situations, are prerequisites of identity development. Unpredictable emotional lability leads to unpredictable behavior and cognitive inconsistency, and consequently interferes with identity development. The tendency of dysregulated individuals to try to inhibit emotional responses may also contribute to an absence of a strong sense of identity. The numbness associated with inhibited affect is often experienced as emptiness, further contributing to an inadequate and at times completely absent sense of self. Similarly, if an individual's sense of events is never "correct" or is unpredictably "correct"—the situation in an invalidating environment—then the individual may be expected to develop an overdependence on others.

Effective interpersonal relationships depend on both a stable sense of self and a capacity for spontaneity in emotional expression. Successful relationships also require a capacity for self-regulation of emotions and tolerance of emotionally painful stimuli. Without such capabilities, it is understandable that individuals develop chaotic relationships. When emotion dysregulation is pervasive or severe, it interferes with a stable sense of self and with normal emotional expression. Difficulties controlling impulsive behaviors and expressions of extreme negative emotions can wreak havoc on relationships in many ways; in particular, difficulties with anger and anger expression preclude the maintenance of stable relationships.

Relationship of Emotion Dysregulation to DBT Skills Training[16]

As noted above, many mental disorders can be conceptualized as disorders of emotion regulation, with deficits in both up- and down-regulation. Once you realize that emotions include both actions and action tendencies, you can see the link between emotion dysregulation and many disorders defined as behavior dyscontrol (e.g., substance use disorders). DBT skills are aimed directly at these dysfunctional patterns.

First, dysregulation of the sense of self is common in individuals with severe emotion dysregulation. In both depression and BPD, for example, it is not unusual for individuals to report having no sense of a self at all, feeling empty, and not knowing who they

are. Feelings of being disconnected from others, of contempt for self, and of invalidity or worthlessness are also common. In addition, individuals with high emotion dysregulation often view reality through the lens of their emotions, rather than the light of reality as it is. Thus both judgmental responses and distorted inferences, assumptions, and beliefs are common sequelae. To address such dysregulation of the sense of self, the first DBT skills training module (Chapter 7) aims to teach a core set of "mindfulness" skills—that is, skills having to do with the ability to consciously experience and observe oneself and surrounding events with curiosity and without judgment; to see and articulate reality as it is; and to participate in the flow of the present moment effectively. To address the impact of high emotionality, mindfulness skills also focuses on observing and accurately describing internal and external present events without judgment or distortion of reality. Mindfulness skills are core to all subsequent skills, and thus are reviewed at the beginning of each subsequent skills module.

Second, individuals with emotion dysregulation often experience interpersonal dysregulation. For example, they may have chaotic and intense relationships marked with difficulties. Nevertheless, they may find it extremely hard to let go of such relationships; instead, they may engage in intense and frantic efforts to keep significant individuals from leaving them. More so than most, these individuals seem to do well when they are in stable, positive relationships and to do poorly when they are not in such relationships. Problems with anger and jealousy can ruin intimate relationships and friendships; envy and shame can lead to avoidance of others. A highly anxious individual may need to have a partner around all the time as a safety behavior. In contrast, severe depression may cause difficulties connecting or engaging in relationships. Thus another DBT skills training module (Chapter 8) aims to teach interpersonal effectiveness skills.

Third, difficulties with emotion dysregulation are common in many disorders. These difficulties include problems with recognizing emotions, with describing and labeling emotions, with emotional avoidance, and with knowing what to do when an emotion is on the scene. Therefore, a third DBT skills training module (Chapter 9) aims to teach these and other emotion regulation skills.

Fourth, individuals with high emotion dysregulation often have patterns of behavior dysregulation, such as substance misuse, attempts to injure or kill themselves, and other problematic impulsive behaviors. Impulsive and suicidal behaviors are viewed in DBT as maladaptive problem-solving behaviors resulting from an individual's inability to tolerate emotional distress long enough to pursue potentially more effective solutions. To counter these maladaptive problem-solving and distress tolerance behaviors, a fourth DBT skills training module (Chapter 10) aims to teach effective, adaptive distress tolerance skills.

Table 1.1 lists the specific skills in each of these modules.

TABLE 1.1. Overview of Specific DBT Skills by Module

Mindfulness Skills

Core mindfulness skills
  Wise mind (states of mind)
  "What" skills (observe, describe, participate)
  "How" skills (nonjudgmentally, one-mindfully, effectively)

Other Perspectives on Mindfulness
  Mindfulness practice: A spiritual perspective (including wise mind and practicing loving kindness)
  Skillful means: Balancing doing mind and being mind
  Wise mind: Walking the middle path

Interpersonal Effectiveness Skills

Obtaining objectives skillfully
  Clarifying priorities
  Objectives effectiveness
    DEAR MAN (Describe, Express, Assert, Reinforce; stay Mindful, Appear confident, Negotiate)
  Relationship effectiveness
    GIVE (be Gentle, act Interested, Validate, use an Easy manner)
  Self-respect effectiveness
    FAST (be Fair, no Apologies, Stick to values, be Truthful)
  Whether and how intensely to ask or say no
Supplementary interpersonal effectiveness skills
  Building relationships and ending destructive ones
    Skills for finding potential friends
    Mindfulness of others
    How to end relationships
  Walking the middle path skills
Dialectics
Validation
Behavior change strategies

Emotion Regulation Skills

Understanding and naming emotions
Changing emotional responses
  Checking the facts
  Opposite action
  Problem solving
Reducing vulnerability to emotion mind
  ABC PLEASE (Accumulate positive emotions, Build mastery, Cope ahead; treat PhysicaL illness, balance Eating, avoid mood-Altering substances, balance Sleep, get Exercise)
Managing really difficult emotions
  Mindfulness of current emotions
  Managing extreme emotions

Distress Tolerance Skills

Crisis survival skills
  STOP skill
  Pros and cons
  TIP body chemistry
    (Temperature, Intense exercise, Paced breathing, Paired muscle relaxation)
  Distracting with wise mind ACCEPTS
    (Activities, Contributing, Comparisons, Emotions, Pushing away, Thoughts, Sensations)
  Self-soothing through the senses
    (vision, hearing, smell, taste, touch; body scan)
  IMPROVE the moment
    (Imagery, Meaning, Prayer, Relaxation, One thing in the moment, Vacation, Encouragement)

Reality acceptance skills
  Radical acceptance
  Turning the mind
  Willingness
  Half-smiling
  Willing hands
  Mindfulness of current thoughts

Supplementary distress tolerance skills when the crisis is addiction:
  Dialectical abstinence
  Clear mind
  Community reinforcement
  Burning bridges and building new ones
  Alternative Rebellion and adaptive denial

The Standard DBT Treatment Program

DBT was originally created for high-risk, multiple-diagnosis clients with pervasive, severe emotion dysregulation; the clinical problems presented by these clients were complicated. It was clear from the beginning that treatment had to be flexible and based on principles, rather than tightly scripted with one protocol to fit all clients. To give some clarity and structure to the inherent flexibility built into the treatment, DBT was constructed as a modular intervention, with components that can be dropped in and pulled out as the needs of each client and the structure of the treatment dictate.

Treatment Functions

DBT clearly articulates the functions of treatment that it is designed: (1) to enhance an individual's capability by increasing skillful behavior; (2) to improve and maintain the client's motivation to change and to engage with treatment; (3) to ensure that generalization of change occurs through treatment; (4) to enhance a therapist's motivation to deliver effective treatment; and (5) to assist the individual in restructuring or changing his or her environment in such a way that it supports and maintains progress and advancement toward goals (see Figure 1.2).

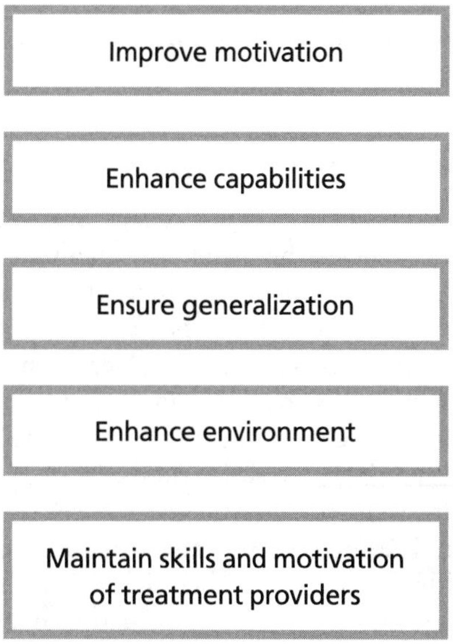

Treatment Modes

To accomplish these functions effectively, treatment is spread among a variety of modes: individual therapy or case management, group or individual skills training, between-session skills coaching, and a therapist consultation team (see Figure 1.3). Each of the modes has different treatment targets, and also different strategies available for reaching those targets. It is not the mode itself that is critical, but its ability to address a particular function. For example, ensuring that new capabilities are generalized from therapy to a client's everyday life might be accomplished in various ways, depending on the setting. In a milieu setting, the entire staff might be taught to model, coach, and reinforce use of skills; in an outpatient setting, generalization usually occurs through telephone coaching. The individual therapist (who is always the primary therapist in standard DBT), together with the client, is respon-

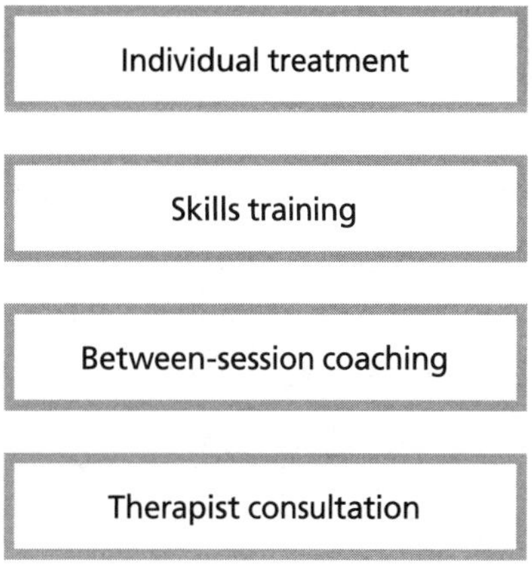

FIGURE 1.2. Functions of comprehensive treatment. Adapted from Lungu, A., & Linehan, M. M. (2015). Dialectical behaviour therapy: A comprehensive multi- and trans-diagnostic intervention. In A. Nezu & C. Nezu (Eds.), *The Oxford handbook of cognitive behavioural therapies*. New York: Oxford University Press. Copyright 2014 by The Guilford Press. Adapted by permission of The Guilford Press and Oxford University Press.

FIGURE 1.3. Modularity of treatment modes. Adapted from Lungu, A., & Linehan, M. M. (2015). Dialectical behaviour therapy: A comprehensive multi- and trans-diagnostic intervention. In A. Nezu & C. Nezu (Eds.), *The Oxford handbook of cognitive behavioural therapies*. New York: Oxford University Press. Copyright 2014 by The Guilford Press. Adapted by permission of The Guilford Press and Oxford University Press.

sible for organizing the treatment so that all functions are met.

DBT Skills Modules

The skills taught to clients reflect a key dialectic described earlier—the need for clients to accept themselves as they are, and the need for them to change. Hence there are sets of acceptance skills as well as change skills. For any problem encountered, effective approaches can include acceptance as well as change (see Figure 1.4). Skills are further divided into the four skills modules by the topics they address: mindfulness, emotion regulation, interpersonal effectiveness, and distress tolerance. Each skills module is further divided into a series of sections, and then further divided into a series of separate skills that are ordinarily taught in sequence but can also be pulled out separately for teaching and review. Clients can work on a single skill or set of skills at a time; this helps keep them from being overwhelmed by all the things they need to learn and change. Once clients have made progress in a set of skills, they can incorporate those skills into work on a new skills module. Some of the more complex skills, such as the interpersonal assertiveness skills (i.e., the "DEAR MAN" skills described in Chapter 8), are also made up of smaller parts to increase comprehension and accessibility.

Roles of Skills Trainer and Individual Therapist

As described earlier in this chapter, the theoretical model on which DBT is based posits that a combination of capability deficits and motivational problems underlies emotion dysregulation. First, individuals with severe and pervasive emotion dysregulation, including those with BPD, lack important self-regulation, interpersonal, and distress tolerance skills. In particular, they are unable to inhibit maladaptive mood-dependent behaviors, or to initiate behaviors that are independent of current mood and necessary to meet long-range goals. Second, the strong emotions and associated dysfunctional beliefs learned in the original invalidating environment, together with current invalidating environments, form a motivational context that inhibits the use of any behavioral skills a person does have. The person is also often reinforced for inappropriate and dysfunctional behaviors. Therefore, attention needs to be paid to increasing both a person's repertoire of skills and his or her motivation to employ those skills. However, as my colleagues and I developed this treatment approach, it quickly became apparent that (1) behavioral skills training to the extent we believe necessary is extraordinarily difficult, if not impossible, within the context of a therapy oriented to reducing the motivation to die and/or act in a highly

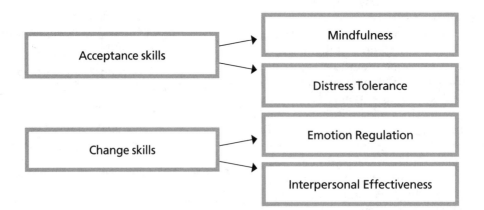

FIGURE 1.4. Modularity of acceptance and change skills. Adapted from Lungu, A., & Linehan, M. M. (2015). Dialectical behaviour therapy: A comprehensive multi- and trans-diagnostic intervention. In A. Nezu & C. Nezu (Eds.), *The Oxford handbook of cognitive behavioural therapies.* New York: Oxford University Press. Copyright 2014 by The Guilford Press. Adapted by permission of The Guilford Press and Oxford University Press.

emotionally reactive fashion; and (2) sufficient attention to motivational issues cannot be given in a treatment with the rigorously controlled therapy agenda needed for skills training. From this dilemma was born the idea of splitting the therapy into two components: one that focuses primarily on behavioral skills training, and one that focuses primarily on motivational issues (including the motivation to stay alive, to replace dysfunctional behaviors with skillful behaviors, and to build a life worth living).

The role of the skills trainer in standard outpatient DBT with severely dysregulated clients is to increase clients' abilities by teaching DBT skills and eliciting practice. The role of the individual therapist is to manage crises and help a client to apply the skills he or she is learning to replace dysfunctional behaviors. The individual therapist provides telephone coaching of skills to the client as needed. Furthermore, as noted above and in Figure 1.3, an integral component of standard DBT is the therapist consultation team: Skills trainers and individual therapists meet on a regular basis not only to support each other, but also to provide a dialectical balance for each other in their interactions with clients.

Individual therapy for chronically suicidal individuals and others with severe disorders may be needed for several reasons. First, with a group of serious and imminently suicidal clients, it can at times be extraordinarily difficult for the skills trainers to handle the crisis calls that might be needed. The caseload is simply too large. Second, in a skills-oriented group that meets only once a week, there is not much time to attend to individual process issues that may come up. Nor is there time to adequately help each individual integrate the skills into his or her life. Some clients need much more time than others do on particular skills, and the need to adjust the pace to the average needs makes it very likely that without outside attention, individuals will fail to learn at least some of the skills.

What kind of individual psychotherapy works best with skills training? Our research findings to date are mixed. In our first study on the topic, we found that skills training plus DBT individual therapy is superior to skills training plus non-DBT individual therapy.[17] In a second study, we tested skills training plus a version of intensive case management that may also be effective for some clients, whereas for others standard DBT with DBT individual therapy may be better.[18] In DBT, "case management" refers to helping the client manage his or her physical and social environment so that overall life func-

tioning and well-being are enhanced, progress toward life goals is facilitated, and treatment progress is expedited.[3] Clients' individual therapists often can serve as case managers, helping the clients to interact with other professionals or agencies, as well as to cope with problems of survival in the everyday world. In this study, however, case management replaced individual DBT therapy. In this version of case management, caseloads were very small (six clients). Case managers met weekly with their teams; used the DBT Suicidal Behavior Strategies Checklist (see Chapter 5, Table 5.2); were available for phone coaching of clients during work hours, and had access to a community crisis line at other times; and applied many of the acceptance elements of DBT (validation, environmental intervention) that balanced the change focus of many DBT skills.

Therapists conducting skills training, however, may not always have control over the type of individual psychotherapy their clients get. This is especially likely in community mental health settings and inpatient or residential units. In settings where DBT is just being introduced, there may not be enough DBT individual therapists to go around. Or a unit may be trying to integrate different approaches to treatment. For example, a number of psychiatric inpatient units have attempted an integration of DBT skills training with individual psychodynamic therapy. Acute inpatient units may structure psychosocial treatment primarily around milieu and skills training, with individual therapy consisting of supportive therapy as an adjunct to pharmacotherapy. The next chapter discusses issues for skills trainers in managing non-DBT individual therapists.

Modifications of Cognitive and Behavior Therapy Strategies in DBT

DBT as a whole and DBT skills training in particular apply a broad array of cognitive and behavior therapy strategies. Like standard cognitive-behavioral therapy (CBT) programs, DBT emphasizes ongoing assessment and data collection on current behaviors; clear and precise definition of treatment targets; and active collaboration between the therapist and the client, including attention to orienting the client to the intervention and obtaining mutual commitment to treatment goals. Many components of DBT (e.g., problem solving, skills training, contingency management, exposure, and cognitive modification) have been prominent in cognitive and behavior therapies for years.

Although DBT borrows many principles and procedures from standard cognitive and behavioral therapies, the development and evolution of DBT over time came about as I tried—and in many ways failed—to get standard CBT to work with the population of clients I was treating. Each modification I made came about as I was trying to solve specific problems I could not solve with the standard CBT interventions available at the time. These modifications have led to DBT's emphasizing 10 areas that, though not new, had not previously received as much attention in traditional CBT applications. The treatment components that DBT has added to CBT are listed below. Many, if not most, of these are now common in many CBT interventions.

1. Synthesis of acceptance with change.
2. Inclusion of mindfulness as a practice for therapists and as a core skill for clients.
3. Emphasis on treating therapy-interfering behaviors of both client and therapist.
4. Emphasis on the therapeutic relationship and therapist self-disclosure as essential to therapy.
5. Emphasis on dialectical processes.
6. Emphasis on stages of treatment, and on targeting behaviors according to severity and threat.
7. Inclusion of a specific suicide risk assessment and management protocol.
8. Inclusion of behavioral skills drawn primarily from other evidence-based interventions.
9. The treatment team as an integral component of therapy.
10. Focus on continual assessment of multiple outcomes via diary cards.

Whether these differences between DBT and standard CBT approaches are fundamentally important is, of course, an empirical question. In any event, CBT interventions have expanded their scope since DBT first appeared, and components of DBT have made their way into many standard interventions. The differences between them and DBT have eroded. This is most clearly evident in the increasing attention to the synthesis of acceptance and change and to the inclusion of mindfulness in many current treatments (e.g., Mindfulness-Based Cognitive Therapy, Acceptance and Commitment Therapy); it can also be seen in the emphasis on attending to in-session behaviors, particularly to therapy-interfering behaviors (e.g., Functional Analytic Psy-

chotherapy). Although researchers to date have not found that the therapeutic relationship necessarily mediates outcomes in behavior therapy, the field as a whole nonetheless puts a greater emphasis now on developing and maintaining a collaborative interpersonal relationship. Chapters 4 and 5 discuss the DBT strategies listed above, as well as how to apply CBT strategies within DBT's skills training context.

Effectiveness of Standard DBT

An overview of randomized controlled trials (RCTs) examining the effectiveness of standard DBT is presented in Table 1.2. As noted previously, standard DBT includes individual DBT therapy, DBT skills training, between-session coaching, and DBT team. For updates on research go to the Linehan Institute (*www.linehaninstitute.org/resources/fromMarsha*).

Standard DBT as a Treatment for BPD

There have now been a large number of studies evaluating the effectiveness of standard DBT as a treatment for high-risk individuals with severe and complex mental disorders. Most but not all of this research has focused on individuals meeting criteria for BPD—primarily because individuals with BPD have high rates of suicide and pervasive emotion dysregulation, and ordinarily present with a complex range of serious out-of-control behaviors. It is just the complexity that arises from such dysregulation that DBT was originally designed to treat. At present DBT is the only treatment with enough high-quality research to be evaluated as effective for this population by the Cochrane Database of Systematic Reviews, a highly regarded independent review group in Great Britain.[19]

Standard DBT as a Treatment for Suicidal Behaviors

In adults diagnosed with BPD and at risk for suicide, standard DBT has yielded significantly higher improvements on measures of anger outbursts, hopelessness, suicidal ideation, and suicidal behavior, as well as reduced admissions to emergency departments and inpatient units for suicidality, when compared to treatment as usual (TAU)[1, 17, 20, 21, 22, 23, 24] and to treatment by community experts.[23, 25] In the latter study, the expert therapists were nominated by mental health leaders in Seattle as the best

TABLE 1.2. RCTs of Standard DBT

Treatment/diagnosis/study population	Comparison group	Significant outcomes
DBT for BPD: **44 females**	Treatment as usual (TAU)	**DBT decreased** risk for suicidal behavior, use of services, dropout **DBT and TAU decreased** suicidal ideation, depression, hopelessness[1, 17, 65]
DBT for BPD: **58 females**	TAU	**DBT decreased** suicide attempts **DBT decreased** nonsuicidal self-injury (NSSI); **TAU increased** NSSI **DBT and TAU decreased** substance use[20, 21]
DBT for BPD: **101 females**	Community treatment by experts (CTBE)	**DBT decreased** suicide attempts, emergency department and inpatient admissions for suicidality, dropout **DBT produced** significant reduction in substance use disorders; significant changes in self-affirmation, self-loving, and self-protecting; and less self-attacking throughout treatment and follow-up **DBT and CTBE decreased** suicidal ideation, depression **DBT and CTBE increased** remission from major depression, anxiety, and eating disorders **CTBE produced** significant treatment interaction for therapist affirmation/therapist projection **DBT increased** introject affiliation[42]
DBT for BPD: **73 females**	TAU + wait list	**DBT and TAU decreased** NSSI, hospital admissions or length of stay in hospital, quality of life, disability[64]
DBT for veterans with BPD: **20 females**	TAU	**DBT decreased** NSSI, hospitalizations, suicidal ideation, dissociation, hopelessness, depression, anger suppression/expression[22]
DBT for veterans with BPD: **20 females**	TAU	**DBT decreased** NSSI, suicidal ideation, depression (self-report), hopelessness, anger expression **DBT and TAU decreased** service use, depression, anxiety, anger suppression[23]
DBT for BPD with current drug dependence: **28 females**	TAU	**DBT decreased** substance abuse **DBT and TAU decreased** anger outcomes[34]
DBT + levo-alpha-acetyl-methadol (LAAM; an opiod agonist medication) for BPD with current opiate dependence: **23 females**	Comprehensive validation therapy with 12-Step group (CVT-12s) + LAAM	**DBT and CVT-12s decreased** psychopathology, opiate use; however, participants in CVT-12s increased their use of opiates in last 4 months[35]
DBT for Cluster B personality disorders: **42 adults**	TAU	**DBT decreased** self-reported risk behavior **DBT and TAU decreased** NSSI reductions, use of services, aggression anger expression, depression, irritability[24]
DBT + medication for at least one personality disorder, high depression score: **35 adults**	Medication only	**DBT produced faster** remission from major depressive disorder[37]
DBT for BPD: **180 adults**	General psychiatric management (GPM)	**DBT and GPM decreased** suicidal behavior, use of crisis services, depression, anger, distress symptoms[66]

(cont.)

TABLE 1.2 (*cont.*)

Treatment/diagnosis/study population	Comparison group	Significant outcomes
DBT for 18- to 25-year-old college students with current suicidal ideation: **63** individuals	Supervision by experts in psychodynamic treatment (SBE)	**DBT decreased** NSSI, use of psychotropic medication, suicidality, self-reported depression **DBT increased** life satisfaction[31]
Inpatient DBT for PTSD: **74** females	TAU + wait list	**DBT increased** PTSD remission[32]
Inpatient DBT for BPD: **60** females	TAU + wait list	**DBT increased** abstinence from NSSI, **decreased** depression and anxiety **DBT and TAU decreased** anger[26]
DBT for any eating disorder and substance abuse/dependence: **21** females	TAU	**DBT decreased** dropout rate, dysfunctional eating behaviors/attitudes and severity of use of substances at post compared to pre **DBT increased** ability to cope and regulate negative emotions at post compared to pre[33]

Note. Data from Neacsiu, A. D., & Linehan, M. M. (2014). Borderline personality disorder. In D. H. Barlow (Ed.), *Clinical handbook of psychological disorders* (5th ed., pp. 394–461). New York: Guilford Press.

(nonbehavioral) therapists in the area. The aim of the research was to find out whether DBT works because of its own unique characteristics or because it is just a standard good therapy. In other words, the question was "Are all treatments equal?" The answer was "No." In comparison to treatment by community experts, DBT cut suicide attempts by half, admissions to hospital emergency departments for suicidality by half, and inpatient admissions for suicidality by 73%. Bohus and colleagues obtained similar findings for a 12-week inpatient DBT adaptation for females with BPD and a history of suicidal behavior.[26] More patients receiving DBT abstained from self-injurious behaviors at posttreatment than patients receiving TAU (62% vs. 31%).

Standard DBT as a Treatment for Mood and Other Disorders

Among individuals meeting criteria for BPD, outcomes across DBT studies indicate that DBT is an effective treatment for a number of disorders other than BPD. During 1 year of treatment, those in DBT have improved significantly in reductions of depression, with remission rates from major depression and substance dependence as good as those found in evidence-based CBT and pharmacological interventions.[27] DBT participants also reported significant improvements in developing a more positive introject (a psychodynamic construct we measured to test the view that DBT only treats symptoms). Those in DBT developed significantly greater self-affirmation, self-love, and self-protection, as well as less self-attack, during the course of treatment; they maintained these gains at a 1-year follow-up.[42]

DBT as a treatment for suicidality is not limited to adults. Research with suicidal adolescents[28, 29, 30] and suicidal college students[31] has also found significant reductions in use of psychotropic medications, depression, and suicidal behaviors, as well as increases in life satisfaction, when DBT is compared to control conditions.

Standard DBT as a General Treatment

Although DBT was originally developed for high-risk, out-of-control individuals with complex difficulties, the modular makeup of the treatment allows therapists to "rev up" or "rev down" the number of components actively used in treatment at a given time. To date, adaptations of DBT have been shown to be effective for posttraumatic stress disorder (PTSD) due to childhood sexual abuse;[32] eating disorders comorbid with substance abuse;[33] drug dependence comorbid with BPD;[34, 35, 36] eating disorders alone;[39, 40] Cluster B personality disorders;[24] PTSD with and without comorbid BPD;[41] and depression in older adults.[37, 38] Taken as a whole, these studies suggest that DBT is a broadly efficacious treatment.

This modular flexibility also allows us to bring into the treatment new interventions and strategies to replace old strategies that are less effective. Thus, as time goes on, it is likely that the utility of DBT will expand as the research base expands.

DBT Skills Training as a Stand-Alone Treatment

DBT skills training is rapidly emerging as a stand-alone treatment. Although the majority of research on DBT efficacy consists of clinical trials on standard DBT, many sites over the years have provided DBT skills alone, usually because of insufficient resources to provide the entire treatment. As these programs multiplied, research to determine whether such programs provided effective treatment got started. This growing area of research is suggesting that skills training alone can be very effective in many situations.

Evidence for the Effectiveness of DBT Skills as a Stand-Alone Treatment

An overview of RCTs examining the effectiveness of DBT skills training without individual therapy is presented in Table 1.3. Additional non-RCT studies examining the effectiveness of DBT skills alone are presented in Table 1.4.

As can be seen in Table 1.3, in clinical RCTs, DBT skills training without concurrent individual therapy has been found effective in a number of areas. It was found to reduce depression in nine separate studies;[38, 42, 45, 47, 48, 49, 51, 52, 54] anger in four studies;[43, 46, 52, 53] and emotion dysregulation,[38, 51] including affective instability[43] and emotional intensity,[44] in four studies. Adaptations of DBT skills have also been found to be an effective treatment for eating disorders in three studies,[39, 45, 46] as well as for drinking-related problems[51] and attention-deficit/hyperactivity disorder (ADHD).[50] Among incarcerated women, DBT skills have been effective at reducing PTSD symptoms, depression, and interpersonal problems.[54] Among men and women in correctional facilities, DBT skills have been shown to decrease aggression, impulsivity, and psychopathology.[55] Skills have also reduced intimate partner violence potential and anger expression among those with histories of such violence. Among individuals in vocational rehabilitation with severe mental disorders, DBT skills have decreased depression, hopelessness, and anger, and have increased number of hours working as well as job satisfaction.[52]

As can be seen in Table 1.4, studies of DBT skills training in pre–post research designs (where there is no control condition to which to compare outcomes) have findings similar to the RCTs. These studies have shown decreased depression [57, 58, 60, 61, 62] and ADHD symptoms,[61] as well as increased global functioning[60] and social adjustment coping.[62] Three studies have been conducted of DBT skills training with families of troubled individuals,[56, 57, 58] and all three showed reduction in grief and a sense of burden. Very few studies have been published of skills training for children; however, in the case of children with oppositional defiant disorder (ODD), DBT skills training was associated with reductions in externalizing and internalizing depression, a reduction in problematic behaviors, and an increase in positive behaviors.[60]

The majority of these studies offered only the skills training component of DBT. Two exceptions were presented by Lynch and colleagues.[37] In the first study, DBT skills and DBT phone coaching were added to antidepressants and compared to antidepressants alone for an elderly, depressed sample. In the second study, standard DBT with medication was compared to medication alone for an elderly, depressed sample with comorbid personality disorders. In both studies, the authors found that the depression remitted much faster when individuals were treated with DBT and medication than when they were treated with medication alone

The eating disorder studies used skills-only adaptations of DBT. Several of these studies did not report which DBT skills they used, making it difficult to determine which skills were important in bringing about clinical change. Although skills training has been linked to the reduction of emotion dysregulation in general,[63] we will need more research to determine exactly which skills are necessary and which can be discarded.

The next chapter addresses key issues in planning to conduct skills training, including suggestions for planning a skills training curriculum.

References

1. Linehan, M. M., Armstrong, H. E., Suarez, A., Allmon, D., & Heard, H. L. (1991). Cognitive-behavioral treatment of chronically parasuicidal bor-

TABLE 1.3. RCTs of DBT Skills Training Only

Diagnosis/study population	Comparison group	Significant outcomes
BPD: **49 women, 11 men**	Standard group therapy	**DBT skills decreased** depression, anxiety, irritability, anger, affective instability, treatment drop-out[43]
BPD: **29 women, 1 man**	Control video	**DBT skills increased** DBT skills knowledge, confidence in skills **DBT skills decreased** in emotional intensity[44]
Bulimia nervosa: **14 women**	Wait-list control	**DBT skills decreased** bingeing/purging behavior, depression[45]
Binge eating disorder: **101 men and women**	Active comparison group therapy	**DBT skills decreased** binge eating[39]
Binge-eating disorder: **22 women**	Wait-list control	**DBT skills decreased** anger, weight, shape and eating concerns **DBT skills increased** abstinence from bingeing behavior[46]
Major depressive disorder: **24 men and women**	Control condition	**DBT skills decreased** scores on depression **DBT skills increased** emotion processing[47]
Major depressive disorder: **29 women and 5 men over 60**	DBT + medication management vs. medication management only	**DBT skills decreased** self-rated depression scores **DBT skills increased** full remission of depressive symptoms/dependency, adaptive coping[38]
Major depressive disorder: **18 women, 6 men**	Wait-list control	**DBT skills increased** emotional processing associated with **decreases** in depression[48]
Bipolar disorder: **26 adults**	Wait-list control	**DBT skills decreased** depression, fear toward reward **DBT skills increased** mindful awareness, emotion regulation[49]
ADHD: **51 adults**	Loosely structured discussion group	**DBT skills decreased** ADHD symptoms[50]
Problem drinking: **87 women, 58 men (all college age)**	BASICS[a]; control	**DBT skills decreased** depression, drinking-related problems **DBT skills increased** emotion regulation, positive mood[51]
Vocational rehab. for severe mental illness: **12 adults**	TAU	**DBT skills decreased** depression, hopelessness, anger **DBT skills increased** in job satisfaction, number of hours worked[52]
Intimate partner violence: **55 men**	Anger management program	**DBT skills decreased** intimate partner violence potential, anger expression[53]
Incarcerated women with histories of trauma: **24 women**	No-contact comparison	**DBT skills decreased** PTSD, depression, and problems in interpersonal functioning[54]
Correctional facility inmates: **18 women, 45 men**	Case management	**DBT skills decreased** aggression, impulsivity, and psychopathology **DBT skills increased** coping[55]

[a]Brief Alcohol Screening and Intervention for College Students (a harm reduction approach).

TABLE 1.4. Non-RCTs of DBT Skills Training Only

Diagnosis/study population	Comparison group	Significant outcomes
Family members of individuals with BPD: **44** men and women	No comparison group; pre–post design	**DBT skills decreased** grief, burden **DBT skills increased** mastery Changes greater in women[56]
Family members of suicide attempters: **13** men and women	Pre–post design	**DBT skills decreased** anxiety, perceived family member burden, emotional overinvolvement **DBT skills increased** global psychiatric health[57]
Self-injurious behavior: **32** women, **2** men	Pre–post design	**DBT skills decreased** number of inpatient hospitalizations, outpatient appointments, general psychopathology[58]
Convicted offenders with diagnosed intellectual disability: **7** women and men	Pre–post design	**DBT skills decreased** dynamic risk **DBT skills increased** relative strengths, coping skills, and global functioning[59]
ODD: **54** male and female adolescents	Pre–post design	**DBT skills decreased** depression, negative behaviors **DBT skills increased** positive behaviors (e.g., productive behaviors)[60]
ADHD: **8** male and female adults?	Pre–post design	**DBT decreased** ADHD symptoms and depression[61]
Victims of interpersonal violence: **31** women	Pre–post design	**DBT skills decreased** depression, hopelessness, general distress **DBT skills increased** in social adjustment[62]

derline patients. *Archives of General Psychiatry, 48,* 1060–1064.

2. Kring, A. M., & Sloan, D. M. (2010). *Emotion regulation and psychopathology: A transdiagnostic approach to etiology and treatment.* New York: Guilford Press.

3. Linehan, M. M. (1993). *Cognitive-behavioral treatment of borderline personality disorder.* New York: Guilford Press.

4. Goldberg, C. (1980). The utilization and limitations of paradoxical interventions in group psychotherapy. *International Journal of Group Psychotherapy, 30,* 287–297.

5. Heller, A. S., Johnstone, T., Shackman, A. J., Light, S. N., Peterson, M. J., Kolden, G. G., et al. (2009). Reduced capacity to sustain positive emotion in major depression reflects diminished maintenance of fronto-striatal brain activation. *Proceedings of the National Academy of Sciences USA, 106,* 22445–22450.

6. Cisler, J. M., Olatunji, B. O., Feldner, M. T., & Forsyth, J. P. (2010). Emotion regulation and the anxiety disorders: An integrative review. *Journal of Psychopathology and Behavioral Assessment, 32,* 68–82.

7. Kring, A. M., & Werner, K. H. (2004). Emotion regulation and psychopathology. In P. Philippot & R. S. Feldman (Eds.), *The regulation of emotion* (pp. 359–408). Mahwah, NJ: Erlbaum.

8. Ekman, P. E., & Davidson, R. J. (1994). *The nature of emotion: Fundamental questions.* New York: Oxford University Press.

9. Tooby, J., & Cosmides, L. (1990). The past explains the present: Emotional adaptations and the structure of ancestral environments. *Ethology and Sociobiology, 11*(4), 375–424.

10. Crowell, S. E., Beauchaine, T. P., & Linehan, M. M. (2009). A biosocial developmental model of borderline personality: Elaborating and extending Linehan's theory. *Psychological Bulletin, 135*(3), 495–510.

11. Ogata, S. N., Silk, K. R., Goodrich, S., Lohr, N. E., Westen, D., & Hill, E. M. (1990). Childhood sexual and physical abuse in adult patients with borderline personality disorder. *American Journal of Psychiatry, 147*(8), 1008–1013.

12. Wagner, A. W., & Linehan, M. M. (1994). Relationship between childhood sexual abuse and topography of parasuicide among women with borderline personality disorder. *Journal of Personality Disorders, 8*(1), 1–9.

13. Messman-Moore, T. L., & Long, P. J. (2003). The role of childhood sexual abuse sequelae in the sexual revictimization of women: An empirical review and

theoretical reformulation. *Clinical Psychology Review, 23*(4), 537–571.

14. Zanarini, M. C., Frankenburg, F. R., Reich, D. B., Hennen, J., & Silk, K. R. (2005). Adult experiences of abuse reported by borderline patients and Axis II comparison subjects over six years of prospective follow-up. *Journal of Nervous and Mental Disease, 193*(6), 412–416.

15. Maccoby, E. E. (1980). *Social development: Psychological growth and the parent–child relationship.* New York: Harcourt Brace Jovanovich.

16. Neacsiu, A. D., Bohus, M., & Linehan, M. M. (2014). Dialectical behavior therapy: An intervention for emotion dysregulation. In J. J. Gross (Ed.), *Handbook of emotion regulation* (2nd ed., pp. 491–507). New York: Guilford Press.

17. Linehan, M. M., Heard, H. L., & Armstrong, H. E. (1993). Naturalistic follow-up of a behavioral treatment for chronically parasuicidal borderline patients. *Archives of General Psychiatry, 50*(12), 971–974.

18. Linehan, M. M., Korslund, K. E., Harned, M. S., Gallop, R. J., Lungu, A., Neacsiu, A. D., McDavid, J., Comtois, K. A., & Murray-Gregory, A. M. (2014). *Dialectical Behavior Therapy for high suicide risk in borderline personality disorder: A component analysis.* Manuscript submitted for publication.

19. Stoffers, J. M., Vollm, B. A., Rucker, G., Timmer, A., Huband, N., & Lieb, K. (2012). Psychological therapies for borderline personality disorder. *Cochrane Database of Systematic Reviews, 2012*(8), CD005652.

20. van den Bosch, L., Verheul, R., Schippers, G. M., & van den Brink, W. (2002). Dialectical behavior therapy of borderline patients with and without substance use problems: Implementation and long-term effects. *Addictive Behaviors, 27*(6), 911–923.

21. Verheul, R., van den Bosch, L. M., Koeter, M. W., de Ridder, M. A., Stijnen, T., & van den Brink, W. (2003). Dialectical behaviour therapy for women with borderline personality disorder: 12-month, randomised clinical trial in The Netherlands. *British Journal of Psychiatry, 182*(2), 135–140.

22. Koons, C. R., Robins, C. J., Lindsey Tweed, J., Lynch, T. R., Gonzalez, A. M., Morse, J. Q., et al. (2001). Efficacy of dialectical behavior therapy in women veterans with borderline personality disorder. *Behavior Therapy, 32*(2), 371–390.

23. Koons, C. R., Chapman, A. L., Betts, B. B., O'Rourke, B., Morse, N., & Robins, C. J. (2006). Dialectical behavior therapy adapted for the vocational rehabilitation of significantly disabled mentally ill adults. *Cognitive and Behavioral Practice, 13*(2), 146–156.

24. Feigenbaum, J. D., Fonagy, P., Pilling, S., Jones, A., Wildgoose, A., & Bebbington, P. E. (2012). A real-world study of the effectiveness of DBT in the UK National Health Service. *British Journal of Clinical Psychology, 51*(2), 121–141.

25. Linehan, M. M., Comtois, K. A., Murray, A. M., Brown, M. Z., Gallop, R. J., Heard, H. L., et al. (2006). Two-year randomized controlled trial and follow-up of dialectical behavior therapy vs. therapy by experts for suicidal behaviors and borderline personality disorder. *Archives of General Psychiatry, 63*(7), 757–766.

26. Bohus, M., Haaf, B., Simms, T., Limberger, M. F., Schmahl, C., Unckel, C., et al. (2004). Effectiveness of inpatient dialectical behavioral therapy for borderline personality disorder: A controlled trial. *Behaviour Research and Therapy, 42*, 487–499.

27. Harned, M. S., Chapman, A. L., Dexter-Mazza, E. T., Murray, A., Comtois, K. A., & Linehan, M. M. (2009). Treating co-occurring Axis I disorders in recurrently suicidal women with borderline personality disorder. *Personality Disorders: Theory, Research, and Treatment*, (1), 35–45.

28. Katz, L. Y., Cox, B. J., Gunasekara, S., & Miller, A. L. (2004). Feasibility of dialectical behavior therapy for suicidal adolescent inpatients. *Journal of the American Academy of Child and Adolescent Psychiatry, 43*(3), 276–282.

29. McDonell, M. G., Tarantino, J., Dubose, A. P., Matestic, P., Steinmetz, K., Galbreath, H., & McClellan, J. M. (2010). A pilot evaluation of dialectical behavioural therapy in adolescent long-term inpatient care. *Child and Adolescent Mental Health, 15*(4), 193–196.

30. Rathus, J. H., & Miller, A. L. (2002). Dialectical behavior therapy adapted for suicidal adolescents. *Suicide and Life-Threatening Behavior, 32*(2), 146–157.

31. Pistorello, J., Fruzzetti, A. E., MacLane, C., Gallop, R., & Iverson, K. M. (2012). Dialectical behavior therapy (DBT) applied to college students: A randomized clinical trial. *Journal of Consulting and Clinical Psychology, 80*(6), 982–994.

32. Bohus, M., Dyer, A. S., Priebe, K., Krüger, A., Kleindienst, N., Schmahl, C., et al. (2013). Dialectical behaviour therapy for post-traumatic stress disorder after childhood sexual abuse in patients with and without borderline personality disorder: A randomised controlled trial. *Psychotherapy and Psychosomatics, 82*(4), 221–233.

33. Courbasson, C., Nishikawa, Y., & Dixon, L. (2012). Outcome of dialectical behaviour therapy for concurrent eating and substance use disorders. *Clinical Psychology and Psychotherapy, 19*(5), 434–449.

34. Linehan, M. M., Schmidt, H., Dimeff, L. A., Craft, J. C., Kanter, J., & Comtois, K. A. (1999). Dialectical behavior therapy for patients with borderline personality disorder and drug-dependence. *American Journal on Addictions, 8*(4), 279–292.

35. Linehan, M. M., Dimeff, L. A., Reynolds, S. K., Comtois, K. A., Welch, S. S., Heagerty, P., et al. (2002). Dialectical behavior therapy versus comprehensive validation therapy plus 12-step for the treat-

ment of opioid dependent women meeting criteria for borderline personality disorder. *Drug and Alcohol Dependence*, 67(1), 13–26.

36. Linehan, M. M., Lynch, T. R., Harned, M. S., Korslund, K. E., & Rosenthal, Z. M. (2009). *Preliminary outcomes of a randomized controlled trial of DBT vs. drug counseling for opiate-dependent BPD men and women.* Paper presented at the 43rd Annual Convention of the Association for Behavioral and Cognitive Therapies, New York.

37. Lynch, T. R., Cheavens, J. S., Cukrowicz, K. C., Thorp, S. R., Bronner, L., & Beyer, J. (2007). Treatment of older adults with co-morbid personality disorder and depression: A dialectical behavior therapy approach. *International Journal of Geriatric Psychiatry*, 22(2), 131–143.

38. Lynch, T. R., Morse, J. Q., Mendelson, T., & Robins, C. J. (2003). Dialectical behavior therapy for depressed older adults: A randomized pilot study. *American Journal of Geriatric Psychiatry*, 11(1), 33–45.

39. Safer, D. L., & Jo, B. (2010). Outcome from a randomized controlled trial of group therapy for binge eating disorder: Comparing dialectical behavior therapy adapted for binge eating to an active comparison group therapy. *Behavior Therapy*, 41(1), 106–120.

40. Safer, D. L., & Joyce, E. E. (2011). Does rapid response to two group psychotherapies for binge eating disorder predict abstinence? *Behaviour Research and Therapy*, 49(5), 339–345.

41. Bohus, M., Dyer, A. S., Priebe, K., Krüger, A., Kleindienst, N., Schmahl, C., Niedtfeld, I., & Steil, R. (2013). Dialectical behaviour therapy for post-traumatic stress disorder after childhood sexual abuse in patients with and without borderline personality disorder: A randomised controlled trial. *Psychotherapy and Psychosomatics*, 82(4), 221–233.

42. Bedics, J. D., Atkins, D. C., Comtois, K. A., & Linehan, M. M. (2012). Weekly therapist ratings of the therapeutic relationship and patient introject during the course of dialectical behavioral therapy for the treatment of borderline personality disorder. *Psychotherapy*, 49(2), 231–240.

43. Soler, J., Pascual, J. C., Tiana, T., Cebrià, A., Barrachina, J., Campins, M. J., et al. (2009). Dialectical behaviour therapy skills training compared to standard group therapy in borderline personality disorder: A 3-month randomised controlled clinical trial. *Behaviour Research and Therapy*, 47(5), 353–358.

44. Waltz, J., Dimeff, L. A., Koerner, K., Linehan, M. M., Taylor, L., & Miller, C. (2009). Feasibility of using video to teach a dialectical behavior therapy skill to clients with borderline personality disorder. *Cognitive and Behavioral Practice*, 16(2), 214–222.

45. Safer, D. L., Telch, C. F., & Agras, W. S. (2001). Dialectical behavior therapy for bulimia nervosa. *American Journal of Psychiatry*, 158(4), 632–634.

46. Telch, C. F., Agras, W. S., & Linehan, M. M. (2001). Dialectical behavior therapy for binge eating disorder. *Journal of Consulting and Clinical Psychology*, 69(6), 1061–1065.

47. Harley, R., Sprich, S., Safren, S., Jacobo, M., & Fava, M. (2008). Adaptation of dialectical behavior therapy skills training group for treatment-resistant depression. *Journal of Nervous and Mental Disease*, 196(2), 136–143.

48. Feldman, G., Harley, R., Kerrigan, M., Jacobo, M., & Fava, M. (2009). Change in emotional processing during a dialectical behavior therapy-based skills group for major depressive disorder. *Behaviour Research and Therapy*, 47(4), 316–321.

49. Van Dijk, S., Jeffrey, J., & Katz, M. R. (2013). A randomized, controlled, pilot study of dialectical behavior therapy skills in a psychoeducational group for individuals with bipolar disorder. *Journal of Affective Disorders, 145,* 386–393.

50. Hirvikoski, T., Waaler, E., Alfredsson, J., Pihlgren, C., Holmström, A., Johnson, A., et al. (2011). Reduced ADHD symptoms in adults with ADHD after structured skills training group: Results from a randomized controlled trial. *Behaviour Research and Therapy*, 49(3), 175–185.

51. Whiteside, U. (2011). *A brief personalized feedback intervention integrating a motivational interviewing therapeutic style and DBT skills for depressed or anxious heavy drinking young adults.* Unpublished doctoral dissertation, University of Washington.

52. Koons, C. R., Chapman, A. L., Betts, B. B., O'Rourke, B., Morse, N., & Robins, C. J. (2006). Dialectical behavior therapy adapted for the vocational rehabilitation of significantly disabled mentally ill adults. *Cognitive and Behavioral Practice*, 13(2), 146–156.

53. Cavanaugh, M. M., Solomon, P. L., & Gelles, R. J. (2011). The Dialectical Psychoeducational Workshop (DPEW) for males at risk for intimate partner violence: A pilot randomized controlled trial. *Journal of Experimental Criminology*, 7(3), 275–291.

54. Bradley, R. G., & Follingstad, D. R. (2003). Group therapy for incarcerated women who experienced interpersonal violence: A pilot study. *Journal of Traumatic Stress*, 16(4), 337–340.

55. Shelton, D., Sampl, S., Kesten, K. L., Zhang, W., & Trestman, R. L. (2009). Treatment of impulsive aggression in correctional settings. *Behavioral Sciences and the Law*, 27(5), 787–800.

56. Hoffman, P. D., Fruzzetti, A. E., Buteau, E., Neiditch, E. R., Penney, D., Bruce, M. L., et al. (2005). Family connections: A program for relatives of persons with borderline personality disorder. *Family Process*, 44(2), 217–225.

57. Rajalin, M., Wickholm-Pethrus, L., Hursti, T., & Jokinen, J. (2009). Dialectical behavior therapy-based skills training for family members of suicide attempters. *Archives of Suicide Research*, 13(3), 257–263.

58. Sambrook, S., Abba, N., & Chadwick, P. (2007). Evaluation of DBT emotional coping skills groups for people with parasuicidal behaviours. *Behavioural and Cognitive Psychotherapy, 35*(2), 241–244.

59. Sakdalan, J. A., Shaw, J., & Collier, V. (2010). Staying in the here-and-now: A pilot study on the use of dialectical behaviour therapy group skills training for forensic clients with intellectual disability. *Journal of Intellectual Disability Research, 54*(6), 568–572.

60. Nelson-Gray, R. O., Keane, S. P., Hurst, R. M., Mitchell, J. T., Warburton, J. B., Chok, J. T., et al. (2006). A modified DBT skills training program for oppositional defiant adolescents: Promising preliminary findings. *Behaviour Research and Therapy, 44*(12), 1811–1820.

61. Hesslinger, B., van Elst, L. T., Nyberg, E., Dykierek, P., Richter, H., Berner, M., et al. (2002). Psychotherapy of attention deficit hyperactivity disorder in adults. *European Archives of Psychiatry and Clinical Neuroscience, 252*(4), 177–184.

62. Iverson, K. M., Shenk, C., & Fruzzetti, A. E. (2009). Dialectical behavior therapy for women victims of domestic abuse: A pilot study. *Professional Psychology: Research and Practice, 40*(3), 242–248.

63. Neacsiu, A. D., Rizvi, S. L., & Linehan, M. M. (2010). Dialectical behavior therapy skills use as a mediator and outcome of treatment for borderline personality disorder. *Behaviour Research and Therapy, 48*(9), 832–839.

64. Carter, G. L., Willcox, C. H., Lewin, T. J., Conrad, A. M., & Bendit, N. (2010). Hunter DBT project: Randomized controlled trial of dialectical behaviour therapy in women with borderline personality disorder. *Australian and New Zealand Journal of Psychiatry, 44*(2), 162–173.

65. Linehan, M. M., Tutek, D. A., Heard, H. L., & Armstrong, H. E. (1994). Interpersonal outcome of cognitive behavioral treatment for chronically suicidal borderline patients. *American Journal of Psychiatry, 151*(12), 1771–1775.

66. McMain, S., Links, P., Gnam, W., Guimond, T., Cardish, R., Korman, L., & Streiner, D. (2009). A randomized trial of dialectical behavior therapy versus general psychiatric management for borderline personality disorder. *American Journal of Psychiatry, 166*(12), 1365–1374.

Chapter 2

Planning to Conduct DBT Skills Training

Behavioral skills training is necessary when the skills needed to solve problems and attain desired goals are not currently in an individual's behavioral repertoire. That is, under ideal circumstances (where behavior is not interfered with by fears, conflicting motives, unrealistic beliefs, etc.), the individual cannot generate or produce the behaviors required. The term "skills" in DBT is used synonymously with "abilities" and includes in its broadest sense cognitive, emotional, and overt behavioral (or action) skills together with their integration, which is necessary for effective performance. Effectiveness is gauged by both direct and indirect effects of the behaviors. Effective performance can be defined as those behaviors that lead to a maximum of positive outcomes with a minimum of negative outcomes. Thus "skills" is used in the sense of "using skillful means," as well as in the sense of responding to situations adaptively or effectively.

The emphasis on integration of behaviors to produce a skillful response is important. Very often (indeed, usually), an individual has the component behaviors of a skill but cannot put them together coherently when necessary. For example, an interpersonally skillful response requires putting together words the person already knows into effective sentences, together with appropriate body language, intonation, eye contact, and so forth. The parts are rarely new; the combination, however, often is. In the terminology of DBT, almost any desired behavior can be thought of as a skill. Thus coping actively and effectively with problems, and avoiding maladaptive or ineffective responses, are both considered using one's skills. The central aim of DBT as a whole is to replace ineffective, maladaptive, or nonskilled behavior with skillful responses. The aim of DBT skills training is to help the individual acquire the needed skills. The steps for planning to conduct DBT skills training are outlined in Table 2.1 and discussed in more detail next. How to integrate DBT skills into non-DBT interventions is described at a later point in the chapter.

Forming (or Joining) a DBT Team[1]

DBT assumes that effective treatment, including skills training, must pay as much attention to the behavior and experience of providers working with clients as it does to the clients' behavior and experience. Thus treatment of the providers is an integral part of any DBT program. This is just as important for those teaching skills as it is for all other DBT providers. No matter how well adjusted clients may be, skills training can at times be enormously challenging and/or stressful, and staying within the DBT frame can be difficult. The roles of consultation are to hold the providers within the DBT frame and to address problems that arise. The fundamental team targets relevant to skills trainers are increasing adherence to DBT principles and accuracy of teaching

---

TABLE 2.1. Organizing DBT Skills Training in Your Practice

1. Form (or join) a DBT team.
2. Select skills training members of your team.
3. Select skills modules and specific skill sets.
4. Plan a skills training curriculum.
5. Decide on:
   a. Massed versus spaced practice in a 1-year program.
   b. Individual versus group skills training.
   c. Open versus closed groups.
   d. Heterogeneous versus homogeneous groups.
6. Clarify the roles of skills trainers, individual therapists, case managers, nurses and line staff, and pharmacotherapists in a skills training program.

---

and coaching skills; providing ideas for enhancing teaching of skills; troubleshooting problems that arise in the course of skills training; increasing and maintaining skills trainers' motivation; and giving support when providers' limits are crossed (and even when these are not crossed!).

DBT consultation groups require at least two people who meet weekly in person if both are in the same locality; when in-person meetings are not possible, team members may meet in an online learning community or via Internet applications. Because the primary focus of a DBT team is on the treatment providers, *not* the skills training recipients, providers do not have to be treating the same clients. For example, a client could be in individual treatment in one clinic and in a skills training group taking place in another clinic, each clinic with its own DBT team. Coordination of interventions, however, is greater if individual therapists, case managers, pharmacotherapists, and skills trainers are on the same team. (See Sayrs & Linehan, in press, for more discussion of how to set up, run, and solve problems in a DBT consultation team.[2])

Selecting Skills Training Members of Your Team: Necessary Qualifications and Characteristics

Skills training can be conducted by psychotherapists, counselors, case managers, social workers, milieu staff (in residential settings), and psychiatric nurses (in inpatient settings). Prescribing psychiatrists and nurse practitioners can be very effective skills coaches. For individuals without identified mental disorders, skills training can also be conducted by anyone (teachers, parents, family members, volunteers, and professional trainers) who is well trained in the principles of skills training and in the skills themselves. Clergy, pharmacotherapists, and other health care providers (e.g., psychiatrists, physicians, nurse practitioners, nurses, occupational therapists, and other medical staff in outpatient settings), when trained in the skills, often make excellent skills coaches. In addition, charismatic individuals who themselves have gone through skills training and have overcome their own difficulties can also make excellent co-trainers and skills peer counselors, again, when trained in the skills.

We know in DBT that to do the treatment effectively, skills trainers need to be well trained in what they are doing. They must have a very good grasp of DBT skills, practice the skills themselves, and know how to teach them. They need to know and be able to use basic behavior therapy techniques (such as behavior analysis, solution analysis, contingency management, exposure procedures, and the basics of skills building) and DBT treatment strategies (such as dialectical strategies, validation and problem-solving strategies, irreverent and reciprocal communication strategies, consultation to the patient, and environmental intervention strategies) as well as DBT protocols, particularly the suicide protocol. These strategies and protocols are described in full in the main DBT text and are reviewed in Chapter 5 of this manual. At this time, we have no evidence that type of academic degree is a critical factor in improving skills training outcomes.

Skill trainers' attitudes toward clients are also very important. Clients who fail to behave skillfully, and claim not to know how to behave differently, are viewed by some therapists as resistant (or at least as governed by motives outside awareness). These clinicians see giving advice, coaching, making suggestions, or otherwise teaching new behaviors as encouraging dependency and need gratification that gets in the way of "real" therapy. Other therapists and skills trainers fall into the trap of believing that clients can hardly do anything. At times they even believe that the clients are incapable of learning new, more skillful behaviors. Acceptance, nurturance, and environmental intervention compromise the armamentarium of these clinicians. Not surprisingly, when these two orientations coexist within a client's treatment team, conflict and "staff splitting" often arise. A dialectical approach would suggest looking for the synthesis, as I discuss more fully in Chapter 13 of the main DBT text.

When a DBT team is being started, the criteria for membership on the team are the same for all participants. Each participant must be on the team voluntarily, must agree to attend team meetings, must be committed to learning and applying DBT, and must be equally vulnerable to team influence. The last criterion means that all participants will bring to the team any difficulties and issues related to their attempts to apply DBT principles and interventions (including skills interventions) with the clients they are working with.

Selecting Skills Modules and Specific Skills to Teach

As noted in Chapter 1, there are four separate DBT skills modules: Mindfulness, Interpersonal Effectiveness, Emotion Regulation, and Distress Tolerance. Each module is divided into core sections and supplementary sections with specialized, optional, or advanced skills. The latter sections can be dropped if they do not meet the needs of specific client populations or if time demands it. Sections and specific skills can also be taught separately. (See Table 1.1 for which skills are core and which are supplementary.) A set of general handouts is given out during orientation before the start of each Mindfulness skills module, if there are new members in the group. A set of supplementary skills teaching behavioral analyses is also included in the general skills. In standard DBT, skills training is conducted in groups of 6–8 (10 at the most) participants plus 2 group leaders, once a week for 2.5 hours (2 hours with adolescents). Participants complete one full cycle of core skills through all the modules in 6 months. In a 1-year treatment program, participants then repeat the cycle for a total of 12 months. The core skills modules are each designed to take from 5 to 7 weeks (Interpersonal Effectiveness, 5 weeks; Distress Tolerance, 6 weeks; Emotion Regulation, 7 weeks). The Mindfulness module is designed to take two weeks and is repeated, along with a brief orientation, before the start of each new module. This basic cycle is outlined in Table 2.2. See the Appendices to Part I for a more detailed outline, along with session-by-session outlines of different DBT skills training programs for various disorders, time periods, and settings.

There are no empirical data to suggest how to order the modules. Since the core mindfulness skills are woven throughout the other training modules, Mindfulness obviously has to be the first module presented. In our current program, the Interpersonal Effectiveness, Emotion Regulation, and Distress Tolerance modules follow in that order, and that is their order in this manual.

The Interpersonal Effectiveness module focuses on how clients can decrease pain and suffering by effectively interacting with their social environment both to elicit changes in others and (when warranted) to resist unwanted influence from others. The Emotion Regulation module assumes that even though a situation (interpersonal or otherwise) may generate pain and suffering, an individual's responses also have to change and can be changed. The Distress Tolerance module assumes that even though there may be a lot of pain and suffering, it can be tolerated, and life can be accepted and lived in spite of pain. Surely this is a difficult lesson for anyone. One can, however, make a reasonably good

TABLE 2.2. Standard Core DBT Skills Training Schedule: Cycling Twice through All Modules over 12 Months

Orientation + Mindfulness module:	2 weeks
Interpersonal Effectiveness module:	5 weeks
Orientation + Mindfulness module:	2 weeks
Emotion Regulation module:	7 weeks
Orientation + Mindfulness module:	2 weeks
Distress Tolerance module:	6 weeks
	(24 weeks, 6 months)
Orientation + Mindfulness module:	2 weeks
Interpersonal Effectiveness module:	5 weeks
Orientation + Mindfulness module:	2 weeks
Emotion Regulation module	7 weeks
Orientation + Mindfulness module:	2 weeks
Distress Tolerance module:	6 weeks
	(48 weeks, 12 months)

case for any order of modules. In many clinics, clients are given the crisis survival strategies handouts (part of the Distress Tolerance module) during the first meeting. These skills are more or less self-explanatory, and many clients find them extremely helpful. They are then reviewed in detail when the Distress Tolerance module is taught. For some clients, their dysregulation and lack of understanding of emotions are so great that a case can be made for starting with the Emotion Regulation module. This is often the case, for example, in our multifamily adolescent groups.

Suggestions for Planning a Skills Training Curriculum

Instructional material in skills training, especially in a group context, should be presented at a pace adapted to the level of participants' understanding. Since the pace of each session will differ, as will the overall pace for particular individuals or groups, the instructional content in Chapters 6–10 of this book is not divided into segments within particular sessions. In my experience, however, the first time trainers teach these skill modules, the amount of material feels overwhelming. New skills trainers tend to spend too much time on early parts of a module and then have too little time later to cover other material that may be more important. What actually is important will necessarily vary with different individuals or groups, depending on their experience and skill levels. In order to facilitate the coverage of all the material by the end of the time scheduled for the particular module, the skills training leaders should construct lesson plans for each session and should attempt to cover the designated material during the session time allotted. Curricula for 11 different skills programs are outlined in the Appendices to Part I. Most of these are based on outlines that have been used in various research studies using DBT skills. The best strategy the first time through a module is to follow the steps below.

1. Decide how many total weeks your skills training program will last, and how long each session will be. The length of your program and of sessions will depend on whether participants do or do not have mental disorders, the severity of their disorders or other problems, the goals of your treatment program (e.g., stabilization, treatment, skills building), staff availability, financial resources, research data on outcomes of various lengths of treatment, and factors unique to your treatment setting.

2. Decide which skills you definitely want to teach and which skills you want to include as ancillary. Content of skills should be based on the research data for the disorders/problems you are addressing and, when there are few research data to guide your choice, on your beliefs about which skills are most appropriate for your clients. The curricula in the Appendices are organized by the number of weeks each program lasts and by the population each program is intended to treat. Look these over and select the skills curriculum that fits your situation best.

3. Decide which handouts and worksheets you want to use (see *www.guilford.com/skills-training-manual*). Do not use them without first reviewing them. Worksheets are associated with handouts; the worksheets for each handout are listed after the number of each handout, and vice versa. Descriptions of the relevant handouts and worksheets are given in the overview box for each skill or set of skills in the teaching notes.

There are several types of worksheets. Overview worksheets cover several skills and can be used when you want to focus primarily on practice of a group of skills, rather than focusing intensively on just the skills taught in a particular session. These worksheets are the first ones in each section and are linked to the handouts that overview each section.

Specific skills worksheets focus on a particular skill or small skills set. In some cases, multiple worksheets focus on the same set of skills (and are given the same worksheet number), but they differ in the amount of practice they provide for. The letters a, b, and c following the worksheet number generally indicate different demands the worksheets put on participants. For example, some of these ask participants to practice a particular skill once or twice between sessions; others ask that each skill in a set be practiced between sessions; and still others ask for daily practice of a skill or set of skills. There are also calendar worksheets for some skills that ask the participants to write about the skills they use each day between sessions.

4. The first time you teach skills, divide each module arbitrarily into sections corresponding to the exact number of weeks available, and try to get through as much of each section as possible. This experience will dictate how to time the modules the second time, and so on. When I teach therapists how to do DBT skills training, I usually recommend that trainers copy the teaching notes covering the skills they will teach in a specific session, and then highlight the main points they plan to cover in that session. With this strategy, it can be useful first to teach the material in the skills modules in the order given in this manual. After the first run-through, modifications in content and order can be made to suit your style or a particular situation.

Massed versus Spaced Practice in a 1-Year Program

Although each training module is designed to take 5–7 weeks to cover, up to a year could be spent on each. The content for each skills area is comprehensive and complex for such a short period of time. Covering the skills training material in this brief number of weeks requires very strict time management. Therapists also have to be willing to go on when some (or even all) clients have not acquired the skills that are currently being taught. Participants are sometimes overwhelmed by the amount of information the first time they go through each module. In a 1-year program, why not expand each module to a series of three 10- to 14-week modules (starting each with 2 weeks of mindfulness skills), rather than two sets of three 5- to 7-week modules? In other words, why not go for massed practice (the first choice) rather than spaced practice (the second choice)? There are several reasons for the present format.

First, all individuals—but particularly those who have trouble regulating their emotions—can be variable in their mood and functionality. They may go through periods of several weeks where they may miss meetings or, when present, pay attention minimally (if at all). Presenting material twice increases the probability that each person will be present, both physically and psychologically, at least once when a particular segment is covered.

Second, different participants have different needs; thus the modules are differentially relevant and preferred by various individuals. Having to sit through a disliked module for 10–14 weeks is very difficult. Sitting through 5–7 weeks of a disliked module is also hard, but not as hard.

Third, in a 10- to 14-week format, the modules scheduled second and third get less practice time than in a 5- to 7-week format taught twice. If I could make a case that one module is indeed the most important and needs the most practice, this would not be a liability. However, I have no controlled empirical data to use in choosing which module that would be. In addition, it is doubtful that one module would be best for all clients. The central premise of a behavioral skills-oriented approach is that acquisition of new skills requires extensive practice. Even though the material often feels overwhelming the first time when presented in the 5- to 7-week format, clients nonetheless seem able to practice the skills in their everyday lives. Thus presenting each module once during the first 6 months of treatment leaves a minimum of 6 months for continued practice before skill training ends.

Fourth, going over the material after clients have had a chance to practice the skills for several months can be beneficial. The material makes more sense. And it offers the chance for the participants to learn that problems that seem really hard at one point may not always seem so hard if they persevere in their attempts to overcome them.

Finally, my experience has been that when 10–14 weeks are allotted to cover a treatment module, it is far easier to divert therapy time to attending to individual participants' crises and process issues. It is easy for the leaders to start thinking that they have plenty of time for digressive topics. Although some attention must be given to these issues, it is easy to drift out of skills training and toward supportive process therapy, when time is not of the essence. In my experience, once this has happened, it is extremely difficult to get back control of the therapy agenda.

Individual versus Group Skills Training

Successful DBT skills training requires discipline by both participants and skills trainers. In skills training, the session agenda is set by the skills to be learned. In typical psychotherapy and in DBT individual therapy, by contrast, the agenda is usually set by a client's current problems. When current problems are pressing, staying with a skills training agenda requires the skills trainers to take a very active role, controlling the direction and focus of the session. Many therapists and skills trainers are not trained to take such a directive role; thus, despite their good intentions, their efforts at skills training often peter out as participants' problems escalate. Inadequate attention to the actual teaching of skills, and the resulting drift in focus, are particularly likely in individual as opposed to group skills training.

Even trainers who are well trained in directive strategies have great difficulty keeping to a directive agenda when participants have pressing problems or crisis situations and want immediate help or advice. The inevitable crises and high emotional pain of such clients constitute a major and continuing problem. It is difficult for the participants, and consequently for their skills trainers, to attend to anything but the current crises during sessions. It is particularly difficult to stay focused on skills when a participant threatens to commit suicide or otherwise quit if his or her current problem is not taken seriously. Taking it seriously (from the participant's point of view) usually means forgoing the day's skills training agenda in favor of resolving the current crisis.

Other participants may be less demanding of session time and energy, but their passivity, sleepiness, fidgetiness, and/or lack of interest in skills training may pose a formidable roadblock. It is easy in such a case for a therapist or skills trainer to get worn out with the client and just give up the effort, especially if a trainer is not a firm believer in skills training anyway. Skills training can also be relatively boring for those doing it if participants are nonresponsive, especially for trainers who have done considerable skills training with other participants. It is like a surgeon's doing the same operation over and over and over. Clients' fluctuating moods from week to week and within the skills training sessions (a characteristic of individuals who have trouble regulating their emotions), together with therapists' wavering interest, can create havoc with the best-laid skills training plans.

Skills training is difficult with clients who have multiple problems, serious difficulties regulating their emotions, frequent crises, or intense desire to change the behavior of another person. Trying to conduct skills training with such an individual is like trying to teach a person how to put up a tent in the middle of a hurricane. Nonetheless, it is also the case that if participants had more effective skills in their repertoires, they would be able to cope much better with crisis situations. And this is the dilemma: How does a trainer teach the skills necessary to cope, when a participant's current inability to cope is so great that he or she is not receptive to acquiring new behavioral responses? In individual treatment, there is often nothing beyond the two participants to keep therapy on track. If both participant and skills trainer want to switch to something else, they can do it easily.

Keeping skills training on track can also be extremely difficult when the participants are friends and family members of other people who are having very serious difficulties. This is particularly the problem when participants are parents or spouses/ partners of individuals who are at high risk for suicide or are engaging in dysfunctional behavior patterns that the participants are having extreme difficulties tolerating. In groups for friends and family members, it is very important for the leaders to make it clear during orientation that the focus of skills training is always on increasing the skills of the *participants*. The focus is *not* on how to change other people. This can be a particular problem for any relative who is in skills training principally to get consultation on how to manage a family member, with the expectation that the relative will be able to help the other person change. A similar problem can occur when any group member insists on help with changing another person (a boss, an employee, etc.). If the difficulty is persistent or is interfering with skills training for others, we have found that one or two individual consultation meetings can be helpful. Clearly, some DBT skills are aimed at influencing others. The DBT interpersonal effectiveness skills

focus on developing influential behavior with others, including effective assertiveness with others and behavioral skills such as reinforcement, extinction, flooding, and punishment aimed at increasing or decreasing the behaviors of others. The line between this focus on participants' interpersonal skills and ability to influence others on the one hand, and a focus on changing specific others, may be thin—but it is important nonetheless. Staying dialectical can be critical here in managing these two polarities.

For many of the reasons discussed above, the standard mode of skills training in DBT is a group intervention. In a group, other participants—or at least therapists' sense of obligation to other participants—keeps skills trainers on track, even when one participant wants to change course. When one participant in group skills training is not in the mood for learning skills, others may be. The reinforcement these other clients give the skills trainers for continuing skills training can be more powerful than the punishment delivered by the participant who is not in the mood.

The crux of the problem is this: Skills training with an individual who does not see its benefits right away is often not immediately reinforcing for either the participant or the person teaching the skills. For many individuals, there is not a sense of immediate relief or problem solving. Skills training is like teaching tennis: A student does not usually win the first game after the first lesson. Winning takes practice, practice, practice. Nor is behavioral skills training as interesting as having "heart-to-hearts," a topic I have discussed in Chapter 12 of the main DBT text. Skills training requires much more active work for both client and therapist. Thus, for individual skills training to work, special precautions must be made for arranging events so that *both* therapist and client will find it reinforcing enough to continue.

Individual Skills Training

A number of circumstances may make it preferable or necessary to conduct skills training with an individual client rather than in a group. In a private practice setting or a small clinic, there may not be more than one client needing skills training at any one time, or you may not be able to organize more than one person at a time for skills training. Some clients are not appropriate for groups. Although in my experience this is very rare, a client who cannot inhibit overt aggressive behavior toward other group members should not be put into a group until this behavior is under control. It is also usually preferable to treat social anxiety disorder (social phobia) before asking a client to join a skills training group. Some clients may have already participated in 1 year or more of a skills training group, but need further focused attention to one category or set of skills.

Finally, a client may not be able to attend the offered group sessions. In primary care settings, or when skills training is being integrated into individual therapy, skills may be taught during individual therapy sessions. In these situations, having the skills handouts and worksheets readily available will make it easiest for the individual practitioners to slip skills training into the fabric of ongoing individual care. In such a case, the therapist can make continuous efforts to incorporate the skills training procedures in every session. A problem with this approach is that the rules are not clear: It is often not apparent to the client what contingencies are operating at any given time in an interaction. The client who wants to focus on an immediate solution to an immediate crisis, therefore, has no guidelines as to when insisting on such attention is appropriate and likely to be reinforced and when it is not. A problem for the therapist is that it is extremely difficult to remain on track. My own inability to do just this was one of the important factors in the development of DBT as it is today.

A second alternative is to have a second therapist do individual skills training with each client. The rules for client and therapist behavior in this case are clear. In this format, general behavioral skills are learned with the skills trainer; crises management and individual problem solving, including the application of skills learned to particular crisis or problem situations, are the focus of sessions with the primary therapist or case manager. This approach seems especially advantageous in certain situations. For example, in our university clinic a number of students are eager to obtain experience in working with individuals with severe disorders who need long-term therapy, but the students are not able to commit to longer-term individual therapy. Conducting focused skills training for a period of time is a good opportunity for these students, and in my experience it has also worked out well for the clients. This would be an option in any setting where residents, social workers, or nurses are in training. In a group clinical practice, therapists may conduct skills training for each other; a large practice may hire some therapists with specific talents in this

area. The treatment model here is somewhat similar to a general practitioner's sending a client to a specialist for specialized treatment.

Individual therapists who have no one to refer clients to for skills training, or who want to do it themselves, should make the context of skills training different from that of usual psychotherapy. For example, a separate weekly meeting devoted specifically to skills training may be scheduled, or skills training and individual therapy can alternate weekly. The latter choice is particularly likely to work when the client does not need weekly individual sessions focused on crises and problem solving. If possible, the skills session should be conducted in a room different from that used for individual psychotherapy. Other possibilities include switching chairs; moving a table or desk near (or between) the therapist and the client to put the skills training materials on; using a blackboard; turning up the lighting; having skills training sessions at a different time of day than psychotherapy sessions, or for a shorter or longer time period; arranging for audio or video recordings of the sessions if this is not done in individual psychotherapy, or vice versa; and billing differently. For a therapist with a particularly difficult client, participation in a supervision/consultation group is important in keeping up motivation and focusing on skills. Even for those individuals who are in group skills training, a task of individual therapists is to reinforce the use of skills and also to teach skills "ahead of time," so to speak, as needed. Many therapists in our clinic also give clients skills homework assignments related to current problems, using the DBT skills training worksheets.

Group Skills Training

The chief advantage of group skills training is that it is efficient. A group can include as few as two people. In our clinic, with very dysfunctional clients, we try to have six to eight persons in each group. Group treatment has much to offer, over and above what any individual therapy can offer. First, therapists have an opportunity to observe and work with interpersonal behaviors that show up in peer relationships but may only rarely occur in individual therapy sessions. Second, clients have an opportunity to interact with other people like themselves, and the resulting validation and development of a support group can be very therapeutic. DBT encourages outside-of-session relationships among skills group clients, as long as those relationships—including any conflicts—can be discussed inside the sessions. Third, clients have an opportunity to learn from one another, thus increasing avenues of therapeutic input. Fourth, groups typically reduce the intensity of the personal relationship between individual clients and the group leaders; in dynamic terms, the transference is diluted. This can be very important, because the intensity of therapy sometimes creates more problems than it solves for clients who have problems regulating their emotions. Fifth, if a norm of practicing skills between sessions can be established, such a norm can increase skills practice in individuals who on their own might be much less likely to do the skills homework practice ordinarily assigned weekly. Finally, skills groups offer a relatively nonthreatening opportunity for individual clients to learn how to be in a group.

In my ongoing DBT research programs, we have offered a variety of different treatment programs. In our 1-year standard DBT program, clients in individual therapy also participate in group skills training. In our 1-year DBT case management program, clients have a DBT case manager as well as group skills training. In our adolescent program, each adolescent sees an individual therapist, and the parents or other caregivers and the adolescent attend the skills group. We also offer a 6-month skills training program for friends and family members of individuals who either are difficult to be with or have difficult mental disorders. We have offered a similar skills training group for individuals with emotion dysregulation.

A number of issues need to be considered in setting up a skills group—whether to have open or closed groups; whether groups should be heterogeneous or homogeneous; and how many group leaders or trainers there should be and what these persons' roles should be. I discuss these issues next.

Open versus Closed Groups

In an open group, new members can enter on a continuing basis. In a closed group, the group is formed and stays together for a certain time period; new members are not allowed once the group composition is stable. Whether a group is open or closed will often depend on pragmatic issues. In many clinical settings, especially inpatient units, open groups are a necessity. In outpatient settings, however, it may be possible to round up a number of people who want skills training and who will agree to stay together for a period of time. If a choice is available, which type of group works better?

I have tried both types of groups and believe that open groups work better for skills training. There are two reasons. First, in a closed group it becomes progressively easier to deviate from the skills training agenda. Process issues frequently become more prominent as members get more comfortable with one another. The group as a whole can begin to drift away from a focus on learning behavioral skills. Although process issues may be important and cannot be ignored, there is a definite difference between a behavioral skills training group and an interpersonal process group. Periodically adding new skills training group members, who expect to learn new behavioral skills, forces the group to get back on task.

Second, in an open group new clients have the capacity to reenergize a group or allow a change of norms when needed. In addition, for individuals with difficulty with change and/or trust, an open group allows clients an opportunity to learn to cope with change in a relatively stable environment. A somewhat controlled but continual rate of change allows therapeutic exposure to change in a context where clients can be helped to respond to it effectively.

Heterogeneous versus Homogeneous Groups

DBT skills training group members in my clinic are largely (but not completely) homogeneous with respect to diagnosis. Depending on the training needs of my students or the research studies currently in progress, we have restricted entry to individuals who (1) meet criteria for BPD; (2) have BPD and are highly suicidal; (3) have BPD with serious anger problems; (4) have BPD and substance use disorders; (5) have BPD and PTSD; (6) are suicidal adolescents together with their parents; (7) have disordered emotion regulation; or (8) are friends or family members of individuals with serious disorders. In most groups, we will also allow in one or two participants who are being treated in our clinic but meet criteria for other disorders (e.g., depression, anxiety disorders). Group members are not particularly homogeneous in other ways. Ages range from 13 to 18 years in the adolescent groups and from 18 up in other groups; some groups include clients of both sexes. Socioeconomic, education, marital, and parental statuses vary.

With the exception of groups designed for friends and families and for adolescents and their families, we prohibit sexual partners from being in the same skills training group. Sexual partners are placed into different groups at intake. If a sexual relationship develops among two members of a group, we have a rule that one must drop out. Such relationships can create enormous difficulties for the partners.

For many of our clients so far, our group represents their first experience of being with other individuals sharing very similar difficulties. Although from my perspective a homogeneous group is an asset in doing group skills training, the choice obviously has pros and cons.

Arguments against a Homogeneous Group

There are a number of rather strong arguments against a homogeneous group of clients who have severe disorders, including severe emotion dysregulation, suicidal behaviors, or behaviors that might elicit contagion. First, such a group for suicidal and/or highly impulsive individuals can be risky on an outpatient basis. Any kind of therapy, individual or group, can be very stressful for clients with disordered emotion regulation. Extreme emotional reactivity all but ensures that intense emotions will be aroused, requiring skillful therapeutic management. A therapist has to be very good at reading and responding to nonverbal cues and indirect verbal communications—a difficult task under the best of circumstances. Therapeutic comments can be misinterpreted, or interpreted in a way that the therapist did not mean, and insensitive comments can have a strong impact.

These problems are compounded in group therapy. It is impossible for therapists to track and respond individually to each group member's emotional responses to a therapy session. With more clients and a faster pace than in individual therapy, there are more opportunities for therapists to make mistakes and insensitive remarks, as well as for clients to misconstrue what is going on. In addition, it is more difficult for clients to express their emotional reactions to a group therapist in front of other group members. Thus the possibility for clients leaving in turmoil, with emotional responses they cannot handle, is greatly increased in group over individual therapy.

A second, related drawback to homogeneous groups has to do with the tendency of clients with high emotion regulation problems to become emotionally involved with one another's problems and tragedies. These clients often become anxious, angry, depressed, and hopeless not only about the problems in their own lives, but about the problems of those close to them. Thus just listening to others' life descriptions can precipitate intense, painful emotional responses. This has also been a very difficult issue for our staff members; we also have to listen to painful story after story from our clients. Imagine how much more difficult it is for individuals who have little capacity to modulate their responses to emotionally charged information.

Another argument against homogeneous groups of clients who have trouble regulating their emotions or impulses is based on the notion that in such a group there will be no one to model appropriate, adaptive behaviors—or, similarly, that there will be extensive modeling of inappropriate behaviors. I have simply not found this to be the case. In fact, I am frequently amazed at the capacity of our clients to be helpful to one another in coping with life's problems. In difficult therapy protocols such as exposure-based procedures, it is not unusual for clients to help each other cope with getting through the treatment. The one area where an absence of appropriate modeling does seem to exist is in the area of coping with extreme negative feelings. Especially with suicidal individuals at the beginning of treatment, it is often necessary for the group leaders to take much of the responsibility for modeling how to cope with negative emotions in a nonsuicidal manner (see Chapter 5 of this manual).

A fourth argument against homogeneous groups—particularly with individuals who have BPD or major depression—has to do with their passivity, their ability to "catch" other's moods and behavior, and their inability to act in a mood-independent fashion. Contagion of suicidal behavior can be a particularly difficult problem. At times, if one group member comes to a session in a discouraged or depressed mood, all members of the group will soon be feeling the same way. If group leaders are not careful, even they can sink down with the members. One of the reasons why we have two leaders for each group in our clinic is that when this happens, each therapist will have someone to keep him or her functioning at an energetic level. It can be very difficult.

Finally, it is sometimes said that some client populations (e.g., adolescents or those with BPD) are more prone to "attention seeking" than are other clients, and that this tendency will be disruptive to any group process. Once again, I have not found this to be the case.

Arguments for a Homogeneous Group

From my perspective, there are two powerful arguments for a homogeneous group. First, homogeneity allows the group leaders to tailor the skills and theoretical conceptions they offer to the specific problems of group members. Most of the skills taught are applicable for many client populations. However, a heterogeneous group requires a much more generic presentation of the skills, and the application of the skills to each person's central problems has to be worked out individually. With a homogeneous group, examples can be given that reflect their specific problems and situations. A common conceptual scheme would be difficult to present in a heterogeneous group unless it was very general.

A second argument for a homogeneous group is the opportunity for clients to be with a group of individuals who share the same problems and concerns. In my experience, this is a very powerful validating experience for our clients. Many have been in other groups but have not had the experience of being around others like themselves. For those with BPD and other severe disorders, they may have finally found others who actually understand the often inexplicable urges to injure themselves, the desire to be dead, the inability to regulate anger, the power of urges to use drugs, the inability to pop out of a depressed mood, the frustration of being unable to control emotions and behavior, or the pain of emotionally invalidating experiences. Adolescents have found others who understand their difficulties with parents, the pain of being bullied, their intense desire to be acceptable, and their beliefs that they are not. In a group for friends and family members, clients share the pain of having loved ones suffering and the frequent sense of desperation and helplessness.

A factor that can complicate the advantage of having an entire group of individuals with the same disorder or problem has to do with different rates of individual progress in treatment. When one client is engaging in dysfunctional behaviors, it is very validating to have other group members struggling with the same issue. However, once the client has stopped such behaviors, it can be very hard if others are still engaging in the same behaviors. Hearing about others' out-of-control behavior seems to cause a greater urge to do the same thing; this is, of course, a threatening experience for a person who is working hard at avoiding dysfunctional patterns of behavior. In addition, we have found that as clients progress in therapy, they often begin to change their self-image from that of "person with a disorder" to that of "normal person." Especially if they are very judgmental, they can find it very hard to stay in a group defined as a group for disordered individuals. These two issues—the urge to imitate dysfunctional behavior, and the need to change one's self-image from "disordered" to "not disordered"—must be dealt with effectively by the group leaders if an individual is to continue with the group.

Clarifying Providers' Roles

Skills Group Leaders

In standard DBT groups, we use a model of a primary group leader and a co-leader. The functions of the two leaders during a typical session differ. The primary leader begins the meetings, conducts the initial behavioral analyses of homework practice, and presents new material about skills. The primary group leader is also responsible for the timing of the session, moving from person to person as time allows. Thus the primary group leader has overall responsibility for skills acquisition.

The co-leader's functions are more diverse. First, he or she mediates tensions that arise between members and the primary leader, providing a balance from which a synthesis can be created. Second, while the primary group leader is looking at the group as a whole, the co-leader keeps a focus on each individual member, noting any need for individual attention and either addressing that need directly during group sessions or consulting with the primary leader during breaks. Third, the co-leader serves as a co-teacher and tutor, offering alternative explanations, examples, and so on. The co-leader may move his or her seating around the group as needed to assist participants in finding the right handouts or worksheets or to provide needed support. The co-leader is often the person who keeps track of the homework assignments. This is especially important when special individual assignments are given to one or more participants in the group. In these cases, it is also the co-leader who is charged with remembering the various assignments.

Generally, if there is a "bad guy," it is the primary group leader, who enforces the group norms; if there is a "good guy," it is the co-leader, who always tries to see life from the point of view of a person who is "down." More often than not in a group meeting, though not always, the person who is "down" is a group member; thus, the "good guy" image emerges for the co-leader. As long as both leaders keep the dialectical perspective of the whole, this division of labor and roles can be quite therapeutic. Obviously, it requires a degree of personal security on the part of both therapists if it is to work.

The DBT consultation strategies can be especially important here. The DBT consultation team serves as the third point providing the dialectical balance between the two co-leaders, much as the co-leader does between the primary leader and a group member in a group session. Thus the function of the DBT consultation team is to highlight the truth in each side of an expressed tension, fostering reconciliation and synthesis.

Over the years, many DBT teams have tried to convince me that one skills leader is all that is needed for most groups. I remain unconvinced. With highly dysregulated and/or suicidal individuals, a co-leader is invaluable as a person who can leave the room if needed to block a suicidal person from carrying out a suicide threat, go and get an ice pack for a person with extreme arousal, validate a person who feels attacked by the leader, or coach one person during a break while the leader coaches another. In a multi-family group, the co-leader can coach the adolescent while the leader nudges a parent to practice his or her skills with the adolescent. In groups for friends and family members, as well as other groups where participants have no identified mental disorders, it is surprising how helpful a co-leader can be in attending to the process issues that often arise. In sum, managing a group in skills training is a complex task. Finally, there is no substitute for having an observer of one's own behavior and skills as a group leader or co-leader. For example, due to my work schedule and one skills training group's meeting in the evening, I was coming into group sessions as the primary leader with very little energy, looking tired and sounding uninteresting. Naturally, this did not bode well for a successful skills training session. My co-leader brought it up with me, and we decided on a plan to "rev me up" each week (drinking a cold cola right before group). Now my co-leader not only reminds me each week, but also gives me feedback at break if I need to make a greater effort at "coming alive."

Individual Skills Trainers

In individual skills training, the skills trainer plays the role of both the skills leader and the co-leader as described above. It is extremely important in individual work that the skills trainer stick to the role of teaching skills, while balancing teaching with necessary troubleshooting of problems in learning skills and skills use that arise. Although an individual skills trainer is not an individual therapist, it is appropriate for such a trainer to suggest specific skills for problems that clients present, such as opposite action when a client is avoiding something or cope ahead when a client is afraid of failing at something. That said, it is important for an individual skills trainer not to fall into the role of being an individual therapist. The best way to avoid this is always to keep in mind the mantra of "What skills can you use?"

DBT Individual Therapists

An individual therapist for a person in skills training is the primary treatment provider and as such is responsible for overall treatment planning; for management of crises, including suicidal crises; for taking as-needed coaching and crisis calls or arranging for another provider to take these calls; and for making decisions on modifications to treatment, including how many complete rounds of skills training the individual should be in, whether admission to a higher level of care is necessary, and so forth. Except in a crisis to avoid serious injury or death, skills trainers turn crisis management over to individual therapists.

The task of the therapist with an individual in skills training also includes applying the lens of behavioral skills to helping clients generate solutions to their problems. Indeed, when confronted with a client's problem, a well-trained clinical provider can find an approach to problem solving by using skills from each skills module. Thus, when Distress Tolerance is the current treatment module (or a distress tolerance skill is what the therapist wishes the client to practice), problems may be viewed as ones where distress tolerance is needed. If interpersonal effectiveness is the focus, then the individual provider may ask how the problem (or the solution) might be related to interpersonal actions. Generally, problems become "problems" because the events are associated with aversive emotional responses; one solution may be for the client to work on changing emotional responses to a situation. An effective response may also be cast in terms of radical acceptance or core mindfulness skills.

DBT Case Managers

If a client has no individual psychotherapist, a DBT case manager is the primary provider and is responsible for all the tasks outlined above for the individual therapist. In addition, although both psychotherapists and case managers focus on clinical assessment, planning, and problem solving, case managers are ordinarily more active in facilitating care in the client's living environment. Thus the case manager's role also includes identification of service resources, active communication with service providers, care coordination, and advocacy for options and services to meet an individual's and family's needs. In this role, the case manager not only helps identify appropriate providers and facilities throughout the continuum of services, but also actively works with the client to ensure that available resources are being used in a timely and cost-effective manner. In sum, in contrast to a DBT therapist, a case manager does much more environmental intervention. As a DBT case manager, however, the task is to move more to the center and increase use of "consultation-to-the-patient" strategies (see below). The idea here is to coach clients to actively engage in the tasks that the case managers ordinarily do for the clients—in other words, to teach the clients to fish rather than catch the fish for them. This then involves coaching the clients in the interpersonal, emotion regulation, distress tolerance, and mindfulness skills necessary to be successful.[3]

DBT Nurses and Line Staff

The primary role of DBT nurses and line staff is to manage contingencies on inpatient and residential units, to coach clients in the use of skills, and to use DBT skills to problem-solve difficulties. Their role in skill strengthening and generalization is often critical in milieu-based treatment programs. These providers often make extensive use of the chain analysis skill (described in Chapter 6), as assisting patients with understanding the factors that prompt and drive their behaviors is typically accomplished with more accuracy in the situation where the behaviors occur. From this analysis, a nurse or line staff member can more effectively provide suggestions for a more skillful response or can more clearly intervene in the contingencies surrounding the behavior.

DBT Pharmacotherapists

The primary duties of a pharmacotherapist (whether a psychiatrist or a nurse practitioner) are to provide evidence-based medications matched to the needs of each client, and to monitor compliance with the prescribed medication regimen as well as outcomes and side effects. For a DBT pharmacotherapist, a further essential task is to coach the client whenever possible in relevant DBT skills. DBT skills aimed at treating physical illness, insomnia/nightmares, poor nutrition, effects of drugs and alcohol, and lack of exercise may seem to fit the role best, but it is equally important to focus on the wide array of other DBT skills as well. Like other providers, the pharmacotherapist (except in emergencies) also turns crisis intervention over to the primary provider (therapist or case manager), but until then often asks, "What skills can you use until you get hold of him [or her]?" In some settings, when there is no individual therapist or case manager, the DBT pharmacotherapist assumes the role of primary provider responsible for the tasks outlined above. In other settings, particularly when contact with the pharmacotherapist is infrequent and clients are not known to have serious disorders, the skills leader assumes the role of primary therapist. It is important that these roles be discussed and clarified within the DBT team.

Skills Trainers' Responsibilities with Primary Care Providers

The ability to apply any one of the behavioral skills to any problematic situation is at once important and very difficult. Individual providers must themselves know the behavioral skills inside and out, and must be able to think quickly in a session or a crisis. Given this role of the individual therapist, it is the responsibility of the skills trainers to be sure that the individual therapist has access to skills the client is being taught. When an individual provider is not familiar with the skills being taught, the solution is to do what is possible to inform the therapist. Generally this information, along with attendance and any other important clinical information, is provided to all DBT therapists at the weekly DBT team meetings. Strategies for this are discussed below.

Consultation between DBT Individual Providers and Skills Trainers

Communication between individual DBT providers and skills trainers is exceptionally important. If the expectations of each group of providers for the other are not spelled out and frequently reviewed, it is very likely that the two treatments will not enhance each other. Among the most important aspects of DBT are the DBT consultation team strategies (described in Chapter 13 of the main DBT text). These strategies require all DBT therapists to meet on a regular basis. The goals of these meetings are to share information and to keep therapists within the framework of DBT.

In my clinic, a consultation meeting is held each week for 1–1.5 hours. During the meeting, skills trainers review for the team which skills are the current focus of group sessions. When necessary, the skills trainers actually teach the other team members the skills. In this context, it is helpful for clients if their primary providers and skills trainers share a common language in discussing application of behavioral skills. This also decreases the potential for confusion. Although consistency and conformity between various treating agents are not particularly valued in DBT, such consistency here can be useful, since the number of new skills to be learned is quite large. The weekly meetings increase this communality. In addition, any problems individual clients may be having in applying skills and/or interacting in skills training group meetings are mentioned. A client's primary provider consults with the skills trainers and takes such information into account in planning the individual treatment.

My emphasis on the importance of meetings between individual therapists and skills trainers may seem to contradict "consultation-to-the-patient" strategies, which are also integral to DBT. First, I must point out that these consultation strategies do require DBT therapists to walk a very fine line. The issues are somewhat complex. When the therapeutic unit is defined as a group of people, such as a DBT team, a clinic, an inpatient unit, or some such entity where multiple therapists interact with and treat particular clients in a single coordinated treatment program, then consultation between therapists is essential, provided that the clients are informed of and consent to such collaboration. Applying the consultation strategies in these cases simply requires that therapists refrain from intervening with each other

on *behalf* of a client. Thus therapists must be careful not to fall into the trap of serving as intermediaries for a client. (See Chapter 13 of the main DBT text for a discussion of consultation-to-the-patient strategies; they are also discussed briefly in Chapter 5 of this manual.)

When the Primary Provider Is a Skills Trainer

It is not uncommon that skills trainers are also individual therapists or case managers for some of the clients in a skills training group. Less often, a pharmacotherapist may also be a skills trainer for his or her clients. When either of these is the case, it is important to keep roles clear. In other words, when one is teaching skills it is important to focus on skills, and to wait until after the skills session ends to revert to one's other role. This is not only because of time constraints in a skills class, but also because as soon as skills trainers start managing crises, individual clients (particularly those whose lives involve constant crises) are likely to bring up more crises to discuss and problem-solve. Focusing on learning new behaviors can take a lot more effort than sitting back and discussing the crises of life.

DBT Skills Training outside Standard DBT

Standard DBT combines skills training with individual therapy or intensive case management, plus phone coaching by the individual provider and weekly treatment team meetings. When DBT skills training is offered without the individual provider component, some modifications in the conduct of skills training may be necessary. For example, without an individual therapist, skills trainers may decide to provide phone, text, or e-mail coaching between sessions. There may also be a greater emphasis on use of DBT smartphone coaching apps and other DBT apps and websites. (To locate these, type "DBT self-help" in your search engine.) At times, skills trainers may offer individual consultation sessions to group members. This may be particularly necessary in groups for friends and family members, at times when group members are extremely distraught about a friend or relative and want and need more coaching in use of skills than can occur in a single group session.

Clarifying Individual Therapists' versus Skills Trainers' Roles in Suicidal Crises

Standard DBT—including individual therapy, skills training, as-needed phone coaching/crisis intervention, and the DBT consultation team—was designed specifically for highly suicidal individuals with high emotion dysregulation. Reduction of suicidal and other maladaptive behaviors is *not* the immediate goal of DBT skills training. Instead, skills training is focused on teaching *general* skills that the clients can apply to current problems in living. Application of these skills to current suicidal behavior, to behaviors interfering with therapy progress (except on occasion behaviors interfering with skills training), and to other severely dysfunctional behaviors is not necessarily attempted by skills trainers.

In fact, as I discuss later, discussion of current self-injurious behavior, substance use, and other contagious behaviors is actively discouraged in skills training. Reports of suicidal ideation, prior self-injury, and other maladaptive behaviors/behaviors interfering with therapy—including extreme problems with skills training—are ordinarily relegated to individual therapists, primarily because of time constraints in conducting skills training.

Problems maintaining this skills training orientation arise when an individual therapist sends his or her clients to DBT skills training because of the strong data on DBT as an effective intervention for highly suicidal individuals. Our non-DBT therapist colleagues know that therapists trained in DBT are also trained in assessment and management of suicidal behavior. Thus a non-DBT therapist may start mistakenly relying on a DBT skills trainer to manage high-risk suicidal behavior, at least when the skills trainer is present or available by phone. Unfortunately, a skills training therapist in DBT is relying on an individual therapist in a similar manner. In some cases a DBT skills trainer, if not trained in DBT as a whole treatment, may not even be trained in management of suicidal behaviors. And therein lies the problem: Skills trainers teach skills.

Managing Working with Clients of Non-DBT Individual Therapists

When a DBT skills client is in therapy (or case management) with a non-DBT therapist, it is particularly important for the skills trainer(s) to have a very clear agreement with the individual therapist. In my clinic, we only agree to accept a client with high suicidality and/or severe disorders if the client's individual therapist agrees to the following:

1. The provider or a designated backup individual therapist must agree to resist the temptation to rely on the skills trainer to conduct interventions aimed at reducing current suicidal and other severely dysfunctional behaviors. This means that the individual therapist must agree to be available for crisis calls from the skills trainer and/or the client during and following skills training sessions. This agreement is intended to ensure that the individual therapist, rather than the skills trainer, makes treatment decisions about the client when problems or crises arise. In essence, a skills trainer calls the individual therapist if a crisis arises, and then follows treatment directions. This policy is based on the presumption that the individual therapist knows the client much better than the skills trainer, and that this knowledge is essential in making decisions about crisis management. The individual therapist must be made aware of this policy, and must also be willing to be responsible for treatment management and decision making about treatment. Although a skills trainer may make sure that a client actually gets to the local hospital emergency department, this is very different from deciding that such a move should be made in the first place. An exception to this policy is made when a client is highly suicidal, and the skills trainer believes medical treatment or emergency evaluation for inpatient treatment is needed, but the individual therapist either disagrees without an adequate rationale or refuses to make the necessary treatment management decision. Individual therapists should be advised also that skills therapists are not available for crisis calls from their clients.

2. The individual therapist must agree to coach the client on use of DBT skills in everyday life. We ordinarily give second copies of all the DBT skills handouts and worksheets to our clients and ask them to give these copies to their individual therapists. To be successful, an individual psychotherapist needs to elicit from a client sufficient information about the skills taught in skills training to be able to help the client apply the skills in troublesome areas. The therapist also needs to know (or learn) the skills and be able to apply the skills him- or herself; this is not as simple as it might seem. It is important also to advise therapists that skills trainers do not do telephone coaching on skills, as that is viewed as the role for the individual therapist.

3. Therapists must understand and agree that skills trainers will not give them reports about their client's behaviors in group sessions or reports on group attendance. If a therapist wants such reports and a client agrees, a skills trainer may agree to give periodic reports to the client, who can then give such reports to the therapist. The principle here is contained within the consultation-to-the-patient strategy, which promotes the patient as a credible source of information who can intervene effectively on his or her own behalf within the health care network. (See Chapter 13 of the main DBT text.)

In our clinic, we use the agreement in Figure 2.1 and ask each non-DBT individual therapist to sign it. The experience in my clinic has been that most individual therapists in private practice will agree to these stipulations to get their clients into our skills groups. However, we have had some therapists who initially agreed to these points but, when serious crises arose, insisted that we make the clinical decisions about their clients. We have also had clients who were seeing therapists who refused to take after-hours calls themselves, and instead used our area crisis line as their "backup therapist." Unfortunately, many crisis clinics are staffed by volunteers with little or no formal clinical training, and so a skills trainer cannot usually turn client responsibility over to a crisis line volunteer. It is critical, therefore, that skills trainers who do not want to take responsibility for managing crises (particularly suicidal crises) discuss crisis management with clients' individual therapists before beginning skills training, and also

clarify who will be on call for the clients during and after skills training sessions. Thus we also ask each client's primary therapist to fill out a crisis plan. A form for obtaining a crisis plan and other essential information from a primary therapist is shown in Figure 2.2.

When Individual Psychotherapists Do Not Incorporate Skills Coaching into Psychotherapy

Active intervention and skills coaching may not be compatible with the individual psychotherapy a particular therapist is willing to engage in. Some therapists, for example, view helping clients learn new skillful behaviors as treating the "symptoms" instead of the "illness." In one setting, individual psychotherapists (who were physicians) told clients to get coaching from the nurses in how to replace maladaptive behaviors with skills. This sent the message that the new skills were not important, since the "real therapy" was taking place with their individual therapists. Clients with such therapists will need extra help in using the skills they are learning.

Skills trainers can make a number of optional modifications to address these issues. They might set up an extra weekly skills training meeting where clients can get help in figuring out how to use their skills in troublesome life situations. But people often need help at the moment they are in crisis. Skills training is like teaching basketball: Coaches not only conduct practice sessions during the week, but also attend the weekly game to help the players

---

Client Name: _____

Provider Name: _____ Date (yyyy/mm/dd): _____

I am the primary individual ❑ psychotherapist ❑ case manager ❑ pharmacotherapist for the client referred to above. I understand that my client will not be eligible to participate in the DBT Skills Training Program at _____ unless he or she attends regular individual treatment sessions on an ongoing basis. As the primary provider for this client, I agree that I will:

1. Assume full clinical responsibility for my client.
2. Handle or provide backup services to manage client clinical emergencies.
3. Be available by phone or provide a backup provider phone number to call during skills training sessions of my client.
4. Provide and keep updated the Crisis Plan and Information from Primary Therapist form [Figure 2.2] attached.
5. Help my client apply DBT skills to his or her clinical problems.

FIGURE 2.1. Primary individual provider agreement for clients in DBT skills training.

This must be completed with your client's full awareness of all parties with whom this information may be shared.

Please fill this form out on paper and have client return to the group leaders, or fill out digital copy at: _____ and e-mail to one of the group leaders at: _____

Group Leader's Name: _____ E-mail: _____

Date (yyyy/mm/dd): _____

Client's Name: _____ Clinical ID: _____ DOB (yyyy/mm/dd): _____

Your client's group meets on: _____ at: _____

Primary Therapist:

Name: _____ Phone (Office): _____ Phone (Cell): _____ Fax: _____

E-mail: _____ Available Hours: _____

Address: _____

If your client is at high suicide risk or in crisis requiring immediate intervention and you are unavailable, who should be called?

Your Backup Therapist (when you are in town):

Name: _____ Phone (Day): _____ Phone (Eve): _____ Phone (Cell): _____

Address: _____

Your Backup Therapist (when you are in town):

Name: _____ Phone (Day): _____ Phone (Eve): _____ Phone (Cell): _____

Address: _____

Pharmacotherapist/Primary Care Physician/Nurse Practitioner (if applicable):

Name: _____ Phone (Day): _____ Phone (Eve): _____ Phone (Cell): _____

Case Manager (if applicable):

Name: _____ Phone (Day): _____ Phone (Eve): _____ Phone (Cell): _____

Significant Others (to call in an emergency):

Name: _____ Phone: _____ City: _____

Name: _____ Phone: _____ City: _____

CRISIS PLAN

How can you be reached during a crisis if disposition planning is needed?

_____

_____

Who should be called for disposition planning if you are unavailable?

_____

_____

(cont.)

FIGURE 2.2. Crisis plan and information from primary therapist (confidential).

1. Brief history of client's suicidal behavior.

_____

_____

2. Recent status of client's suicidal behavior (last 3 months). Please describe the most recent and most severe self-injury/suicide attempt. Describe the form, date, circumstances and what intervention resulted, if any (e.g., ER, medical ward, ICU).

_____

_____

_____

3. **Crisis plan:** Describe crisis plan you and client have agreed to for management of suicidal behavior. Describe the typical emotions, thoughts, and behaviors that may precede self-injury/suicide attempts, and the strategies that a client has used successfully in the past.

(EXAMPLE: My client states that if she gets angry or feels helpless, this causes emotion dysregulation. This then triggers the urge to hurt herself by burning herself. She states that if she has this urge, she has successfully coped with these by using these distraction strategies: calling her mother, playing with her dogs, going for a walk to the park, crocheting, having a bath, doing vigorous physical exercise, listening to loud music, or praying. As a last resort, she will call me or my backup therapist and discuss ways for her to get through the moment. When she calls, she says that she finds it really helpful when I help her to find a means of distraction, remind her that she has tolerated urges like this before, and help her try to solve the problem that may be leading to her feeling this way. This plan was developed with my client.)

_____

_____

_____

_____

4. If your client is assessed as in imminent risk of suicidal behavior, self-injury, or violence, and neither you nor your backup can be immediately contacted, how should the skills trainers or other professional staff manage your client?

_____

_____

_____

_____

_____

5. Describe any history of violence and use of weapons. Also specifically describe any occasions of violence and use of weapons in the last 3 months. Describe any current plans that you and the client have to deal with this behavior.

_____

_____

_____

6. Describe any history of substance use. Also specifically describe substance misuse history in the last 3 months. Describe any current plans that you and the client have to deal with this behavior.

_____

_____

_____

7. Client medications: Weight (lbs/kg) _____ Height (inches/cm) _____

Medications	Dose	For	Medications	Dose	For
_____	_____	_____	_____	_____	_____
_____	_____	_____	_____	_____	_____

FIGURE 2.2 *(cont.)*

use what they were practicing all week. With outpatients, this is usually best done via telephone calls. In standard DBT, where clients have individual DBT psychotherapists, phone calls to skills training therapists are severely limited; almost all calls for help are directed to the clients' individual therapists. If an individual therapist does not take calls or give coaching, however, a skills trainer may decide to accept them, at least when the reason for calling is to get such coaching.

On an inpatient unit, milieu staff members should learn the behavioral skills along with the clients. The staff members can then serve as coaches for the clients. One inpatient unit offers weekly skills consultation meetings. The meetings are run like academic office hours; clients can come at any time during office hours for coaching. Ideally, clients can also call on one another for help. In another inpatient setting, one therapist teaches new skills; nursing staff members conduct regular homework review groups, where clients meet together to go over their attempts to practice new skills and get help with areas of difficulty; and individual therapists reinforce the clients' use of skills. In residential settings, it can be useful to offer advanced skills groups where group members help each other apply skills in daily situations.

Skills generalization can also be greatly enhanced if individuals in a client's environment—such as family members—also learn the skills and then help with coaching the client every day.[4] A skills trainer or individual therapist can then assist a family member in coaching the client. Adolescent skills training ordinarily includes both an adolescent and at least one parent, so each can coach the other. Parole officers can be taught the skills so they can coach the parolees on their caseloads. Primary care providers can be taught skills so they can coach their patients. A skills curriculum has been developed for use in school settings, where teachers and school counselors can coach students.[4, 5]

Integrating Skills Training into Non-DBT Individual Therapy

Many non-DBT psychotherapists, counselors, case managers, pharmacotherapists, other mental health providers, nurses, doctors, and other professionals in general medical practice will find it useful at times to integrate DBT skills into their treatment of clients. Providers may want to use only one skill or a variety of skills across different modules. Strategies for incorporating skills into ongoing therapy are as follows. First, carefully read the treatment notes for each of the skills to be used. What is important here is that providers know the skills and know what skills go with what problem or set of problems. Second, decide whether to use a handout and/or worksheet in teaching the skill, or to teach it orally without these materials. If you are planning on occasionally using handouts and/or worksheets, copy them and keep them handy in your office or nearby. When the occasion arises to teach a particular skill, discuss the idea of learning a new skill with the client. Use the orienting strategies discussed in Chapter 6 of this manual, if necessary, to sell the skill you want to teach. Giving a copy of the handout to the client and keeping one yourself, review the skill using the skills training procedures described in Chapter 6. Practice the skill with the client if possible, and give an assignment or suggestion that the client practice the skill before the next visit. As far as possible, be open to the client's calling you between sessions for skills coaching. Be sure to ask about the client's practice in the next visit. Periodically check in with the client to see whether he or she is still using the skills you have taught. Encourage continued skillful behavior. Although it may seem that the directive quality of DBT skills training would be incompatible with psychoanalytic and supportive treatments, the fact that so many nonbehavioral and analytic therapists teach and/or integrate DBT skills into their therapies suggests that this is not the case (enter "psychoanalytic DBT skills" in your search engine for examples).

References

1. Neacsiu, A. D., & Linehan, M. M. (2014). Borderline personality disorder. In D. Barlow (Ed.), *Clinical handbook of psychological disorders* (5th ed., pp. 394–461). New York: Guilford Press.
2. Sayrs, J. H. R., & Linehan, M. M. (in press). *Developing therapeutic treatment teams: The DBT model.* New York: Guilford Press.
3. Case Management Society of America. (n.d.). Retrieved from *www.cmsa.org/Home/CMSA/WhatisaCaseManager/tabid/224/Default.aspx*
4. Miller, A. L., Rathus, J. H., & Linehan, M. M. (2007). *Dialectical behavior therapy with suicidal adolescents.* New York: Guilford Press.
5. Mazza, J. J., Dexter-Mazza, E. T., Murphy, H. E., Miller, A. L., & Rathus, J. H. (in press). *Dialectical behavior therapy in schools.* New York: Guilford Press.

Chapter 3

Structuring Skills Training Sessions

In this chapter, I discuss how to structure various types of DBT skills training sessions, including the pretreatment sessions that should be accomplished before an individual starts skills training. These initial sessions cover preliminary orientation and commitment to DBT training. Once these sessions are completed, several specific types of skills training sessions follow, including (1) sessions that build alliance and orient new participants to skills training; (2) ongoing skills training sessions; and (3) last sessions when one or more individuals are ending their DBT skills training program.

Pretreatment Sessions: Tasks to Complete before Skills Training Begins

"Pretreatment" in DBT refers to all sessions and conversations occurring between a client and a provider until both parties have agreed that DBT is an appropriate intervention for the client's goals and wishes, and both parties have agreed to work together.

There are five pretreatment tasks (outlined in Table 3.1): (1) conducting a pretreatment assessment and deciding the appropriateness of skills training for the client; (2) deciding on the intensity of treatment and type of skills training needed for this particular client; (3) orienting the client to the specifics of skills training; (4) developing a collaborative commitment to do skills training together; and (5) beginning to develop an alliance. Each of these steps should be gone through during the initial individual interviews with each client before he or she is admitted to skills training, and Steps 3–5 should be

repeated during skills orientation, which precedes each iteration of the Mindfulness module.

Conducting a Pretreatment Assessment

Evaluation for skills training should begin with a clinical assessment, including assessment of presenting problems and goals, past and present life-threatening behaviors, diagnostic evaluation as needed, and evaluation of reading and language deficits (if the client's skills in these areas seem questionable). The assessor should also take a general history and ask about history of previous DBT and DBT skills training. These assessments can be done either informally, or formally with structured behavioral assessments. Depending on your setting, it might be advisable to conduct a phone screening interview before scheduling an in-person interview. We have found this particularly important for our friends-and-family groups and for groups aimed at treating individuals with specific problems (e.g., substance use disorders) or diagnoses. The assessor should also decide whether skills training, either individually or in a group, appears appropriate for this client.

TABLE 3.1. Pretreatment Tasks: Tasks to Complete before Skills Training Begins

- Conduct pretreatment assessment.
- Determine intensity and treatment type needed.
- Orient client to specifics of skills training.
- Develop collaborative commitment.
- Begin developing alliance.

Determining the Intensity of Treatment and Type of Skills Training Needed

A major function of the assessment sequence described above is to determine whether the individual client needs a more comprehensive treatment than stand-alone DBT skills training. In other words, does the person need something more than DBT skills? Many options and intensities of care can be considered, such as standard outpatient DBT; DBT skills training plus intensive case management; DBT skills integrated into individual DBT; DBT added to non-DBT case management or psychotherapy; and inpatient, residential, and day treatment DBT. (See Dimeff and Koerner's book for descriptions of various models of DBT intervention.[1]) The number and type of additional treatment components will depend for the most part on the client's "level of disorder," which is defined by the current presence of mental disorder and (if present) the severity, pervasiveness, and complexity of the disorder, as well as the disability and imminent threat to life it creates for the client. The level of disorder is linked to one of four stages of treatment in DBT. Stages of treatment are, in turn, linked to goals and specific targets of behavior to increase and decrease. Table 3.2 is a guide to making this series of decisions.

Generally, the criteria for putting a client in Stage 1 are a current severe mental disorder, behavioral dyscontrol, and/or imminent threat to life. Any of these conditions will prohibit working on any other goals before behavior and functioning come under better control. As Mintz suggested in discussing treatment of the suicidal client, all forms of psychotherapy are ineffective with a dead client.[2] In the subsequent stages (2–4), the treatment goals are to replace "quiet desperation" with nontraumatic emotional experiencing (Stage 2); to achieve "ordinary" happiness and unhappiness, and to reduce ongoing disorders and problems in living (Stage 3); and to resolve a sense of incompleteness, and to achieve a sense of freedom and joy (Stage 4). Not all clients enter therapy at the same stage of disorder; not all clients go through all of the stages; and clients can vacillate between stages.

As noted in Chapter 1, DBT skills training is now being offered as a stand-alone treatment for several mental disorders and for an array of other specific problems; as a preventive intervention in school systems; and as a set of interpersonal, mindfulness, and resiliency skills for the general public. Thus assessment is critical to selecting the right kind of skills program for the client. At this writing, however, there is very little research on how to match individuals seeking DBT to level of care needed. Thus the recommendations in Table 3.2 are based on my own clinical experience and that of others rather than on firm data.

Once the level of care is determined, the next thing that has to be decided is what skills training curriculum best fits the client. As far as possible, this decision should be based on the research that has been conducted to date and the problems presented by the clients. Unfortunately, many research reports do not list the specific skills used. In our clinics we always teach the DBT core skills, and other components, such as the addiction skills, are based on the specific problems of the clients we are treating. I have tried to offer some assistance with these choices in the Part I Appendices, following Chapter 5.

Finally, it is important to decide how you will evaluate progress in treatment. Many people use the DBT diary card (see Chapter 4 of this manual) as a method of tracking increases and decreases in problem behaviors, as well as changes in mood, self-efficacy, use of skills, and the client's beliefs that skills are helping. However, because the diary card was developed as a means for a client and therapist to track behavior on a weekly basis to inform weekly therapy, the diary is not set up in a way that is optimal for data analysis. Using the diary card as a way to track progress over time ordinarily means transferring the data to some sort of database or recording system and then analyzing them for changes over time in each variable you are interested in. This can be done by using statistics and/or by drawing graphs that depict change over time.

In our clinics, and in many clinics providing behavioral interventions, we also use assessment measures that are free or inexpensive and that have acceptable psychometric properties. A list of the measures we use is provided in Table 3.3. If you use assessments from this list, it will be important to select those that will measure outcomes that are important to your client population. In a 6-month treatment, it can be useful to give questionnaires at pretreatment, at 3 months, and at 6 months. For a 1-year treatment, you might want to give them at pretreatment and at 4, 8, and 12 months.

TABLE 3.2. Determining Treatment Intensity and Type of Treatment Needed

Client characteristics/treatment targets	Suggested interventions[a]

DBT Stage 1

1. Life-threatening behaviors—for example:
   a. Suicide attempts
   b. Suicide crisis behaviors
   c. Deliberate self-harm
   d. Other imminent life-threatening behavior
2. Serious therapy-interfering behaviors—for example:
   e. Noncollaborative behaviors
   f. Noncompliance
   g. Nonattending behaviors
   h. Behaviors that interfere with other patients
   i. Behaviors that interfere with therapists' ability to treat
3. Severe quality-of-life-interfering behaviors—for example:
   j. Incapacitating and/or severe mental disorder
   k. Extreme poverty/deprivation/homelessness
   l. Criminal behaviors with high imminent risk of jail
   m. Domestic violence
   n. Behavior dyscontrol with serious consequences
4. Severe Skills Deficits

Standard DBT: Outpatient
   DBT skills training +
   Skills coaching between sessions +
   DBT consultation team +
   DBT individual therapy . . . or

Intensive case management + DBT suicide protocol + Crisis plan with area crisis line . . . or

Standard DBT: Inpatient, residential, day treatment programs
   DBT skills training +
   Skills coaching between sessions +
   DBT individual therapy +
   DBT team . . . or

DBT skills training while on waiting list
   + DBT consultation team

DBT Stage 2

1. PTSD
2. Residual mental disorders with moderate severity not treated in Stage 1—for example:
   a. Anxiety disorders
   b. Eating disorders
   c. Mood disorders
3. Emotion dysregulation/dysfunctional intensity or duration of emotions—for example:
   d. Shame, guilt, sensitivity to criticism
   e. Anger, disgust, envy, jealousy
   f. Loneliness, inhibited grieving
   g. Emptiness, excessive sadness
   h. Fear

Standard DBT: Outpatient (see above) +

DBT PTSD protocol + prolonged exposure or other evidence-based PTSD treatment

DBT skills training curriculum for:
   Eating disorders
   Emotion dysregulation
   Treatment-resistant depression

DBT Stage 3

1. Problems in living—such as:
   a. Mild-severity disorders
   b. Difficulties in setting and/or achieving life goals
   c. Difficulties with problem solving
   d. Low self-efficacy/self-esteem
   e. Inadequate quality of life
   f. Relationship/marital distress
   g. Employment difficulties/distress
   h. Mild emotion dysregulation
   i. Indecision/desire for consultation
   j. Need for check-ins, checkups, tuneups

DBT skills training + DBT team + as-needed individual treatment (DBT or non-DBT) and/or as-needed skills coaching

DBT Stage 4

1. Incompleteness—for example:
   a. Desire for spiritual fulfillment/spiritual direction
   b. Desire for peak experiences/experience of reality as it is
   c. Boredom
   d. End of life issues

DBT reality acceptance and mindfulness skills training + DBT team and/or mindfulness retreats with participants (*under development*)

---

[a]It is important to recognize that the suggestions I give here are based both on my experience and on research to date. Research on DBT, however, is expanding at a rapid rate, and it is important for the reader to keep up with research as it is reported. These recommendations are likely to change over time and as new research findings are obtained.

TABLE 3.3. Assessment Instruments Used with Potential DBT Participants at the Behavioral Research and Therapy Clinics, University of Washington

Measures for adults

Borderline Symptom Checklist–23 (BSL-23)
Bohus, M., Kleindienst, N., Limberger, M. F., Stieglitz, R., Domsalla, M., Chapman, A. L., et al. (2009). The short version of the Borderline Symptom List (BSL-23): Development and initial data on psychometric properties. *Psychopathology, 42*(1), 32–39.
http://blogs.uw.edu/brtc/publications-assessment-instruments

DBT Diary Card[a]
(See Chapter 4) *http://blogs.uw.edu/brtc/publications-assessment-instruments/*

Demographic Data Scale (DDS)[a]
Linehan, M. M. (1994). Unpublished measure, University of Washington.
http://blogs.uw.edu/brtc/publications-assessment-instruments/

Dialectical Behavior Therapy Ways of Coping Checklist[a]
Neacsiu, A. D., Rizvi, S. L., Vitaliano, P. P., Lynch, T. R., & Linehan, M. M. (2010). The Dialectical Behavior Therapy Ways of Coping Checklist (DBT-WCCL): Development and psychometric properties. *Journal of Clinical Psychology, 66*(1), 1–20.
http://blogs.uw.edu/brtc/publications-assessment-instruments/

Difficulties in Emotion Regulation Scale (DERS)
Gratz, K. L., & Roemer, L. (2004). Multidimensional assessment of emotion regulation and dysregulation: Development, factor structure, and initial validation of the Difficulties in Emotion Regulation Scale. *Journal of Psychopathology and Behavioral Assessment, 26,* 41–54.
chipts.ucla.edu/downloads/299

Dissociative Experiences Scale (DES)
Bernstein, E. M., & Putnam, F. W. (1986). Development, reliability, and validity of a dissociative scale. *Journal of Nervous and Mental Disease, 174,* 727–735.
serene.me.uk/tests/des.pdf

Hamilton Anxiety Scale (HAM-A)
Hamilton, M. (1959). The assessment of anxiety states by rating. *British Journal of Medical Psychology, 32,* 50–55.
www.psychiatrictimes.com/clinical-scales-anxiety/clinical-scales-anxiety/ham-hamilton-anxiety-scale

Hamilton Depression Scale (HAM-D)
Hamilton, M. (1960). A rating scale for depression. *Journal of Neurology, Neurosurgery and Psychiatry, 23,* 56–62.
healthnet.umassmed.edu/mhealth/HAMD.pdf

Lifetime Suicide Attempt Self-Injury Count (S-SASI)[a]
Linehan, M. M., & Comtois, K. A. (1996). Unpublished manuscript, University of Washington.
http://blogs.uw.edu/brtc/publications-assessment-instruments

Patient Health Questionnaire–9 (PHQ-9)
Kroenke, K., & Spitzer, R. L. (2002). The PHQ-9: A new depression and diagnostic severity measure. *Psychiatric Annals, 32,* 509–521.
www.integration.samhsa.gov/images/res/PHQ%20-%20Questions.pdf

Posttraumatic Stress Disorder Checklist
Weathers, F. W., Litz, B. T., Herman, D. S., Huska, J. A., & Keane, T. M. (1993). *The PTSD Checklist (PCL): Reliability, validity, and diagnostic utility.* Paper presented at the 9th annual conference of the International Society for Traumatic Stress Studies, San Antonio, TX.
www.bhevolution.org/public/document/pcl.pdf

Reasons for Living Inventory (RFL)
Linehan, M. M., Goodstein, J. L., Nielsen, S. L., & Chiles, J. A. (1983). When you are thinking of killing yourself: The Reasons for Living Inventory. *Journal of Consulting and Clinical Psychology, 51*(2), 276–286.
http://blogs.uw.edu/brtc/publications-assessment-instruments

Suicidal Behaviors Questionnaire (SBQ)[a]
Linehan, M. M. (1981). Unpublished manuscript, University of Washington.
http://blogs.uw.edu/bttc/publications-assessment-instruments

Suicide Attempt Self-Injury Interview (SASII)[a]
Linehan, M. M., Comtois, K. A., Brown, M. Z., Heard, H. L., & Wagner, A. (2006). Suicide Attempt Self-Injury Interview (SASII): Development, reliability, and validity of a scale to assess suicide attempts and intentional self-injury. *Psychological Assessment, 18*(3), 303–312.
http://blogs.uw.edu/brtc/publications-assessment-instruments

State–Trait Anger Expression Inventory (STAXI)
Spielberger, C. D., Jacobs, G. A., Russell, S., & Crane, R. S. (1983). Assessment of anger: The State–Trait Anger Scale. *Advances in Personality Assessment, 2*(2), 1–47.
Contact Psychological Assessment Resources, 800-331-8378, *www4.parinc.com*

(cont.)

[a]Developed at the University of Washington; copying and distribution to clients allowed.

TABLE 3.3 (*cont.*)

Measures for adults (*cont.*)

Structured Clinical Interview for DSM-IV, Axis I (SCID)

First, M. B., Spitzer, R. L., Gibbon, M., & Williams, J. B. W. (1995). *Structured Clinical Interview for Axis I DSM-IV Disorders—Patient Edition (SCID-I/P)*. New York: Biometrics Research Department, New York State Psychiatric Institute.

Contact Biometrics Research for a research version of the SCID, 212-960-5524

Structured Clinical Interview for DSM-IV, Axis II Personality Disorders (SCID-II)

First, M. B., Gibbon, M., Spitzer, R. L., Williams, J. B. W., & Benjamin, L. (1996). *User's guide for the Structured Clinical Interview for DSM-IV Axis II Personality Disorders (SCID-II)*. New York: Biometrics Research Department, New York State Psychiatric Institute.

Contact American Psychiatric Press, Inc., 800-368-5777, *www.appi.org/index.html*

UCLA Loneliness Scale

Russell, D., Peplau, L. A.. & Ferguson, M. L. (1978). Developing a measure of loneliness. *Journal of Personality Assessment, 42*, 290–294.

www.fetzer.org/sites/default/files/images/stories/ pdf/selfmeasures/Self_Measures_for_Loneliness_and_ Interpersonal_Problems_UCLA_LONELINESS.pdf

University of Washington Risk Assessment Protocol (UWRAP)[a]

Reynolds, S. K., Lindenboim, N., Comtois, K. A., Murray, A., & Linehan, M. M. (2006). Risky assessments: Participant suicidality and distress associated with research assessments in a treatment study of suicidal behavior. *Suicide and Life-Threatening Behavior, 36*(1), 19–33.

http://blogs.uw.edu/brtc/publications-assessment-instruments

University of Washington Risk Assessment & Management Protocol (UWRAMP)[a]

Linehan, M. M., Comtois, K. A., & Ward-Ciesielski, E. F. (2012). Assessing and managing risk with suicidal individuals. *Cognitive and Behavioral Practice, 19*(2), 218–232.

http://blogs.uw.edu/brtc/publications-assessment-instruments

Measures for adolescents

Brief Reasons for Living Inventory for Adolescents (BRFL-A)

Osman, A., Kopper, B. A., Barrios, F. X., Osman, J. R., Besett, T., & Linehan, M. M. (1996). The Brief Reasons for Living Inventory for Adolescents (BRFL-A). *Journal of Abnormal Child Psychology, 24*(4), 433–443.

https://depts.washington.edu/brtc/files/Osman,%20 A.%20(1996)%20The%20Brief%20RFL%20for%20 Adolescents%20(BRFL-A).pdf

Schedule for Affective Disorders and Schizophrenia for School-Age Children (Kiddie-SADS)

Endicott, J., & Spitzer, R. L. (1978). A diagnostic interview: The Schedule for Affective Disorders and Schizophrenia. *Archives of General Psychiatry, 35*(7), 873–844.

www.wpic.pitt.edu/ksads

Suicidal Behaviors Interview (SBI)

Reynolds, W. M. (1990). Development of a semi-structured clinical interview for suicidal behaviors in adolescents. *Psychological Assessment, 2*(4), 382–390.

Contact: *william.reynolds@ubc.ca*

Suicide Ideation Questionnaire—Junior

Siemen, J. R., Warrington, C. A., & Mangano, E. L. (1994). Comparison of the Millon Adolescent Personality Inventory and the Suicide Ideation Questionnaire—Junior with an adolescent inpatient sample. *Psychological Reports, 75*(2), 947–950.

Contact Psychological Assessment Resources, 800-331-8378, *www4.parinc.com*

Note. I use the DSM-IV to assess for borderline personality disorder but am moving to DSM-V to measure other disorders.

Orienting the Client to the Specifics of Skills Training

Following assessment, the therapist should briefly present the skills deficit model of emotional and behavioral dysregulation, which is discussed briefly in Chapter 1 of this manual and in detail in Chapter 2 of the main DBT text. If diagnostic interviewing and commitment to skills training have been thoroughly covered at intake or by the individual therapist in standard DBT, the pretreatment meeting with the skills leader or co-leader can be much briefer. In my clinic, each individual in our standard DBT program first has a thorough intake (including diagnostic interviews), and then meets with the individual DBT therapist for a thorough discussion of DBT skills training. Clients then meet with the skills leader or co-leader for 15 or so minutes before their first skills session. Individuals in our skills training groups (with no individual therapy) have an intake session first and then meet with the skills leader or co-leader to evaluate whether skills training is appropriate for each client's goals. Initial commitment for skills training is obtained at this meeting.

The individual pretreatment interview with the skills trainer should orient the client to the specifics of skills training. This includes how the group (if there is a group) will function, what the client's and the trainer's roles in skills training are, and how skills training is different from other types of therapy

In standard DBT (which includes an individual provider), these discussions ordinarily take place between a client and an intake coordinator (if there is one), and then between the client and the individual provider. In standard DBT, the skills trainer usually calls and then meets new clients for 5–15 minutes before their first skills training session. If skills training is a stand-alone intervention or if skills are being integrated into ongoing individual therapy, then the skills trainer performs all the tasks that an individual provider would normally provide.

Orienting Clients to Skills Training versus Other Types of Therapy

It is essential that the leaders discuss the difference between a skills training group and other group or individual psychotherapies. Many individuals look forward to a group where they can share with individuals like themselves. Although there is much sharing in the group, it is not unlimited—and it is focused on practicing skills, not on whatever crises may have occurred during the week. Many participants have never been in any kind of behavior therapy, much less a skills-oriented group. My experience is that the difference cannot be stressed too much. Often clients have had an enormous amount of nonbehavioral therapy in which they have been taught various "necessary ingredients" for therapeutic change—ingredients that skills training often does not address extensively. In every group we have conducted so far, one or more clients have gotten angry about their inability to talk about "what is really important" in the group. For one client, talking about whatever comes to mind was so firmly associated with the process of therapy that she refused to acknowledge that skills training could be a form of therapy. Needless to say, there was much friction with her in the group. I discuss orienting to skills training in more detail in this manual's Chapters 4 and 6.

Developing a Collaborative Commitment to Do Skills Training

Once you have decided to accept a person into skills training, it is important that you yourself make a commitment to treating the individual. Entering a treatment with reluctance, reserve, or antagonism, or on unwanted commands from others, can markedly impair your chances of developing a strong and collaborative relationship with your skills training participants. It is also important to talk with potential clients about any pressures from family members that may be the main impetus for their coming to DBT or to skills training specifically—particularly with adolescents coming to treatment with their parents. Because standard DBT requires both individual therapy and skills training, it is altogether possible that an individual therapist is also pressuring a client to attend skills training. For DBT to be effective, individuals must participate voluntarily; thus, you may need to work with the potential clients to see the pros and not just the cons of coming to skills training and learning the DBT skills offered. Remember, participation can be pressured and voluntary at the same time. At this point, if you accept a reluctant but mostly willing client for treatment, the practice of radical acceptance and opposite action will be particularly important. Working with your DBT team will also be important for strengthening your personal commitment to the task. Follow all of the DBT guidelines on obtaining an initial therapy commitment from skills training participants. These are outlined and discussed in Chapters 9 and 14 of the main DBT text. It is impossible to get too much commitment! A skills trainer should not assume that other therapists (e.g., the individual psychotherapist or the intake interviewer in a clinic setting) have gotten the commitment needed. This is a mistake my colleagues and I made early in our program, and we paid a dear price for it. The pretreatment session is also a good opportunity to begin developing a personal therapeutic alliance with the client (the fifth pretreatment task; see Chapters 14 and 15 of the main DBT text for more on this topic).

Beginning to Develop the Alliance

Use of standard DBT therapeutic relationship strategies, such as relationship acceptance and relationship enhancement, is particularly important at the start of skills training (see below). In a group context, one of the first tasks of the group leaders is to enhance the bonding between group clients and the leaders, and to begin the process of building group cohesion. We have found it useful to have the leaders call each new group member a few days before the first skills training meeting to remind him or her of the session, clarify directions, and communicate looking forward to meeting him or her. It is also a good time for the leaders to address last-minute fears and plans to drop out before even starting. Individuals joining an ongoing group are also invited to come early to their first session for a brief orientation to the basics of DBT skills training. At the session before new members join, we usually discuss the importance of encouraging and welcoming new members. Clients starting a module late are, in addition, given a brief review of skills already taught.

The leaders should arrive a few minutes early before each group meeting, especially the first meeting of a new group, to greet clients and interact briefly with group members. For reluctant and/or fearful clients, this can be a soothing experience. It also offers an opportunity for leaders to hear concerns and refute plans to leave early. We try to confine individual interactions to the context of group mingling, in order to keep the essential identity of group rather than individual therapy. This issue is discussed further below.

As might be expected, group members are very timid and fearful during the first meeting. Appropriate behavior is not clear, and the trustworthiness of group clients is doubtful. We generally begin by going around the group and asking each person to give his or her name, to say how he or she heard about the group, and to give any information about him- or herself the person cares to share. The group leaders also give information about themselves and how they came to be leading the group.

The next task of skills trainers is to help clients see the relevance of a skills training model to their own lives. An overview of the skills training treatment year is given (see Table 2.2 in Chapter 2); a theory of disordered emotion regulation that stresses the role of inadequate skills is presented; and the format for the upcoming sessions is described. If the group is homogeneous with regard to disorder or problem type (e.g., substance use disorders, suicidal behavior, eating disorders), then a similar skills deficit model of the specific problem behavior is also provided. Discussion is elicited at each point about the relevance of the material to the client's own experiences. A handout (General Handout 1) illustrat-

ing the relationship between the characteristics of disordered emotion regulation and the goals of skills training is distributed and discussed (see Chapter 6 of this manual for details); usually I also write this on the whiteboard in the therapy room.

It is essential here for the skills trainer to communicate an expectancy that the treatment will be effective at helping the clients improve the quality of their own lives. The treatment must be "marketed" to clients. (See Chapters 9 and 14 of the main DBT text for further discussion of marketing therapy to clients and eliciting commitments.) At this time I usually make the point that DBT is not a suicide prevention program (or substance abstinence or symptom improvement program), but a life enhancement program. It is not our idea to get people to live lives not worth living, but rather to help them build lives they actually want to live. Dialectical and validation strategies (see Chapters 8 and 9 of the main DBT text, and Interpersonal Effectiveness Handouts 15–19a) are the primary treatment vehicles here.

Relationship Acceptance

Relationship acceptance strategies in group skills training require that leaders experience and communicate acceptance of group members in several different spheres. First, the clinical progress of each client must be accepted as it is. Relationships between leaders and group members, between members and other therapists, between and among individual members, between the group leaders themselves, and between the group as a whole and the group leaders must also be accepted. The sheer complexity of the situation can make acceptance difficult, because it is easy to get overwhelmed; rigidity and nonacceptance usually follow. It is essential to try not to pave over or quickly truncate conflict and difficult emotions in the group. Many clients who have trouble regulating their emotions also have great difficulty with group skills training. Some are in it only because it is required, and they feel uncomfortable and are unable to interact effectively in this atmosphere. For others, skills seem unimportant, juvenile, or silly. Still others quickly become demoralized by unsuccessful attempts to master the skills.

Group skills training with clients who have difficulties regulating their emotions does not have the naturally occurring reinforcement for leaders that most groups have. Skills training leaders are faced with dead silences; noncompliance; inappropriate and sometimes extreme responses to the slightest deviation from perfect sensitivity; and a group atmosphere that at times can be uncommunicative, hostile, unsupportive, and unappreciative. The potential for mistakes in leading such a group is vast. A leader can expect not only to make many mistakes, but also to be acutely aware of the many mistakes the other group leader makes. Reality acceptance skills are crucial if mistakes are to be responded to in a nondestructive manner.

Leaders' attacking group members or threatening them is almost always a result of a failure in relationship acceptance. Acceptance requires a nonjudgmental attitude that sees all problems as part of the therapeutic process—"grist for the mill," so to speak. Leaders simply have to see that most problematic responses on the part of the group derive from emotionally dysregulated response patterns. In other words, if clients didn't present with the problems that drive leaders crazy, they wouldn't need a skills training group. To the extent that leaders fail to recognize this fact, they are likely to engage in rejecting, victim-bashing behaviors that may be too subtle to be seen for what they are, but nonetheless have an iatrogenic effect. In other words, an "easy" leader disposition has to be either innate or cultivated.

Relationship Enhancement

Relationship enhancement strategies involve behaviors by skills trainers that increase the therapeutic values of the relationship. In other words, they are behaviors that make the relationship more than simply a helpful friendship. A positive, collaborative interpersonal relationship is no less important in skills training than it is in any other type of therapy. However, the development of such a relationship is considerably more complex in group skills training, because of the increased number of individuals involved in the relationship. The question for the group leaders is how to establish such a relationship between group members and leaders, as well as among the members themselves.

All of the DBT strategies are designed in one way or another to enhance the collaborative working relationship. The strategies discussed here are those intended primarily to establish the group leaders as experts, as creditable, and as efficacious. Thus the goal of these strategies is to communicate to the group members that the leaders indeed know what they are doing and have something to offer that will

probably be helpful to the group members. This is no easy task. The task is made even more difficult by the fact that group members often share with one another their previous failures in individual and other group therapies, and comment about the hopelessness of their situations and the meagerness of any help that can be offered. Group members often portray their problems as Goliath and the treatment as David, but without David's Old Testament success. The task of the leaders is to convey the story as it indeed occurred.

Expertise, credibility, and efficacy can be conveyed in a variety of ways. Skills trainers' neatness, professionalism, interest, comfort, self-confidence, speech style, and preparation for therapy sessions are no less useful in skills training than in individual psychotherapy. It is especially important in conducting groups to have the group room prepared before the group members arrive: Handouts and worksheets should be distributed; chairs should be in place; and the refreshments should be made and available (if refreshments are provided). The key to the credibility problem, in my experience, is that many clients—particularly those with severe and chronic disorders—simply do not believe that learning the skills presented will in fact be helpful. This disbelief detracts from any positive motivation to learn the skills, and unless clients learn the skills and obtain positive rewards, it is difficult to change this attitude. Indeed, this dynamic can become a vicious circle.

Leaders must come up with a way to break this vicious circle if the clients are to move forward. The most helpful approach is for the leaders to tell group members that in their experience, these skills have been helpful to some people some of the time. This, of course, can only be said if it is indeed the leaders' experience; leaders who have never taught these skills must rely on others' experience. (Our outcome data can form a database for inexperienced skills trainers.) In addition, leaders can share their own experience with skills. For some clients, the most powerful inducement to learn the skills is the knowledge that the leaders have found the skills helpful for themselves.

Credibility is damaged when leaders promise that a particular skill will solve a particular problem. In fact, DBT is something of a shotgun approach: Some of the skills work some of the time for some of the people. I have not had any clients to date who could not benefit from something, but no one benefits from everything. It is crucial to present this information; otherwise, the leaders' credibility is on the line immediately.

Another key issue to address is that of trust and confidentiality. Opportunities to display trustworthiness occur when one member is absent from a group session. At all times, confidences must be kept, and unnecessary information about a group member should not be conveyed when that group member is absent. The absence of a group member, however, can serve as a powerful opportunity for enhancing other group members' trust in the leaders. The manner in which the absent member is discussed conveys information to all other members about how they will be treated when they are absent. Generally, the policy should be to protect group members from negative judgments. For example, if a group member blows up, walks out of a session, and slams the door, the leaders can respond to the event with sympathetic explanations rather than with critical judgments.

This same strategy, of course, can be used when all group members are present. It is not unusual for one group member to behave in a fashion that the leaders know will result in negative judgments by other group members. Or other group members may be quite critical of one another. The leaders' role here is that of protectors of the accused and the judged. This leadership task cannot be overemphasized, especially during the clients' first modules in skills training. Not only does this approach serve to model nonjudgmental observation and description of problematic behavior for group members; but it also conveys to all of the members that when they are attacked, they too will be protected. The most useful way to convey expertness and credibility is, of course, to be helpful. Thus the leaders need to think through skills that have a high likelihood of working with a particular group member. A skill that is working should be highlighted so that the member will also see the benefits.

Skills trainer credibility in standard DBT group skills training is further complicated by the fact that there are two group leaders. In my clinic, the co-leader is usually a trainee who, in fact, does not have the expertise of the primary leader. It is essential that the primary leader not undermine the credibility and expertness of the co-leader. It is important for the inexperienced co-leader to find his or her emotional center and act from there. It is this inner-centeredness, rather than any particular set of therapeutic skills, that is most important. The primary leader and co-leader do not need to have the same set of skills or to convey expertise in the same areas. The dialectical perspective as a whole is what counts.

Presenting Skills Training Guidelines

Make the rules of skills training explicit at the very beginning. Their presentation is an important part of the treatment process, not a precursor to the process and it offers an opportunity for the skills trainers to specify and obtain agreement to the treatment contract from each client. My experience is that the presentation and discussion of rules can usually be accomplished at the beginning of each iteration of the mindfulness module. In an open group, the guidelines should be discussed each time a new member enters the group. Guidelines I have found useful are outlined in General Handout 3 and described below.

1. *Participants who drop out of skills training are NOT out of skills training.* Only clients who miss 4 weeks of scheduled skills training sessions in a row have dropped out of therapy and cannot re-enter for the duration of the time in their treatment contract. For example, if a client has contracted for 1 year, but misses 4 weeks in a row during the sixth month, then he or she is out for the next 6 months or so. At the end of the contracted time, he or she can negotiate with the skills trainer(s) (and the group, if he or she was in one and it is continuing) about readmission. There are no exceptions to this rule. The rule for skills training is thus the same as the rule for individual DBT psychotherapy.

Across multiple studies using this rule, our dropout rates in 1-year DBT programs have been reasonably low. I suspect that our emphasis on a time-limited commitment and the clarity of the rules about how to drop out are crucial to our low dropout rate.

2. *Participants who join the skills training group support each other.* There are many ways to be a supportive person in skills training sessions. It is important that skills leaders review what is needed to be supportive. This includes preserving confidentiality, attending regularly, practicing skills between sessions, validating others, giving noncritical feedback, and being willing to accept help from a person (a leader or a fellow client) from whom help is requested.

A good group norm of coming on time and practicing skills between sessions is essential—but admittedly hard at times to develop. Discussing the importance of building norms at the start of each new module can be very helpful. My experience is that most skills training members want such norms to develop. (We have found it very effective to give out stickers to each person who comes to skills training on time that week.)

3. *Participants who are going to be late or miss a session call ahead of time.*

This rule serves several purposes. First, it is a courtesy to let skills trainers know not to wait for latecomers before starting. Second, it introduces an added response cost for being late and communicates to clients that promptness is desirable. Finally, it gives information as to why a client is not present.

4. *Participants do not tempt others to engage in problem behaviors.* This rule asks clients not to come to skills sessions under the influence of drugs or alcohol. However, if drugs or alcohol have already been used, clients are to come to the sessions acting clean and sober. Particularly for those with substance use disorders, a rule saying not to come to skills sessions when using substances just gives individuals with poor self-regulation a good excuse for not coming. Instead, my position is that skills learning is context-dependent, and thus for persons with substance use disorders, learning and practicing skills while under the influence of drugs or alcohol are particularly important. This is definitely the time when skills are needed.

This rule also outlaws descriptions of dysfunctional behaviors, which can be contagious. In my experience, communications about self-injury, substance use, bingeing or purging, and similar behaviors elicit strong imitation effects among individuals with disordered emotion regulation. These urges to imitate can be very difficult to resist. Therefore, just as in individual DBT, clients in skills training must agree not to call or communicate with one another *after* a self-injurious act. At every point in DBT, a major objective is to diminish the opportunity for reinforcement of dysfunctional behaviors. This is particularly true for discussions of suicidal behaviors.

5. *Participants do not form confidential relationships outside of skills training sessions.* The key word in the fifth rule is "confidential." Clients may not form relationships outside the sessions that they cannot discuss in the sessions. DBT encourages outside-of-session relationships among group clients. In fact, the support that members can give one another with daily problems in living is one of the strengths of group DBT. The model here is similar to that of Alcoholics Anonymous and other self-help groups, where calling one another between meetings, socializing, and offering mutual support are viewed as therapeutic. Encouragement of such relationships, however, provides the possibility for interpersonal conflict that is inherent in any relationship. The key is whether interpersonal problems that arise outside the sessions can be discussed in the sessions (or, if that is too difficult or threatens to get out of hand, with the leaders). To the extent that such issues can be discussed and appropriate skills can be applied, a relationship can be advantageous. Troubles arise when a relationship cannot be discussed and problems increase to such an extent that one member finds it difficult or impossible to attend meetings, either physically or emotionally.

Group leaders should assign current sexual partners to different groups at the onset. This rule also functions to alert group members that if they enter into a sexual relationship, one member of the pair will have to drop out. To date we have had several sexual relationships begin among group members; each created enormous difficulties for the partners involved. In one case, the initiating partner broke off the relationship against the wishes of the other, making it very hard for the rejected partner to come to group sessions. Generally, this rule is clear to everyone involved. Without the rule, however, dealing with an emerging sexual relationship between clients is very tricky, since post hoc application of rules is unworkable with individuals who have dysregulated emotions.

There are two exceptions to the rule. In skills training groups for friends and families, where couples, partners, and multiple family members often join the group, it is not reasonable or feasible to outlaw private relationships. A similar situation arises in the multifamily skills groups commonly held with adolescents. In these situations, however, it is important to note that when relationship conflicts threaten the group, the leaders will approach it in a manner similar to that described above.

6. *Participants who are suicidal and/or have severe disorders must be in ongoing individual treatment.* This rule is ordinarily discussed with clients during pretreatment (rather than during a group session), and the requirement to be in individual treatment is laid out at that time. Of note here is that these clients must actually meet with their individual therapists on a regular basis to stay in skills training. If the clients are in individual DBT treatment, then they cannot miss four scheduled individual sessions in a row. If they are in another form of individual therapy, then the attendance guidelines of that treatment must be followed. The exception to this rule is when clients are on a waiting list for therapy. Data collected by a Canadian research team found that skills training alone was effective in reducing suicide attempts in suicidal individuals on a treatment waiting list.[3]

This early emphasis on the likely need of highly dysregulated and/or suicidal participants for extra help in mastering the skills is very important later when the clients run into difficulty. It is all too easy for the skills trainers to overestimate the ease of learning skills; such overestimation sets the clients up for later disillusionment and hopelessness.

DBT skills training does not require that the individual therapist be a DBT therapist. Nonetheless, the requirement for individual therapy can still be quite formidable at times. In our experience, it is not uncommon for individual therapists in the community to get pushed past their limits by clients with dysregulated emotions, and then to terminate therapy precipitously with these clients. When this happens, it can be extraordinarily difficult to find an individual therapist willing to work with such clients, especially with those who are mourning the loss of previous therapists. This is especially problematic when the clients cannot afford to pay the high fees often charged by professionals who are experienced enough to be helpful. Unfortunately, many public health clinics are so understaffed that they cannot provide individual psychotherapy, or clients may have already burned out their local clinics. In these cases, the skills training leaders often must function as short-term backup crisis therapists and assist the clients in finding appropriate individual therapists.

Presenting DBT Assumptions

The assumptions underlying treatment are outlined in General Handout 4 and described below. Along with the skills training guidelines, they are presented and discussed with skills participants during orientation (which is repeated before the start of each Mindfulness skills module) and in person with clients who join a skills group after the first session of a module. An "assumption" is a belief that cannot be proved, but group members agree to abide by it anyway. DBT across the board is based on the following assumptions.

1. *People are doing the best they can.* The idea here is that all people at any given point in time are doing the best they can, given the causes of behavior that have occurred up to this moment.

2. *People want to improve.* The common characteristic of all people is that they want to improve their lives. As noted by the Dalai Lama at a meeting I was part of, a common characteristic of all people is that they want to be happy.

3. **People need to do better, try harder, and be more motivated to change.* The fact that someone is doing the best he or she can and wants to do even better does not mean that this is enough to solve the problem. (The asterisk here means that this is not always true. In particular, when progress is steady and is occurring at a realistic rate, with no let-up or episodic drop in effort, doing better, trying harder, and being more motivated are not needed.)

4. **People may not have caused all of their own problems, but they have to solve them anyway.* People have to change their own behavioral responses and alter their environment for their lives to change. (The asterisk here indicates that with children or disabled persons, others might be needed to solve some problems. For example, young children cannot get themselves to treatment if parents or others refuse to take them.)

5. *New behavior has to be learned in all relevant contexts.* New behavioral skills have to be practiced in the situations where the skills are needed, not just in the situation where the skills are first learned.

6. *All behaviors (actions, thoughts, emotions) are caused.* There is always a cause or set of causes for actions, thoughts, and emotions, even if people do not know what the causes are.

7. *Figuring out and changing the causes of behavior is a more effective way to change than judging and blaming.* Judging and blaming are easier, but anyone who wants to create change in the world has to change the chains of events that cause unwanted behaviors and events.

Format and Organization of Ongoing Skills Training Sessions

The structuring of session time is the major factor differentiating formal DBT skills training from DBT individual psychotherapy. In individual DBT psychotherapy, the agenda is set by a client's behavior since the last session and within the current session; the agenda is open until the client shows up for the session. In skills training, the therapy agenda is set by the behavioral skill to be taught; the agenda is set before a client shows up for the session.

Skills training sessions require at least four sections: (1) a beginning ritual, (2) review of homework practice since the last session, (3) presentation of new material, and (4) a closing "wind-down." In my clinic, skills training sessions for individuals with severe disorders (including BPD) last for 2½ hours, generally with a 15-minute break in the middle. The format is reasonably consistent for the whole year. The sessions begin with a mindfulness exercise, followed by group members' sharing their attempts (or lack of attempts) to practice behavioral skills during the preceding week, followed by a break. The second hour is devoted to presenting and discussing new skills. The last 15 minutes are allotted to a session wind-down, which involves going around the room and having each person share one observation about the session (a practice of the mindfulness skills of observing and describing).

This format varies slightly for the final session of each module. Instead of presenting new material, that session's second half is devoted to a review of all the skills from that module; a review of skills from the previous modules; and a discussion of pros and cons of using the skills and skill generalization across situations and contexts in participants' lives. The session concludes with a wind-down, which can consist of observations about the module as a whole and how the weeks and sessions on the module went.

If any individuals are leaving the skills training group, there is time set aside to say goodbye and discuss termination issues. Generally, we ask those leaving for ideas on snacks for the last meeting, and also let them choose the mindfulness practice at the beginning of the group. We give (standing with the participant by our side) each graduating person a graduation certificate signed by the two co-leaders and a graduation card with personal notes from each leader. Unless there is a good reason for not doing so, we end the session with each person given an opportunity to say a personal good bye. In sum, you want to give departing participants a positive sendoff.

In our friends-and-family program and in skills training for participants with less severe disorders, groups last from 90 minutes to 2 hours. Adolescent groups also last from 90 minutes to 2 hours. Individual skills training sessions ordinarily last 45–60 minutes. In each case, however, the general four-part structure of sessions is the same as outlined in

Table 3.4. Each of the four sections is discussed in more detail below.

Some inpatient settings have split this format in two, holding two weekly sessions—one devoted to homework review and one devoted to new skills. This is a reasonable model on inpatient and day treatment units, where staff members have some ability to persuade clients to attend both weekly sessions. In an outpatient setting, however, there is a danger that clients will not attend homework review sessions when they have not practiced any of their skills during the preceding week. Skills trainers will want to prevent that from occurring.

Other settings have shortened the session time, usually from 2½ to 1½ hours. In my clinic's experience with adults with severe behavioral and emotional dyscontrol, 1½ hours is not enough time for a group session. Even with 2½ hours, 50–60 minutes for homework review with eight group members gives each member about 6–8 minutes of group attention—not very much. Nor is 50–60 minutes for new material much time, either. Although group leaders can present a lot of material in that time, they also need time to do in-session practice of new skills, to discuss questions about the week's new content, to check skill comprehension with each member, and to go over new homework sheets to be sure that clients understand how to do the practice and how to record it. Individual skills training can be accomplished in weekly 45- to 50-minute sessions.

Session Room Setup and Materials

It is important to set up the room for skills training sessions differently from what is usually done for traditional group or individual therapy. To the degree possible, the aim should be to elicit a sense of being in a classroom. We conduct our group sessions in a conference room around a table, with a whiteboard for the skills trainers to write on. For

TABLE 3.4. Standard Skills Training Session Format

- Beginning ritual (mindfulness exercise)
- Review of homework practice
- Break
- Presentation of new material/skills
- Closing wind-down

individual skills training, we bring in a small desk for the client to sit at; if this is not possible, we teach individual skills in a room different from the individual therapy room. Skills training handouts and worksheets for all modules to be taught are given out in three-ring binders with pockets in front and back. Handouts are printed on one color of paper, and worksheets on another color. Generally, we try not to use white paper, as it makes it more difficult for those with dyslexia to read. We also use labeled dividers between sections and between handouts and worksheets within sections. In the front binder pockets, we put forms to track weekly practice assignments; in the back pockets, we put a supply of DBT diary cards. The diary card lists the most important DBT skills taught. Next to each skill on the card is a space for recording whether or not the client actually practiced the skill on each day during the week. (See Chapter 4 and Figure 4.1 for more details about the diary card, as well as Chapter 6 of the main DBT text.) Pencils/pens for taking notes are available on the table. Clients are instructed to bring in their binders each week. Loaner binders are available if they forget their own.

Other materials to bring to the session include a small bell that can be rung to start and end mindfulness practices, and a selection of distress tolerance tools (e.g., cold gel pack, rubber ball with spikes, balance board) for use by people who may be in danger of dissociating during the sessions. It can also be useful to record sessions on video, if the necessary equipment is available. (For more on this, see the discussion in Chapter 4 on managing the homework review.)

At our group sessions, we serve decaffeinated coffee and tea (and usually snacks as well). Before the beginning ritual, members get coffee or tea and a snack and get settled. In our groups, if people want to bring their own snacks, then they have to bring enough to share with everyone.

Session-Beginning Ritual

We begin with the session leader or co-leader leading a mindfulness practice. An effort is made to vary the practices so that over the weeks we practice each of the mindfulness skills. Mindfulness practices are listed on Mindfulness Handouts 4a–4c and 5a–5c. We start each practice by ringing the mindfulness bell three times, and end it by ringing the bell once. Then we go around the room and ask each participant (including the leader and co-leader) to share

his or her experience with the group. This sharing is very important, as it does not take much time and gives the leader or co-leader a chance to provide corrective feedback if needed. If members have missed one or more previous sessions, they are given a chance to tell the group where they have been. If missing sessions is a problem for a person, attention (no more than 5 minutes or so) can be paid to analyzing what interferes with coming and how to overcome it. If there are group issues (e.g., announcements; not calling when missing; or coming late), they are dealt with at the beginning of the session. This brief attention to therapy-interfering behaviors is very important and should not be dropped.

A therapist who is conducting individual skills training should follow the session-beginning guidelines in Chapter 14 of the main DBT text—greeting the client with warmth; attending, if only briefly, to the client's current emotional state; and repairing relationship difficulties at the beginning of a session if needed. Only a limited amount of time should then be spent on beginning strategies. If possible, the therapist should help the client use his or her distress tolerance crisis survival strategies (see Chapter 10 of this manual) to manage current emotions if extreme and distract from the need for further repair, do skills training, and get back to repair at the end of the session or at the next individual psychotherapy meeting.

Review of Homework: Sharing of Homework Practice Efforts

The next phase of treatment is the sharing of between-session efforts to practice the specific behavioral skills (mindfulness, interpersonal effectiveness, emotion regulation, distress tolerance) being taught. In our group sessions, the primary group leader goes around the circle and asks each member to share with the group what he or she has practiced during the preceding week. In my experience, waiting for members to volunteer takes up too much time. However, I may let members decide who to start with in going around the circle. Vocabulary can be very important here. Behaviorists are used to calling practice "homework," and therefore to asking clients about their "homework practice." Some of our clients like this terminology and prefer to think of skills training as a class they are taking, much like a college course. Others feel demeaned by the words, as if they are being treated like children in school and once again having to report to adults.

A discussion of the semantics at the very beginning of treatment can be successful in defusing this issue.

The weekly sharing of homework practice efforts is an essential part of skills training. The sure knowledge that not only will each client be asked about his or her efforts to practice skills, but that not practicing will be analyzed in depth, serves as a powerful motivation for at least attempting to practice skills during the week. The norm of weekly *in vivo* practice is set and maintained during the sharing. Every client should be asked to share his or her experiences, even those who communicate extreme reluctance or aversion to the task. This part of the session is so important that its completion takes precedence over any other group task. To finish the sharing in the 50–60 minutes allotted takes very good time management skills on the part of the primary leader, as noted above. However, the usual absence of one or more clients, together with the equally usual tendency of one or two each week to refuse to interact more than briefly, adds considerably to the time per person available for sharing. Managing homework practice is discussed further in Chapter 4 of this manual.

Break

Most clients get restless after about an hour of a group session. We usually take a 10- or 15-minute break at about the halfway mark. Members can get a refill of coffee or tea, and a snack if snacks are provided. Most clients go outside for fresh air. This part of the session is important, because it provides an unstructured period of time for group clients to interact. Generally the group leaders stay near but somewhat apart from group clients during the break. Group cohesion, independent of the leaders, is thus fostered. If a member needs individual attention from a leader, however, it is given at this point. One of our main problems has been that clients having a hard time at a session often leave during the break. We have found it advisable to be particularly alert to anyone who may be leaving, so that intervention can be attempted before he or she walks out.

Presentation of New Material

The hour after the break is devoted to the presentation and discussion of new skills or, if necessary, the review of ones already covered. The material in Chapters 7–10 is presented in this part of the session.

The first 30 minutes of each *new* skills training module (remember that there are four) is spent in discussing the rationale for that particular module. (In an ongoing group, the time devoted to homework review is cut short during the first session of each iteration of the Mindfulness module.) The leaders' task here is to convince the clients that the skills to be covered in the upcoming module are relevant to their lives; that if they improve these particular skills their lives will improve; and, most importantly, that they can actually learn the skills. The leaders often have to be creative in demonstrating how particular sets of skills apply to particular problems. The specific rationales for each module are described in Chapters 7–10.

Closing Wind-Down

Allotting time at the end of a group skills training session for winding down is very important for clients with emotion dysregulation. These sessions are almost always emotionally charged and painful for some. Individuals who have difficulties regulating their emotions are acutely aware of the negative effects of their own skill deficits. Without emotion regulation skills of their own, clients can be in great emotional difficulty after a session, especially if nothing is done to help them regulate their affect and end or "close up" the session, so to speak.

A wind-down period also provides a time for clients who have dissociated during the session, usually because of painful memories, to come back into the session before parting. I was alerted to this need during my first DBT skills training group. After several months, it came up in a group discussion that almost every member of the group was going out drinking after the meetings as a means of affect control. Skills trainers will often find that topics that seem very innocuous are actually very stress-provoking for individuals with disordered emotion regulation. For example, a group member once became extremely emotional and disorganized as I was introducing the Interpersonal Effectiveness module and the fact that one task of the module would be to learn to say no effectively. She was currently enmeshed in a group of drug dealers who frequently raped her. She didn't say no because the group was her meal ticket.

Wind-downs should last from 5 to (at most) 15

minutes. I have used several wind-down methods. The most popular with our group members is the "observe and describe" wind-down. Each member describes one thing he or she observed during the session. The observation can be of liking or disliking an event that occurred during group (e.g., "I liked the mindfulness exercise today"), something someone else did (e.g., "Suzy came on time and stayed the whole time"), or a description of a self-observation (e.g., "I felt really sad when talking about my father"). The idea in this exercise is for the leaders to coach the clients in how to describe just the facts they observed, without adding assumptions and interpretations to the facts. For example, instead of saying, "I noticed I did better this week than last," a client might be coached to say, "The thought arose in my mind that I did better this week than last." Instead of "I noticed that Bill was really angry this week," the client might say, "I noticed thinking that Bill was really angry this week." A therapist who is conducting skills training individually should follow the session-closing strategies in Chapter 14 of the main DBT text.

With more advanced groups, a process-observing wind-down can be used. In this method, we spend between 5 and 15 minutes sharing our observations of how things went in the session. Members may offer observations about themselves, one another, the leaders, or the group as a whole. Although the leaders may have to model such observations at the beginning, members usually pick up on the method rapidly. As time passes and the group progresses, we find that members usually become quite astute observers and describers of one another's behavior, progress, mood changes, and apparent difficulties. At times, the leaders may facilitate more in-depth observations and comments by asking general questions about observations (e.g., "What do you make of that?"). Or the leaders may encourage a member to check out an observation, especially when an observation involves an inference about another's feelings, mood state, or opinion. Another important leader task is to draw out members who do not spontaneously offer an observation. During wind-down, each member should be encouraged to offer at least one observation, even if that observation is simply that it is difficult to offer an observation. An observing wind-down is also an opportunity to utilize insight (interpretation) strategies in a group setting. It is particularly useful for the group leaders to comment on patterns of group interactions and

group changes that they have noticed. Such insights highlight and foster the growth of dialectical thinking. In a group context, comments about group members' behavior not only communicate to the individuals in question, but give information to all members about how they can evaluate and interpret their own behavior.

Although the process-observing wind-down may be very useful, it is also the type of wind-down with the most potential for creating problems. These problems almost always happen when the observation period gets out of the leaders' control and ends in overly critical observations, in escalating responses to critical feedback, and occasionally in members' storming out and refusing ever to come back. This can be a particular problem when more experienced or advanced clients (e.g., those who have gone through several skills training modules) are mixed with those who are just beginning skills training. The more advanced clients may be ready for much more process than new clients can tolerate. The process-observing wind-down is a natural place for advanced clients to begin to try out more confrontational comments. I discuss the problems of too much process work in first-year skills training groups more thoroughly in Chapter 5 of this manual. In both these types of "observe and describe" wind-downs, it is important that the group leaders go last. When necessary, this gives the leaders a chance to make an observation that pulls the group together and repairs any damage that might have been done by others' observations.

Other wind-downs might consist of clients' bringing in music that is soothing and uplifting. (No music extolling drug use or suicide!) Each member can say what he or she is going to be doing for the next week. Any current news or sports event can be discussed if it is relevant to most if not all the group members. Any topic (favorite movies, animals, movie stars, books, foods, etc.) can be discussed. The list of topics is up to group leaders' imagination and common sense.

Observing Limits

DBT does not generally believe in *setting* limits, but instead favors *observing* naturally occurring limits. In skills training, however, a number of limits are set by the therapy itself. These limits are arbitrary, in that I could conceivably have developed different rules. Other limits that must be observed are those of the skills trainers as individuals and (in a group context) of the group as a whole.

Limits of Skills Training Itself

The key limitation of DBT skills training is that the skills trainers do not function as individual therapists during skills training sessions. The role of skills trainers is clearly defined and limited to teaching behavioral skills and dealing with the interpersonal relationships that arise in sessions. A skills trainer is like a university professor or a high school teacher. "Personal" calls texts, or e-mails to skills training leaders are acceptable only under certain conditions: Clients may contact the skills trainers if they will not be able to attend a group session for some reason, or if they have a serious interpersonal problem with a trainer or group member that cannot be resolved in a session.

There are three exceptions to these coaching limits. The first is when a skills training client is also receiving DBT individual psychotherapy from another therapist in the same clinical setting. In these instances, a skills training leader serves as a backup therapist for the individual therapist. Thus, when the individual psychotherapist is out of town, it is appropriate for the client to call the skills trainer under the same circumstances that he or she would call the individual therapist. When the reason for the call is to discuss interpersonal relationships in the skills training, there are some limits. These limits are the natural limits of the skills training leader, and thus the ordinary strategies of observing limits in individual therapy apply. It is essential that a skills training leader in this situation understand these phone limits and communicate them clearly to the clients. The second exception is in multifamily skills training for adolescents who are also in individual DBT. In these situations, the adolescent calls the individual therapist for coaching, and the parent or other family member in skills training can call the skills trainer for coaching. The reason for this is that often coaching is needed for managing the relationship with one of the other persons in the treatment (i.e., the adolescent with a parent, or vice versa). A conflict arises when the same person is coaching both parties and disagreements arise. The third exception is when a skills trainer is teaching skills on an inpatient or residential unit and is also a milieu skills coach before and after sessions. In these situations, the skills trainer may give ad hoc coach-

ing as needed during his or her shift, or (as is done in some settings) may have regular office hours for skills coaching on the unit.

In my experience, the best way to communicate phone limits is by discussing the important role of the individual psychotherapist in the total DBT program, and pointing out that skills trainers do not duplicate the individual psychotherapist's job. In our experience, clients grasp this rule very quickly and rarely violate it. If a client is in a skills-only program and does not have an individual therapist, then calling the local crisis line should be recommended, as these services are ordinarily very good. If necessary and possible, you might want to provide the crisis line personnel with a coaching plan for specific clients. We have done that in our clinic with very good results. Most phone calls, texts, and e-mails other than session cancellations revolve around their relationships with skills trainers or (in a group context) with other group members. At times, a client may make contact to find out whether a trainer hates him or her and wants the client out of skills training. At other times, a client may call to discuss how it is completely impossible to continue in skills training any longer, since sessions are so painful. Relationship problem-solving strategies must be implemented by the skills training leaders during such phone calls. These are discussed in detail in Chapter 15 of the main DBT text and in Chapter 5 of this manual. In a skills-only group, such as the friends-and-family group in our clinic, phone calls to the skills trainers to discuss life problems and repeated requests for individual time with the skills trainers surrounding skills training sessions should alert the skills trainers that such clients may need more help than can be given in skills training. In these cases, individual therapy may be recommended and referrals given.

A second limit during the first year of DBT skills training is that personal crises are generally not discussed in skills training sessions. This limit is made crystal clear for the first several sessions and is reclarified thereafter when clients wish to discuss their current crises. If a crisis is extreme, of course, skills training leaders may choose to violate the rule. To cite a very extreme example, when a group member in our clinic was raped on her way to a group session, we of course discussed it. A death in the family, a divorce, a breakup of a relationship, or a rejection by a therapist may be reported and briefly discussed at the beginning of sessions.

The key to getting individuals with disordered emotion regulation to follow this rule is the way in which crises are dealt with. Generally, any topic can be discussed if the focus is on how the client can use the skills being learned to cope with the crisis. Thus, although at first glance it would appear that the "crisis of the week" cannot be discussed, at second glance it is obvious that it can be, as long as it is discussed within the context of DBT skills. This orientation, however, is not always the orientation that a person is hoping for. Rather than giving clients free rein to discuss their problems and to share all the details, skills training leaders very quickly intervene to highlight the relationship of these problems to the particular skill module of the moment.

For example, if an individual psychotherapist has terminated a client or a client has been fired, this can be dealt with in terms of the interpersonal effectiveness skills the client can use to find out why, to find a new therapist or new job, or to get the therapist or job back. It can also be approached from the standpoint of how hurt the client is feeling in response to the rejection and how the client can use emotion regulation skills to feel better. If core mindfulness skills are the focus, the client can be encouraged to observe and describe the event and his or her responses. The client can also be helped to notice any judgmental thoughts and how to focus on what works rather than on revenge. Finally, the problem can be approached in terms of how the person is going to survive it or tolerate it without engaging in impulsive destructive behaviors. Most problems lend themselves to an analysis in terms of each of the skill modules. Noninterpersonal situations, which at first glance may seem inappropriate for the Interpersonal Effectiveness module, can be looked at as opportunities for finding friends to share with and for obtaining the social support the client needs to cope with the problem. Skills trainers must be vigilant in always bringing the crisis back to the skills. When the skills seem ineffective or insufficient for the problem, clients in individual therapy should be encouraged to talk with their therapists.

A third limit is that skills training sessions are focused on increasing the skills of the individuals attending the sessions. The focus is not and cannot be on how to change other people in clients' lives. Although interpersonal effectiveness skills are often aimed at changing what other people do, the focus even there is on the clients' learning the skills and being able to use them, not on how effective they are at changing people the clients want to change. This is a particularly critical limit in our friends-and-family groups. Here the individuals come to skills training because they have very difficult people in their lives. It is natural for them to think that a skills class can teach them how to get those difficult persons to be less difficult. Although this very likely may be a result of the individuals' learning the skills taught in skills training, it is not the focus.

It is often helpful here to tell the "rainmaker" story. A Native American tribe was in the fifth year of a terrible drought. All the crops were failing, and the people were in danger of starving. The tribe invited a rainmaker to come to bring the rain. When the rainmaker arrived, he went into the tepee set up for him. After the first night had passed, the people expected him to come out and start his rainmaking, but he did not. After 3 days, he still had not come out. The elders of the tribe then went into the tepee and asked, "When are you going to start making the sky bring down rain?"

The rainmaker said, "I am bringing myself into order. When I come into order, the tribe will come into order. When the tribe comes into order, the fields will come into order. When the fields come into order, the sky will come into order. And when the sky comes into order, it will rain."

This story has always reminded me of a woman who took our skills training class. She had a daughter who had very severe BPD. The mother met me some time later and said, "When I learned the DBT skills, I was transformed, and when I was transformed, my daughter was transformed." It is this point of view that skills trainers must continue to explain and support.

Finally, the limits of structured skills training may have to be observed in regard to process issues. The group leaders need to carefully communicate the limits on process issues, individual crises, and general life discussions in a skills training program versus a psychotherapy process group. (The tendency to favor process discussions and work on individual crises is, as I have noted previously, much more pronounced when skills training is conducted individually; this is a principal reason for conducting skills training in groups.)

Personal Limits of Skills Training Leaders

The observing-limits approach with respect to the skills training leaders is no different in DBT skills training than it is in other components of DBT. Essentially, it is the task of the leaders to observe their own limits in conducting the treatment. In my experience, the crucial limit that must be observed has to do with phone calls. Skills trainers must track their own ability to handle lengthy interpersonal discussions with clients and must communicate their limits clearly to the clients.

Limits of a Group as a Whole

The key limit of DBT skills training groups when clients have severe problems with emotion regulation is that they cannot tolerate hostile attacks in sessions. My colleagues and I have had to make it very clear to group members that behaviors such as throwing things, destroying property, and attacking or harshly criticizing other group members are proscribed. When a group member engages in hostile behavior, the group member is encouraged to work on the problem with his or her individual psychotherapist (if the person has one) or with a skills trainer after the group session. However, it is preferable for an individual to leave a group session (even if only temporarily) than to engage in these behaviors. The group leaders, of course, have to be careful in this situation not to punish the member for leaving on the one hand, and to punish him or her for staying on the other. Dialectical balance is crucial, since the leaders also want to encourage the member to stay at a session and inhibit maladaptive behaviors as long as possible.

References

1. Dimeff, L. A., & Koerner, K. (Eds.). *Dialectical behavior therapy in clinical practice*. New York: Guilford Press.
2. Mintz, R. S. (1968). Psychotherapy of the suicidal patient. In H. L. P. Resnik (Ed.), *Suicidal behaviors: Diagnosis and management* (pp. 271–296). Boston: Little, Brown.
3. McMain, S. F., Guimond, T., Habinski, L., Barnhart, R., & Streiner, D. L. (2014). *Dialectical behaviour therapy skills training versus a waitlist control for self harm and borderline personality disorder*. Manuscript submitted for publication.

Chapter 4

Skills Training Treatment Targets
and Procedures

As discussed in Chapter 3, DBT organizes treatment by levels of disorder and stages of treatment. Within each stage of treatment, DBT focuses on a hierarchy of behavioral targets highlighting behaviors to increase and behaviors to decrease. The hierarchy helps ensure that the most important behaviors are attended to first. When clients enter skills training in standard DBT, and when DBT skills training is combined with other modes of treatment (such as milieu treatment), treatment targets are divided among the modes of treatment. For example, when a Stage 1 client presents with life-threatening behaviors, severe therapy-interfering behaviors, and/or severe quality-of-life-interfering behaviors, then decreasing these behavioral patterns would be the primary treatment targets of the individual therapist or case manager. PTSD and other serious mental disorders would ordinarily be treated also by an individual provider. In all stages of treatment (see Table 3.2), the task of the skills trainer is to increase skillful behavioral patterns. This chapter begins with a discussion of skills training targets and continues with a discussion of skills training strategies used to achieve those targets. A detailed discussion of how to manage the homework review portion of the session ends the chapter.

"Strategies" are coordinated activities, tactics, and procedures that a skills trainer employs to achieve treatment goals—in this case, the acquisition and use of behavioral skills. "Strategies" also include coordinated responses that the provider should give to a particular problem presented by a client. These, along with other DBT procedures, are how skills trainers address skills training targets. In the context of DBT as a whole, skills training procedures constitute one of four sets of change procedures; the other three are contingency man-

agement, exposure-based, and cognitive modification procedures. Skills training procedures, as their name suggests, will be the "meat" of interventions in behavioral skills training. However—and this is important—it is impossible to do a competent job in skills training without an understanding of how to make contingencies work with a client (contingency procedures); how to manage exposure to threatening material and situations (exposure-based procedures); and how to deal with maladaptive expectancies, assumptions, and beliefs (cognitive modification procedures). In most senses, these procedures cannot be pulled apart from the implementation of skills training procedures; I do so here in this chapter only for the sake of exposition. The next chapter describes the other three sets of change procedures, along with other DBT strategies.

Skills Training Behavioral Targets

Skills training behavioral targets, in order of importance, are (1) stopping behaviors that are very likely to destroy therapy; (2) skill acquisition, strengthening, and generalization; and (3) reducing therapy-interfering behaviors. The agenda for skill acquisition, strengthening, and generalization is presented in Chapters 7–10 of this manual. Although this agenda is the impetus for skills training in the first place, it must be set aside when behaviors emerge that are likely to destroy the treatment, either for a specific person or (in a group context) for the group as a whole. In contrast to DBT individual psychotherapy, however, behaviors that slow down progress in therapy (rather than threaten to destroy it altogether) are last rather than second in the hierarchy. As noted in Chapter 3, the primary target behaviors for individual psychotherapy in DBT are (1) decreasing suicidal and other life-threatening behaviors; (2) decreasing therapy-interfering behaviors; (3) decreasing quality-of-life-interfering behaviors; and (4) increasing behavioral skills. A comparison of this hierarchy with that for skills training indicates the role of skills training in the total scheme of things. A therapist who is conducting both the individual psychotherapy and skills training for a particular client must be very clear about which targets take priority in which treatment modes. Maintaining the distinction between skills training and individual therapy is one of the keys to successful DBT.

Successfully addressing skills training behavioral targets requires an integration of almost all the DBT treatment strategies. This can be extremely difficult in Stage 1 of DBT (see Chapter 3 of this manual and Chapter 6 of the main DBT text for a discussion of stages), because often both clients and trainers do not want to attend to skills training. Work on the therapeutic process, having "heart-to-heart" talks, resolving real-life crisis, and so forth can all be more reinforcing (for both trainers and clients) than the sometimes mundane task of working on general behavioral skills. However, a trainer who ignores the target hierarchy is not doing DBT skills training. That is, in DBT *what* is discussed is as important as *how* it is discussed. Difficulties in getting a client to go along with the targets should be treated as problems to be solved. A trainer who is having trouble following the target hierarchy (a not unlikely problem) should bring up the topic in the next therapist consultation team meeting. The following discussion addresses each target in the skills training hierarchy.

Priority 1: Stopping Behaviors Likely to Destroy Skills Training

The highest-priority target is stopping client behaviors that, when and if they occur, pose a serious threat to the continuation of therapy. The emphasis here is a simple matter of logic: If therapy is destroyed, other targets cannot be achieved. The object is to maintain the skills training sessions. The behavior has to be *very serious* to be considered this high in priority. Included in this target are violent behaviors, such as throwing objects, pounding loudly or destructively on things, and hitting or verbally attacking other clients during group therapy sessions. (Verbal attacks on the skills trainers are not considered therapy-destroying behavior.) Other

target behaviors are self-injurious acts (e.g., cutting or scratching wrists, picking off scabs so that bleeding starts, taking excessive medications) and suicide crisis behaviors during group sessions, including breaks (e.g., threatening suicide in a credible manner and then storming out of the session). Also included are behaviors that make it impossible for anyone to concentrate, focus, or hear what is going on (e.g., yelling, hysterical crying, loud moaning, or constant out-of-turn talking). At times, an interpersonal problem among group members or between members and leaders, or a structural problem in the way skills training is delivered, may be so serious that skills training will fall apart if it is not attended to. For example, one member may not be able to come back to skills training because of an interpersonal clash, hurt feelings, excessive hopelessness, or the like. In these cases, repairing the problem should be the priority. A therapist may attend to an individual problem by phone between sessions or before or after sessions, if not in the session itself. Finally, a united rebellion of the clients against the trainers is also considered a top-priority target, as is a rebellion of the trainers against the clients.

The skills trainer's goal is to stop therapy-destructive behaviors and repair "rips" in the therapeutic "fabric" as quickly and efficiently as possible. For clients in standard DBT, further work on the destructive behaviors is left for the individual therapist to handle. With or without an individual therapist, an individual meeting before or after a skills training session may be called for. Although teaching clients interpersonal effectiveness, emotion regulation, distress tolerance, or mindfulness skills may be useful in reducing the destructive behavior, a number of other treatment strategies may be necessary to bring these behaviors under control quickly (e.g., use of both positive and aversive contingencies).

When a client is engaging in behaviors that are clearly destructive to skills training, the skills trainers must respond promptly and vigorously. A modified version of the therapy-interfering behavior protocol described in Chapter 15 of the main DBT text can be applied here; the strategies, modified for use in a skills training setting, are listed in Table 4.1.

Managing Suicidal Behaviors

When suicide crisis behaviors occur (which by definition suggest a high likelihood of impending suicide), skills trainers do the absolute minimum crisis intervention necessary and then, as quickly as pos-

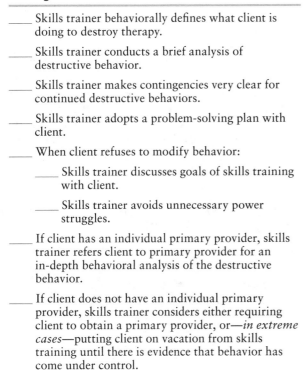

TABLE 4.1. Therapy-Destroying Behavior Strategies Checklist

____ Skills trainer behaviorally defines what client is doing to destroy therapy.

____ Skills trainer conducts a brief analysis of destructive behavior.

____ Skills trainer makes contingencies very clear for continued destructive behaviors.

____ Skills trainer adopts a problem-solving plan with client.

____ When client refuses to modify behavior:

    ____ Skills trainer discusses goals of skills training with client.

    ____ Skills trainer avoids unnecessary power struggles.

____ If client has an individual primary provider, skills trainer refers client to primary provider for an in-depth behavioral analysis of the destructive behavior.

____ If client does not have an individual primary provider, skills trainer considers either requiring client to obtain a primary provider, or—*in extreme cases*—putting client on vacation from skills training until there is evidence that behavior has come under control.

Note. Adapted from Table 15.5 in Linehan, M. M. (1993). *Cognitive-behavioral treatment of borderline personality disorder.* New York: Guilford Press. Copyright 1993 by The Guilford Press. Adapted by permission.

sible, turn the problem over to the individual therapist or to area crisis services. Except to determine whether immediate medical care is needed, reports of previous self-injurious acts are given almost no attention during a skills training session. "Remember to tell your therapist" is the modal response for those in individual psychotherapy. (As noted in Chapter 3, suicidal individuals and those with severe disorders must have an individual therapist to participate in skills training.) The one exception, as noted above, is when these behaviors become destructive to the continuation of therapy for other group members. They are then targeted directly in the skills training group sessions. The general principle is that skills trainers treat a client in a suicidal crisis like a student who gets deathly ill in school. The nearest relative (in this case, the individual therapist or case manager) is called. A skills trainer who is also the individual client's therapist should turn to the problem *after* the skills training session. Unless it is impossible to do otherwise, skills train-

ing should not be interrupted to attend to a suicidal crisis.

Attention to suicidal ideation and communications during skills training is limited to helping the client figure out how to apply the DBT skills currently being taught to the suicidal feelings and thoughts. During mindfulness training, the focus may be on observing and describing the urge to engage in self-injury or thoughts of suicide as these come and go. During distress tolerance training, the emphasis may be on tolerating the pain or using crisis intervention skills to cope with the situation. During emotion regulation training, the focus may be on observing, describing, and trying to change the emotions related to suicidal urges. In an interpersonal effectiveness framework, the emphasis may be on saying no or asking for help skillfully. The same strategy is used when the client discusses life crises, problems interfering with quality of life, or previous traumatic events in his or her life. Everything is grist for the skill application mill, so to speak. Strategies for assessment and management of suicide risk when individual therapists are not available are outlined in Chapter 5 of this manual (see especially Table 5.2).

Managing Skills Trainers' Desire to Get Rid of Difficult Clients

It is not infrequent that skills trainers decide that the solution to dealing with difficult clients is to kick them out of skills training. In a very friendly group, for example, you may have a new member who is loudly grumpy or sulks most weeks, taking up a lot of your time. A person may be hostile to you and other group members, or may routinely say insensitive and mean things to others. In a group where most do homework, one person may refuse to do homework and complain about the need to do homework, requiring you to analyze the missing homework on a weekly basis. Others may routinely insist on talking about complicated personal problems, and may accuse you of being insensitive or uncaring when you try to reframe the problem in terms of skills that could be used. A client may frequently sob, yell, or bang the table so loudly in group sessions that it is difficult to proceed. Clients may put their feet on the table and refuse to put them down, loudly empty purses or backpacks on the table every week to clean them out, bring in alcohol disguised as cola, and argue vehemently with every point you try to make. In over 30 years of conducting DBT skills groups, I have never kicked out a group member. I have nevertheless many times felt sure that a group would go better if I could just get rid of one or two participants. When a troublesome person finally does leave a group, however, someone else in the group usually then becomes a problem. In other words, I have never seen a group improve by getting rid of a member. In the majority of cases, I have found that my ability to manage a difficult group participant with equanimity and a lightness of tone has allowed other group members not only to cope with disturbance, but also to find ways of appreciating the contributions that the difficult member often does manage to make.

Managing Skills Trainers' Desire to Attack Difficult Clients

Skills trainers often have an intense desire for group skills training to go well for everyone. When one person threatens this desire, it is natural for group leaders' anxiety to increase, along with their attempts to control the offending group member. When efforts to control disruptive behaviors fail, it is easy to become overprotective of the other participants. When that happens, anger and judgmentalness can increase, and when this happens, you suddenly are at risk of therapy-interfering behavior yourself. There have been many groups where I have held onto the table legs to keep myself from storming out of the room, or cursing group members for being so ungrateful for my hard work. In these difficult situations, it can be very hard to teach without being judgmental, and "emotion mind" is easy to fall into. What to do at these points? Attack or withdraw? If ever there is a time for skills trainers to use their own DBT skills, this is the time. All of your skills can be helpful. Here are just a few examples:

1. Observe what a difficult client is actually doing, and describe it nonjudgmentally in your own mind before commenting on the behavior.
2. Practice radical acceptance of clients who engage in repetitively annoying behaviors, but who are corrigible if you make the effort.
3. Practice opposite action with a matter-of-fact or light tone of voice when you want to withdraw.
4. Practice opposite action, using irreverence or humor with a light tone of voice, to avoid at-

tacking and to lower tension between you and the individual and in the room.
5. Use the DEAR MAN, GIVE FAST skills (see Interpersonal Effectiveness Handouts 5, 6, and 7) to ask a person to stop behaviors that distract you or others. Use the "broken record" and negotiate (Interpersonal Effectiveness Handout 5) if necessary.
6. Put problem behaviors on an extinction schedule (see Interpersonal Effectiveness Handout 21), and plunge in where angels fear to tread by acting as if clients are cooperating even when they are not.

Priority 2: Skill Acquisition, Strengthening, and Generalization

With very few exceptions, most of the skills training time is devoted to acquisition, strengthening, and generalization of the DBT behavioral skills: core mindfulness, distress tolerance, emotional regulation, and interpersonal effectiveness. Active practice and use of behavioral skills are extremely difficult for individuals with highly disordered emotion regulation, since these require them to regulate their own behavior in the service of practicing skills. Thus, if passive and/or dysregulated behavior is followed by a group leader's shifting attention to another member (in a group context) or by a discussion of how the client is feeling or why he or she doesn't want to participate, this risks reinforcing the very behavior (passivity or dysregulation) that skills training is intended to reduce. At times, trainers can simply drag clients through difficult moments in skills training; such an approach, however, requires the trainers to be very sure of their behavioral assessments. The key point is that such an approach should be strategic rather than simply insensitive. For example, there are times when it is more skillful to leave a skills participant alone for a while. This is particularly true for brand-new group members; for individuals with known social anxiety disorder (social phobia); or at times for individuals who have asserted skillfully that they are willful now, intend to be willful throughout the group, and clearly are sticking to their guns. Some effort to engage such clients may be useful, but excessive efforts may backfire. If necessary, skills trainers can meet with distressed clients during break or after sessions to discuss and problem-solve the clients' dysregulated or interfering behaviors.

Priority 3:
Reducing Therapy-Interfering Behaviors

Behaviors that interfere with therapy, but do not destroy it, are not ordinarily addressed systematically in skills training. This decision is based primarily on the fact that if therapy-interfering behaviors were a high-priority treatment target for individuals with high emotion dysregulation, trainers might never get around to the designated skills training. Skills training does not address the therapy process itself, except as an avenue for teaching and practicing the skills being taught. When therapy-interfering behaviors are occurring, effective strategies are (1) to ignore the behavior, if it is brief; or (2) in a matter-of-fact but firm tone, ask the client to stop the behavior and then resolutely focus (no matter what) on teaching the skills in the module at hand. This is almost always the strategy employed with the less serious therapy-interfering behaviors. Sometimes these behaviors offer a particularly good opportunity for practicing the skills currently being taught. At most, these behaviors are commented on in a way that communicates the desirability of change, while at the same time letting the client know that very little time can be devoted to problems unrelated to the skills being taught. Thus mood-dependent passivity, restlessness, pacing around the room, doodling, sitting in odd positions, attempts to discuss the week's crisis, oversensitivity to criticism, or anger at other clients will be ignored at times. The client is treated (ingeniously, at times) as if he or she is not engaging in the dysfunctional behaviors.

At other times, a skills trainer may instruct or urge such a client to try to apply behavioral skills to the problem at hand. For example, a client who gets angry and threatens to leave may be instructed to try to practice distress tolerance skills or the emotion regulation skill of opposite action (i.e., acting opposite to the action urge of anger). A client who is refusing to participate may be asked whether he or she is being willful. If the response is "yes," the trainer may ask whether the client is willing to practice the skill of willingness. I often ask, "Any idea of when you will be willing to practice willingness?" A client who is withdrawn and dissociating may be urged to practice crisis survival skills (e.g., cold gel pack across the eyes, paced breathing). In our groups, we keep a number of rubber balls with spikes, a balance board, and cold gel packs available for use by people who are in danger of dissociating during skills train-

ing sessions. Skills trainers matter-of-factly suggest their use when appropriate. The key point here is that if skills trainers allow skills training sessions to become focused on the therapy process or on clients' life crises—including suicidal behaviors and quality-of-life-interfering behaviors—then training in skills will be forfeited.

As I have discussed in Chapter 3 of this manual, there is a wind-down period at the end of each skills training session. This is an appropriate time to observe therapy-interfering behaviors or, even more importantly, improvement in previous interfering behaviors. As long as everyone gets a chance to voice an observation, this time can be used as therapy process time. One of the advantages of an observing wind-down is that it provides a time and place for discussing behaviors that are interfering with therapy. (Cautions about process-observing wind-downs have also been discussed in Chapter 3.)

Skills Training Procedures: How to Meet Skills Training Targets

During skills training, and more generally throughout DBT, skills trainers and clients' individual treatment providers must insist at every opportunity that clients actively engage in the acquisition and practice of skills needed to cope with life as it is. In other words, they must directly, forcefully, and repeatedly challenge the passive problem-solving style of individuals with emotion dysregulation. The procedures described below are applied by every DBT provider across all modes of treatment where appropriate. They are applied in a formal way in the structured skills training modules.

There are three types of skills training procedures. Each type focuses on one of the Priority 2 target behaviors: (1) skill acquisition (e.g., instructions, modeling); (2) skill strengthening (e.g., behavioral rehearsal, feedback); and (3) skill generalization (e.g., homework assignments and homework review, discussion of similarities and differences in situations). In skill acquisition, a trainer is teaching new behaviors. In skill strengthening and generalization, the trainer is trying both to fine-tune skilled behaviors and to increase the probability that the person will use the skilled behaviors already in his or her repertoire in relevant situations. Skill strengthening and skill generalization, in turn, require the application of contingency procedures, exposure, and/or cognitive modification. That is, once the trainer is sure that a particular response pattern is within the client's current repertoire, then other procedures are applied to increase the client's effective behaviors in everyday life. It is this emphasis on active, self-conscious teaching, typical of many approaches to CBT, that differentiates DBT from many psychodynamic approaches to treating clients with disordered emotion regulation. Some skills training procedures, however, are virtually identical to those used in supportive psychotherapy. The targets of skills training are determined by the parameters of DBT; the emphasis on certain skills over others is determined by behavioral analysis in each individual case.

Skill Acquisition

The second half of each skills training session is primarily focused on teaching new material, generally through lectures, discussions, practice, and role-plays. Each skills training module contains a number of specific behavioral skills. One or sometimes two skills are taught in each session, or three if some of the skills are very easy to learn. Although it is usually not a good idea to present a lot of individual skills to be learned (the idea being that it is better to learn a few skills well than a lot of skills poorly), I have found that presenting many skills counteracts two problems with individuals who have difficulties regulating their emotions. First, presenting many skills suggests that the trainer is not oversimplifying the problems to be solved. Second, teaching a large quantity of skills works against clients' being able to say credibly that absolutely nothing works. If one thing doesn't work, the trainer can always suggest trying a different skill. With many skills to draw from, the client's resistance usually runs out before the trainer's ability to offer new skills to try does.

Orienting and Committing to Skills Training: Task Overview

Skills acquisition begins with orienting and commitment strategies. Orienting is a skills trainer's chief means of selling the new behaviors as worth learning and likely to work. Skills training can only be accomplished if a person actively collaborates with the treatment program. In addition, knowing exactly what the task is, what one's role is, and what one can expect from the other person facilitates learning enormously. Orientation is called for with each specific skill and with each homework assignment.

Some clients have skill deficits and are fearful about acquiring the new skills. It can be useful to point out here that learning a new skill does not mean actually having to use the skill. That is, a person can acquire a skill and then choose in each situation whether to use it or not. Sometimes clients do not want to learn new skills because they feel hopeless that anything will really help. I find it useful to point out that every skill I teach has helped either me or people I know. However, a skills trainer cannot prove ahead of time that particular skills will actually help a given individual. Thus I also point out that no skill is likely to be useful to every person.

Before teaching any new skill, the trainer should give an overall rationale (or draw it in Socratic fashion from the client) for why the particular skill or set of skills might be useful. At times, this may only require a comment or two; at other times, it may require extensive discussion. At some point, the skills trainer should also explain the rationale for his or her methods of teaching—that is, a rationale for the DBT skills training procedures. The most important point to make here, and to repeat as often as needed, is that learning new skills requires practice, practice, practice. Equally important is that practice has to occur in situations where the skills are needed. If these points do not get through to a client, there is not much hope that he or she will actually learn anything new. Once oriented, the client needs to make a recommitment to learning each skill and each skill module, as well as a commitment every week to practice new skills between sessions.

Assessing Clients' Abilities

Skill acquisition procedures are aimed at remediating skill deficits. DBT does not assume that all, or even most, of the problems that a person with emotion dysregulation has are motivational in nature. Instead, the emphasis is on assessing the extent of the person's abilities in a particular area; skill acquisition procedures are then used if skill deficits exist. It can, however, be very difficult to determine whether clients with high emotion dysregulation are incapable of doing something, or are capable but emotionally inhibited or constrained by environmental factors. Although this is a complex assessment question with any client population, it can be particularly hard with these individuals because of their inability to analyze their own behavior and abilities. For example, they often confuse being *afraid* of doing something with not being *able* to do it. In addition, there are often powerful contingencies mitigating against their admitting having any behavioral capabilities. (I have reviewed many of these in Chapter 10 of the main DBT text.) Clients may say that they do not know how they feel or what they think, or that they can't find words, when in reality they are afraid or too ashamed to express their thoughts and feelings. As many of them say, they often do not want to be vulnerable. Some clients have been taught by their families and therapists to view all of their problems as motivationally based, and have either bought that story entirely (and thus believe they can do anything, but just do not want to) or have rebelled completely (and thus never entertain the possibility that motivational factors might be as important as ability-related factors). These therapy dilemmas are discussed more fully in the next chapter.

To assess whether a behavioral pattern is within a client's repertoire, the skills trainer has to figure out a way to create ideal circumstances for the client to produce the behavior. For interpersonal behaviors, an approximation to this is role playing during the skills training session—or, if the client refuses, asking the client to indicate what he or she would say in a particular situation. Alternatively, one client can be asked to coach another during a role play. I am frequently amazed to find that individuals who appear very interpersonally skilled cannot put together reasonable responses in certain role-play situations, whereas individuals who seem passive, meek, and unskilled are quite capable of responding skillfully if the role play can be made comfortable enough. In analyzing distress tolerance, the trainer can ask what techniques the client uses or thinks helpful in tolerating difficult or stressful situations. Emotion regulation can sometimes be assessed by interrupting an exchange and asking whether the client can change his or her emotional state. Self-management and mindfulness skills can be analyzed by observing clients' behavior in sessions, especially when they are not the focus of attention, and questioning them about their day-to-day behavior.

If a client produces a behavior, the skills trainer knows it is in the person's repertoire. However, if the client does not produce it, the trainer cannot be sure; as in statistics, there is no way to test the null hypothesis. When in doubt, it is usually safer to proceed with skill acquisition procedures just in case, and then observe any consequent change in behavior. Generally there is no harm in doing so, and most of the procedures also affect other factors related to skilled behavior. For example, they may work because they give the individual "permission" to behave in a certain way, and thus reduce inhibitions, rather than because they add to the individual's behavioral repertoire. The principal skill acquisition procedures are instructions and modeling.

Instructions

In DBT, "instructions" are verbal descriptions of the skill components to be learned. This direct teaching constitutes didactic strategies. Instructions can vary from general guidelines ("When you are checking whether your thoughts fit the facts, be sure to check out the probability that the dire consequences will occur") to very specific suggestions as to what the client should do ("The minute an urge hits, go get a cold gel pack and hold it in your hand for 10 minutes") or think ("Keep saying over and over to yourself, 'I can do it'"). Especially in a group setting, instructions can be presented in a lecture format with a blackboard or whiteboard as an aid. Instructions can be suggested as hypotheses to be considered, can be set forth as theses and antitheses to be synthesized, or can be drawn out in a Socratic method of discourse. In all cases, a trainer must be careful not to oversimplify the ease of behaving effectively or of learning the skill. With adolescents, it can be very useful to let them read sections of the skills handouts out loud before you launch into specific instructions and examples. In my groups, hands ordinarily shoot up when I suggest this. With individuals who have already learned a skill once, you can ask for volunteers to describe it, including how it might be used and for what. You can add comments and examples as necessary.

As the skills are taught, it is critical to attempt to link each skill to its intended outcome. For example, in teaching relaxation, skills trainers should describe not only how relaxation works but when it works, why it works, and what it works for. It is also useful to discuss when it doesn't work, why it may not work, and how to make it work when it seems not to be working. The more trouble trainers can predict in advance, the better clients are likely to learn the skill.

It is particularly important to remember that immediate emotional relief is not the goal of every skill taught in DBT skills training. This distinction is often not grasped by either clients or new skills trainers. In fact, when clients say that something didn't work, they almost always mean that it didn't make them feel better immediately. Thus the relationship of skills to long-term goals versus short-term goals, and to long-term relief versus immediate relief, has to be discussed over and over. It is particularly important not to be pulled into always trying to show how a skilled behavior will make a person feel better right away. First, it isn't usually true; second, even if it were true, it is not necessarily beneficial.

USING THE HANDOUTS

The skills training handouts available on the special website for this manual (*www.guilford.com/skills-training-manual*) provide written instructions. It is important, however, to note that you do not have to repeat every word on each handout during a skills session. The written handouts function as cues for your teaching and as reminders for clients of what and how to practice the skillful behaviors when they are not in skills sessions. For example, many participants have commented that they carry their skills binders with them, so that when they forget what skill to use or how to use a skill, they can look it up on the handouts. One of our clients once told his wife during an argument that she had to wait a minute while he went out to check his skills book. Within sessions, many of the handouts are designed to encourage participants to check off goals and the new behaviors they plan to practice. Handouts also provide a place for clients to take notes. For many clients, this latter function is particularly important. When I have updated handouts and tried to replace old handouts with new ones, clients routinely want to keep their old ones (as well as their old, filled-out worksheets).

Modeling

Modeling can be provided by trainers, other clients, or other people in a client's environment, as well as by audio or video recordings, films, or printed material. Any procedure that provides a client with examples of appropriate alternative responses is a form of modeling. The advantage of a skills trainer's providing the modeling is that the situation and materials can be tailored to fit a particular client's needs.

There are a number of ways to model skilled behavior. In-session role playing (with the skills trainer as a participant) can be used to demonstrate appro-

priate interpersonal behavior. When events between a trainer and the client arise that are similar to events the client encounters in his or her natural environment, the trainer can model handling such situations in effective ways. The skills trainer can also use self-talk (speaking aloud) to model coping self-statements, self-instructions, or restructuring of problematic expectations and beliefs. For example, the trainer may say, "OK, here's what I would say to myself: 'I'm overwhelmed. What's the first thing I do when I'm overwhelmed? Break down the situation into steps and make a list. Do the first thing on the list.'" Telling stories, relating historical events, or providing allegorical examples (see Chapter 7 of the main DBT text) can often be useful in demonstrating alternative life strategies. Finally, self-disclosure can be used to model adaptive behavior, especially if a skills trainer has encountered problems in living similar to those a client is currently encountering. Particularly useful are well-told dramatic and/or humorous teaching stories based on a skills trainer's running into a problem and then figuring out how to use skills to solve the problem. In our experience, clients love these stories, tell them to others, and—because they often remember a skills trainer's stories better than the handouts—use the stories to remind themselves of how to use the skills. As I have said many times in my program, "If you want to get to know our skills trainers really well, just watch them teach skills. You will find out how they used skills to overcome almost all problems in their lives." This tactic is discussed at length in Chapter 12 of the main DBT text, and careful attention to the guidelines listed there is recommended.

All of the modeling techniques described above, of course, can also be used in a group context by members modeling for one another. The ideal is for one group member to demonstrate in front of the whole group how to handle a situation skillfully. The more comfortable group members are with one another and with the group leader, the easier it is to induce them to act as models. Humor and flattery can be great aids here.

In addition to in-session modeling, it can be useful to have clients observe the behavior and responses of competent people in their own environments. The behaviors that they observe can then be discussed in sessions and practiced by everyone. The skills training handouts provide models of how to use specific skills. Biographies, autobiographies, and novels about people who have coped with similar problems provide new ideas as well. It is always important to discuss with the clients any behaviors modeled by the skills trainers or other clients, or presented as models outside of therapy, to be sure that the clients are observing the relevant responses.

One goal of the skills training sessions is to impart information about particular coping strategies to participants. A second, equally important goal is to elicit from the participants rules and strategies for effective coping that they have learned in the particular situations they encounter. Thus skills training should be taught so that the instructional material is augmented as a result of each discussion. Participants should be encouraged to take notes and to expand the handouts and worksheets furnished during sessions with their own and other participants' ideas. Whenever a particularly good strategy is presented in a session, all (including the skills training leaders) should be instructed to write it down in the appropriate space on their handouts or worksheets. The strategy should then be included in practice and review, just as are strategies presented initially by the leaders.

Skill Strengthening

Once skilled behavior has been acquired, skill strengthening is used to shape, refine, and increase the likelihood of its use. Without reinforced practice, a skill cannot be learned; this point cannot be emphasized too much, since skill practice is effortful behavior and directly counteracts the tendencies of individuals with disordered emotion regulation to employ a passive behavior style.

Behavioral Rehearsal

"Behavioral rehearsal" is any procedure in which a client practices responses to be learned. This can be done in interactions with trainers or other clients, and in simulated or *in vivo* situations. Any skilled behaviors—verbal sequences, nonverbal actions, patterns of thinking or cognitive problem solving, and some components of physiological and emotional responses—can, in principle, be practiced.

Practice can be either "overt" or "covert." Covert practice is practicing the requisite response in imagination and is discussed further below. Overt practice is behavioral rehearsal; various forms are possible. For example, in a group context, group members may role-play problematic situations (together or with the leaders), so that each member can practice responding appropriately. To learn to control physiological responses, clients may practice relaxing during a session. When clients are learning the skill of checking the facts, the leaders can start a round robin and ask each client to generate a new interpretation of facts about an event. When specific problems are presented, clients can be encouraged to problem-solve and/or to describe how they would cope ahead with the problem situation. When clients are learning radical acceptance, they can be instructed to write down the important and less important things in their lives they need to accept on the worksheet provided, and then share what they have written with the group.

Covert response practice may also be an effective form of skill strengthening. It may be more effective than overt methods for teaching more complex skills, and it is also useful when a client refuses to engage in overt rehearsal. Whereas clients can be asked to practice emotion regulation generally, "emotional behavior" cannot be practiced directly. That is, clients cannot practice getting angry, feeling sad, or experiencing joy. Instead, they have to practice specific components of emotions (changing facial expressions, generating thoughts that elicit or inhibit emotions, changing muscle tension, etc.). In my experience, adults with emotion dysregulation rarely like behavioral rehearsal, especially when it is done in front of others. Thus a fair amount of cajoling and shaping will be needed. If a client won't role-play an interpersonal situation, for example, a skills trainer can try talking him or her through a dialogue ("Then what could you say?"). The client can also be asked to try practicing just part of a new skill, so that it is not overwhelming. The essence of the message is that in order to *be* different, people must practice *acting* differently. Some trainers do not like behavioral rehearsal either, especially when it requires them to role-play with the clients. For trainers who feel shy or uncomfortable, the best solution is for them to practice role playing with members of their DBT therapist consultation team. At other times, trainers resist role playing because they do not want to push rehearsal on clients. These trainers may not be aware of the wealth of data indicating that behavioral rehearsal is related to therapeutic improvement.

Response Reinforcement

Trainers' reinforcement of clients' responses is one of the most powerful means of shaping and strengthening skilled behavior. Many individuals have lived in environments that overuse punishment. They often expect negative, punishing feedback from the world in general and their therapists in particular, and apply self-punishing strategies almost exclusively in trying to shape their own behavior. Over the long run, skill reinforcement by trainers can modify the clients' self-image in a positive manner, increase their use of skilled behavior, and enhance their sense that they can control positive outcomes in their lives. One of the benefits of group therapy over individual therapy is that when a group leader actively and obviously reinforces a skilled behavior in one group member, the same behavior is vicariously reinforced among all other group members (if they are attending). In other words, this provides "more bang for the buck." Moreover, group therapy can be very powerful when group members become adept at reinforcing skilled behaviors in one another.

The techniques of providing appropriate reinforcement are discussed extensively in Chapter 10 of the main DBT text. Those principles are very important and should be reviewed thoroughly. Note that "reinforcement" refers to all consequences or contingencies that increase the probability of a behavior. Although reinforcers are typically thought of as generally positive, desirable, or rewarding events, they need not be. A reinforcer is anything an individual will change his or her behavior to get or to have removed. A positive reinforcer is a positive event that is added, and a negative reinforcer is a negative event that is taken away. Reinforcers can be naturally occurring consequences of behavior, or arbitrary events determined by the individual providing the reinforcement, or (better yet) negotiated with the individual who is being reinforced. Identification of concrete reinforcers is necessary for each individual client. In our groups, we use both natural and arbitrary reinforcers. For example, individuals who complete worksheets between sessions get one sticker (an arbitrary positive reinforcer) per page, and if they use the skill but don't write it down on the worksheet they get half of a sticker; two half stickers get one complete sticker. If they complete all of the worksheets assigned for homework, they also avoid being asked assessment questions about the missing homework. In our experience, many clients will work at homework just to avoid being questioned about how it was that they did not do the homework. We also reinforce participants with one sticker if they arrive on time for skills training. Generally we keep on hand a large number of stickers of all kinds; we provide favored stickers if

financially feasible. We have no research data on our sticker strategy, but we have definitely noticed an improvement in homework completion since we put the policy in place.

What is important is that once you have outlined specifically and clearly what behaviors are required for specific reinforcers, you must stick to your decisions and not reinforce behavior that does not meet the criteria you have clearly identified. It is equally important not to skip analyzing failures to do homework because you are worried about how an individual will react. See the section on managing homework review later in this chapter for more on this topic. If no one or only a few individuals consistently meet criteria for reinforcement, then you need either to change your criteria for it or to consider switching to shaping as a strategy.

Skills trainers need to stay alert and notice client behaviors that represent improvement, even if these make the trainers rather uncomfortable. For example, teaching clients interpersonal skills to use with their parents, and then punishing or ignoring those same skills when the clients use them in a training session, is not therapeutic. Encouraging clients to think for themselves, but then punishing or ignoring them when they disagree with a trainer, is not therapeutic. Stressing that "not fitting in" in all circumstances is not a disaster and that distress can be tolerated, and then not tolerating clients when they do not fit comfortably into a trainer's schedule or preconceived notions of how individuals with emotion dysregulation act, is not therapeutic.

Feedback and Coaching

"Feedback" is the provision of information to clients about their performance. Feedback should pertain to performance, not to the motives presumably leading to the performance. This point is very important. An unfortunate factor in the lives of many individuals with severe emotion dysregulation is that people rarely give them feedback about their behavior that is uncontaminated with interpretations about their presumed motives and intent. When the presumed motives do not fit, the individuals often discount or are distracted from the valuable feedback they may be getting about their behavior. Feedback should be behaviorally specific; that is, a skills trainer should tell the client exactly what he or she is doing that seems to indicate either continuing problems or improvement. Telling clients that they are manipulating, expressing a need to control, overreacting, clinging, or acting out is simply not helpful if there are not clear behavioral referents for the terms. This is, of course, especially true when a trainer has pinpointed a problem behavior correctly but is making inaccurate motivational inferences. Many arguments between clients and trainers arise out of just this inaccuracy. The role and use of interpretation in DBT are discussed extensively in Chapter 9 of the main DBT text. Learning to tell the difference between behaviors observed and interpretations about behavior is also an important part of the mindfulness "what" skill of describing (see Mindfulness Handout 4 for a description of the "what" skills).

A skills trainer must attend closely to a client's behavior (within sessions or self-reported) and select those responses on which to give feedback. At the beginning of skills training, the client may do little that appears competent; the trainer is usually well advised at this point to give feedback on a limited number of response components, even though other deficits could be commented upon. Feedback on more may lead to stimulus overload and/or discouragement about the rate of progress. A response-shaping paradigm should be used, with feedback, coaching, and reinforcement designed to encourage successive approximations to the goal of effective performance (see Interpersonal Effectiveness Handout 20, as well as Chapter 10 of the main DBT text). Individuals with disordered emotion regulation often desperately want feedback about their behavior, but at the same time are sensitive to negative feedback. The solutions here are for trainers to surround negative feedback with positive feedback, to normalize skills deficits by telling stories about themselves or others who have had the same problems, and/or to cheerlead with encouraging statements. Treating clients as too fragile to deal with negative feedback does them no favor. An important part of feedback is giving clients information about the effects of their behavior on their skills trainers; this is discussed more extensively in Chapter 12 of the main DBT text.

"Coaching" is combining feedback with instructions. It is telling a client how a response is discrepant from the criterion of skilled performance and how it might be improved. Clinical practice suggests that the "permission" to behave in certain ways that is implicit in coaching may sometimes be all a client needs to accomplish changes in behavior. Coaching is ordinarily integrated into homework review. It is also used when trainers are helping clients apply skills they are learning to their everyday lives, and

when problem behaviors show up during skills training sessions.

Skill Generalization

DBT does not assume that skills learned in therapy will necessarily generalize to situations in everyday life outside of therapy. Therefore, it is very important that skills trainers actively encourage this transfer of skills. There are a number of specific procedures that skills trainers can use as well, as described below.

Between-Session Consultation

If clients are unable to apply new skills in their natural environment, they should be encouraged to get consultation from their individual therapists, case managers, counselors, or from supportive family members (particularly if family members are also learning DBT skills); and from one another between sessions. Skills trainers can give these individuals lessons on how to provide appropriate coaching. In some areas, crisis line personnel may also be able to coach DBT skills. On residential, inpatient, and day treatment units, clients can be encouraged to seek assistance from staff members when they are having difficulty. Another technique is to provide a unit behavioral consultant with regular office hours. This consultant's task is to help clients apply their new skills to everyday life.

Review of Session Video Recordings

If possible, video recordings of skills training sessions should be made. The videos can then be reviewed by clients between sessions if there is a room available where they can come and watch them. (Because of confidentiality concerns, it is important for clients not to take videos out of your clinical setting.) There are several benefits to clients in watching video sessions. First, clients are often unable to attend to much of what transpires during skills training sessions because of substance use prior to sessions, high emotional arousal during sessions, dissociation, or other concentration difficulties accompanying depression and anxiety. Thus clients may improve their retention of material offered during the sessions by viewing the session videos. Second, clients may gain important insights from viewing themselves and their interactions with others. Such insights often help clients understand

and improve their own interpersonal skills. Third, many clients report that watching a skills training video can be very helpful when they are feeling overwhelmed, panicked, or unable to cope between sessions. Simply watching a video, especially if the client can watch one of a session where a needed skill was taught, has an effect similar to that of having an additional session. Skills trainers should encourage use of the videos for these purposes.

Use of DBT Web-Based Resources, DVDs, and DBT Skills Apps

Over the years I have developed a series of skills training videos that clients can either buy or borrow to take home and watch. My experience teaching DBT skills has been that even when I am the skills leader, participants often also like watching me teach the same skill on a video. At times watching them, I have thought my own videos are better than me. There are now many self-help websites for DBT skills; many of these give DBT skills instructions, as well as examples of using them in daily life. Smartphone apps on DBT are proliferating as well; most of these apps are set up to provide mobile coaching in skills use. Look up DBT apps on your carrier.

My online video and audio recordings can be found in a number of places. Try the video page of the Behavioral Tech website (*http://behavioraltech. org/products/list.cfm?category=Videos*), or look up "Linehan DBT videos" and "DBT self-help" on your search engine, on YouTube, or on iTunes.

In Vivo Behavioral Rehearsal: Homework Assignments

Homework assignments are keyed to the specific behavioral skills currently being taught. It is advantageous if a skills trainer or a client can also get the client's individual therapist to use some of the homework assignments and accompanying worksheets throughout therapy, or on an as-needed basis. This is always done in standard DBT. For example, one worksheet focuses on identifying and labeling emotions and takes clients through a series of steps to help them clarify what they are feeling. The individual therapist may suggest that a client use this form whenever he or she is confused or overwhelmed by emotions. The website for this book (*www.guilford. com/skills-training-manual*) contains multiple worksheets covering each of the DBT behavioral skills but skills trainers and individual therapists

can also revise these to fit either their clients' or their own personal preferences and needs.

Use of Assignment Worksheets and Diary Cards

The first half of every skills training session is devoted to review of homework, as described in Chapter 3. This is how trainers check on clients' behavioral progress (or lack of it) between sessions and provide necessary feedback and coaching. It is essential that homework review, including providing individualized feedback and coaching, not be skipped. When review is skipped, clients are not reinforced for their practice, and over time practice is likely to drop off. When review is limited to what skills were practiced, and individual feedback and coaching on skills use are skipped, little may be learned. This is equivalent to a piano teacher's checking to see that the student practiced during the week, but never listening to the student play the piece that was practiced. Little progress can be expected when such is the case. The primary method of tracking skills practice is by reviewing the worksheets assigned at the previous session. DBT diary cards should also be reviewed when clients are in DBT skills training only (i.e., are not in an individual therapy where skills use is routinely evaluated). The DBT diary card (Figure 4.1) lists the most important DBT skills taught. The top half of the diary card is reviewed in individual therapy, and the bottom half can be reviewed in both individual therapy and skills training sessions. For clients in a skills-only program and for parents in a multifamily skills group, use only the bottom half of the diary card, which covers some of the most important skills. Next to each skill is a space for daily recording of whether or not the client actually practiced the skill that day. (See Table 4.2 for instructions in helping a client to use the diary cards.) If multiple members of a family are filling out the diary card each week, it can be useful for them to attach the cards to the kitchen refrigerator or some other public place. In addition, diary sheets can be created for each skills training module and given to clients as the need arises. A weekly review of the diary card is important, because if only the previous week's homework is reviewed, there is a danger that skills taught previously will drop off the client's radar and not be practiced. Not bringing in the diary card (when diary cards are reviewed), or reporting no practice effort or skills application, is viewed as a problem in self-management and is ana-

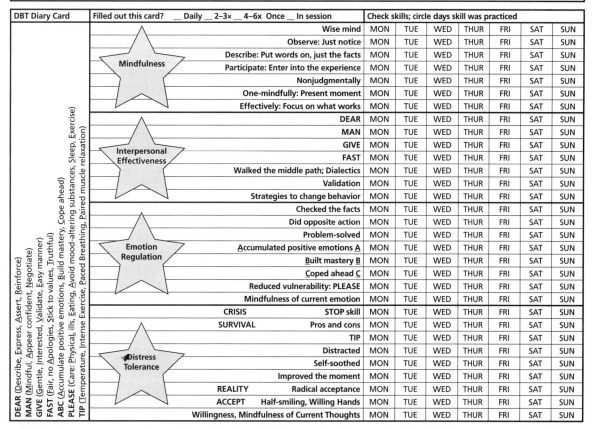

Dialectical Behavior Therapy Diary Card — Name: ___ Filled Out in Session? Y N — How Often Did You Fill Out? __ Daily __ 2–3x __ 4–6x __ Once — Last Day Filled Out: Month __ Year __ Day __

Circle Start Day / Day of week	Highest Urge To:			Highest Rating for Each Day			Drugs/Medications							Actions			Emotions	Optional
	Commit Suicide	Self-Harm	Use Drugs	Emotion Misery	Physical Misery	Joy	Alcohol		Illegal Drugs		Meds. as Prescribed	p.r.n./Over-the-Counter Meds.		Self-Harm	Lied	Used Skills*		
	0–5	0–5	0–5	0–5	0–5	0–5	#	What?	#	What?	Y/N	#	What?	Y/N	#	0–7		
MON																		
TUE																		
WED																		
THUR																		
FRI																		
SAT																		
SUN																		

Med. Change This Week

Homework Assigned and Results This Week:

*Used Skills
0 = Not thought about or used
1 = Thought about, not used, didn't want to
2 = Thought about, not used, wanted to
3 = Tried but couldn't use them
4 = Tried, could do them but they didn't help
5 = Tried, could use them, helped
6 = Automatically used them, didn't help
7 = Automatically used them, helped

Urges to:	Coming into Session (0–5)	Belief I Can Change or Regulate My:	Coming into Session (0–5)
Quit Therapy		Emotions	
Use Drugs		Actions	
Commit Suicide		Thoughts	

Skills Focus This Week:

DBT Diary Card	Filled out this card? __ Daily __ 2–3x __ 4–6x Once __ In session	Check skills; circle days skill was practiced						
Mindfulness	Wise mind	MON	TUE	WED	THUR	FRI	SAT	SUN
	Observe: Just notice	MON	TUE	WED	THUR	FRI	SAT	SUN
	Describe: Put words on, just the facts	MON	TUE	WED	THUR	FRI	SAT	SUN
	Participate: Enter into the experience	MON	TUE	WED	THUR	FRI	SAT	SUN
	Nonjudgmentally	MON	TUE	WED	THUR	FRI	SAT	SUN
	One-mindfully: Present moment	MON	TUE	WED	THUR	FRI	SAT	SUN
	Effectively: Focus on what works	MON	TUE	WED	THUR	FRI	SAT	SUN
Interpersonal Effectiveness	DEAR	MON	TUE	WED	THUR	FRI	SAT	SUN
	MAN	MON	TUE	WED	THUR	FRI	SAT	SUN
	GIVE	MON	TUE	WED	THUR	FRI	SAT	SUN
	FAST	MON	TUE	WED	THUR	FRI	SAT	SUN
	Walked the middle path; Dialectics	MON	TUE	WED	THUR	FRI	SAT	SUN
	Validation	MON	TUE	WED	THUR	FRI	SAT	SUN
	Strategies to change behavior	MON	TUE	WED	THUR	FRI	SAT	SUN
Emotion Regulation	Checked the facts	MON	TUE	WED	THUR	FRI	SAT	SUN
	Did opposite action	MON	TUE	WED	THUR	FRI	SAT	SUN
	Problem-solved	MON	TUE	WED	THUR	FRI	SAT	SUN
	Accumulated positive emotions A	MON	TUE	WED	THUR	FRI	SAT	SUN
	Built mastery B	MON	TUE	WED	THUR	FRI	SAT	SUN
	Coped ahead C	MON	TUE	WED	THUR	FRI	SAT	SUN
	Reduced vulnerability: PLEASE	MON	TUE	WED	THUR	FRI	SAT	SUN
	Mindfulness of current emotion	MON	TUE	WED	THUR	FRI	SAT	SUN
Distress Tolerance — CRISIS SURVIVAL	STOP skill	MON	TUE	WED	THUR	FRI	SAT	SUN
	Pros and cons	MON	TUE	WED	THUR	FRI	SAT	SUN
	TIP	MON	TUE	WED	THUR	FRI	SAT	SUN
	Distracted	MON	TUE	WED	THUR	FRI	SAT	SUN
	Self-soothed	MON	TUE	WED	THUR	FRI	SAT	SUN
	Improved the moment	MON	TUE	WED	THUR	FRI	SAT	SUN
REALITY	Radical acceptance	MON	TUE	WED	THUR	FRI	SAT	SUN
ACCEPT	Half-smiling, Willing Hands	MON	TUE	WED	THUR	FRI	SAT	SUN
	Willingness, Mindfulness of Current Thoughts	MON	TUE	WED	THUR	FRI	SAT	SUN

Left margin legend:
DEAR (Describe, Express, Assert, Reinforce)
MAN (Mindful, Appear confident, Negotiate)
GIVE (Gentle, Interested, Validate, Easy manner)
FAST (Fair, no Apologies, Stick to values, Truthful)
ABC (Accumulate positive emotions, Build mastery, Cope ahead)
PLEASE (Care: Physical ills, Eating, Avoid mood-altering substances, Sleep, Exercise)
TIP (Temperature, Intense Exercise, Paced Breathing, Paired muscle relaxation)

FIGURE 4.1. Front (top) and back (bottom) of a DBT diary card. The entire back half of the card is used in skills training sessions; the front half is used in individual therapy except for the "Used Skills" column, which is also employed in skills training. Should be printed on 4" × 6" card stock (front and back).

TABLE 4.2. Instructions for Helping a Client Complete the DBT Diary Card

1. *Name*: Put here the client's name, initials, or clinical ID.

2. *Filled Out In Session?* If the card was filled out during the session, have the client circle "Y" for "yes"; otherwise circle "N" for "no."

3. *How Often Did You Fill Out [This Side]?* In the past week, did the client fill out the card daily, 2–3 times, or once?

4. *Date Started*: Ask the client to note the first date the card was started, including year.

5. *Day of Week*: Instruct the client to record information for each day of the week.

6. *Using the 0–5 Rating Scale*: You'll notice that many of the columns require the client to record a numerical value from 0 to 5. This is a subjective, continuous scale intended to communicate the client's experience along a variety of behaviors or experiences. The anchor point 0 represents the absence of a particular experience (e.g., no urge); the anchor point 5 refers to the strongest degree of the experience (e.g., strongest urges imaginable).

7. *Urges to . . .* : The "*Commit Suicide*" column refers to any urges to commit suicide. The "*Self-Harm*" column refers to urges to engage self-harm or in any self-injurious behaviors. The "*Use Drugs*" column refers to use of any drug of *abuse* (e.g., over-the-counter meds., prescription meds., street/illicit drugs)—or, for clients not using drugs to any urge to escape.

8. *Highest Ratings* refers to ratings of intensity of emotional misery, intensity of physical misery or pain, and degree of joy (or happiness) experienced during the day. Have the client rate each emotion daily, using the 0–5 rating scale.

9. *Drugs/Medications*: For alcohol, have the client put down how many drinks and what type of alcohol (e.g., "3" for 3 beers). For illegal drugs, have the client specify the type of drug used (e.g., heroin) and how much was used. For p.r.n./over-the-counter medications, have the client put down how many doses and what type of medication was taken. For meds. as prescribed, if taken as prescribed, have the client put a "Y" for yes; if not taken as prescribed (either too much or too little, or some medications but not others), have the client put down an "N" for no.

   - Write "ditto" marks in subsequent specify boxes, to indicate use is the same as the previous day.
   - An Easier Way: The client can use horizontal lines through rows and vertical lines through columns to indicate no use. For instance, if the

client didn't use any prescription meds. this week, a vertical line down the "Y/N" column under "Meds. as Prescribed" is OK. Or if the client didn't use alcohol, over-the-counter meds., or prescription meds. on Wednesday, then a horizontal line may be drawn through the corresponding boxes for Wednesday.

10. *Actions . . .* : The column "**Self-Harm**" refers to any intentional self-harm or suicide attempt. The "Lied" column refers to all overt and covert behaviors that mask telling the truth. It's important for the client to assume a nonjudgmental stance in completing this. Instruct the client to put the number of lies told per day in the column, and place an * in this column to signify lying on the diary card. The *Used Skills* (0–7) column is used to report the highest skill usage for the day. When making this rating, the client should refer to the 0–7 "*Used Skills*" table just under the columns.

    The last two columns are optional. Two columns are for tracking specific emotions, and two are for any other behaviors you and the client want to track. Note that there is not a rating scale for these, so when you and the client are deciding what to track, also decide how to track it—for example, with a "Y," "N," a 0–5 or 0–7 scale, or by describing what and how much (i.e., "What?" and #).

11. *Med. Change This Week*: Instruct the client to write down any changes in prescribed medications. These changes may consist of modifications in the dosage (increase or decrease) of the medications (e.g., increase from 5 mg to 10 mg; a decrease from 20 mg to 10 mg), the dropping of a medication, or the addition of a new medication. If there is insufficient room, the client should describe these on a separate piece of paper.

12. *Homework Assigned and Results This Week*: Have the client record any behaviors assigned for the week, describe what was done, and indicate what the results were.

13. *Urges to Use (0–5) and Urges to Quit Therapy (0–5)*: Have the client rate the intensity of *current* urges to engage in these behaviors, at the beginning of the session.

14. *Skills Focus This Week*: Instruct the client to write down any skills that are specifically focused on, used, or practiced during the week. This space can also be used to write down what skills need more focus during the week.

15. *Belief I Can Change or Regulate . . .* : Using the same 0–5 rating scale, rate your belief regarding your ability to change or regulate your *emotions*, *actions*, and *thoughts* as you start your therapy session.

lyzed and discussed as such. The problem should be framed in such a way that whatever skills are currently being taught can be applied.

Creating an Environment That Reinforces Skilled Behavior

Individuals differ in styles of self-regulation. On the continuum whose poles are internal self-regulation and external environmental regulation, many individuals with high dysregulation of emotions and associated actions and thoughts are near the environmental pole. Many therapists seem to believe that the internal self-regulation pole of the continuum is inherently better or more mature, and spend a fair amount of therapy time trying to make individuals with emotion dysregulation more self-regulated. Although DBT does not suggest the converse—that environmental regulation styles are preferable—it does suggest that going with the clients' strength is likely to be easier and more beneficial in the long run. Thus, once behavioral skills are in place, clients should be taught how to maximize the tendency of their natural environments to reinforce skilled over unskilled behaviors. This may include teaching them how to create structure, how to make public instead of private commitments, how to find communities and lifestyles that support their new behaviors, and how to elicit reinforcement from others for skilled rather than unskilled behaviors. (See Distress Tolerance Handouts 19 and 20.) This is not to say that clients should not be taught self-regulation skills; rather, the types of self-regulation skills taught should be keyed to their strengths. Written self-monitoring with a prepared diary form, for example, is preferable to trying to observe behavior each day and make a mental note of it. Keeping alcohol out of the house is preferable to trying a self-talk strategy to inhibit getting out the bottle. It is easier to diet if a client eats at home rather than out at restaurants that serve yummy but huge meal portions. Using an alarm to wake up can be more effective than counting on oneself to wake up when needed.

A final point needs to be made here. Sometimes clients' newly learned skills do not generalize because out in the real world clients punish their own behavior. This is usually because their behavioral expectations for themselves are so high that they simply never reach the criteria for reinforcement. This pattern must change if generalization and progress are to occur. Problems with self-reinforcement and self-punishment are discussed more extensively in Chapters 3, 8, and 10 of the main DBT text; the behavioral validation strategies described in that text's Chapter 8 and in this manual should be used in skills training as well (see also Interpersonal Effectiveness Handouts 18 and 19). I discuss these topics further in the skills module content chapters of this manual (Chapters 7–10).

Family and Couple Sessions

One way to maximize generalization is to have individuals from the clients' social community learn the DBT skills. Usually, these will be members of the clients' families or their spouses or partners. In adolescent DBT programs, for example, as noted previously, skills training ordinarily includes parents or other family care providers. Trainers can give clients copies of the skills handouts to take home to teach their family members and/or friends the skills. Thus all members of a family can be learning the same sets of skills, and can practice together and coach each other. Family members of clients with emotion dysregulation have been very receptive to this type of therapy. Skills training can also be offered for friends and family members of adults who are in the DBT treatment program. In these situations, clients and their family members may be in separate groups.

Use of Fading Principles

At the beginning of skills training, the trainers model, instruct, reinforce, give feedback, and coach the clients for using skills both within the therapy sessions and in the natural environment. If skillful behavior in the everyday environment is to become independent of the trainers' influence, however, the trainers must gradually fade out use of these procedures, particularly instructions and reinforcement. The goal here is to fade skills training procedures to an intermittent schedule, such that the trainers are providing less frequent instructions and coaching than clients can provide for themselves, and less modeling, feedback, and reinforcement than clients obtain from their natural environments.

Managing Review of Skills Practice Homework

It is important to remember that DBT is a problem-focused treatment with two core intervention strategies: validation and problem solving. Both are important in managing homework review. When trainers are reviewing homework, the strategy is to validate when the assigned skills are practiced correctly and effectively—and to problem-solve when no homework is done, the skills are not practiced correctly and/or effectively, and/or problems in using the skills are identified. Even for clients who are eager to learn, who read the skills book at home, and who practice the skills religiously, problems in correctly and effectively using the skills can arise. Thus it is important not to cut this review time in favor of more time for teaching new skills in the second half of the session.

Problem solving is a two-stage process: (1) understanding the problem at hand (behavioral analysis) and (2) attempting to generate new, effective use of the skills (solution analysis). Understanding the problem at hand requires defining problems in using the skills, highlighting patterns and implications of current skills use, and developing hypotheses about factors interfering with effective use of the skills. The second stage, that of targeting change, requires providing feedback on correct implementation of skills when needed; developing solutions to the problems that have arisen in using skills; and encouraging efforts to practice the skills by providing the rationale for using skills and troubleshooting implementation of solutions. The aim of this repeated focus on analyzing and problem-solving difficulties is not only to get clients to begin using the skills effectively, but also to get clients to begin using the problem-solving strategies with one another and eventually with themselves.

To a large extent, skills training is a general case of solution analysis. Skills are presented as practical solutions to life's problems, and the potential effectiveness of various skills in particular situations is discussed during each meeting. Perhaps more than any other set of strategies, solution analysis utilizes the power of a group context. Each member should be encouraged to offer solution ideas to other group members and to help develop strategies to solve the problems described. For example, a member who is having trouble paying attention during group sessions and getting homework assignments into short-term memory can be helped to think of ways to attend more closely. The group as a whole can almost always be counted on to come up with many solutions to not remembering to practice during the week. Difficulties in selecting the right skill to use or

in applying a skill in a particular situation are further opportunities for group solution analysis. Almost always, someone will already have solved the problem at hand for him- or herself; thus the group leaders should be especially careful in the solution analysis phase not to jump in with solutions before eliciting possible solutions from other group members. However, they should not be reluctant to offer a solution or a particular application of a skill, even if other group members have offered other ideas.

Managing the sharing of between-session practice requires enormous sensitivity on the part of the leaders. The tasks here are to prod each client gently to analyze his or her own behavior; to validate difficulties; and to counter tendencies toward judging negatively and holding the self to impossibly high standards. At the same time, leaders help clients develop more effective skill strategies for the coming week if needed. The leaders must be adept at alternating attention between the previous week's behaviors and in-session attempts to describe, analyze, and solve problems. Shame, humiliation, embarrassment, self-hatred, anger, and fear of criticism or looking "stupid" are common emotions interfering with the ability to engage in and profit from homework review. Deft handling of these emotions is the key to using practice sharing therapeutically; it involves combining validating strategies with problem-solving strategies, and irreverent communication with reciprocal communication. (See Chapter 5 of this manual for more on validation and communication strategies.)

The first step in practice sharing is for each group member to share with the group the particular skills he or she used (and the success or failure of these efforts), as well as the situations the skills were used in during the previous week. Clients will inevitably present their situations and/or skill use in very general and vague terms at first. They will also often describe their inferences of others' motives or emotions, or their judgmental beliefs, as if these inferences and beliefs are facts. The task of a skills trainer is to engage a client in the strategy of behavioral analysis. In other words, the task is to get a client to describe (using the mindfulness "what" skill of describing) the particular environmental and behavioral events leading up to the problem situation and to the successful or unsuccessful attempt to use the skills.

Obviously, providing such a description requires that a client be able to observe during the week. Often clients have great difficulty describing what happened because they are not astute observers; however, with repeated practice and repeated reinforcement over the weeks, their observation and description skills tend to improve. A minute description allows a trainer to assess whether a client in fact used the skills appropriately. If the client has practiced and the skills have worked, he or she should be supported and encouraged by the leaders. The client models for other clients how they can use those same skills for similar problems. Thus the leaders should try briefly to elicit from other group members examples of either similar problems or similar skill usage to foster this generalization. Client-to-client praise and encouragement are reinforced. It is very important to get each client to describe in detail his or her use of the skills in that particular week's problematic situations. The same amount of attention to detail must be given to the week's successes as to the week's difficulties. In addition, over time the leaders can use such information to identify the client's patterns in skill usage.

The insight strategies can also be used. During homework sharing, it is very important to look carefully for patterns in situational problems, as well as typical responses to such problems. Highlighting idiosyncratic patterns can be especially helpful in future behavioral analyses. This is especially important if a client is consistently reporting only one skill strategy. For example, in one of my groups I had a client who always tried to change problem situations as his primary method of emotion regulation. Although his skills at problem-solving situations were excellent and commendable, nonetheless it was also important for him to learn other methods (e.g., tolerating the situation, distracting himself). Skills trainers should comment on any rigid patterns that they see, as well as on effective patterns or skills that the clients use. Clients' observations and comments about their own or one another's skillful patterns should, of course, be noted and reinforced. (It is essential to follow the guidelines provided in the insight section in Chapter 9 of the main DBT text.)

Not every problem situation can be changed. My experience is that when given a limited amount of time to share, clients with disordered emotion regulation will almost always share their successes in using skills, and will rarely want to describe their problems and failures. Thus listening carefully to the successes is even more important than it might be with other populations.

When the Skills Did Not Help

If a client could not use the skills being taught, or reports using the skills but not getting any benefits from them, the leaders use problem-solving strategies such as behavioral analysis to help the client analyze what happened, what went wrong, and how he or she could use the skills better next time. It is extremely important at this point to lead the client through a detailed examination of just what did occur. This can be torturous, because almost always (especially during the first several months of therapy) clients are fearful of skills trainers' and other members' judgments, and are also judging themselves in negative ways. Thus they can be expected to be very inhibited. Sometimes a client will jump right in with a notion of why a skill didn't work or why he or she couldn't apply it, without examining the actual events. These explanations are frequently pejorative and involve name calling (e.g., "I am just stupid"). Or a client may accept without question the premise that his or her situation is hopeless and skills will never help. Emotionally dysregulated people are rarely able to analyze objectively and calmly what led up to a particular problem, especially when the problem is their own behavior. Obviously, if they cannot conduct such an analysis, attempts to solve the problem are probably doomed from the start. Many are unable to see the critical role of environmental context in behavior and persist in viewing all behavior as a function of internal motives, needs, and the like. (It is, of course, essential that skills trainers not collude with this view.) Thus the skills trainer's task here is to engage the client in a behavioral analysis; to model nonpejorative, nonjudgmental behavioral evaluations; and (in a group context) to get both the individual and the group engaged in the process so that the same skills can be used in other problem situations. (How to do this, where to start and stop, and roadblocks to avoid are described in detail in Chapter 9 of the main DBT text.)

Over time, it is important to encourage and reinforce clients in helping one another analyze and solve difficult problems.

When a Client Has Difficulty with Homework

During sharing, a client will often report that he or she did not practice at all during the preceding week. It would be an error to take this comment at face value. On close examination, we often find that the client did practice; he or she just did not actually solve the problem. The discussion then turns to the issue of shaping and setting appropriate expectations. Often we find that the client does not have a complete understanding of how to practice the skill assigned. Or we may find that the person does not understand many of the skills discussed previously, but has been afraid to ask questions. In these instances, both the self-censoring of questions and the problem in homework practice should be discussed. Whenever possible, it is useful to ask other clients to help the person having difficulty. In the case of interpersonal effectiveness, we may ask another client to role-play how he or she would cope with the situation. Emotion regulation and distress tolerance do not lend themselves to demonstration, but other clients can share how they have coped (or would cope) with similar situations.

Sometimes a client reports that he or she tried to use the skills but could not carry them out. Chaos in the environment, lack of skills, or not understanding the assignment or instructions can be important influences. For example, a client may enter an interpersonal situation with every intent of applying some of the interpersonal effectiveness skills learned previously, but then may get confused and forget what to say or how to respond to a particular remark by the other person. At other times, a client may report using the skill appropriately, except that it didn't work. Even the most skilled negotiator cannot always get what he or she wants; relaxation exercises, even when used correctly, do not always lead to reduction of anxiety and tension. In these instances, it is essential to get precise information about what happened. A client and a trainer may both be tempted to skip this and decide that this particular skill is not useful for this particular client. Although this may be true, it may also be true that the client is not applying the skill in the correct way. At each point in the analysis, the trainer should be open to almost any problem. No matter what, the trainer should treat each problem as one to be solved and jump immediately to "How could you solve that?"

Finally, sometimes a client who says he or she did not practice actually did practice, but either did not realize it or used skills learned outside skills training. This information can be missed completely if the patient's experiences during the week are not explored in enough depth.

In general, what works for whom is very individual. Leaders must be cautious, however, in assuming a skill doesn't fit the particular client. Inexperienced leaders often give up on a skill too easily. They may assume that the specific skill is not a good match for a specific group member when, in actuality, the client has not been applying the skill properly.

When a Client Did Not Do Any Homework Practice

Almost all incidents of noncompliance with homework assignments (i.e., refusing or forgetting to practice skills) and of refusal or failure to engage in skills training activities should elicit an immediate movement into behavioral analysis with the client involved. The clients' tendency to offer simple solutions and answers must be counteracted. Common reasons given by clients for not practicing include not wanting to, not remembering, and not having an occasion to practice. Rarely can they identify the situational factors influencing their lack of motivation, failure to remember, or inability to observe practice opportunities. Individuals with disordered emotion regulation tend to use punishment, commonly in the form of self-denigration, as a form of behavior control. It is, of course, important that the leaders resist the temptation to collude with clients in punishing themselves for not practicing. Members who have not attempted to practice during the preceding week will often not want to discuss the reason for not practicing and will ask the leaders to go on to the next person. It is essential that the leaders not be convinced to do this. The analysis of not doing homework can be very important. In the case of a person who is avoiding the topic because of fear or shame, it offers a chance to practice opposite action, a skill taught in the emotion regulation module. It also offers other group members an opportunity to practice their own behavior management and problem-solving skills within the context of the group.

The first step is to get a precise definition of the behaviors missing, followed by problem solving to avoid the same problem in the future. (See missing links analyses in Chapter 6 of this manual for step-by-step instructions.) Ask the following questions in order:

1. "Did doing your homework get into short-term memory?" This means "Were you aware of the assignment?" If the answer is no, there is no point in trying to solve any other problem. Non-awareness may be due to inattention in the session, absence from the session, and/or not reading or getting the reminder of the homework. If this is the problem, solutions for how to find out and know the assignment must be found. If the client says yes, move to the next question.

2. *"Were you willing to do the needed or expected effective behavior?"* If the answer to this question is no, ask what got in the way of willingness to do effective behaviors. Ideas might include willfulness, feeling inadequate, or feeling demoralized. Problem-solve what got in the way of willingness— for example, to practice radical acceptance, do pros and cons, or practice opposite action. If the client says yes, move to the third question.

3. *"Did the thought of doing your homework ever come into your mind?"* If no, work on developing ways to get the thought of homework to come into mind. (Get the group to generate lots of ideas.) If the answer is yes, move to the fourth question.

4. *"What got in the way of doing your homework once you thought of it?"* If "I'll do it later" showed up, ask whether the thought of doing the homework returned at a later point. If not, as above, work on how to get the idea to show up again. If yes, analyze what happened then. If willfulness showed up ("No! I'm not going to do it!"), work on solving that problem. (Be open to the likelihood that willfulness may stay around for a while.) Don't use willfulness to treat willfulness.

Analyzing Motivation to Complete Homework Practice

A frequent comment that requires careful analysis is "If I didn't do it, I must not have wanted to do it." Motivational interpretations are often learned in previous therapies, even when they have little to do with reality. Even if the problem *is* one of motivation, the question of what is interfering with motivation must be addressed. The most important thing to remember here is to offer nonpejorative hypotheses and communicate to the client a nonjudgmental attitude; the client is usually judgmental enough. Hypotheses that are particularly worthy of exploration include hopelessness that the skills will do any good; hopelessness that the client can ever learn the skills; beliefs that he or she doesn't need the skills and already has them; and beliefs that he or she should have learned these skills earlier, and therefore is inadequate or stupid for having to learn them now. Such beliefs probably lead to negative emotional re-

actions, which the client then flees from. It is very important to communicate to clients that it is OK to have hopeless beliefs, and that the skills trainers will not feel invalidated if the clients do not have perfect trust in them. Although each of these beliefs may be perfectly reasonable (and should be validated), holding on to the beliefs is probably not useful, and thus cheerleading (see Chapter 8 of the main DBT text), cognitive modification (see Chapter 11 of the main DBT text), and solution analysis (see Chapter 5 of this manual) are in order.

Failures in motivation and in memory offer important opportunities for the leaders to teach principles of behavioral management and learning. (See this manual's Chapter 8, especially Section XVII.) The goal over time is to use these principles to replace the judgmental theories based on willpower and mental illness that individuals with emotion dysregulation often hold. Failure to practice is a problem to be solved.

Improving Compliance with Between-Session Skills Practice

I have found the following strategies useful in helping group members improve the frequency of skills practice between sessions.

1. *Give specific assignments.* When you are assigning homework, give very specific assignments. In addition, provide a homework assignment calendar for clients to write down assignments, and worksheets for clients to write down the results of their practice. Send e-mails, text messages, or other reminders during the week to remind everyone of the assignments.

2. *Give clients a choice of worksheets.* On the website for this book, there are usually at least two worksheets for each assignment. I have found that clients have very specific likes and dislikes when it comes to worksheets. Some like to write a lot, and some don't. I have developed a series of worksheets for almost every skills handout, so that clients can have a greater sense of control over what they actually practice and write down.

3. *Reinforce completion of homework.* This can be done by giving out a tangible reward that fits the group you are teaching. We give out one sticker for each worksheet a client completes between sessions. If for some reason a client did not have access to the assignment, then filling out any worksheets will be given the same number of stickers. A secondary outcome of this strategy is that it cuts off almost any good reason for not doing any homework skills practice. If you want to give an arbitrary reinforcer for homework, such as a sticker, you have to be specific in telling clients exactly how much practice is needed to get the reward. Awarding stickers has had a remarkable effect on increasing homework compliance in our clinic and in other clinics we know of. As noted previously, clients in our groups love the stickers and often bring in their favorites to add to our stock. They put them on the outside of their skills binders. Other groups give out candy. Vouchers that can be exchanged for a range of tangible rewards can also be effective. As in programs for substance use disorders, you might be able to get community merchants to donate to a gift locker to use in these programs.

4. *Do not give the reward if the client did not complete the requisite homework*. This point is critical. Many clients will become very distressed, angry, sad, or tearful when they do not get a reward. It may seem much easier just to give the reward anyway, but this is a mistake. Once you do this several times, the function of the stickers as contingent on doing homework practice will be lost. Those doing their homework for stickers may then become distressed. If you want to reinforce other behaviors (e.g., trying hard), you can give out other rewards. For example, I give out a verbal "10,000 gold stars" (and sometimes an extravagant "12,000 or 13,000") at intervals whenever someone engages in behavior I want to be sure to reinforce. Although the stars are purely verbal, clients seem very willing to work for them. I began doing this in skills groups when a client petulantly said in a group session that she had heard I give out gold stars in other settings, and she wanted to know why I never gave them out in the skills group.

5. *Start the review of homework with one or two who haven't done it*. Ask at the beginning of the session who has and has not done the homework. Start with those who have not done it, and ask the series of questions listed above. For the average client, the analysis of *not* doing homework is somewhat aversive, despite your efforts to do it in a nonaversive manner. This aversive review of homework noncompletion, however, can be very motivating and should not be skipped, no matter how much the clients try to get you to skip it. However, you can at times end the review as soon as you determine that the clients' refusal to proceed or willfulness about it will make it difficult to proceed. In general, my policy is to go to the next person or topic whenever a client refuses to respond. What I do not do is skip asking the client to respond (always in a tone of voice that implies I have forgotten that they do not want to be asked). In essence, I put clients' requests that I skip them on an extinction schedule. The exception here is the person who has made it abundantly clear that he or she is *not* participating in homework review or in the group as a whole. With such an individual, I might say in homework review, "Are you still not doing homework [or not sharing homework]?" Or I might say, "Are you still on strike?" If there is no answer or the answer is yes, I might go on or I might say, "Well, I want you to know my hope springs eternal."

6. *Jump to those who have done homework after analyzing one or two who haven't*. Do this when more than two out of eight clients have not done their homework. Be sure to reinforce any and all homework done. Listening to homework reports and getting others in the group to listen are crucial here. Give needed feedback, and try to involve other group members in discussing homework. Relate one person's use of skills or difficulties to those of others in the group when possible.

Application of Fundamental DBT Strategies in Behavioral Skills Training

The overarching strategy in DBT is the emphasis on dialectics at every turn in treatment. As can be seen in Figure 5.1, core DBT strategies are designed in pairs, representing acceptance on the one hand and change on the other. There are five major strategy categories: (1) the overarching dialectical strategies; (2) core strategies (problem solving vs. validation); (3) communication style strategies (irreverent vs. reciprocal); (4) case management strategies (consultation-to-the-patient vs. environmental intervention); and (5) integrative strategies. The core strategies of problem solving and validation,

together with the dialectical strategies, form the essential components of DBT. Communication strategies specify interpersonal and communication styles compatible with the therapy. Case management strategies specify how the therapist interacts with and responds to the social network in which the client is enmeshed.

As can be seen in Figure 5.2, DBT is a modular treatment. The key characteristic of a modular treatment is that the treatment provider can move the treatment strategies within various treatment modules in and out of treatment as needed. Skills

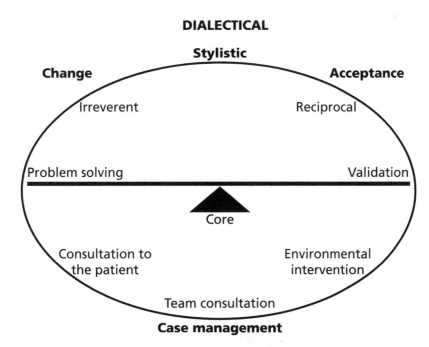

FIGURE 5.1. Treatment strategies in DBT. From Linehan, M. M. (1993). *Cognitive-behavioral treatment of borderline personality disorder.* New York: Guilford Press. Copyright 1993 by The Guilford Press. Reprinted by permission.

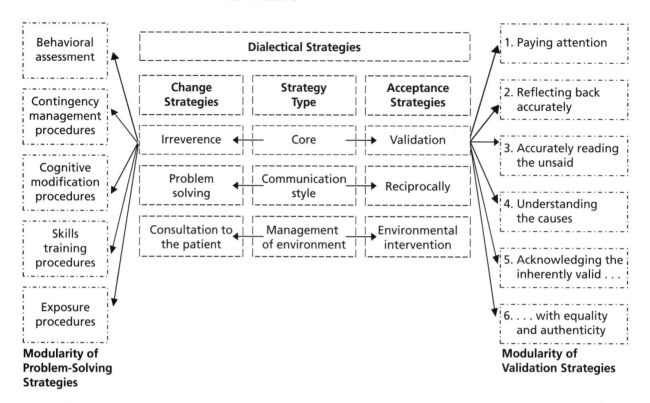

FIGURE 5.2. Example of modularity of strategies and procedures.

training procedures are part of the problem-solving change strategies. Although not exhaustive, the modules shown in Figure 5.2 represent treatment strategies that skills trainers routinely use and are described in more detail later in this chapter. The focus in skills training is for the client to learn and put into action new skillful means of responding to problems in living. Although the skills taught can be divided into change skills and acceptance skills (see Figure 5.3), learning and using new skills nevertheless represents a change on the part of the client.

Integrative strategies outline how to handle specific problem situations that may come up during skills training, such as problems in the therapeutic relationship, suicidal behaviors, therapy-destroying behaviors, and ancillary treatments. Some of these strategies have already been discussed in Chapters 3 and 4. A number of therapist strategies have also been translated into skills for clients and are discussed further in Chapters 6–10. All the strategies are discussed in detail in the main DBT text. Skills trainers need to know them all in order to respond flexibly to new problems that arise. This chapter reviews the basic DBT strategies and procedures; it also addresses some of the problems that may arise

specifically in skills training, as well as some of the modifications of strategies I have found useful, particularly in a group context.

Dialectical Strategies: Maintaining Therapeutic Balance

The dialectical focus in DBT occurs at two levels of therapeutic behavior. At the first level, a skills trainer must be alert to the dialectical balance occurring within the treatment environment. In a group setting, each group member (including each leader) is in a constant state of dialectical tension at many levels and in many directions. The first set of tensions consists of those between each individual member and the group as a whole. From this perspective, the group has an identity of its own, and each member can react to the group as a whole. Thus, for example, a member may be acting in dialectical tension with the group's norms, its beliefs or attitudes, or its "personality." In addition, insofar as the identity of the group as a whole is both the sum of and more than its parts, the identity of each individual in the group is in some aspect defined by his or her relationship to the group. Because both the identity of the group and the identity of each individual change over the skills training year, identification of members with the group and the struggles that evolve with this identity provide a dialectical tension that can be harnessed for the sake of therapeutic progress.

A second set of tensions consists of those between each individual pair within the group—tensions that can become active at any moment when two group members interact. A drawback of allowing members to interact with one another outside the group is that relationships between members can develop outside the public arena of the group. Thus the dialectical tensions between one member and another will often not be apparent to the leaders or other group members. Overlaying and interfacing with these two levels, so to speak, is a third set of dialectical tensions between each individual and his or her unique environment—a context brought into the treatment situation via long-term memory.

The group leaders must be aware of the multiple tensions impinging on a skills training session at any given time. Maintaining a therapeutic balance and moving the balance toward reconciliation and growth are the tasks of the skills trainers. It is essential here for each trainer to remember that he or she is also a group member—and thus is also in dialectical tension with the group as a whole, with the other leader, and with each individual member.

Clearly, the dialectical framework that is necessary here is that of a dynamic, open system. The system includes not only those present, but also all external influences that are brought into group

sessions via long-term memory and established behavioral patterns. This framework will help the group leaders avoid the mistake of always interpreting members' behavior from the point of view of a closed system, which assumes that all responses are a direct reaction to events within sessions. It is far more common, however, for a group activity or event to precipitate the remembering of events that have occurred outside sessions. Clients with disordered emotion regulation are often quite unable to put aside cognitive processing of very stressful events, to stop ruminating, or to focus on one thing in the moment. It is also a mistake, on the other hand, for the leaders never to attribute client behavior to in-session events. It is this dialectical tension between and among influential events that the leaders must be attuned to.

The second level of dialectical focus is on teaching and modeling dialectical thinking as a replacement for dichotomous, either–or, black-and-white thinking. It is important for both leaders and co-leaders to be facile with an array of dialectical techniques.

Specific Dialectical Strategies

Dialectical strategies are described in simple language in the skills handouts on dialectics (Interpersonal Effectiveness Handouts 15 and 16), and all of the dialectical strategies are described in detail in Chapter 7 of the main DBT text. Although trainers will use all of the dialectical strategies at one time or another, some are particularly useful in skills training.

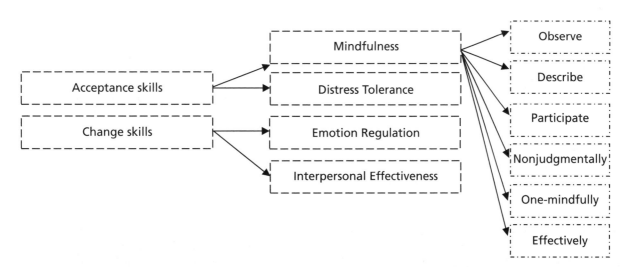

FIGURE 5.3. Example of modularity of DBT skills.

The most common dialectical strategies in DBT are storytelling and metaphors. The teaching notes for each skill (Chapters 6–10 of this manual) provide a number of examples but are by no means exhaustive. For example, at the very start of skills training, the opportunity arises to enter the paradox of how it can be that everyone is doing the best they can and simultaneously everyone needs to do better. Entering the paradox here requires the trainers to refrain from providing rational explanations; in order to achieve understanding and to move toward synthesis of the polarities, each person needs to resolve the dilemma for him- or herself.

Playing the devil's advocate is another key strategy. A trainer presents a propositional statement that is an extreme version of one of a client's own dysfunctional beliefs, and then plays the role of devil's advocate to counter the client's attempts to disprove the extreme statement or rule. It is an important strategy for helping clients let go of ineffective myths about emotions and about using interpersonal skills. Almost any disaster or crisis is an opportunity to practice not only particular skills, but the strategy of making lemonade out of lemons (i.e., finding the positives in a negative situation).

As I have noted in Chapter 2 of this manual, conducting an open (rather than closed) group offers an opportunity to allow natural change—yet another dialectical strategy. Dialectics are critically important in the two most important characteristics of skills training: assessing use of skills and teaching new skills. Assessing dialectically involves openness to being incorrect in one's analysis and understanding of clients' difficulties with skills. It is always asking the question "What is being left out here?" A group setting, in particular, offers a rich environment for demonstrating the futility of approaching problem solving with a "right versus wrong" cognitive set. No matter how brilliant a solution to a particular problem may be, it is always possible for a group member to come up with another strategy that may be equally effective. And every problem solution has its own set of limitations; that is, there is always "another side of the story." It is extremely important for the group leaders not to get into a battle of trying to prove that the skills being taught are the only right way to handle every situation, or even any particular situation. Although the skills may be very effective for some purposes, they are not more "right" than other approaches. Thus the leaders' task is to ask this question repeatedly:

"How can we all be right, and how can we test the effectiveness of our strategies?"

Typical Dialectical Tensions

Feelings and Beliefs versus Wise Mind

The strategy of "wise mind" is the first core mindfulness skill taught (see Chapter 7 of this manual) and should then be encouraged throughout skills training. When a client makes a statement representing an emotional or feeling state (e.g., "I feel fat and unlovable") as if the feeling state provides information about the empirical reality ("I am fat and unlovable"), it is effective at times simply to question the client: "I'm not interested right now in what you believe or think. I am interested in what you know to be true in your wise mind. What do you know to be true? What does wise mind say is true?" The dialectical tension is between what the client believes in "emotion mind" and what he or she thinks to be true ("reasonable mind"); the synthesis is what she knows to be true in wise mind. The push toward wise mind can be easily abused, of course, especially when a trainer confuses wise mind with what the trainer believes to be the case. This can be particularly difficult when the trainer overvalues the wisdom of his or her own knowledge or opinions. The value of therapeutic humility cannot be overstated. When such divergences arise, the trainer's task is to ask, "What is being left out of my own position?" while simultaneously looking for a synthesis. In DBT, one of the major functions of the consultation team is to provide a balance to the arrogance that can easily accompany a therapist's or trainer's powerful position.

Willingness versus Willfulness

The tension between "willingness" and "willfulness" is an important one in skills training. Although I discuss it much more fully in Chapter 10 of this manual, the essential tension is between responding to a situation in terms of what the situation needs (willingness) and responding in a way that resists what a situation needs or responding in terms of one's own needs rather than those of the situation (willfulness). Thus willfulness encompasses both trying to "fix" the situation and sitting passively on one's hands, refusing to respond at all.

Many forms of this tension can arise during skills training. A key one arises in a group context when the leaders are interacting with one member or the group as a whole, and the member or group is withdrawing and refusing to interact. The tension is between the leaders' attempting to influence the member or group and allowing themselves to be influenced by the member or group. The essential question, framed somewhat more directly, is this: How far should the leaders push, and how far should the group member or the group as a whole resist? Use of the terms "willfulness" and "willingness" can be quite helpful in this dilemma. I have found myself on many occasions discussing who is being willful with a client. Is it me, the client, or both of us? Of course, the answer to the question revolves around what is needed in the situation, and it is at this point that skill becomes important. It is also, however, a matter of perspective or dialectical focus. The group leaders must keep in mind the member's or group's needs at the moment and in the long term—current comfort versus future gain—and balance these respective goals. If this balance is missed, then the leaders are in danger of being willful. It is all too easy to get into a power struggle with group members, in which the needs of the leaders to make progress, to feel effective, or to create a more comfortable atmosphere come into conflict with the needs of the members.

The problem of willfulness versus willingness is nowhere more apparent than when a skills trainer is juggling the needs of an individual group member and those of the group as a whole. This most commonly occurs when one member is refusing to interact; is hostile; or otherwise is behaving in a way that influences the mood, comfort, and progress of the entire group. In my experience, such a threat to the group's good can bring out the tendency to be willful in a skills trainer. Generally the tension here is between two types of willfulness. On the one hand, a trainer can be willful by actively controlling or attacking the errant member or his or her behavior. Because group members are often singularly unskilled at coping with negative affect, when one member creates conflict, other group members may withdraw. As the mood of the group becomes increasingly tense or hopeless, the skills trainer naturally wants to turn it around; thus the attempt to control the member initiating the conflict ensues. In contrast, the skills trainer can be equally willful by ignoring the conflict and tense mood and responding in a passive way. Passivity in this case actually masquerades as activity, since ignoring the tension is generally manifested by the trainer's continuing to push and escalate the conflict.

The synthesis of willfulness on each side is willingness. It is critically important to remember that no matter how aversive a client's behavior may be, willfulness cannot be fought with willfulness. Thus it is critical that skills trainers respond to willfulness with willingness. For example, I have often found it useful to ask (in a light voice) a client who appears willful, "Are you by chance feeling willful right now?" If the client answers yes, I ordinarily ask, "How long do you think you are going to be willful?" With or without an answer, I "allow" the willful client to continue to be willful and ask only that he or she let me know when willingness returns. With adolescents who are willful in skills training, I have asked, "Hmm, are you by chance on strike?" If the answer is yes, I say "OK," and keep on with the rest of the group.

Good Guy versus Bad Guy

In a group setting, keeping group members working together collaboratively is often very hard work for the leaders. Variations in individual members' moods when they arrive for a session, as well as reactions to in-session events, can have a tremendous effect on any given individual's willingness to work collaboratively during a particular group meeting. It is not atypical that an entire group may be "not in the mood" for working at a particular meeting. When this happens, the leaders must continue to interact with the group members in an attempt to get them working collaboratively again. However, this attempt to interact with the members is often viewed by the members as "pushing," and the leader doing the work (usually the primary group leader) is viewed as the "bad guy" by the group members. At this point it is often helpful for the co-leader to validate the group members' experience. As they are pushed by the primary leader, they often not only retreat but become more rigid in their refusal to interact. Validation from the co-leader can reduce the negative affect and enhance their ability to work. When this occurs, however, the co-leader may then be viewed as the "good guy." Thus the dialectical tension builds between the leaders. This scenario is closely related to the psychodynamic concept of "splitting."

The danger is that the leaders will allow themselves to become "split," so to speak, acting as independent units rather than a cohesive whole. This is most likely to happen if either of the leaders begins to see his or her position as "right" and the other leader's position as "wrong." Once this happens, the leaders pull away from one another and disturb the balance that might otherwise occur. This will not go unnoticed, because group members watch the relationship between the leaders closely. I often refer to group skills training as a recreation of family dinners. Most members have many experiences of unresolved conflicts and battles occurring at family dinners. Group skills training is an opportunity for members to experience a wholeness in the resolution of conflict. The leaders' ability to contain the dialectic in their relationship—to stay united and whole, even as they take different roles—is essential for this learning. Of course, being the "good guy" can be quite comfortable, and being the "bad guy" can be quite uncomfortable. Thus it takes some skillfulness and personal feelings of security for the primary leader to take the role of the "bad guy." (I should be careful to note here that it is not always the primary leader who is the "bad guy"; at times, either leader can take this role.)

Another dialectical tension that may build is that between the skills training leaders and clients' individual psychotherapists. Here the skills trainers can either be the "good guys" or the "bad guys," and the individual therapists can play the corresponding role. In my experience, during the first year of a standard comprehensive DBT treatment program, the skills trainers are more often the "bad guys" and the individual therapists are the "good guys"; however, on occasion the roles are switched. In fact, this is one of the great assets of separating skills training from individual therapy in DBT: It allows a client to have a "bad guy" and a "good guy" simultaneously. Thus the client is often able to tolerate staying in therapy more readily.

The function of the "good guy" is often to hold the client in therapy while he or she resolves conflicts with the "bad guy." Many individuals with disordered emotion regulation do not have the experience of staying in a painful relationship long enough to work a conflict out and then to experience the reinforcement of conflict resolution. DBT, therefore, offers perhaps a unique context in which this can be done. In a sense, clients always have a benign consultant to help them deal with conflicts with the other providers. The essential ingredient is that whoever is the "good guy" must always be able to hold in mind the therapeutic relationships as a whole, rather than allowing them to resolve into "right versus wrong" and true "good guy versus bad guy." It is the skills trainers' ability to hold these

relationships as a whole that will eventually allow their clients to learn to do the same. As the trainers model balance, clients will learn to balance themselves.

Content versus Process

As noted previously, group process issues are not attended to systematically during group skills training, except when negative process threatens to destroy the group. For this to go smoothly, it is critical that skills trainers orient participants to the difference between a skills training group and a therapy process group. Those who have been in the latter often have difficulties with the concept of learning skills versus discussing and working on interpersonal processes. When interpersonal conflicts arise in a group, or emotions become so dysregulated that it is difficult to make progress, the tension that immediately arises is between a decision to proceed with teaching content versus a decision to stop and attend to the process in the group.

Attending to process can be fraught with difficulties, particularly when clients are highly dysregulated. More than a few minutes of process is often more than these clients can handle. The danger is that a conflict beginning in one session may not be resolved, because clients walk out or the session ends. When this happens and the conflict is serious, the skills leaders may need to spend time talking with clients individually to help them work through the issues. If possible, it is best to put these discussions off until a session break, or to hold them after the session, by phone between sessions (if the conflict is severe), or before the next session. To highlight that these discussions are not individual therapy, I conduct them somewhere in the hallway—or, if it is necessary to go into a room to talk, I keep the door open. On the other hand, if content alone is attended to without any attention to process, a group can eventually break down. This is particularly the case when the leaders have not been able to establish a norm of coming to group skills training on time, of doing homework assignments, of paying attention in group sessions, and of treating others with respect. In these cases, holding the balance between content and process is essential.

In my experience, some skills training leaders do better with content and find it easy to ignore process, whereas other leaders do well with process and find it easy to ignore content. It is rare that a leader will find achieving this critical balance an easy task.

Perhaps the key is recognizing that individuals with low distress tolerance pull toward making every moment they are in comfortable. Their inability to put discomfort on a shelf and attend to a task poses a formidable obstacle to continuing with content when process issues are in the foreground. We have found it necessary, time and again, to forge ahead. Forging ahead generally requires the trainers to ignore some or even most of the process issues, and to respond as if clients are collaborating even when they are not. It is a delicate balance that can only be mastered with experience.

Following the Rules versus Reinforcing Assertiveness

As noted in Chapter 3 of this manual, DBT skills training has a number of rules. These rules are not unimportant, and some of them are unequivocal and unbendable. On the other hand, a primary target in DBT is teaching interpersonal skills, including the ability to assert oneself. If skills trainers are doing their job well, a tension arises over time between maintaining the rules (regardless of clients' assertions and requests to the contrary) and reinforcing clients' growing assertive skills by bending the rules when requested in an appropriate manner. The ability to balance "giving in" and "not giving in" is essential. It is here that the trainers' attitude of compassionate flexibility must be balanced with unwavering centeredness (qualities discussed in Chapter 4 of the main DBT text).

What is required is clear thinking on the part of the skills trainers. Giving in for the sake of giving in is as rigid as holding to rules for their own sake. The simple fact that a client requests that a rule be bent or broken in an appropriate manner, however, is not sufficient for reward. Clearly, appropriate requests are not always met with a gracious response in the real world. In fact, one of the key misconceptions of many individuals I treat is that if they ask appropriately, the world will (or should) always give them what they need or want. Learning to deal with the fact that this does not always happen is essential for growth and is one of the goals of distress tolerance training (see Chapter 10 of this manual). On the other hand, the attempt to teach this fundamental lesson should not be confused with arbitrary refusals to make exceptions when the situation requires it. Once again, the notion of willingness can be viewed as the synthesis, and thus as the path for the trainers to follow.

Willingness, however, requires clarity on the skills trainers' part. The clarity needed has to do with the ultimate goals of therapy for an individual member (or for the group, in a group setting) and the means of achieving the goals. The tension that most often exists is that between current comfort and learning to deal with discomfort. Skills trainers must straddle these two aims in coming to a decision about what is the most effective response to a client's assertive behavior.

The task is much easier, of course, if the skills trainers can see emerging client assertiveness as progress rather than as a threat. However, life becomes much more difficult for the trainers when clients begin interacting as peers rather than as "clients." The "one up, one down" relationship that so often exists in therapy is threatened as the clients make progress. To the extent that the skills trainers can take delight in the clients' emerging abilities to outreason and outmaneuver them, therapy progress will be enhanced and not threatened. Essential in a group context, of course, is respecting the other group members' point of view. It is also essential for the trainers to recognize when they are up against a brick wall and are not going to win their point anyway. At these times, the willingness to bend the rules and agree to a client's assertive request can sometimes radically change the nature of the therapeutic relationship.

The use of two leaders in conducting group treatment offers further avenues for setting up dialectic, as noted earlier. In essence, each group leader's style can function as one element in the dialectical opposition. For example, a "good cop, bad cop" strategy, in which one leader focuses on content while the other focuses on process, can be used. Or one leader can help the other leader and a group member synthesize a tension or conflict. While one leader presents one side of the whole, the other leader presents the contrasting side.

Core Strategies: Validation and Problem Solving

Validation

The validation strategies (representing core acceptance) are essential to DBT. As noted previously, it was the necessity of combining validation—a set of acceptance strategies—with problem-solving and other change strategies that first led me to develop a "new" version of CBT. Problem solving must be intertwined with validation. As in individual DBT, validation strategies are used in every skills training session in DBT. They involve a nonjudgmental attitude and a continual search for the essential validity of each client's responses (and, in a group context, those of the group as a whole). In group settings, both the leaders and the group as a whole function as the opposing pole to the invalidating environments commonly experienced by individuals with disordered emotion regulation.

The first general task in validating during skills training is to help clients observe and accurately describe their own emotions, thoughts, and overt behavior patterns. Much of DBT behavioral skills training—in particular, mindfulness training—is aimed at just this. Second, skills trainers communicate empathy with clients' emotional tone, indicate understanding of (though not necessarily agreement with) their beliefs and expectancies, and/or make clear observations of their behavioral action patterns. In other words, the trainers observe and describe the clients' behavior accurately. Third, and most importantly, the trainers communicate that the clients' emotional responses, beliefs/expectancies, and overt behaviors are understandable and make sense in the context of their lives and the current moment. It is particularly important for the skills trainers to validate normative behaviors and those that fit the facts of the clients' situations. In each instance, the trainers look for the nugget of gold in the cup of sand—the validity within what may otherwise be a very dysfunctional response. This is the reverse of the invalidating environment's approach. The components of validation are outlined in Figure 5.2 and are discussed further below and in detail in Interpersonal Effectiveness Handouts 17 and 18, as well as Chapter 8 of the main DBT text.

In both group and individual skills training, almost constant cheerleading is necessary. The skills trainers' biggest problem here will probably be maintaining the energy necessary to cajole, prod, sweet-talk, and cheer on the clients' very slow movement in adopting new, more skillful behaviors. The tensions between "I can't; I won't," and "You can; you must," can drain even the most energetic trainer. Each group leader must rely on the other to provide fresh energy when one is losing steam or when one needs to be bailed out of a willful dialogue with members.

It is equally important in group skills training to elicit and reinforce clients' validation of one another. The ability to validate others is one of the skills

taught in the Interpersonal Effectiveness module. Individuals with high emotion dysregulation are very often exceptional in their ability to empathize with and validate one another. They are also capable of highly judgmental responses. (In some groups, this can become a special problem if the wind-down at the end of session includes individual observations.) They can find it very difficult to understand and validate emotional patterns they have not experienced, thought patterns they are not familiar with, and behaviors they have not exhibited. My experience, however, is that group members bend over backward to validate one another, and that a greater problem is for the leaders to draw out their critical observations that might provide valuable feedback to others. Peace at all costs—a typical objective in some invalidating environments—should not be the norm in group skills training. Other clients, of course, grew up with the norm of no peace at any cost; once again, a dialectic emerges.

In group skills training sessions, validation means that the leaders should always point out the truth inherent in clients' comments and group experiences, even while simultaneously demonstrating the contradictory point of view. Conflict within the group or between an individual group member and a leader is dealt with by validating both sides of the conflict and arriving at a resolution that finds the synthesis of both points of view, rather than invalidating one side or the other.

A "How To" Guide for Validation

The essence of validation is this: The skills trainers communicate to the clients that their responses make sense and are understandable within their current life context or situation. The trainers actively accept clients and communicate this acceptance to clients. Clients' responses are taken seriously and are not discounted or trivialized. Validation strategies require the skills trainers to search for, recognize, and reflect to the clients and/or the group as a whole the validity inherent in their responses to events. With unruly children, parents have to "catch them while they're good" in order to reinforce their behavior; similarly, skills trainers have to uncover the validity within clients' responses, sometimes amplify this validity, and then reinforce it.

Two things are important to note here. First, validation means the acknowledgment of that which is valid. It does not mean "making" valid. Nor does it mean validating that which is invalid. The skills trainers observe, experience, and affirm, but do not create validity. Second, "valid" and "scientific" are not synonyms. Science may be one way to determine what is valid, logical, sound in principle, and/or supported by generally accepted authority. However, an authentic experience or apprehension of private events is also a basis for claiming validity—at least, when it is similar to the experiences of others or when it is in accord with other, more observable events.

Validation can be considered at any one of six levels. Each level is correspondingly more complete than the previous one, and each level depends on the previous levels. Taken as a whole they are definitional of DBT and are required in every interaction with the client. I have described these levels most fully in a 1997 publication.[1]

■ *At Level 1 of validation, the skills trainers listen to and observe what clients are saying, feeling, and doing.* They also make corresponding active efforts to understand what is being said and observed. The essence of this step is that both the skills leader and co-leader stay awake and interested in clients, paying attention to what they say and do in the current moment. The trainers notice the nuances of response in the interaction. Validation at Level 1 communicates that the client per se, as well as the client's presence, words, and responses in the session, have "such force as to compel serious attention and [usually] acceptance."[2] Although both trainers are charged with Level 1 validation, paying attention to nuances of responses across the entire group is a special responsibility of the co-leader, as noted in Chapter 2.

■ *At Level 2 of validation, the skills trainers accurately reflect back to the clients the clients' own feelings, thoughts, assumptions, and behaviors.* The skills trainers convey an understanding of the client by hearing what the clients have said, and seeing what the clients do and how they respond. Validation at Level 2 sanctions, empowers, or authenticates that each individual is who he or she actually is. At Level 2, the skills trainers are always checking to be sure that their reflections are accurate, and are always willing to let go of their previous understanding in favor of a new understanding.

■ *At Level 3 of validation, the skills trainers articulate the unverbalized.* The skills trainers communicate understanding of aspects of the clients' experience and response to events that have not been communicated directly by the clients. The trainers

"mind-read" the reasons for the clients' behavior and figure out how the clients feel and what they are wishing for, thinking, or doing, just by knowing what has happened to the clients. The skills trainers can make the link between precipitating events and behaviors without being given any information about the behaviors themselves. The trainers can also articulate emotions and meanings the clients have not expressed. Level 3 validation is most important in the review of homework and in responding to clients' difficulties in learning, accepting, or practicing new skills.

■ *At Level 4, behavior is validated in terms of its causes.* Validation here is based on the notion that all behavior is caused by events occurring in time; thus, in principle, it is understandable. The skills trainers validate (this validation is not to be confused with "approval" or "excusing") the clients' behavior by showing that it is caused by past events. Even though information may not be available to determine all the relevant causes, the clients' feelings, thoughts, and actions make perfect sense in the context of the clients' current experiences, physiology, and lives to date. At a minimum, what "is" can always be justified in terms of sufficient causes; that is, what is "should be," in that whatever was necessary for it to occur had to have happened.

■ *At Level 5, skills trainers validate in terms of present context or normative functioning.* Skills trainers communicate that behavior is justifiable, reasonable, well grounded, meaningful, and/or efficacious in terms of current events, normative biological functioning, and/or clients' ultimate life goals. The skills trainers look for and reflect the wisdom or validity of clients' responses (and often those of the group as a whole), and communicate that the responses are understandable. The skills trainers find the relevant facts in the current environment that support clients' behaviors. The clients' dysfunction does not blind the skills trainers to those aspects of response patterns that may be either reasonable or appropriate to the context. Thus the skills trainers search the clients' responses for their inherent reasonableness (as well as commenting on the inherent dysfunction of various aspects of these responses, if necessary).

■ *Level 6 of validation requires radical genuineness on the part of the skills trainers.* The task is to recognize each person as he or she is, seeing and responding to the strengths and capacities of the client, while keeping a firm empathic understanding of his or her actual difficulties and incapacities. The skills trainers believe in each client and his or her capacity to change and move toward ultimate life goals, just as they may believe in a friend or family member. The trainers respond to the client as a person of equal status, due equal respect. Validation at the highest level is the validation of the individual "as is." The skills trainers see more than the role—more than a "client" or a "disorder." Level 6 validation is the opposite of treating a client in a condescending manner or as overly fragile. It is responding to the individual as capable of effective and reasonable behavior rather than assuming that he or she is an invalid. Whereas Levels 1–5 represent sequential steps in validation of a kind, Level 6 represents change in both level and kind.

Two other forms of validation should also be mentioned here:

■ *Cheerleading strategies* constitute a further form of validation and are the principal strategies for combating active passivity and tendencies toward hopelessness in many clients with serious emotion dysregulation. In cheerleading, skills trainers communicate the belief that clients are doing their best and validate clients' ability to eventually overcome their difficulties (a type of validation that, if not handled carefully, can simultaneously invalidate clients' perceptions of their helplessness). In addition, skills trainers express a belief in the therapy relationship, offer reassurance, and highlight any evidence of improvement. Within DBT, cheerleading is used in every therapeutic interaction. Although active cheerleading should be reduced as clients learn to trust and to validate themselves, cheerleading strategies always remain an essential ingredient of a strong therapeutic alliance.

■ *Functional validation* is yet another form of validation that is used regularly in DBT. It is a form of nonverbal or behavioral validation that, at times, may be more effective than verbal validation. For example, if a skills trainer drops a 50-pound block on the client's foot, it would be considered invalidating if the trainer's response is to do nothing except say, "Wow, I can see that really hurts! You must be in a lot of pain." Functional validation would entail the trainer's removing the block from the client's foot.

See Chapter 8 of the main DBT text for more on validation.

Problem Solving

A number of the core problem-solving strategies have been discussed in Chapter 4 (behavioral analysis, insight, didactic strategies, solution analysis, and orienting/commitment strategies). In this section, I review several additional and important problem-solving procedures as outlined in Figure 5.2: contingency management, exposure-based procedures, and cognitive restructuring. These procedures are each aimed at change and are basic components of all major CBT approaches. It's important not only for therapists to be adept at using these procedures, but also for clients to know them; elements of each procedure have been translated into DBT skills. Contingency management procedures are taught in the Interpersonal Effectiveness module (Chapter 8, Section XVII; see also Interpersonal Effectiveness Handouts 20–22). The skill of opposite action (Emotion Regulation Handouts 9–11) is based on exposure procedures long known to be effective treatments for anxiety and phobias. In DBT, these principles have been expanded to apply to all problem emotions. The skill of checking the facts (Emotion Regulation Handouts 8–8a) is a translation of cognitive restructuring into a skill. These procedures are also covered in Chapter 10 of the main DBT text.

Contingency Management Procedures

Every response within an interpersonal interaction is potentially a reinforcement, a punishment, or a withholding or removal of reinforcement. "Contingency management" is the provision of consequences for specific behaviors, aimed at increasing or maintaining behaviors that are wanted and decreasing behaviors that are not wanted. Although natural consequences are preferred (see below), they often do not occur frequently or immediately enough to be effective in changing client behavior patterns. Thus contingency management requires skills trainers to organize their behavior strategically, so that client behaviors that represent progress are reinforced, while unskillful or maladaptive behaviors are extinguished or punished.

Orientation to contingency management in skills training starts with the first session. When the rules of DBT skills training are introduced in the first orientation session, the major therapeutic contingencies are discussed. However, only two of the rules involve clear contingencies: Missing 4 consecutive weeks of scheduled skills training sessions, or not meeting with one's individual DBT therapist for four consecutive scheduled sessions (if a client is in standard DBT) or as required by the specific skills program (if a client is in a non-DBT treatment), will result in termination of therapy. There are no clearly stated contingencies for violation of the other rules. In my experience, it is never a good idea to tell clients that they will be terminated from skills training if they break the other rules. However, there are contingent consequences. The main ones are trainer and/or member disapproval, leader and group attention to the rule breaking, and more interpersonal distance.

The basic idea in contingency management is that a client's adaptive functional behavior results in reinforcement, whereas negative maladaptive behavior results in either aversive consequences or no discernible consequences that could reinforce the behavior. A "reinforcer," by definition, is any behavioral consequence that increases the probability of the behavior's occurring again. "Extinction" is reducing the probability of a behavior's occurring by removing the behavioral reinforcer(s). "Punishment" is any behavioral consequence that decreases the probability of the behavior's occurring again.

APPLYING REINFORCING CONTINGENCIES

As noted, *any* consequence that increases the probability of a behavior is a reinforcer. The most important point is not to assume that any particular response to a client's behavior is a positive reinforcer without checking. For example, in our clinic, not only do we use stickers as reinforcers for doing skills homework and for coming to skills training on time; we also let participants tell us what stickers they want, and we pay close attention to whether using stickers is working to increase and maintain the targeted behaviors. Ordering pizza for the group if all members were present, for example, did not work in our substance dependence program. As I have mentioned in Chapter 4, when a client said in one of my groups that she did not think it was fair that I gave out "12,000 gold stars" to people outside of group (as she had heard), I immediately started giving out "10,000–13,000 gold stars" for any skillful behavior that appeared to be particularly difficult for participants to do. Because the gold stars were completely imaginary, it had not occurred to me that they would work with skills participants. Work, however, they did.

It is important to note that praise of skills use may or may not reinforce clients' skillful behaviors. For example, if an individual's history involves many instances in which praise and acknowledgment of skill and strength have led to an absence of further help and/or higher expectations, praise may be aversive instead of rewarding. It is not a good idea, however, to stop praising skillful behaviors altogether, for two reasons. First, a client can interpret the absence of praise as never being able to do anything right— in other words, as implied criticism. Second, praise in most settings is meant as a reinforcer, and it is important for praise to become a reinforcer for clients. So what is the synthesis? The best strategy is not to go overboard with excessive praise, but to give clear feedback about skillful behavior (i.e., to comment that the behavior is skilled if it is, and constitutes progress if it does), and when necessary to follow this immediately with recognition that this does not mean the client can solve all of his or her problems or has no more problems to be solved. In this way, the praise is freed from the expectancy that competence will result in loss of any further help. It is also important to remember to balance praising effective use of skills with praising effort even when it is not effective. Praise of effort is particularly important when new behaviors are being shaped. Use (and misuse) of praise as a reinforcer is discussed in more detail in Chapter 10 of the main DBT text.

NATURAL REINFORCERS

As far as possible, skills trainers should try to provide natural reinforcers for clients' adaptive behavior. "Natural reinforcers" are consequences that clients can expect in everyday life. Thus, if clients are taught assertion skills, and trainers never reward assertive behaviors by giving clients what they request, then it is unreasonable to expect those behaviors to continue. Similarly, if clients' attempts at regulating intense anxiety precipitated by being asked to talk in skills training sessions are met with trainers' making them talk even longer, then it is unreasonable to expect the clients to continue regulating their anxiety. If clients improve their tolerance of aversive events during sessions, and this is followed by the trainers' allowing sessions to become more aversive, then it is unreasonable to expect further distress tolerance. The point is that as clients begin to apply the skills being taught, skills trainers must be careful to respond in a manner that will reinforce such improvement. Although shaping principles require the trainers eventually to "up the ante," so to speak, by requiring even more skillful behavior, these increases in demands must be kept gradual. Otherwise, clients will always feel that they cannot do enough to please the trainers or get their needs met. It can also be useful to pair natural reinforcement with praise.

SHAPING

In "shaping," gradual approximations to the target behavior are reinforced. Shaping requires a skills trainer to break the desired behavior down into small steps and to reinforce each of these steps sequentially. It has to do with what behaviors a trainer expects from clients and is willing to reinforce. Trying to extract an adaptive behavior from clients without reinforcing small steps on the way to the goal behavior usually does not work. Without shaping, both skills trainers and clients would become so frustrated and distressed that skills training could not proceed. Inevitably, individuals with pervasive and severe disordered emotion regulation have no self-shaping skills. Unreasonable expectations for immediate perfection (by the clients, their family members, or their therapists) can interfere with their ability to learn the skills gradually. Thus it is crucial that skills trainers continually model shaping principles. Not only should they be discussed openly and explained, but trainers' expectations of clients should also follow shaping principles. What group leaders sometimes forget, however, is that these same principles apply to the entire group. In my experience, one of the greatest difficulties in conducting DBT group skills training is that skills trainers' expectations for the group as a whole are often far higher than the group can deliver.

EXTINCTION AND PUNISHMENT

As important as reinforcement is the withholding of reinforcement for behaviors targeted for extinction. In theory, this may seem obvious, but in practice, it can be quite difficult. The problematic behaviors of emotionally dysregulated clients are often quite effective in obtaining reinforcing outcomes or in stopping painful events. Indeed, the very behaviors targeted for extinction have often been intermittently reinforced by mental health professionals, family members, and friends. Contingency management at times requires the use of aversive consequences similar to "setting limits" (punishment) in other treatment modalities, as well as the systematic and tenacious withdrawal of usual reinforcers (extinction).

Three guidelines are important in using aversive consequences. First, punishment should "fit the crime," and a client should have some way of terminating its application. For example, a detailed analysis when skills practice assignments are not done is ordinarily aversive for most clients. Once it has been completed, however, a client's ability to pursue other topics should be restored without further comment about the client's not completing the week's assignment. Second, it is crucial that skills trainers use punishment with great care, in low doses, and very briefly, and that a positive interpersonal atmosphere be restored following any client improvement. If a client is banging on the table, but stops when a firm request is made to "cut it out," a warm interaction with the client should follow. Third, punishment should be just strong enough to work. Although the ultimate punishment is termination of skills training, a preferable fallback strategy for egregious behavior that threatens to destroy the group is putting clients on "vacations from training." This approach is considered when a situation is so serious that it is impossible to carry on effective group skills training, and all other contingencies and interventions have failed. Examples of such instances might include property destruction during group sessions, stealing important property of others from the clinic and refusing to return it, continued selling of drugs on the clinic's front porch, putting confidential information obtained in group sessions on Facebook, buying guns for other group members to commit suicide with, or threatening a skills trainer in front of his or her children. It does not include all the very irritating and often dysfunctional emotional behaviors that many clients engage in. Learning how to tolerate irritation is one of the important goals of skills training. It can be equally important for skills trainers to learn it. When utilizing the vacation strategy, the trainers clearly identify what specific new behaviors are required, what behaviors have to be changed, and what conditions must be met for the client to return. The trainers maintain intermittent contact by phone or letter, and provide a referral or backup while the client is on vacation. (In colloquial terms, the trainers kick the client out, then pine for his or her return.)

Generally, aversive procedures should be used when a client is avoiding difficult activities such as coming to skills training sessions, doing homework, practicing in sessions, or engaging in active problem solving. In these cases, it is essential to intervene immediately and push clients, instead of ignoring them and allowing the avoidance to continue. In other words, the avoidance response must be short-circuited. The idea is to make the immediate consequences of avoiding more aversive than those of not avoiding. When clients miss a session, for example, our policy is to call them immediately (using an unknown phone number if necessary) and try to cheerlead them into coming to the session. During such calls, skills trainers use various strategies (e.g., the DEAR MAN, GIVE skills, including broken record, easy manner, and negotiating) taught to clients in the Interpersonal Effectiveness module. (I usually have a bus schedule handy when I call.) An exception to this policy, discussed later, is made when calling reinforces missing sessions.

Another common pattern in a group context is for a member who did not do any homework practice to try to avoid discussing it in the session. If the group leaders skip over that member and go on to the next person, then the avoidance has worked. The best strategy, discussed in detail in Chapter 4, is to move immediately, in a nonjudgmental and warm fashion, to analyze not doing the homework. If the member still refuses after some pushing, a leader might move toward analyzing why he or she doesn't want to talk—or, if this is too aversive, it can be discussed privately during a break. The point is that avoidance should not be rewarded.

Positive maladaptive behaviors (e.g., attempts to get attention, sobbing, hostile behavior, attempts to discuss weekly life crises) should be put on an extinction schedule. A skills trainer ignores the client's maladaptive behaviors and continues to interact with the client as if he or she is not producing such behaviors. Or, if the behaviors cannot be ignored, the trainer can make a brief comment suggesting that the client cope by using some of the skills being taught in the current (or a past) skills module. Thus a client who begins crying can be encouraged to practice distress tolerance or mindfulness skills. If a client is storming out of the room, a trainer can suggest calmly the use of emotion regulation skills; once calm, the client can come back into the session. With few exceptions (e.g., the skills trainers have clear reasons to believe that a client is leaving to commit suicide, or the client is brand-new and is clearly overwhelmed), skills trainers should not routinely follow clients when they leave skills training sessions precipitously. Even if it would not reinforce these clients' leaving, it might serve as vicarious re-

inforcement for others' leaving. However, leaving (and thus avoiding skills training) should not be reinforced unchecked. Thus, if the client is in individual therapy, a trainer should alert the therapist, so that the behavior can be dealt with in individual therapy as an instance of therapy-interfering behavior, or the precipitous leaving can be discussed in the next session. If the client is not in individual therapy, one of the skills trainers should discuss the problem with the client before, after, or during a break in a subsequent session.

It is very important to remember to soothe clients whose behavior is on an extinction schedule and those who are receiving aversive consequences. (In my experience, the ability to put a client's behavior on an extinction schedule and simultaneously soothe the person is one of the hardest tasks for new skills trainers to learn.) In each case, the behavior is what is being punished, not the person. Especially in group skills training, leaders need to develop the ability to ignore many behaviors and to come back to the members with a soothing comment after the behaviors stop. Or, even while the dysfunctional behaviors are going on, leaders can soothe members while at the same time insisting that they practice their skills anyway. To a member crying about a relationship breakup, a leader might say something to this effect: "I know this is really difficult for you, but try your best to distract yourself from your troubles. Be mindful to the task, and tell me about your efforts to practice your skills this week." After listening to a few other group members, the leader might go back to this member and ask briefly but warmly, "How are you doing with your attempt to be mindful to group? . . . Keep trying."

OBSERVING LIMITS

"Observing limits" constitutes a special case of contingency management involving the application of problem-solving strategies to client behaviors that threaten or cross a trainer's personal limits. Such behaviors interfere with the trainer's ability or willingness to conduct the therapy. Trainers must take responsibility for monitoring their own personal limits and for clearly communicating them to clients. Trainers who do not do this eventually burn out, terminate therapy, or otherwise harm their clients. DBT favors natural over arbitrary limits. Thus limits vary among therapists, over time, and over circumstances. Limits should also be presented as for the good of trainers, not for the good of clients.

What the clients are arguing is in their best interests may not ultimately be good for their skills trainers.

For example, I am very easily distracted when teaching new skills. I have stopped many skills training sessions to ask various members to stop squeaking a chair, throwing popcorn, or talking to their neighbors. When one client said, "Marsha, you are so easily distracted!", I said, "Yes, I am, so cut it out, please." When clients are repeatedly late, I may point out how demoralized I am that they have not figured out how to get there on time. After one client said, "Marsha, you are always demoralized," I replied, "And I would stop being demoralized if you would get here on time."

An important limit in standard DBT is that a group skills trainer takes calls when a client wants to find out what the homework was or to say that the client will not attend or will be late, but the trainer does not take coaching calls. The individual therapist takes these calls. In our multifamily skills groups, however, a skills leader takes coaching calls from a parent (and the adolescent's therapist takes calls from the adolescent). Otherwise, as noted above, limits vary among providers, over time, and over circumstances, and often the DBT team may have to help skills trainers expand their limits. See Chapter 10 of the main DBT text for more on observing limits.

Exposure-Based Procedures

Structured exposure procedures, (e.g., prolonged exposure for PTSD), are not used in DBT skills training. DBT skills training, however, can be effectively combined with exposure-based protocols, and many principles of exposure are woven throughout DBT skills. For example, as noted earlier, Opposite Action is a variation on exposure treatments. Others that also elicit exposure include: Mindfulness of current emotions; observing sensations; participating; the distress tolerance skills of paired muscle relaxation, body scan meditation, improving the moment (which is opposite action for many), radical acceptance, and mindfulness of current thoughts; and the emotion regulation skills of the sleep hygiene protocol and mindfulness of current emotions. DBT skills in these cases can help clients cope with urges to use dysfunctional means to end emotion pain and regulate and reduce the anger, shame, or humiliation that victims of trauma often experience. Less structured exposure-based procedures, however, are consistently used in skills training. First, exposure

to the cue that precedes a problem behavior must be nonreinforced. For example, if a client is fearful that admitting to not doing the skills homework will lead to his or her being rejected and starts coming late after skills review, the skills trainers must not reinforce the client's shame by addressing the absence of skills practice in a judgmental voice tone or otherwise communicate rejection. Second, clients' avoidance of topics, procedures, and process discussions (when process is the focus) is almost always blocked. Third, clients are instructed over and over about the value of exposure. After several months in well-run DBT skills training, every client should be able to give a very good rationale for why and when avoidance makes things worse and why, and when exposure improves them. Thus, when clients employ exposure to difficult tasks or feared situations during homework practice, the skills trainers should note and reinforce it.

Cognitive Modification Procedures

COGNITIVE RESTRUCTURING

There are a number of structured exercises throughout the skills training program for helping clients check the facts of a situation (see this manual's Chapter 9, Section VIII, and Emotion Regulation Handout 8 for this skill) and modify dysfunctional assumptions and beliefs. The mindfulness skills of describing and being nonjudgmental focus intensely on teaching clients how to describe what is observed, and how to tell the difference among observing an event in the environment, a thought about the event, and an emotion about the event (see this manual's Chapter 7, Sections V and VII, and Mindfulness Handouts 4 and 5 for these skills). However, formal cognitive restructuring plays a much smaller role in DBT than in other forms of CBT, and cognitive techniques play only a small role in DBT treatment of disordered emotion regulation in particular. This topic is discussed extensively in Chapters 8 and 11 of the main DBT text.

CONTINGENCY CLARIFICATION

The task in contingency clarification is to help clients clarify the "if–then" contingency relationships in their lives and in the learning of skills. Contingency clarification can be distinguished from the didactic strategies. The didactic strategies stress general contingency rules that hold for all or most people;

contingency clarification always looks for the contingencies operating in an individual client's life. It is looking for the pros and cons of one set of behaviors versus another set of behaviors. It is important for everyone to access pros and cons when deciding what to do in a situation, and this is why there is emphasis on pros and cons at the start of every skills module. In skills training, it is important to discuss the pros and cons of learning and practicing each new skill, and to analyze what happens when dysfunctional behaviors are replaced with new skills. The idea here is to help clients learn to better observe the contingent relationships occurring in their everyday lives. Individuals with disordered emotion regulation often have great difficulty observing these natural contingencies. When it comes to observing the effects of using new behavioral skills, they may miss the benefits. One of the skills trainers' tasks is to demonstrate to clients that the contingencies formerly favoring dysfunctional behaviors are not currently operating.

Homework practice always includes trying a new skill and observing its outcome. The idea is not to prove preconceived beliefs of the skills trainers or of the clients about contingent relationships, but rather to explore the actual contingent relationships existing in the clients' everyday lives. It will often become clear in the process that the contingencies, or rules, for one person may not apply to another. Furthermore, rules that operate in one context may not operate in another situation for the very same person.

Figuring out the rules of the game, so to speak, is intimately related to the behavioral skill of being effective or focusing on what works—one of the core mindfulness skills. Doing what works means engaging in behaviors where contingent outcomes are the desired outcomes. This approach is often a new one for individuals with emotion dysregulation, since they are more experienced at looking at behaviors in moral terms of "right" or "wrong" rather than in terms of outcomes or consequences. Contingency clarification strategies are a step in moving these individuals toward more effective behavior.

Stylistic Strategies

DBT balances two quite different styles of communication that refer to how the therapist executes other treatment strategies. The first, "reciprocal communication," is similar to the communication style advocated in client-centered therapy. The sec-ond, "irreverent communication," is quite similar to the style advocated by Carl Whitaker in his writings on strategic therapy.[3] Reciprocal communication strategies are designed to reduce a perceived power differential by making the therapist more vulnerable to the client. In addition, they serve as a model for appropriate but equal interactions within an important interpersonal relationship. Irreverent communication is usually riskier than reciprocity; however, it can facilitate problem solving or produce a breakthrough after long periods when progress has seemed thwarted. To be used effectively, irreverent communication must balance reciprocal communication, and the two must be woven into a single stylistic fabric. Without such balancing, neither strategy represents DBT. I discuss stylistic strategies briefly below; a fuller discussion is provided in Chapter 12 of the main DBT text.

Reciprocal Communication Strategies

Responsiveness, self-disclosure, warm engagement, and genuineness are the basic guidelines of reciprocal communication. Reciprocal communication is a friendly, affectionate style reflecting warmth and engagement in the therapeutic interaction. Self-involving self-disclosure in individual therapy consists of a therapist's immediate, personal reactions to a client and his or her behavior. Reciprocal communication in the context of skills training requires that trainers make themselves vulnerable to their clients and express this vulnerability in a manner that can be heard and understood by the clients. As always, there is a question of balance here, and the fulcrum on which this balance is based is the welfare of the clients. Thus reciprocity is in the service of the clients, not for the benefit of the skills training leaders. Leaders' expressions of vulnerability in sessions not only address the power imbalance that all clients experience, but also can serve as important modeling events. Such expressions can teach clients how to draw the line between privacy and sharing, how to experience vulnerable states without shame, and how to cope with their own limitations. In addition, they provide glimpses into the world of so-called "normal" people, thus normalizing vulnerability and life with limitations.

One of the easiest ways to use reciprocal communication in skills training is for the skills trainers to share their own experiences in using the skills being taught. In my experience, one of the benefits of leading skill groups is that it gives me an opportunity to keep working on improving my own skills. If group leaders can share their own attempts (and especially their failures) with drama and humor, so much the better. Sometimes the trick is for the leaders to label their own experiences as relevant to the skills the group is attempting to learn. For example, when I am teaching how to say no to unwanted requests, I almost always discuss my own difficulties in saying no to group members' pressures to get me to do things I don't think are therapeutic. Since resisting their intense attempts at persuasion usually requires me to use all of my own skills, the example covers quite a bit of the material we teach in skills training. By now, all of my skills groups know about my efforts to deal with my unreasonable fear of heights when I go hiking (focusing on one thing in the moment, distraction, self-encouragement); with back pain on meditation retreats (focusing on one thing, radical acceptance); with my sudden fear of tunnels (opposite action, coping ahead with various severities of earthquakes); with trying to find my way after getting lost while driving in Israel (radical acceptance [after hours of nonacceptance] that a road that ended at the edge of a cliff the first time would not be the correct road out the next time, even if it was the only road going the right direction); and with other assorted life dilemmas I encounter from week to week. Co-leaders of mine have discussed their troubles in learning to meditate, difficulties with asking for things, problems in coping with bosses and professors, the process of mourning losses, and so on. The point is that sharing one's own use of skills being taught can provide valuable modeling both in how to apply skills and in how to respond to one's own vulnerability in a nonjudgmental fashion. The use of self-disclosure is an important part of DBT. In skills training, modeling uses of skills and ways of coping with adversity is the most frequent form of self-disclosure. The primary rule is that disclosure must be in the interest of the clients, not the interest of the skills trainers. That said, most clients love hearing good stories from the leaders. My clients often say when I ask them if they have already heard a specific story, "Yes, we have, but tell us again, Marsha." The good news here is that, like a parent telling bedtime stories, a leader can often tell a good story over and over.

Reciprocal communication can be difficult to practice in a group setting as opposed to a one-to-one setting. It can feel like many against one or two. This difficulty, of course, should give group leaders more empathy for the group members, who usu-

ally experience the very same problem. Nonetheless, sharing the difficulty does not make it go away. It can also be very difficult to respond in a manner appropriate to each member, when members are in many different places (psychologically speaking) at once. The time it takes to find out where even one member is may preclude efforts to explore the current psychological state of other members. And, to the extent that group leaders attend to such within-session process issues, they are veering away from the goals of skills training anyway. By contrast, an individual skills trainer can titrate responses to fit the individual client; timing and attention to various topics can be geared to the state of the one person at hand. In group sessions, it is very difficult to strike a response that meets each member's needs. Thus it is often much more difficult to move the group forward (or anywhere but down, it often seems). This frustration may act to make group leaders want to pull away and close up, or, at other times, to pull close enough to attack. Either way, the frustration reduces the experience of warmth and engagement. In such a stressful atmosphere, it is sometimes difficult to relax. And it is difficult for leaders to be responsive when they are not relaxed.

Great care must be taken to observe the effects of self-disclosure on group members. To a certain extent, their ability to accept such a stance is variable. In a group setting, however, individual differences may be harder to detect than in the individual setting, where the focus is always on the individual client. Difficulties are easy to camouflage and easy to overlook. It is reasonably safe to say, however, that all members will have difficulties with the leaders' expressing their frustration and/or anger with the group; thus extraordinary care must be taken in doing so.

Irreverent Communication Strategies

Irreverent communication is used to push a client "off balance," get the client's attention, present an alternative viewpoint, or shift the client's affective response. It is a highly useful strategy when the client is immovable, or when therapist and client are "stuck." It has an "offbeat" flavor and uses logic to weave a web the client cannot escape. Although it is responsive to the client, irreverent communication is almost never the response the client expects. An important value of irreverence is that unexpected information is more deeply processed cognitively than expected information is.[4, 5] For irreverence to be effective, it must both be genuine (vs. sarcastic or judgmental) and come from a place of compassion and warmth toward the client. Otherwise, the client may become even more rigid. When using irreverence, a therapist or trainer highlights some unintended aspect of the client's communication or "reframes" it in an unorthodox manner. For example, if the client storms out of skills training saying, "I am going to kill myself," the skills trainer might say when catching up with the client, "I thought you agreed not to drop out of skills training." Irreverent communication has a matter-of-fact, almost deadpan style that is in sharp contrast to the warm responsiveness of reciprocal communication. Humor, a certain naiveté, and guilelessness are also characteristic of the style. A confrontational tone can be irreverent as well, by communicating "bullshit" to responses other than the targeted adaptive response. For example, the skills trainer might say, "Are you out of your mind?" or "You weren't for a minute actually believing I would think that was a good idea, were you?" The irreverent skills trainer also calls the client's bluff. For the client who says, "I'm quitting therapy," the skills trainer might respond, "Would you like a referral?" The trick here is to time the bluff carefully, with the simultaneous provision of a safety net; it is important to leave the client a way out.

Irreverence has to be used very carefully in group skills training, although it can be used quite liberally when skills training is conducted individually. This is because irreverence requires a skills trainer to observe very closely its immediate effects and move to repair any damage as quickly as possible. It is very difficult to be that astute and attentive to each individual in a group setting. The person a group leader is talking to may be very receptive to an irreverent statement, but another group member, listening in, may be horrified. Once leaders get to know their clients fairly well, they can be more comfortable using irreverence. As noted above, specific examples and the rationale for irreverent communication (as well as reciprocal communication) are discussed in Chapter 12 of the main DBT text.

The main place for irreverence, in a group context, is usually in the individual work with each client during the first hour of a session (the homework practice-sharing component). In irreverence, problematic behavior is reacted to as if it were normal, and functional adaptive behavior is reacted to with enthusiasm, vigor, and positive emotionality. Dysfunctional plans or actions may be overreacted to in a humorous fashion or viewed as a fabulous opportunity for skills practice (turning the "lemon" of problem behavior into lemonade). Behaviors or communications may be responded to in a blunt, confrontational style. The aim of irreverence is to jolt the individual client, or the group as a whole, into seeing things from a new, more enlightened perspective. Irreverent communication should help clients to make the transition from seeing their own dysfunctional behavior as a cause of shame and scorn to seeing it as inconsequential and even funny and humorous. To do this, a skills trainer can only be a half step ahead of clients; timing is of the essence. An irreverent attitude is not an insensitive attitude; nor is it an excuse for hostile or demeaning behavior. A group leader always takes suffering seriously, albeit matter-of-factly, calmly, and sometimes with humor.

Case Management Strategies

Consultation-to-the-Client Strategies

In general, DBT requires a skills trainer to play the role of a consultant to the client rather than that of a consultant to other people in the client's social or health care network, including other therapists the client may have. DBT assumes that the client is capable of mediating between various therapists and health care providers. Thus the skills trainer does not play a parental role, and does not assume that clients are unable to communicate in a straightforward manner with those in their own treatment network. When safety is an immediate issue, or it is very obvious that a client cannot or will not serve as his or her own intermediary, the skills trainer should move from the "consultation-to-the-client" strategies to the "environmental intervention" strategies (see below). The rationale, strategies, and rules for when to use which of these two groups of strategies are clearly laid out in Chapter 13 of the main DBT text. The consultation strategies are quite different from how providers may have learned to relate to other professionals treating their clients.

The one exception to these rules occurs when the skills trainers and a client's individual therapist are all in a DBT program and consult weekly in the therapist consultation team. The role of the skills trainers in these consultations is to give the individual DBT therapist information about how the client is doing in skills training; they alert the therapist to problems that may need work in individual psychotherapy, and share insights that are being given in the skills training sessions.

These consultations are limited to sharing of information and joint treatment planning. It must, of course, be clear to the clients from the very beginning that they are being treated by a team of therapists who will coordinate therapy at every opportunity. The interaction of the two therapy modalities is stressed by both the individual therapist and the skills trainers. DBT skills trainers, however, do not serve as intermediaries for individual clients with their individual therapists. If clients are having problems with their individual therapists, the skills trainers usually consult with clients on how they might address these problems with their individual therapists. Generally, the task of the skills trainers is to help clients use the skills they are learning to work on the problem.

If a client is in individual therapy that is independent of the DBT program (i.e., individual work with another therapist in a different treatment setting), the consultation-to-the-client approach may involve some contact with the individual therapist. These consultations ordinarily should be conducted with the client present. The material taught in skills training can and usually should be shared with the individual psychotherapist. The skills trainers' task in this case is to help the client do this effectively. A client in skills training only may be seeing other care providers, such as a pharmacotherapist or other type of health care provider. In these cases, the skills trainers interact with them as needed in the same manner that they interact with non-DBT therapists. That is, skills trainers consult to the client on how to work with the other care providers, and the client is present for any interactions of skills trainers with these care providers.

Difficulties that individual clients experience with other therapists and clinical agencies can be dealt with in the skills training sessions if those difficulties can be made relevant to the skills being taught. For example, in the Interpersonal Effectiveness module, an individual client may be helped to communicate more effectively with other professionals treating him or her. In the Emotion Regulation module, clients can be helped to modulate their emotional reactions to these professionals. During the Distress Tolerance module, they can be assisted in accepting and tolerating the behaviors of other professionals that they find problematic. Generally, problems with treatment professionals brought up in skills training sessions are dealt with in precisely the same manner that any other interpersonal problem is dealt with.

Environmental Intervention Strategies

Strategies for intervening directly in the client's environment are rarely used by skills trainers. Clients will often want much more environmental intervention from skills trainers than the trainers should be willing to give. One example (which occurs frequently with highly suicidal clients) has to do with getting a pass from an inpatient unit to come to a session. It can often be difficult for a client to talk a hospital into giving such a pass. The client may then want a skills trainer to call the hospital on his or her behalf. The trainer's first response should be to emphasize that it is the client's responsibility to behave in such a way that inpatient treatment personnel will want to allow him or her to leave the hospital on a pass for skills training. My one concession to the politics of inpatient hospitalization is that if it appears absolutely necessary, I will call the inpatient personnel to let them know that I do indeed expect inpatients to get themselves out on a pass to come to skills training sessions. I do not, however, try to convince them to let a particular client out. Over and over in skills training sessions, trainers must stress that their job is to teach clients environmental intervention skills so that clients can do environmental interventions for themselves. New clients may be shocked at first with this confidence that they will eventually succeed in learning these skills. But the shock is balanced with an emerging pleasure at being treated as adults who can run their own lives.

Integrative Strategies

There are six integrative strategies in DBT for responding to the following specific issues and problems in treatment: (1) ancillary treatments, (2) crises, (3) suicidal behaviors, (4) therapeutic relationship issues, (5) telephone calls, and (6) therapy-interfering or -destroying behaviors. Telephone calls and therapy-interfering or -destroying behaviors have already been discussed in Chapters 3 and 4 of this manual, respectively. In the remainder of this chapter, I briefly review the strategies for ancillary treatments, crises, suicidal behaviors, and relationship problem solving as they apply to skills training. All these strategies are discussed in greater detail in Chapter 15 of the main DBT text.

Ancillary Treatments

There is nothing in standard DBT (skills training, DBT individual treatment, DBT team) that proscribes ancillary health care, including mental health care, as long as these programs are clearly ancillary to DBT and not the primary treatment. The basic idea here is that for clients in DBT, there can only be one primary therapist responsible for the overall care of the client. In standard DBT, the individual DBT therapist is the primary treatment provider; overall treatment planning, crisis and suicide management, case management, and decisions about ancillary treatments are in the hands of this therapist. As noted in Chapter 2 of this manual, a similar stance is taken when an individual in DBT skills training has a non-DBT individual therapist or case manager instead of a DBT therapist. In both cases, management of crises, suicidal behaviors, and ancillary treatment (e.g., emergency department or inpatient admission) is handled by the skills trainers only until the primary therapist can be contacted. Once this therapist is contacted, client management will be turned over to him or her—or, if necessary, the skills trainer will carry out treatment directions given by the primary therapist.

If a client is in DBT skills training only, with no other mental health treatment provided, it is the responsibility of the skills leaders to manage crises, suicidal behaviors, and any other client problems that arise in treatment. Depending on the skills of the skills trainers and the needs of the client, these events may be managed completely by the skills trainers, or the client may be referred for ancillary individual treatment. If they are managed by the skills trainers, this will ordinarily require individual sessions. Management of client suicidality or of individual or family crises is extremely difficult in a group setting—particularly crises that are recurrent, such as difficulties with a suicidal or drug-dependent spouse or child.

Crisis Strategies

When a skills training client in crisis is also in individual therapy, skills trainers should (1) refer the client to the individual therapist and assist him or her in making contact if necessary; and (2) help the client apply distress tolerance skills until contact is made. The crisis strategies described in Chapter 15 of the main DBT text should be used in a modified version. If the client has no individual therapist, all of the crisis strategies used in individual therapy should be used; following resolution of the crisis, the client should be referred to individual DBT, other appropriate therapy, or intensive case management.

Just as clients can be in a state of individual crisis, a group can also be in a state of crisis. A group in crisis is functioning in a state of emotional overload. Usually this will be the result of a common trauma, such as a group member's committing suicide, a hostile act directed at the entire group, or a trainer's leaving. In these instances, group leaders should employ all of the crisis strategies used in individual crisis intervention; they are simply applied to the entire group instead of to one client. The steps are summarized in Tables 5.1 and 5.2.

Suicidal Behavior Strategies

If the risk of suicide is imminent and the client is also in individual therapy, a skills trainer should call the individual therapist immediately for instructions on how to proceed. As noted in Chapter 2 of this manual, individual therapists (both DBT and non-DBT) of skills training clients agree at the start to be available by phone; to provide a backup provider's phone number to call if necessary during their clients' skills training sessions; and to provide an up-to-date crisis plan. If neither a client's individual therapist nor a backup therapist can be located, the skills trainer must do crisis intervention until contact can be made with the individual therapist. If the client does not have an individual therapist, the skills trainer does crisis intervention and then refers the client for individual therapy if needed (in combination with continued skills training). As a general rule, a skills trainer should be much more conservative in the treatment of suicidal risk than is the individual therapist. The crisis plan is a good place to start. Steps for intervention when a client is threatening imminent suicide or self-injury, or is actually engaging in self-injurious behavior during contact (or has just engaged in it), are discussed in detail in the main DBT text and are outlined in Table 5.2.

Relationship Problem Solving

Relationship problem solving is the application of general problem-solving strategies to the therapeutic relationship. In individual skills training, that relationship is between the trainer and the client. In group skills training, however, at least four relationships may require problem solving: (1) member ver-

TABLE 5.1. Crisis Strategies Checklist

_____ Skills trainer attends to emotion rather than content.

_____ Skills trainer explores the problem now.

    _____ Skills trainer focuses on immediate time frame.

    _____ Skills trainer identifies key events setting off current emotions and sense of crisis.

    _____ Skills trainer formulates and summarizes the problem.

    _____ Skills trainer focuses on problem solving.

    _____ Skills trainer gives advice and makes suggestions.

    _____ Skills trainer frames possible solutions in terms the skills group is learning.

    _____ Skills trainer predicts future consequences of action plans.

    _____ Skills trainer confronts group maladaptive ideas or behavior directly.

    _____ Skills trainer clarifies and reinforces group's adaptive responses.

    _____ Skills trainer identifies factors interfering with productive plans of action.

_____ Skills trainer focuses on affect tolerance.

_____ Skills trainer helps group commit itself to a plan of action.

_____ Skills trainer assesses group members' suicide risk (if necessary).

_____ Skills trainer anticipates a recurrence of the crisis response.

Note. Adapted from Table 15.1 in Linehan, M. M. (1993). _Cognitive-behavioral treatment of borderline personality disorder._ New York: Guilford Press. Copyright 1993 by The Guilford Press. Adapted by permission.

sus group leaders, (2) group versus group leaders, (3) member versus member, and (4) leader versus leader. Not only are there more relationships to balance, but there are also many more issues coming into play. The public nature of the relationships is particularly important. Individuals who have difficulties regulating their emotions are exquisitely sensitive to any threat of rejection or criticism; when that rejection or criticism is public, they may experience such overwhelming and intense shame that it completely cuts off any chance of adequate problem solving. Thus leaders have to be correspondingly sensitive in dealing with relationship problems in treating such individuals. The relationship problem solving typical of process therapy groups is simply not possible with individuals who are sensitive to rejection, emotionally dysregulated, and without interpersonal skills. Therefore, some of this problem solving has to be conducted individually and outside the group sessions. Otherwise, problems may not be resolved and may escalate to such an extent that members find it impossible to continue in the group.

Member versus Group Leader

It is essential for clients with high suicidality and/or severe emotion dysregulation to form an attached relationship with at least one of the group leaders if they are to continue in skills training. Without such attachments, the trials, tribulations, and traumas that frequently arise in skills training will overwhelm the clients, and they will eventually drop out of therapy. These individual relationships, which are distinct from a leader's relationship to the group as a whole, are enhanced by individual attention given to group members before and after group meetings and during breaks.

Relationship problems between group members and group leaders should not be ignored. Depending on the seriousness of the problem, a problem-solving meeting may take place before, after, or during a break in a skills training session; on the phone; or in a scheduled individual meeting before or after a group meeting. Whenever possible, such an individual meeting should be scheduled near in time to the group session, so that it does not take on the character of an individual psychotherapy session. It is best to hold the meeting in a corner of the group therapy room or somewhere in the hall or waiting area. Also, the focus should be kept on the member's problems with the group or with the leader.

As a first step, the leader should help the group member observe and describe exactly what the problem is and with whom he or she has the problem. Sometimes the problem will be with one or the other leader. The public light of group sessions seems to enhance members' sensitivity to even slight rejections or insensitive comments on the part of the leaders. Comments that might not lead to trouble in an individual interaction can lead to great problems in group therapy. Thus, if the problem is a leader's behavior, problem solving should be centered around it.

At other times, however, the problem is not with a group leader's behavior, but rather with the notion of attending and working in the group at all. With individuals in ongoing individual therapy, these problems are usually dealt with by the individual therapist. The primary therapist assists the client with all behaviors that interfere with treat-ment, including those that show up in ancillary or collateral treatment. At times, however, a client may also profit from some individual attention from the group leaders. During such a meeting, strategies can be worked out to reduce the stress on the individual member. For example, we have had some group members who simply could not sit through an entire group session without becoming hostile or having a panic attack. In these cases, plans were developed so that when the clients saw that their behavior was about to go out of control, they would get up and leave the session for a few moments' break.

Careful attention must be paid to issues of shaping. Clients who have difficulties regulating their emotions are prone to indirect communication, which at times requires mind reading by the skills

---

TABLE 5.2. DBT Suicidal Behavior Strategies Checklist

When threats of imminent suicide or self-injury are occurring, and skills trainer cannot turn management over to an individual therapist:

_____ Skills trainer assesses the risk of suicide and of self-injury.

    _____ Skills trainer uses known factors related to imminent suicidal behavior to predict imminent risk.

    _____ Skills trainer knows the likely lethality of various suicide/self-injury methods.

    _____ Skills trainer consults with emergency services or medical consultant about medical risk of planned and/or available method(s).

_____ Skills trainer follows the crisis plan already prepared.

_____ Skills trainer removes, or gets client to remove, lethal items.

_____ Skills trainer emphatically instructs client not to commit suicide or engage in self-injurious behavior.

_____ Skills trainer maintains a position that suicide is not a good solution.

_____ Skills trainer generates hopeful statements and solutions for coping.

_____ Skills trainer keeps contact when suicide risk is imminent and high (until client's care is stabilized).

_____ Skills trainer anticipates a recurrence (before care is stabilized).

_____ Skills trainer communicates client's suicide risk to current or new individual therapist as soon as possible.

When a self-injurious act is taking place during contact or has just taken place:

_____ Skills trainer assesses potential medical risk of behavior, consulting with local emergency services or other medical resources to determine risk when necessary.

_____ Skills trainer assesses client's ability to obtain medical treatment on his or her own.

_____ If medical emergency exists, call emergency services.

_____ Skills trainer stays in contact with client until aid arrives.

_____ Skills trainer calls individual therapist (if there is one).

_____ If risk is low, skills trainer instructs client to obtain medical treatment, if necessary, and to call his or her individual therapist (if in therapy).

Note. Adapted from Table 15.2 in Linehan, M. M. (1993). *Cognitive-behavioral treatment of borderline personality disorder.* New York: Guilford Press. Copyright 1993 by The Guilford Press. Adapted by permission.

trainers. How much mind reading should a group skills trainer engage in? How much outreach should be made to a withdrawn group member? The goal is to require group members to reach their capabilities and if possible to go slightly beyond these, without requiring so much that the members fall back in failure. At the beginning of skills training, leaders will often need to telephone group members when they miss sessions or after they storm out of sessions.

The key, however, is not to engage in this behavior so reliably that clients begin to expect it, count on it, and become distressed if a leader does not reach out or call. The best approach is for leaders to be direct in their communications about what they will and won't do. As discussed earlier in this chapter, the DBT policy is to reach out and call group members when such calling is not reinforcing maladaptive behaviors, and to refrain from reaching out when it will reinforce such behaviors. Obviously, such judgments are difficult. It is especially difficult at the beginning of skills training, when leaders have little idea of the group members' respective capabilities; in this case, it is important to make policies clear. In all cases, however, it is essential not to *assume* that a particular response on the part of the leaders is reinforcing. There is no substitute for observing the consequences of various therapeutic actions.

Our general policies are as follows. If a member does not show up for a skills training session, that person is called immediately by one of the leaders and urged strongly to drop everything and come to the group session immediately. This phone call is designed to cut off the person's ability to avoid a group session. Clients with disordered emotion regulation often believe that if they don't come to a group session, they won't have to deal with group issues; calling immediately interferes with the avoidance. The phone conversation should be kept strictly to a discussion of how the person can get to the session, even if he or she arrives for only the last half hour. We have at times even offered to send a leader or a volunteer staff person out to pick up the person when the reason for not coming is lack of transportation. In short, the phone call in this situation serves to cut off reinforcement for avoidance rather than to reinforce the avoidance behavior. (For clients who know our clinic's phone number and refuse to pick up, we often use phones with other, unknown numbers to make our calls.)

If a leader waits a few days to call, or if the phone call addresses the person's problems, then the call may well reinforce the client's tendency to withdraw

rather than confront problems. In this event, the withdrawal leads to positive outreach on the part of the skills trainer, a positive interaction, and sometimes a positive resolution. The dialectical dilemma here is the need to choose between avoiding reinforcement for withdrawal and allowing a member to drop out. A leader simply has to face the fact that many clients who have trouble regulating their emotions cannot engage in problem solving alone. Thus, in the interests of shaping, the leader should call, do problem solving, and then emphasize that the direct discussion of the problem does result in problem resolution. Once this pattern is stabilized, then the leader can gradually decrease the degree of outreach, while simultaneously verbally instructing the individual that he or she is expected to increase outreach to the leaders and to the skills training group. While at the beginning the leader walks all the way over to the client's side of this "teeter-totter," he or she needs to grab the client and begin moving back toward the middle. Without this movement, the very problems that outreach is intended to resolve may be exacerbated.

With highly suicidal and/or dysregulated clients, leaders should expect to spend a considerable amount of time resolving crises related to skills training. The key point is that interventions should be limited to problems in the clients' relationship to the group as a whole or to the group leaders. In other crisis situations, leaders should instruct the clients to call their individual therapists (or refer such a client to an individual therapist if the client does not have one). If a leader suspects that phone calls may be reinforcing a client's problem, outcomes of phone calls should be closely observed, and the possibility should be discussed openly with the client as yet another problem to be solved.

Because there are two leaders in group skills training, each leader should take great care to observe the consultation-to-the-client approach. That is, one leader should not become an intermediary between a client and the other leader. A leader can, however, work with the client on how to resolve a problem with the other leader. In my experience, it is rare for a group member to be having serious problems with both group leaders at the same time. When this occurs, skills trainers must bring the topic up with their DBT therapist consultation team.

The most difficult problem to address—and the easiest to ignore—is that of the group member who comes to every session and stays for the entire session, but either interacts in a hostile manner or withdraws. Once I had a group member who came and fell asleep during most group sessions. What I wanted to do was reciprocally withdraw from the group member. When a leader withdraws from a group member, however, the group member can be expected to withdraw even further and eventually drop out. Addressing these issues directly in group sessions can be threatening, can take up a lot of time, and is usually not a good idea as a first approach. Since the group member is not directly expressing a problem and is not asking for attention, it is the leader's responsibility to approach him or her and set up an individual consultation before or after a group session or during the break.

Failure to initiate an action is usually a sign that a leader is frustrated and, perhaps, is not motivated to keep the member in the group. At these times, having a second leader can be an enormous asset. The one leader can prod the other to address the issue.

Group versus Group Leaders

When the entire group is engaging in therapy-interfering behavior vis-à-vis the group leaders, the problem cannot, of course, be dealt with individually; it is a group problem. When should this problem be addressed directly, and when should it be ignored? An attempt to address the problem directly often backfires. Once group members have withdrawn or begun to interact in a hostile manner, they are often unable to stop the withdrawal in order to process the problem. Any move on the leaders' part to address the problem is viewed as criticizing further or as creating more conflict, and the group simply withdraws further.

It is usually better either to ignore the group withdrawal or hostility, or to comment on it briefly without pushing the issue and then focus on drawing out individual group members. At this point, it is essential to be able to cajole, distract, and otherwise respond to the problem in a relatively indirect manner. If leaders reciprocate with hostility, coldness, and withdrawal, the problem will increase.

This is perhaps one of the most difficult situations that group skills training leaders must face. Unfortunately, it can often happen in the beginning months of a new skills training group, particularly when members are forced to be in the group and really don't want to be there. It is a bit like trying to walk through quicksand—pulling with all one's strength to get one foot up, and then putting it down again in front of the other. Although it is exhaust-

ing and frustrating, the leaders' refusal to give up or give in and reciprocate with hostility or obvious frustration communicates clearly to clients that no matter what they do or how withdrawn they are, the group will progress and continue.

On the other hand, leaders can do only so much with a group if the group members are withdrawn and not talking. In these situations, it is helpful to be able to read the clients' minds. It is sometimes a good idea for the leaders to have a dialogue (out loud) with one another, trying to figure out the problem. Although over time the group members should develop the ability to resolve group stalemates with the leaders via problem solving, at the beginning progress is usually not visible. It is absolutely essential in these situations that leaders *not* let their own judgments and hostile interpretations have free rein. Compassion and empathy are essential. Sharing frustration with the DBT team can be very useful here. Individual therapists may have gathered helpful information about reasons for the group's distress from their own individual clients.

Member versus Member

Not infrequently, there is conflict between individual members in a skills training group. In my experience, encouraging group members to discuss their problems with one another openly in a group session almost always results in disaster. Again, clients who have trouble regulating their emotions often cannot tolerate criticism in a group setting; thus member-to-member problems need to be dealt with privately until the collective ability to solve problems publicly is increased. In private interactions with a distressed group member (before or after a session or during a break), a leader's primary role is to soothe the distressed member and to explain the offending member in a sympathetic manner. If criticisms or member-to-member conflicts arise during a session, a leader's best strategy is to serve as the third point or fulcrum. Rather than suggesting that the conflicting members talk with one another to resolve their differences or hurt feelings, the leader should publicly defend the offending member while simultaneously empathizing with the offended member. If the conflict is over procedural issues, problem solving can go forward in the group session. For example, a conflict arose in one of our skills training groups between one member's need for the window curtains to be closed and other group members' need for the curtains to be open. Such conflicts should be mediated by a group leader, but can be discussed in group sessions. A leader's role in these cases is somewhat like a parent's or teacher's role with a group of quarreling children. The sensitivities of each individual member must be respected; a leader must resist the tendency at times to sacrifice one member for the good of the whole.

Leader versus Leader

Perhaps the most damaging conflict in conducting DBT group skills training is that which can arise between the two group leaders. Smooth coordination can be especially difficult when the leaders have different theoretical perspectives, when they take different views of how groups should be conducted, or when one or both leaders wish for a different role in the skills training than the role assigned. These issues need to be resolved outside the skills training sessions, preferably before the first session. When conflicts arise in sessions, the usual procedure is for the co-leader to defer to the primary leader during the session and argue his or her case afterward.

A particular problem arises when the co-leader is better tuned in to group members and to the unfolding process than the primary leader. This is a situation where the DBT consultation team can be quite useful. No matter what the difference in experience between leaders may be, it is important for them not to fall into the trap of who is "right" and who is "wrong." Not only is this approach dialectically flawed, but it is rarely useful in resolving a conflict.

A related situation can occur when group members complain about an absent leader to the other leader. How should the leader who is present react? The most important thing is not to become split off from the absent leader. The same strategy used when an absent member is being discussed should be employed. That is, the present leader should portray the absent leader in a sympathetic light, while simultaneously validating the concerns of the members present. It is a tricky line to walk, but essential nonetheless.

Relationship Generalization

Leaders must be vigilant in noticing when interpersonal relationships within the group are similar to problems individuals are having outside group sessions. A number of typical problems show up in group skills training. The exquisite sensitivity to criticism of individuals with emotion dysregulation, and the rapid onset of extreme shame, almost

always create problems. The public nature of the group setting simply exacerbates these problems. Problems that individuals have with their families or their children are likely to show up in the group. Many members have problems in coping with authority figures, especially when the authority figures are telling them what to do. Others have problems with being authority figures and voicing their opinions. Therefore, at least some clients will have problems doing homework practice. Some individuals will have problems admitting to progress; others may have difficulties admitting to lack of progress or to not knowing how to use a skill.

The inability of many individuals with high emotion dysregulation to put personal problems on a shelf and attend to the skills training material is similar to their difficulties outside skills training at work, at school, or with their family members. Their inability to remember to practice skills (or to get themselves to practice even when they do remember), and then to punish or berate themselves in a judgmental fashion, is indicative of their general difficulties with self-management. Their tendency to withdraw emotionally and become silent when any conflict occurs during group sessions is typical of their difficulties in dealing with conflict outside the group. An often unstated, but particularly difficult, problem of many group members is their inability to shut themselves off emotionally from other group members' pain. Consequent exacerbation of their own painful emotions can result in either panic attacks, hostile behavior, or complete emotional withdrawal. As can be seen from just this partial list, skills training in a group setting can be counted on to bring up many of the everyday problems that individuals with emotion dysregulation have.

Some group members who ordinarily have reasonably good emotion regulation may have very little regulation when specific topics come up. This is especially true in two types of situations. The first is when a client's main problems are with a relative or close friend who also has a severe disorder, and whom the client cannot seem to help. The second is when the client's family or close friends persistently do things that lead to misery for the client. Trouble arises in such cases when clients become determined to get the group leaders to help them figure out how to change the other persons. These clients may view their own use of skills as relatively hopeless, or may have a blind spot about their own ineffective behaviors. Often the only strategy that can work with these clients is to insist repeatedly that the focus of skills training is on developing their own skills, not those of their relatives or friends. In these cases, it is essential that the skills leaders remain firm. At times an activity may need to be stopped to address the problem before continuing. In one of my groups, for example, I was teaching problem solving. One client (whose problem with her son was the example to be solved) repeatedly insisted that the only possible solutions were new behaviors from her son. All attempts by me to focus on solutions that the mother could implement were met with tears and screams that she was being invalidated. I finally realized I could not use that problem to demonstrate problem solving, said as much, and made up a new example to work with. I then discussed the issue with the client at the end of the group session.

The basic idea of relationship generalization strategies is to help members see when their everyday problems are showing up within the skills training group. However, this can be quite tricky, because it must be done without invalidating clients' real problems with the group or with specific members. It is important that leaders not be overinclined to attribute all within-therapy problems to outside problems, rather than to inadequacies in the group format or to the leaders' application of the treatment.

Clients' difficulties in accepting negative feedback or implied criticism suggest that leaders must be extremely sensitive in applying the relationship generalization strategies. In my own experience, the best way to do this is to take an individual problem, make it into a universal problem, and then discuss it in that context. Astute group members may figure out that they are the ones being talked to, but still it is not a public humiliation.

The first step in relationship generalization is to relate the within-session relationship problem to general problems that need work both in and out of the skills training group. Just making this connection (an insight strategy; see Chapter 9 of the main DBT text) can sometimes be therapeutic. The next step is to use problem-solving strategies to develop alternative response patterns for members to try. The key in relationship generalization is to plan for rather than to assume generalization. Planning, at a minimum, requires discussion with the group members. The discussion should also include developing homework in which clients can practice applying new skills to everyday situations. Since this is the essential idea undergirding skills training and homework practice anyway, relationship generalization is especially compatible with DBT skills training.

The Appendices to Part I, which follow this chapter, provide a wide variety of options for structuring DBT skills training programs. Part II of this manual (Chapters 6–10) presents instructions for how to orient clients to skills training and to teach the four DBT skills training modules. The handouts and worksheets for skills training clients can be found on the special website for this manual (*www.guilford.com/skills-training-manual*) and may be downloaded and printed.

References

1. Linehan, M. M. (1997). Validation and psychotherapy. In A. C. Bohart & L. S. Greenberg (Eds.), *Empathy reconsidered: New directions in psychotherapy* (pp. 353–392). Washington, DC: American Psychological Association.
2. Cayne, B. S., & Bolander, D. O. (Eds.). (1991). *New Webster's dictionary and thesaurus of the English language*. New York: Lexicon.
3. Whitaker, C. A. (1975). Psychotherapy of the absurd: With a special emphasis on the psychotherapy of aggression. *Family Process, 14,* 1–16.
4. Bower, G. H., Black, J. B., & Turner, T. J. (1979). Scripts in memory for text. *Cognitive Psychology, 11*(2), 177–220.
5. Friedman, A. (1979). Framing pictures: The role of knowledge in automatized encoding and memory for gist. *Journal of Experimental Psychology: General, 108*(3), 316–355.

Introduction: Options for Putting Together Your DBT Skills Training Program

There are many ways to put together a skills training program. This manual includes not only the standard skills used in most standard 6-month and 1-year DBT programs, but also a large set of additional skills that you can integrate with the standard skills if you wish. Included are optional skills that expand on the standard skills, and supplementary skills that expand skills training to new areas. You can adapt your skills program to your particular populations and time constraints.

The teaching notes in Chapters 6–10 give instructions on how to use each of the skills, and identify those that are ordinarily optional and those that are supplemental. Whether a skill is standard, optional, or supplementary, however, can change, depending on the type of skills program you are running. For example, validation as a separate skill is optional in the adult program, but standard in the multifamily adolescent program. The skills for addictive behaviors are supplementary with most populations, but standard when the clients being treated are individuals with addictions.

These Appendices present session-by-session schedules for 11 different skills programs. Many of the schedules I have provided have been used in treatment studies where outcomes for DBT were very strong. Other schedules are still being evaluated; they range from the standard 24-week DBT skills program that repeats modules for a full year to a 4-week skills program. The skills schedules are presented in Schedule 1. Descriptions of the schedules are as follows.

■ *Schedule 1: 24 Weeks, Linehan Standard Adult DBT Skills Training (Research Studies, 2006 and After).* This is the schedule I have used in clinical outcome studies since 2006.[1, 2, 3] One cycle through the skills runs 24 weeks, and it is then typically repeated, for a total of 48 weeks. In research, we have used it with individuals who met criteria for BPD and were at high risk for suicide, as well as with suicidal individuals meeting criteria for both BPD and PTSD. Clinically, we use it with suicidal adults meeting criteria for BPD, as well as with our friends-and-family skills groups. Clients in the latter type of group enter with no known diagnosis of mental disorder themselves; they usually attend to learn skills for coping better with difficult people in their lives (e.g., children, partners, parents, or bosses/co-workers).

■ *Schedule 2: 24 Weeks, Linehan Standard Adult DBT Skills Training (before 2006).* This schedule was used in research and clinical skills classes at my clinic at the University of Washington.[4, 5] It was based on the original DBT skills manual, which contained fewer skills. In Schedule 2, I have translated as well as possible the names and numbering of the original skills into their names and numbers in this manual. As you can see, early research used fewer skills than subsequent studies, although in both Schedules 1 and 2, programs have run 48 weeks each (24 weeks, repeated once).

■ *Schedule 3: 12 Weeks, Soler Adult DBT Skills Training; Schedule 4: 20 Weeks, McMain Adult DBT Skills Training; and Schedule 5: 14 Weeks, Neacsiu Adult DBT Emotion Regulation Skills Training.* Schedules 3–5 outline the skills used in three different skills-only treatment programs. Schedule 3 was tested with women meeting criteria for BPD, in research evaluating the efficacy and effectiveness of DBT skills compared to standard group psychotherapy.[6, 7] Schedule 4 was evaluated by McMain as an intervention for individuals with BPD on a wait list for standard DBT.[8] Both of these studies were conducted before the current set of revised skills was available. I have translated as well as possible the names and numbering of the skills used by both Soler and McMain into their names and numbers in this manual. Schedule 5 was evaluated by Neacsiu (using the revised skills) as a treatment for individuals without BPD, but with high emotion dysregulation and at least one mood disorder.[9]

■ *Schedule 6: 25 Weeks, Adolescent Multifamily DBT Skills Training.* This is the multifamily skills program for families of teens high in emotion dysregulation and at high risk for suicide. The skills program is part of a standard DBT program for adolescents. It is in use at the University of Washington and at the University of California at Los Angeles. We have found that teens and their parents have no problems with using the same handouts as our adult clients. The most common feedback we get from teens in our posttreatment interviews is that the skills groups were their favorite parts of the treatment. For further information on conducting skills training with teens (and particularly for in-depth discussion of how to treat teens with DBT), see our book on DBT for treating suicidal adolescents,[10] as well as the new DBT skills book for adolescents.[11]

■ *Schedule 7: Variable Sessions, Inpatient DBT Skills Training (Intermediate Unit and Acute Unit).* Two sets of skills are given here. The first is for individuals on an inpatient unit for an intermediate length of stay; the second is for individuals on an acute unit, ordinarily for 1–2 days.[12] Both skill sets assume a 7-day skills curriculum. If the average intermediate length of stay is 2 weeks, patients can be exposed to each skill twice. For a 2-day stay, one skill might be taught over and over.[13]

■ *Schedule 8: DBT Skills for Addictive Behaviors (to Integrate with Schedule 1 Skills); and Schedule 9: DBT Parenting Skills (to Integrate with Schedule 1 Skills).* Schedules 8 and 9 outline sets of skills that can be integrated into any of the standard sets of skills training.[14, 15] They are presented here as they would be integrated into Schedule 1. Schedule 8 is the set of addiction skills for addictive behaviors that we integrated into standard DBT skills training in the studies we have conducted at the University of Washington for men and women meeting criteria for both BPD and drug dependence and/or opiate addiction. Schedule 9 highlights the behavior change strategies and validation skills so important in parent training.

■ *Schedule 10: Comprehensive DBT Mindfulness Skills Training.* This schedule includes the mindfulness skills from each DBT module. This is a particularly good set of skills if you are offering an "introduction to mindfulness" program. The skills can be taught as laid out in the schedule, or taught in other arrangements that meet the needs and desires of the group you are teaching. If you have a long-term mindfulness program, you can alternate between teaching each skill and having a silent session focused on mindfulness practice (e.g., meditation, mindful walking, or other practices). Consider starting sessions with meditation (use a mindfulness bell for timing, and consider rotating timers). Begin with 5–10 minutes of mindful meditation, increasing it over time to 20–25 minutes. For instructions for mindful meditation, draw upon your own training, ideas from mindfulness handouts, or recording-led mindfulness practices. Consider ending your sessions with brief readings; for example, read one story per session from *The Song of the Bird* by Anthony DeMello.[16] After the reading, give participants time to think about how the reading is relevant to their lives. After 4–5 minutes of reflection, ring your mindfulness bell. Starting with the skills leader, invite participants to share brief comments on the reading. (Be sure to let people say, "I pass.")

■ *Schedule 11: Advanced DBT Skills Training.* This set of skills works well in a DBT advanced class. These are skills that are often not included in the standard skills groups because of time constraints, but are often requested by skills group participants. It is important to note, however, that in advanced classes participants usually want to have a large say in what skills are covered. Participants may want to spend very little time on reviewing old skills or learning new skills, and instead may want to focus the agenda on problem-solving issues that have come up in participants' lives during the week. When this is the case, you can teach new skills when they are appropriate for solving members' problems, and otherwise ask participants to focus on using their own skills to help one another use DBT skills to solve problems. The issues here are often what skill is needed and how to use it effectively. When this is the agenda, skills practice and role playing may occupy much of the group's time. A notebook with *all* the skills can be useful here for participants to use as a sort of dictionary to help them find appropriate skills for specific problems.

In sum, there are many types of DBT skills training programs and many different approaches to teaching the DBT skills. Studies are in progress around the world as I write this. It is useful to keep up on the DBT skills literature. To find skills research, go to Google Scholar (*http://scholar.google.com*) and enter "DBT Skills Training." If you read of programs that you believe would be useful in your environment, get in touch with the authors and ask for a list of the skills they taught.

You can also get new ideas for providing skills training by searching the Internet periodically. For example, you can find videos of me teaching some of the skills on YouTube (search "Marsha Linehan DBT skills"). There are many DBT self-help sites that can also give you good ideas on teaching (search "DBT self-help"). The International Society for the Improvement and Teaching of DBT (ISIT-DBT; *http://isitdbt.net*) has an annual meeting the day before the annual meeting of the Association of Behavioral and Cognitive Therapies (ABCT; *www.abct.org*). Workshops and research on DBT skills are very often available there as well. If you are using a skills set without research data, be sure to keep track of outcomes and client feedback in your own program, and make changes as needed.

References

1. Linehan, M. M., Comtois, K. A., Murray, A. M., Brown, M. Z., Gallop, R. J., Heard, H. L., et al. (2006). Two-year randomized trial + follow-up of dialectical behavior therapy vs. therapy by experts for suicidal behavior and borderline personality disorder. *Archives of General Psychiatry, 63*(7), 757–766.
2. Harned, M. S., Chapman, A. L., Dexter-Mazza, E. T., Murray, A., Comtois, K. A., & Linehan, M. M. (2008). Treating co-occurring Axis I disorders in chronically suicidal women with borderline personality disorder: A 2-year randomized trial of dialectical behavior therapy versus community treatment by experts. *Journal of Consulting and Clinical Psychology, 76*(6), 1068–1075.
3. Linehan, M. M., Korslund, K. E., Harned, M. S., Gallop, R. J., Lungu, A., Neacsiu, A. D., McDavid, J., Comtois, K. A., & Murray-Gregory, A. M. (2014). *Dialectical Behavior Therapy for high suicide risk in borderline personality disorder: A component analysis.* Unpublished manuscript.
4. Linehan, M. M., Armstrong, H. E., Suarez, A., Allmon, D., & Heard, H. L. (1991). Cognitive-behavioral treatment of chronically parasuicidal borderline patients. *Archives of General Psychiatry, 48*, 1060–1064.
5. Linehan, M. M., Heard, H. L., & Armstrong, H. E. (1993). Naturalistic follow-up of a behavioral treatment for chronically parasuicidal borderline patients. *Archives of General Psychiatry, 50*, 971–974.
6. Soler, J., Pascual, J. C., Tiana, T., Cebria, A., Barrachina, J., Campins, M. J., et al. (2009). Dialectical behaviour therapy skills training compared to standard group therapy in borderline personality disorder: A 3-month randomized controlled clinical trial. *Behaviour Research and Therapy, 47*, 353–358.
7. Soler, J., Pascual, J. C., Campins, J., Barrachina, J., Puigdemont, D., Alvarez, E., et al. (2005). Double-blind, placebo-controlled study of dialectical behavior therapy plus olanzapine for borderline personality disorder. *American Journal of Psychiatry, 162*(6), 1221–1224.
8. McMain, S. F., Guimond, T., Habinski, L., Barnhart, R., & Streiner, D. L. (2014). *Dialectical behaviour therapy skills training versus a waitlist control for self-harm and borderline personality disorder.* Manuscript submitted for publication.
9. Neacsiu, A. D., Eberle, J. W., Kramer, R., Wiesmann, T., & Linehan, M. M. (2014). Dialectical behavior therapy skills for transdiagnostic emotion dysregulation: A pilot randomized controlled trial. *Behaviour Research and Therapy, 59*, 40–51.
10. Miller, A. L., Rathus, J. H., & Linehan, M. M. (2007). *Dialectical behavior therapy with suicidal adolescents.* New York: Guilford Press.
11. Rathus, J. H., & Miller, A. L. (2015). *DBT skills manual for adolescents.* New York: Guilford Press.
12. Swenson, C. R., Witterholt, S., & Bohus, M. (2007). Dialectical behavior therapy on inpatient units. In L. A. Dimeff & K. Koerner (Eds.), *Dialectical behavior therapy in clinical practice: Applications across disorders and settings* (pp. 69–111). New York: Guilford Press.
13. Bohus, M., Haaf, B., Simms, T., Schmahl, C., Limberger, M. F., Schmahl, C., et al. (2004). Effectiveness of inpatient DBT for BPD: A controlled trial. *Behaviour Research and Therapy, 42*(5), 487–499.
14. Linehan, M. M., Schmidt, H., Dimeff, L. A., Craft, J. C., Kanter, J., & Comtois, K. A. (1999). Dialectical behavior therapy for patients with borderline personality disorder and drug-dependence. *American Journal on Addictions, 8*, 279–292.
15. Linehan, M. M., Dimeff, L. A., Reynolds, S. K., Comtois, K. A., Shaw-Welch, S., Heagerty, P., et al. (2002). Dialectical behavior therapy versus comprehensive validation plus 12-step for the treatment of opioid dependent women meeting criteria for borderline personality disorder. *Drug and Alcohol Dependence, 67*, 13–26.
16. De Mello, A. (1984). *The song of the bird.* New York: Image Books.

Schedule 1: 24 Weeks, Linehan Standard Adult DBT Skills Training Schedule (Research Studies, 2006 and After)

	Week	Standard Handout(s)	Optional Handout(s)
Repeated at the start of each module: 2 Weeks Orientation, Mindfulness Skills			
Orientation; Goals and Guidelines	1	G1: Goals of Skills Training G3: Guidelines for Skills Training G4: Skills Training Assumptions	G1a: Options for Solving Any Problem
Wise Mind; Mindfulness "What" Skills	1	M1: Goals of Mindfulness Practice M2: Overview: Core Mindfulness Skills M3: Wise Mind: States of Mind M4: Taking Hold of Your Mind: "What" Skills	M1a: Mindfulness Definitions (to hand out for home) M3a: Ideas for Practicing Wise Mind
Mindfulness "How" Skills	2	M4: Taking Hold of Your Mind: "What" Skills (cont.) M5: Taking Hold of Your Mind: "How" Skills	
Module 1		**+6 Weeks Distress Tolerance Skills**	
Crisis Survival; Pros and Cons	3	DT1: Goals of Distress Tolerance DT2: Overview: Crisis Survival Skills DT2: When to Use Crisis Survival Skills DT5: Pros and Cons	DT4: The STOP Skill
TIP skills	4	DT6: Tip Skills: Changing Your Body Chemistry	DT6a: Using Cold Water, Step by Step DT6b: Paired Muscle Relaxation, Step by Step
Distracting; Self-Soothing; Improving the Moment	5	DT7: Distracting DT8: Self-Soothing DT9: Improving the Moment	DT8a: Body Scan Meditation, Step by Step DT9a: Sensory Awareness, Step by Step
Reality Acceptance	6	DT10: Overview: Reality Acceptance Skills DT11: Radical Acceptance DT11b: Practicing Radical Acceptance, Step by Step (or use DTWS 9: Radical Acceptance) DT12: Turning the Mind	DT11a: Radical Acceptance: Factors That Interfere with DTWS9: Radical Acceptance
Willingness; Half-Smiling; Willing Hands	7	DT13: Willingness DT14: Half-Smiling and Willing Hands	DT14a: Practicing Half-Smiling and Willing Hands
Mindfulness of Thoughts	8	DT15: Mindfulness of Current Thoughts DT15a: Practicing Mindfulness of Thoughts	
	9, 10	**2 Weeks Orientation, Mindfulness Skills**	
Module 2		**+7 Weeks Emotion Regulation Skills**	
Understanding and Labeling Emotions	11	ER1: Goals of Emotion Regulation ER2: Overview: Understanding and Naming Emotions ER3: What Emotions Do for You ER4: What Makes It Hard to Regulate Your Emotions ER5: A Model for Describing Emotions ER6: Ways to Describe Emotions	ER4a: Myths about Emotions ER5a: A Brief Model for Describing Emotions
Checking the Facts	12	ER7: Overview: Changing Emotional Responses ER8: Checking the Facts (with ERBWS5: Checking the Facts)	ER8a: Examples of Emotions That Fit the Facts

	Week	Standard Handout(s)	Optional Handout(s)
Opposite Action	13	ER10: Opposite Action (with ERWS6: Figuring Out How to Change Unwanted Emotions) ER11: Figuring Out Opposite Actions (with ERWS7)	ER9: Opposite Action and Problem Solving: Deciding Which to Use
Problem Solving	14	ER12: Problem Solving ER13: Reviewing Opposite Action and Problem Solving	
A	15	ER14: Overview: Reducing Vulnerability to Emotion Mind ER15: Accumulating Positive Emotions in the Short Term ER16: Pleasant Events List	
	16	ER17: Accumulating Positive Emotions in the Long Term ER18: Values and Priorities List	ER20b: Sleep Hygiene Protocol
B, C; PLEASE; Mindfulness of Emotions	17	ER19: Build Mastery and Cope Ahead ER20: Taking Care of Your Mind by Taking Care of Your Body ER22: Mindfulness of Current Emotions	ER20a: Nightmare Protocol, Step by Step ER20b: Sleep Hygiene Protocol ER21: Overview: Managing Really Difficult Emotions ER23: Managing Extreme Emotions ER24: Troubleshooting Emotion Regulation Skills (with ERWS16: Troubleshooting Emotion Regulation Skills) ER25: Review of Skills for Emotion Regulation
	18, 19	**2 Weeks Orientation, Mindfulness Skills**	
Module 3		**+5 Weeks Interpersonal Effectiveness Skills**	
Understanding Obstacles; Clarifying Goals	20	IE1: Goals of Interpersonal Effectiveness IE2: Factors in the Way of Interpersonal Effectiveness IE4: Clarifying Goals in Interpersonal Situations	
DEAR MAN	21	IE5: Guidelines for Objective Effectiveness: Getting What You Want (DEAR MAN)	IE5a: Applying DEAR MAN Skills to a Difficult Current Interaction
GIVE	22	IE6: Guidelines for Relationship Effectiveness: Keeping the Relationship (GIVE)	IE6a: Expanding the V in GIVE: Levels of Validation IE17: Validation IE18: A "How To" Guide to Validation IE18a: Identifying Validation
FAST	23	IE7: Guidelines for Self-Respect Effectiveness: Keeping Respect for Yourself (FAST)	
Evaluating Options	24	IE8: Evaluating . . . Options (with IEWS6: The Dime Game) IE9: Troubleshooting . . . (with IEWS7: Troubleshooting)	

Note. Repeat sequence for 1-year program.

Schedule 2: 24 Weeks, Linehan Standard Adult DBT Skills Training Schedule (Research Studies before 2006)

	Week	Standard Handout(s)
Module 1		**2 Weeks Orientation, Mindfulness Skills**
Orientation; Goals and Guidelines	1	G1: Goals of Skills Training G3: Guidelines for Skills Training
Wise Mind; Mindfulness "What" Skills	1	M3: Wise Mind: States of Mind M4: Taking Hold of Your Mind: "What" Skills
Mindfulness "How" Skills	2	M4: Taking Hold of Your Mind: "What" Skills (cont.) M5: Taking Hold of Your Mind: "How" Skills
Module 2		**6 Weeks Distress Tolerance Skills**
Pros and Cons	3	DT1: Goals of Distress Tolerance DT5: Pros and Cons
Distracting Self-Soothing	4	DT7: Distracting DT8: Self-Soothing
Improving the Moment	5	DT9: Improving the Moment
Reality Acceptance	6	DT11: Radical Acceptance DT12: Turning the Mind
Half-Smiling	7	DT14: Half-Smiling[a]
Willingness	8	DT13: Willingness
	9–10	**Repeat 2 Weeks Orientation, Mindfulness Skills**
Module 3		**6 Weeks Emotion Regulation Skills**
Understanding Emotions	11	ER1: Goals of Emotion Regulation ER3: What Emotions Do for You ER4: What Makes It Hard to Regulate Your Emotions ER4a: Myths about Emotions
Understanding and Labeling Emotions	12	ER5: A Model for Describing Emotions ER6: Ways to Describe Emotions
	13	ER15: Accumulating Positive Emotions in the Short Term ER16: Pleasant Events List
	14	ER17: Accumulating Positive Emotions in the Long Term ER18: Values and Priorities List
	15	ER19: Building Mastery[a] ER20: Taking Care of Your Mind By Taking Care of Your Body ER22: Mindfulness of Current Emotions
Opposite Action	16	ER10: Opposite Action (with WRWS6: Figuring Out How to Change Unwanted Emotions) ER11: Figuring Out Opposite Actions
	17–18	**Repeat 2 Weeks Orientation, Mindfulness Skills**
Module 4		**6 Weeks Interpersonal Effectiveness Skills**
Understanding Obstacles; Clarifying Goals	19	IE1: Goals of Interpersonal Effectiveness IE2: Factors In the Way of Interpersonal Effectiveness
	20	IE4: Clarifying Goals in Interpersonal Situations
DEAR MAN	21	IE5: Guidelines for Objective Effectiveness: (DEAR MAN)
GIVE Skills	22	IE6: Guidelines for Relationship Effectiveness: Keeping the Relationship (GIVE)
FAST Skills	23	IE7: Guidelines for Self-Respect Effectiveness: Keeping Respect for Yourself (FAST)
Evaluating Options	24	IE8: Evaluating Options . . . (with IEWS6: The Dime Game) IE9: Troubleshooting . . . (with IEWS7: Troubleshooting . . .)

Note. Repeat sequence for 1-year program.
[a]These handout titles differ from their present versions because the handouts did not include certain skills.

Schedule 3: 13 Weeks, Soler Adult DBT Skills Training Schedule

	Week	Standard Handout(s)
2 Weeks Orientation, Mindfulness Skills		
Orientation; Wise Mind	2	G1: Goals of Skills Training G3: Guidelines for Skills Training M3: Wise Mind: States of Mind
Mindfulness "What" Skills	1	M4: Taking Hold of Your Mind: "What" Skills
Mindfulness "How" Skills	2	M5: Taking Hold of Your Mind: "How" Skills
3 Weeks Distress Tolerance Skills		
Distracting; Self-Soothing; Improving the Moment	3	DT7: Distracting DT8: Self-Soothing DT9: Improving the Moment
Reality Acceptance	4	DT11: Radical Acceptance DT11b: Practicing Radical Acceptance, Step by Step (or DTWS9, Radical Acceptance) DT12: Turning the Mind
Willingness; Mindfulness of Thoughts	5	DT13: Willingness DT15: Mindfulness of Current Thoughts
4 Weeks Emotion Regulation Skills		
Understanding Emotions	6	ER1: Goals of Emotion Regulation ER3: What Emotions Do for You
Understanding and Labeling Emotions		ER5: Model for Describing Emotions ER6: Ways to Describe Emotions
A	7	ER15: Accumulating Positive Emotions in the Short Term ER16: Pleasant Events List ER17: Accumulating Positive Emotions in the Long Term
B, C; PLEASE; Mindfulness of Emotions	8	ER19: Build Mastery[a] ER20: Taking Care of Your Mind by Taking Care of Your Body ER22: Mindfulness of Current Emotions
Opposite Action	9	ER10: Opposite Action (with ERWS6: Figuring Out How to Change Unwanted Emotions)
4 Weeks Interpersonal Effectiveness Skills		
Understanding Obstacles; Clarifying Goals	10	IE1: Goals of Interpersonal Effectiveness IE2: Factors In the Way of Interpersonal Effectiveness
DEAR MAN	10	IE5: Guidelines for Objective Effectiveness: Getting What You Want (DEAR MAN)
GIVE FAST	11	IE6: Guidelines for Relationship Effectiveness: Keeping the Relationship (GIVE) IE7: Guidelines for Self-Respect Effectiveness: Keeping Respect for Yourself (FAST)
Evaluating Options	12	IE8: Evaluating Your Options (with IEWS6: The Dime Game)

[a]This handout titles differs from its present versions because the handout did not include skills for cope ahead.

Schedule 4: 20 Weeks, McMain Adult DBT Skills Training

	Week	Standard Handout(s)
Orientation; Mindfulness	1	G1: Goals of Skills Training M3: Wise Mind: States of Mind
4 Weeks Distress Tolerance Skills		
Pros and Cons	2	DT1: Goals of Distress Tolerance DT5: Pros and Cons
TIP Skills; Self Soothing	3	DT6: TIP Skills: Changing Your Body Chemistry DT7: Distracting DT8: Self-Soothing
Radical Acceptance; Willingness	4	DT11: Radical Acceptance DT12: Turning the Mind DT13: Willingness DT14: Half-Smiling and Willing Hands
Mindfulness "What" Skills	5	M4: Taking Hold of Your Mind: Mindfulness "What" Skills
5 Weeks Interpersonal: Walking the Middle Path		
Dialectics	6	IE16: How to Think and Act Dialectically IE16a: Examples of Opposite Sides That Can Both Be True IE16b: Important Opposites to Balance
Self-Validation	7	IE17: Validation (focusing on self-validation IE19: Recovering From Invalidation
Validation of Others	8	IE17 Validation (focusing on validating others) IE18: A "How To" Guide to Validation
Behavioral Principles— Positive Reinforcement	9	IE20: Strategies for Increasing the Probability of Desired Behaviors
Mindfulness "How" Skills	10	M5: Mindfulness How Skills
5 Weeks Emotion Regulation Skills		
Rationale; Model of Emotions; Observing and Describing Emotions	11	ER1: Goals of Emotion Regulation ER3: What Emotions Do for You ER5: A Model for Describing Emotions ER6: Ways to Describe Emotions
PLEASE	12	ER20: Taking Care of Your Mind by Taking Care of Your Body
Increasing Positive Experiences (Short-Term and Long-Term); Mastery	13	ER15: Accumulating Positive Emotions in the Short Term ER16: Pleasant Events List ER17: Accumulating Positive Emotions in the Long Term ER18: Values and Priorities List ER19: Build Mastery and Cope Skills
Opposite Action	14	ER9: Opposite Action and Problem Solving: Deciding Which to Use ER10: Opposite Action (with ERWS6: Figuring Out How to Change Unwanted Emotions) ER11: Figuring Out Opposite Actions
Mindfulness in Everyday Life	15	Review and practice mindfulness skills ER22: Mindfulness of Current Emotions
5 Weeks Interpersonal Effectiveness Skills		
Rationale; Priorities	16	IE1: Goals of Interpersonal Effectiveness Skills IE3: Overview: Obtaining Objectives Skillfully IE4: Clarifying Goals in Interpersonal Situations
DEAR MAN	17	IE5: Guidelines for Objective Effectiveness: Getting What You Want (DEAR MAN)
GIVE FAST	18	IE6: Guidelines for Relationship Effectiveness: Keeping the Relationship (GIVE) IE7: Guidelines for Self-Respect Effectiveness: Keeping Respect for Yourself (FAST)
Identifying Obstacles	19	IE2: Factors in the Way of Interpersonal Effectiveness IEWS7: Troubleshooting Interpersonal Effectiveness with Skills
Evaluating Options	20	IE8: Evaluating Options . . . (with IEWS6: The Dime Game)

Schedule 5: 14 Weeks, Neacsiu Adult DBT Emotion Regulation Skills Training

	Week	Standard Handout(s)
2 Weeks Orientation, Mindfulness Skills		
Wise Mind; Observe	1	M3: Wise Mind M4: Taking Hold of Your Mind: Mindfulness "What" Skills
Describe; Participate; Nonjudgmentally; One-Mindfully; Effectively	2	M4: Taking Hold of Your Mind: Mindfulness "What" Skills M5: Taking Hold of Your Mind: Mindfulness "How" Skills
6 Weeks Interpersonal Effectiveness Skills		
Understand, Identify, Label Emotions	3	ER1: Goals of Emotion Regulation ER2: Overview: Understanding and Naming Emotions ER3: What Emotions Do for You ER4: What Makes It Hard to Regulate Your Emotions ER5: A Model for Describing Emotions ER6: Ways to Describe Emotions
Checking the Facts	4	ER7: Overview: Changing Emotional Responses ER8: Checking the Facts (with ERWS5: Checking the Facts
Opposite Action	5	ER10: Opposite Action (with ERWS6: Figuring Out How to Change Unwanted Emotions) ER11: Figuring Out Opposite Actions
Problem Solving	6	ER12: Problem Solving ER13: Reviewing Opposite Action and Problem Solving
Accumulating Positives and Building Mastery	7	ER15: Accumulating Positive Emotions in the Short Term ER17: Accumulating Positive Emotions in the Long Term ER19: Build Mastery and Cope Ahead
Cope Ahead and PLEASE	8	ER19: Build Mastery and Cope Ahead ER20: Taking Care of Your Mind by Taking Care of Your Body
1 Week Review of Mindfulness Skills		
Wise Mind; Observe	9	M3: Wise Mind M4: Taking Hold of Your Mind: Mindfulness "What" Skills
Describe; Participate; Nonjudgmentally; One-Mindfully; Effectively	9	M4: Taking Hold of Your Mind: Mindfulness "What" Skills M5: Taking Hold of Your Mind: Mindfulness "How" Skills
4 Weeks Distress Tolerance Skills		
TIP Skills	10	DT6: TIP Skills: Changing Your Body Chemistry
Distracting, Self-Soothing, Improving the Moment	11	DT7: Distracting DT8: Self-Soothing DT9: Improving the Moment
Radical Acceptance; Turning the Mind	12	DT10: Overview: Reality Acceptance Skills DT11: Radical Acceptance DT11b:Practicing Radical Acceptance, Step by Step (or DTWS: Radical Acceptance) DT12: Turning the Mind
Willingness; Half-Smiling; Mindfulness of Thoughts	13	DT13: Willingness DT14: Half-Smiling and Willing Hands DT15: Mindfulness of Current Thoughts
1 Week Interpersonal Effectiveness Skills		
DEAR MAN, GIVE FAST; Interpersonal Validation Behavioral Principles in Relationships	14	IE5: Guidelines for Objective Effectiveness: (DEAR MAN) IE6: Guidelines for Relationship Effectiveness: Keeping the Relationship (GIVE) IE7: Guidelines for Self-Respect Effectiveness: Keeping Respect for Yourself (FAST) IE17: Validation IE18: A "How To" Guide to Validation IE20: Strategies for Increasing the Probability of Desired Behaviors IE21: Strategies for Decreasing or Stopping Undesired Behaviors IE22: Tips for Using Behavior Change Strategies Effectively

Schedule 6: 25 Weeks, Adolescent Multifamily DBT Skills Training

	Week	Standard Handout(s)	Optional Handout(s)
	**Repeated at the start of each module:** **2 Weeks Orientation, Mindfulness Skills + 1 Week Middle Path Skills**		
Orientation	1	G1: Goals of Skills Training G3: Guidelines for Skills Training G4: Skills Training Assumptions G5: Biosocial Theory (if not reviewed in individual therapy)	G1a: Options for Solving Any Problem G2: Overview: Introduction to Skills Training G7: Chain Analysis (if not taught in individual therapy) G8: Missing-Links Analysis (if not taught as part of homework review)
Mindfulness Goals; Wise Mind; "What" Skills	1	M1: Goals of Mindfulness Practice M3: Wise Mind M4: Taking Hold of Your Mind: "What" Skills	M2: Overview: Core Mindfulness Skills M3a: Ideas for Practicing Wise Mind M4a–c: Ideas for Practicing Observing, Describing, Participating
	2	M5: Taking Hold of Your Mind: "How" Skills	M5a–c: Ideas for Practicing Nonjudgmentalness, One-Mindfulness, Effectiveness
Middle Path; Dialectics	3	IE15: Dialectics IE16: How to Think and Act Dialectically IE16a: Examples of Opposite Sides That Can Both Be True	IE16b: Important Opposites to Balance IE16c: Identifying Dialectics
Module 1		**5 Weeks Distress Tolerance Skills**		
Crisis Survival STOP Skill; Pros and Cons	4	DT1: Goals of Distress Tolerance DT3: When to Use Crisis Survival Skills DT4: The STOP Skill Crisis Survival Skills DT5: Pros and Cons	
TIP Skills	5	DT6: TIP Skills: Change Your Body Chemistry	DT6a: Using Cold Water, Step by Step DT6b: Paired Muscle Relaxation, Step by Step DT6c: Effective Rethinking and Paired Relaxation
Distracting; Self-Soothing; Improving the Moment	6	DT7: Distracting Attention DT8: Self-Soothing DT9: Improving the Moment	DT8a: Body Scan Meditation, Step by Step DT9a: Sensory Awareness, Step by Step
Reality Acceptance	7	DT10: Overview: Reality Acceptance Skills DT11: Radical Acceptance DT12: Turning the Mind DT14: Half-Smiling and Willing Hands	DT11a: Radical Acceptance: Factors That Interfere DT11b: Practicing Radical Acceptance, Step by Step (or DTWS9, Radical Acceptance) DT14: Half-Smiling and Willing Hands
Willingness	8	DT13: Willingness DT21: Alternate Rebellion and Adaptive Denial Review and graduation for those ending skills training	
	9–10	**2 Weeks Orientation, Mindfulness Skills**	
Module 2		**7 Weeks Emotion Regulation Skills**		
Validation	11	IE17: Validation IE18: A "How To" Guide to Validation	IE18a: Identifying Validation
Understanding Emotions	12	ER1: Goals of Emotion Regulation ER2: Overview: Understanding and Naming Emotions ER5: Model for Describing Emotions ER6: Ways to Describe Emotions	ER3: What Emotions Do for You

	Week	*Standard Handout(s)*	*Optional Handout(s)*
Changing Emotions	13	ER7: Overview: Changing Emotional Responses ER8: Check the Facts (with ERWS5: Check the Facts)	ER8a: Examples of Emotions That Fit the Facts
Checking the Facts	14	ER9: Opposite Action and Problem-Solving: Deciding Which to Use ER10: Opposite Action	ER11: Figuring Out Opposite Actions
Problem Solving	15	ER12: Problem Solving ER13: Reviewing Opposite Action and Problem Solving	
Accumulating Positive Emotions	16	ER15: Accumulating Positive Emotions in the Short Term ER16: Pleasant Events List R17: Accumulating Positive Emotions in the Long Term ER18: Values and Priorities List	ER12: Build Mastery and Cope Ahead ER14: Overview: Reducing Vulnerability to Emotion Mind ER17: Accumulating Positive Emotions in the Long Term
Building Mastery Ahead and Coping PLEASE	17	ER 19: Build Mastery and Cope Ahead ER20: Taking Care of Your Mind by Taking Care of Your Body Review and graduation for those ending skills training	ER20a: Nightmare Protocol, Step by Step ER20b: Sleep Hygiene Protocol
	18–19	**2 Weeks Orientation and Mindfulness Skills**	
Module 3		**6 Weeks Interpersonal Effectiveness Skills**	
Clarifying Goals	20	IE1: Goals of Interpersonal Effectiveness IE2: Factors in the Way of Interpersonal Effectiveness IE4: Clarifying Goals in Interpersonal Situations	IE2a: Myths That Interfere with Effectiveness IE3: Overview: Obtaining Objectives Skillfully
DEAR MAN	21	IE5: Guidelines for Objective Effectiveness: Getting What You Want (DEAR MAN)	IE5a: Applying DEAR MAN Skills to a Difficult Current Interaction
GIVE	22	IE6: Guidelines for Relationship Effectiveness: Keeping the Relationship (GIVE)	IE6a: Expanding the V in GIVE: Levels of Validation IE17: Validation (review)
FAST; Validation	23	IE7: Guidelines for Self-Respect Effectiveness: Keeping Respect for Yourself (FAST)	IE18: A "How To" Guide to Validation (review) IE19 Recovering from Invalidation IE19a: Identifying Self-Invalidation
The Dime Game	24	Evaluating Options . . . (with IEWS6: The Dime Game)	
Troubleshooting	25	IE9: Troubleshooting: When What You Are Doing Isn't Working Review and graduation for those ending skills training	

Schedule 7: Variable Sessions, Inpatient DBT Skills Training (Intermediate Unit and Acute Unit)

Module	Intermediate Unit	Acute Unit
Core Mindfulness	M4: Wise Mind M5: Taking Hold of Your Mind: Mindfulness "What" Skills M6: Taking Hold of Your Mind: Mindfulness "How" Skills	M4: Wise Mind M5: Taking Hold of Your Mind: Mindfulness "What" Skills M6: Taking Hold of Your Mind: Mindfulness "How" Skills
Distress Tolerance	DT5: Pros and Cons DT6: TIP Skills: Changing Your Body Chemistry DT7: Distracting DT8: Self-Soothing DT9: Improving the Moment DT11: Radical Acceptance DT12: Turning the Mind DT14: Half-Smiling and Willing Hands DT13: Willingness	DT5: Pros and Cons DT6: TIP Skills: Changing Your Body Chemistry DT7: Distracting DT8: Self-Soothing DT9: Improving the Moment DT11: Radical Acceptance DT12: Turning the Mind
Emotion Regulation	ER5: A Model for Describing Emotions ER6: Ways to Describe Emotions ER10: Opposite Action ER15: Accumulating Positive Emotions in the Short Term ER16: Pleasant Events List	ER6: Ways to Describe Emotions ER10: Opposite Action ER15: Accumulating Positive Emotions in the Short Term ER16: Pleasant Events List
Interpersonal Effectiveness	IE4: Clarifying Priorities in Interpersonal Effectiveness IE5: Guidelines for Objectiveness Effectiveness . . . (DEAR MAN) IE6: Guidelines for Relationship Effectiveness . . . (GIVE) IE7: Guidelines for Self-Respect Effectiveness . . . (FAST)	IE4: Clarifying Priorities in Interpersonal Effectiveness IE5: Guidelines for Objectiveness Effectiveness . . . (DEAR MAN) IE6: Guidelines for Relationship Effectiveness . . . (GIVE)

Note. Adapted from Table 4.5 in Swenson, C. R., Witterholt, S., & Bohus, M. (2007). Dialectical behavior therapy on inpatient units. In L. A. Dimeff & K. Koerner (Eds.), *Dialectical behavior therapy in clinical practice: Applications across disorders and settings* (pp. 69–111). New York: Guilford Press. Copyright 2007 by The Guilford Press. Adapted by permission.

Schedule 8: DBT Skills for Addictive Behaviors (to Integrate with Schedule 1 Skills)

Possible module	Handouts
General	DT16: Overview: When the Crisis Is Addiction DT16a: Common Addictions
Core Mindfulness	DT18: Clear Mind DT18a: Behavior Patterns Characteristic of Addict Mind and of Clean Mind
Distress Tolerance	DT17: Dialectical Abstinence DT17a: Relapse Prevention Planning DT20: Burning Bridges and Building New Ones DT21: Alternative Rebellion and Adaptive Denial
Interpersonal Effectiveness	DT19: Community Reinforcement

Note. You can weave these skills into the modules listed to the left of the handouts list or you can teach them as a group in sequence by their numbers.

Schedule 9: DBT Parenting Skills Behaviors (to Integrate with Schedule 1 Skills)

DEAR MAN	IE20: Strategies for Increasing the Probability of Desired Behaviors IE21: Strategies for Decreasing or Stopping Undesired Behaviors IE22: Tips for Using Behavior Change Strategies Effectively IE22a: Identifying Effective Behavior Change Strategies
GIVE	IE17: Validation IE18: A "How To" Guide to Validation IE18a: Identifying Validation
FAST	IE19: Recovering from Invalidation IE19a: Identifying Self-Invalidation

Note. You can weave these skills into the modules listed to the left of the handouts list or you can teach them as a group in sequence by their numbers.

Schedule 10: Comprehensive DBT Mindfulness Skills Training

	Week	Standard Handout(s)	Optional Handout(s)
Orientation; Goals; Wise Mind	1	M1: Goals of Mindfulness Practice M1a: Mindfulness Definitions M2: Overview: Core Mindfulness Skills M3: Wise Mind: States of Mind	
Mindfulness "What" Skills	2	M4: Taking Hold of Your Mind: Mindfulness "What" Skills	M4a: Ideas for Practicing Observing M4b: Ideas for Practicing Describing M4c: Ideas for Practicing Participating
Mindfulness "How" Skills	3	M5: Taking Hold of Your Mind: Mindfulness "How" Skills	M5a: Ideas for Practicing Nonjudgmentalness M5b: Ideas for Practicing One-Mindfulness M5c: Ideas for Practicing Effectiveness
Spiritual Mindfulness	4	M7: Goals of Mindfulness Practice: A Spiritual Perspective M7a: Wise Mind from a Spiritual Perspective M8: Practicing Loving Kindness to Increase Love and Compassion	
	5	M7: Goals of Mindfulness Practice: A Spiritual Perspective M7a: Wise Mind from a Spiritual Perspective M8: Practicing Loving Kindness to Increase Love and Compassion	
Mindful Meditation	6	DT8a: Body Scan Meditation, Step by Step DT9a: Sensory Awareness, Step by Step	
	7	ER22: Mindfulness of Current Emotions: Letting Go of Emotional Suffering DT15: Mindfulness of Current Thoughts DT15a: Practicing Mindfulness of Thoughts	
Reality Acceptance	8	DT10: Overview: Reality Acceptance Skills DT11: Radical Acceptance DT11a: Radical Acceptance: Factors That Interfere DT11b: Practicing Radical Acceptance, Step by Step (or use DTWS9, Radical Acceptance) DT12: Turning the Mind	DTWS9: Radical Acceptance
Willingness	9	DT13: Willingness DT14: Half-Smiling and Willing Hands	DT14a: Practicing Half-Smiling and Willing Hands
Mindful Action	10	M9: Skillful Means: Balancing Doing Mind and Being Mind	M9a: Ideas for Practicing Balancing Doing Mind and Being Mind
Middle Path	11	M10: Walking the Middle Path: Finding the Synthesis between Opposites IE12: Mindfulness of Others	IE12a: Identifying Mindfulness of Others

Schedule 11: Advanced DBT Skills

	Week	Standard Handout(s)	Optional Handout(s)
Orientation	1	Discuss goals of advanced skills training Develop with group guidelines for skills training G1a: Options for Solving Any Problem	Review skills and decide which skills will be covered in the group
Mindfulness			
Mindfulness Review	2	M3: Wise Mind M4: Taking Hold of Your Mind: Mindfulness "What" Skills M5: Taking Hold of Your Mind: Mindfulness "How" Skills	M7: Goals of Mindfulness Practice: A Spiritual Perspective M7a: Wise Mind from a Spiritual Perspective
Mindfulness	3	M7: Goals of Mindfulness Practice: A Spiritual Perspective M7a: Wise Mind from a Spiritual Perspective M8: Practicing Loving Kindness to Increase Love and Compassion	
Building Relationships			
Building Relationships	4	IE10: Overview: Building Relationships IE11: Finding and Getting People to Like You IE12: Mindfulness of Others	IE11a: Identifying Skills to Find People and Get Them to Like You IE12a: Identifying Mindfulness of Others
Relationships	5	IE17: Validation IE18: A "How To" Guide to Validation	IE18a: Identifying Validation
Relationships	6	IE19: Recovering from Invalidation IE19a: Identifying Self-Validation IE13: Ending Relationships	IE19a: Identifying Self-Validation IE13a: Identifying How to End Relationships
Walking the Middle Path			
Walking the Middle Path	7	IE15: Dialectics IE16: How to Think and Act Dialectically IE16a: Examples of Opposite Sides That Can Both Be True IE16b: Important Opposites to Balance	IE16c: Identifying Dialectics
Walking the Middle Path	8	M9: Skillful Means: Balancing Doing Mind and Being Mind M9a: Practices for Balancing Doing Mind and Being Mind M10: Walking the Middle Path: Finding the Synthesis between Opposites	
Behavior Change Strategies			
Chain Analysis	9	G6: Overview: Analyzing Behavior G7: Chain Analysis (with GWS2, Chain Analysis of Problem Behavior) G7a: Chain Analysis, Step by Step	
Missing-Links Analysis	10	G8: Missing-Links Analysis (with GWS3, Missing-Links Analysis)	

(cont.)

	Week	Standard Handout(s)	Optional Handout(s)
Behavior Change Strategies	11	IE20: Strategies for Increasing the Probability of Desired Behaviors IE21: Strategies for Decreasing or Stopping Undesired Behaviors IE22: Tips for Using Behavior Change Strategies Effectively	IE22a: Identifying Effective Behavior Change Strategies
Develop further curriculum with participants			
	12		
	13		
	14		
	15		
	16		
	17		

Note. Consider teaching this curriculum as a second module, or add to Schedule 1, or let participants choose the skills they would like covered.

PART II

Teaching Notes
for DBT Skills Modules

Chapter 6

General Skills:
Orientation and Analyzing Behavior

There are two sets of general skills. The first set focuses on orientation to skills training, including a handout on the biosocial theory of emotion dysregulation. The second set focuses on how to analyze behavior so that a client can figure out the causes or events that influence the behavior. This allows the client to problem-solve how to change the behavior or how to prevent it in the future.

Orientation

An orientation to skills training takes place during the first session of a new skills group. The purposes of this orientation are to introduce members to one another and to the skills training leaders; to orient members to the structural aspects of skills training (e.g., format, rules, meeting times); to orient them to the leaders' approach and goals; to sell the skills as worth learning and likely to work; and to generate enthusiasm for learning and practicing the skills. This chapter provides an outline of topics to be covered, but their content can be easily modified to reflect your particular circumstances (e.g., format, timing, fees, rules, use of the telephone). An optional section for teaching the biosocial theory of how emotion dysregulation develops is included.

As discussed in Chapter 4, orienting is a skills trainer's chief means of selling the skills to group members. Therefore, important tasks for skills trainers are to highlight the usefulness of the skills, to elicit participants' specific personal goals, and then to link these goals to the skills modules. Specific goals for the skills training you are conducting will depend on the skills that you plan to teach. The

specific goals listed on General Handout 1 and in the teaching notes are general enough to cover most of what might be taught in the average group. Optional goals are noted. Skills training guidelines, or rules, are presented and discussed along with skills training assumptions.

In the teaching notes, I have put a checkmark (✓) next to material I almost always cover. If I am in a huge rush, I may skip everything that is not checked. In the handouts and worksheets (see *www.guilford. com/skills-training-manual*), I have put stars (★) on the standard handouts I almost always use.

After the first orientation session, reorientation may be reviewed with members, or abbreviated if there are no new members starting the group. Make an effort not to skip it, as review can be useful to remind participants of assumptions and guidelines, and it is a good time to discuss whether new guidelines should be added. If there are new members, leaders should try to get old members to conduct as much of the orientation as possible. In either case, if orientation is concluded before the session ends and the optional handouts are not being taught, leaders should proceed to the material for the core mindfulness skills in Chapter 7.

Diary Cards

Diary cards (see Figure 4.1 in Chapter 4) provide spaces for logging practice of all relevant skills. These are usually introduced and reviewed by a client's individual DBT therapist. However, clients who are not in DBT individual treatment should be introduced to the diary card in the orientation session. If the diary card, which includes use of skills, is not

Thanks to Anita Lungu, Debra Safer, Christy Telch, and Eunice Chen.

being reviewed by a participant's individual therapist, the skills portion of the card can be reviewed weekly as part of the homework practice review, in addition to any assigned skills practice worksheets. If only the previous week's homework is reviewed, there is a danger that skills taught previously will drop off the client's radar and not be practiced.

Biosocial Theory

The biosocial theory is often reviewed in individual DBT sessions, and in some programs it is taught in adolescent and multifamily skills programs. The theory is particularly relevant for individuals meeting criteria for BPD and for individuals with pervasive emotion dysregulation. It is important, if you are treating another population, such as one with emotion overcontrol or other disorders, that you teach a biosocial theory appropriate to the population you are treating. The idea that all behavior is a joint product of biology and environment, however, applies to everyone. If group members or individual therapists have reviewed this theory, there may be little to gain by reviewing it again.

Analyzing Behavior

Because many DBT therapists teach their clients how to conduct their own analysis of problematic behaviors, I have added a supplementary set of skills that teach participants how to analyze and problemsolve dysfunctional ineffective behaviors ("chain analyses") and how to identify effective behaviors that are needed but missing ("missing-links analyses"). The chain analysis has been widely used in DBT. I developed the missing-links analysis at the request of both adolescents and parents in our multifamily group.

Chain Analysis

Conducting chain analyses of problem behaviors is a critical part of DBT. There are many ways to teach clients how to do this, and there are many places and times to teach it in the course of therapy. In standard DBT treatment programs, individual therapists teach their clients how to do a chain analysis in the course of individual therapy. DBT treatment teams employ abbreviated chain analyses to assess team-interfering behaviors of team members. In my treatment teams, we always do a brief chain analysis with individuals who are late for team meetings. It is often taught in residential and inpatient treatment programs. It is an important part of skills training for eating disorders[1] and can also be very useful in substance use disorder programs. When participants are not in individual therapy, teaching chain analysis can be incorporated into skills training when there is time and it appears useful. Inclusion of the chain analyses in skills training per se is optional.

Missing-Links Analysis

Whereas a chain analysis breaks down problem behaviors, missing-links analysis is used to identify effective behaviors that are missing. It consists of a systematic set of questions and was originally developed for therapists to conduct rapid assessments of failures to do assigned skills homework in group settings, where there is often limited time to review homework. When missing-links analysis was used for homework review in adolescent multifamily skills groups, parents immediately wanted to learn how to do it to analyze their children's missing effective behaviors. Teens also wanted to use it to analyze their parents' missing behaviors. From there, it became clear that it could be a useful strategic set of questions for any missing effective behavior.

┌─────────────────────────┐
│   **Teaching Notes**   │
└─────────────────────────┘

I. THE GOALS OF SKILLS TRAINING (GENERAL HANDOUTS 1–1A)

> **Main Point:** The overall goal of DBT skills training is to help individuals change behavioral, emotional, thinking, and interpersonal patterns associated with problems in living.
>
> **General Handout 1: Goals of Skills Training.** Use this handout to get clients to think about how they could personally benefit from skills training, to identify which areas they are most interested in, and to identify specific personal goals of behaviors to increase and decrease in their own skills training. For clients who have taken other skills training modules and been through orientation before, this is an opportunity to evaluate the progress they have made on their personal goals since the beginning of the previous module. The idea is to generate some enthusiasm for learning and practicing the skills.
>
> Research on DBT is moving very fast, and data suggest that DBT skills training may be effective for a large variety of goals. If General Handout 1 does not fit the goals of your group or individual client, feel free to adapt or develop an entirely new list of goals for your client(s).
>
> **General Handout 1a: Options for Solving Any Problem** *(Optional).* This optional handout can be used at the start of a skills module, or it can be used at another point when you believe it would be useful. The handout was designed as a reply to participants who responded to offers of help in solving life's problems with a "Yes, but . . . " attitude. It can be particularly helpful to review this handout in those situations. This handout describes the three effective responses to any problem and shows what categories of skills are needed for each. It also serves as a reminder that the only response that needs no skillful behavior is the last option: "Stay miserable."
>
> **General Worksheet 1: Pros and Cons of Using Skills** *(Optional).* This optional worksheet is designed to help participants decide whether they have anything to gain from practicing their DBT skills. It is particularly useful when they are feeling willful or apathetic and don't want to practice. It can be reviewed rather quickly if participants already know how to fill out a pros-and-cons worksheet. If not, review the principles of doing pros and cons. Be sure to instruct participants to fill out pros and cons for both the option of practicing skills and the option of not practicing. It can be useful, if there is time, to have participants fill this out at least partially during the sessions. Suggest that participants carry the sheet with them or post it somewhere at home, so they can easily review it as needed.

A. Introductions

To ease into a first session for newcomers, you can try going around the room and asking members to give their names, tell how they heard about the group, and provide any other information they would like to share. As the group leaders, you should also give information about yourselves and how you came to lead the group.

B. General Goal of Skills Training

The overall goal of skills training is to learn skills for changing unwanted behaviors, emotions, thinking, and events that cause misery and distress.

✓ C. Behaviors to Decrease

Ask participants to read General Handout 1 and check each set of behaviors they would like to decrease. If there is a behavior on a particular list they do not have trouble with, they can cross it out. Alternatively, they can circle the behaviors they think are most important to decrease.

💬 **Discussion Point:** Discuss and share what is checked and circled. Ask participants to fill out personal goals at the bottom of the page. Discuss and share personal goals, including behaviors to decrease and skills to increase.

> **Note to Leaders:** The goals below are organized first by specific module and include supplemental skills that you may or may not be teaching. You can skip describing and discussing supplemental skills if you are not teaching them. In general, these notes are guidelines and should be adapted as needed to fit the specific skills you plan to teach and the characteristics of the people you are working with.

✓ **D. Skills to Increase**

✓ **1. Mindfulness Skills**

Mindfulness skills help us focus attention on the present moment, noticing both what is going on within ourselves and what is going on outside of ourselves and become and stay centered. Mindfulness as a practice has now become widespread, with courses taught in corporations, medical schools, and many other settings.

Present the **mindfulness goals** by types of skills you are teaching:

- **Core mindfulness skills (the mindfulness "what" and "how" skills)** teach us how to observe and experience reality as it is, to be less judgmental, and to live in the moment with effectiveness.
- **(Supplemental) Mindfulness skills from a spiritual perspective (including wise mind from a spiritual perspective and practicing loving kindness)** focus on experiencing ultimate reality, forming an intimate connection with the entire universe, and developing a sense of freedom.
- **(Supplemental) Skillful means: Balancing doing mind and being mind**
- **(Supplemental) Wise mind by walking the middle path**

💬 **Discussion Point:** Discuss goals of mindfulness skills training. Get feedback about individual goals. Ask participants to write down their individual goals on General Handout 1.

✓ **2. Interpersonal Effectiveness Skills**

Interpersonal effectiveness skills help us maintain and improve relationships both with people we are close to and with strangers.

Present the **interpersonal effectiveness goals** by types of skills you are teaching:

- **Core interpersonal effectiveness skills** teach us how to deal with conflict situations, to get what we want and need, and to say no to unwanted requests and demands—all this in a way that maintains our self-respect and others' liking and respect for us.
- **(Supplemental) Building relationships and ending destructive relationships.** These skills enable us to find potential friends, get people to like us, and maintain positive relationships with others. They also show how to build closeness with others on the one hand, and how to end destructive relationships on the other.
- **(Supplemental) Walking the middle path.** These skills help us to walk a middle path in our relationships, balancing acceptance with change in ourselves and in our relationships with others.

💬 **Discussion Point:** Discuss goals of interpersonal effectiveness skills training. Get feedback about individual goals. Ask participants to write down their individual goals on General Handout 1.

✓ **3. Emotion Regulation Skills**

Emotion regulation includes enhancing control of emotions, even though complete emotional control cannot be achieved. To a certain extent we are who we are, and emotionality is part of us. But we can get more control and perhaps learn to modulate some emotions.

Present the **emotion regulation goals** by types of skills you are teaching:

- **Understanding and naming emotions:** These skills enable us to understand emotions in general and understand and identify our own emotions.
- **Changing emotional responses:** These skills help us to reduce the intensity of painful or unwanted emotions (anger, sadness, shame, etc.), and to change situations that prompt painful or unwanted emotions.
- **Reducing vulnerability to emotion mind:** These skills enable us to reduce vulnerability to becoming extremely or painfully emotional, and to increase emotional resilience.
- **Managing really difficult emotions:** These skills help us to accept ongoing emotions and to manage extreme emotions.

Discussion Point: Discuss goals of emotion regulation skills training. Get feedback about individual goals. Ask participants to write down their individual goals on General Handout 1.

✓ 4. **Distress Tolerance Skills**

Distress tolerance is the ability to tolerate and survive crisis situations without making things worse. Also, these skills teach us how to accept and fully enter into a life that may not be the life we hoped for or want.

Present the **distress tolerance goals** by types of skills you are teaching:

- **Crisis survival skills:** These skills enable us to tolerate painful events, urges, and emotions when we cannot make things better right away.
- **Reality acceptance skills:** These skills permit us to reduce suffering by accepting and living a life that is not the life we want.
- **(Supplemental) Skills when the crisis is addiction:** These skills enable us to back down from addiction and live a life of abstinence.

Discussion Point: Discuss goals of distress tolerance skills training. Get feedback about individual goals. Ask participants to write down their individual goals on General Handout 1.

5. **Analyzing Behavior (Supplemental)**

Present these skills if you intend to teach Sections VI and VII of general skills (see below).

- **Chain analysis and missing-links analysis** are ways to figure out the causes of problem behaviors and plan for problem solving.

E. Format of Skills Training

1. Order and Length of Skills Modules

Review the order and length of skills modules, if this has not been discussed in a previous interview. The specifics here will depend on the nature of your particular skills training program and where in the cycle of modules the orientation session falls. (See also Chapter 3 of this manual.)

✓ 2. **Session Format**

Briefly review the overall session format: beginning ritual, review of skills practice since the last session, break, presentation of new material, and a closing wind-down.

F. Options for Solving Any Problem

> **Note to Leaders:** If the optional General Handout 1a is used at orientation, highlight the role of DBT skills in each component of solving life's problems. Remind participants of the options if at a future point they reject all or most suggestions for solving a problem.

Tell clients: "The options for responding to pain are limited. There may be an infinite number of really painful things that can happen to you. But there are not an infinite number of responses you can make to pain. In fact, if you sit back and think about it, there are only four things you can do when painful problems come into your life: You can solve the problem, change your feelings about the problem, tolerate the problem, *or* just stay miserable (and perhaps even make it worse)."

1. Solve the Problem

Say to clients: "First, you can try finding a way to end or change the problem situation, or by figuring out a way to avoid the situation or get out of it for good. This is the first thing you could do—solve the problem." Give these examples as needed:

Example: "If the distress comes from conflict in your marriage, one solution could be to avoid spending time with your spouse; another solution could be to get a divorce and leave the relationship; alternatively, you could get couple counseling and change the relationship so that the conflict is resolved."

Example: "If the problem is that you are afraid of flying, you could solve this by avoiding flying; alternatively, you could find a treatment program aimed at reducing fear of flying."

Give these examples of skills that can help with problem solving:

- Walking the middle path (from interpersonal effectiveness skills)
- Problem-solving skills (from emotion regulation skills)

2. Feel Better about the Problem

Tell clients: "A second way of responding to pain is by changing your emotional responses to it. You could work at regulating your emotional response to the problem or figure out a way to make a negative into a positive." Give these examples as needed:

Example: "Remind yourself that conflict is a normal part of marriage and that it is nothing really to be distressed about. Alternatively, develop more positive relationships outside of your marriage, so that the negative aspects of conflict with you partner are not very important."

Example: "Work on feeling better about having a fear of flying; alternatively, join a phobia support group."

Give these examples of skills that can help with feeling better about the problem:

- Emotion regulation skills
- Mindfulness skills

3. Tolerate the Problem

Say to clients: "When you can't solve the problem that is generating distress and you can't feel better about it, you can still alleviate some of the distress." Give these examples as needed:

Example: "In a marriage full of conflict, you might not be able to solve the problem through divorce or by improving the relationship. You might also not succeed in feeling better about the problem. But you will be less distressed and miserable about it if you practice radical acceptance of the problem."

Example: "If you simply cannot get rid of your flying phobia and also can find no way to like it or feel good about it, then you can reduce the suffering it causes you by radically accepting it: It is what it is."

Give these examples of skills that can help with tolerating the problem:

- Distress tolerance skills
- Mindfulness skills

4. Stay Miserable

Tell clients: "The fourth option is that you can stay miserable. You could, of course, also do something to make matters worse!"*

Give this example of how to stay miserable:

■ Use *no* skills!

II. OVERVIEW: INTRODUCTION TO SKILLS TRAINING (GENERAL HANDOUT 2)

> **Main Point:** Very briefly, describe the topics that will be covered. Let participants know if you are not going to cover the biosocial theory of emotion dysregulation. If you are not covering it, be sure to read it yourself and decide if you want to give the handout to participants. If you do give it out, you might want to suggest that participants read it before the next session, so that you can answer any questions at that time.
>
> **General Handout 2: Overview: Introduction to Skills Training.** This overview handout can be reviewed briefly or skipped, depending on time. Do not teach the material while covering this page unless you are skipping the related handouts.
>
> **Worksheet:** None.

This introduction is aimed at providing a good grasp of the guidelines and rules that are important for your skills training program as well as the assumptions that underlie skills training.

A. Guidelines for Skills Training

This is the first and most important topic. It covers the requirements and the expectations for skills training. This topic and its handout (General Handout 3) may not be as important if you are teaching skills in individual sessions.

B. Skills Training Assumptions

This topic and its handout (General Handout 4) describes the seven assumptions that underpin DBT skills training.

C. Biosocial Theory

This topic and its handout (General Handout 5) provide a detailed review of the biosocial theory that underpins our thinking about emotion dysregulation.

III. ORIENTATION TO SKILLS TRAINING (GENERAL HANDOUTS 3–4)

> **Main Point:** For skills training to go smoothly, each participant should know and understand the guidelines and assumptions that underpin DBT skills training.
>
> **General Handout 3: Guidelines for Skills Training.** When you are discussing these guidelines, it is necessary not only to present them, but also to address possible misconceptions about how to "get around" the guidelines. It is useful to ask participants to take turns in reading the guidelines and explaining how they understand and interpret them.

---

*The fabulous idea of adding on "you can make things worse" was sent to me in an e-mail from a person who had gone through DBT skills training. Unfortunately, I cannot find the e-mail to give proper credit to this person. I hope to hear from her for a correction in the future.

General Handout 4: Skills Training Assumptions. When you are introducing the assumptions of skills training, it is useful to make the distinction between the guidelines in General Handout 3 (which are behavioral standards to be followed while in skills training) and assumptions (which are beliefs that cannot be proved, but that all participants agree to abide by anyway).

General Worksheet 1: Pros and Cons of Using Skills. The worksheet is designed to help participants decide whether they are willing to practice and use the skills you are teaching them. Its major use is to communicate that the goal is to be *effective and skillful* in getting what participants want (i.e., in reaching their own goals). It is not about doing whatever participants want, following rules, giving in, or doing what other people want. This worksheet can also be used as an exercise to improve the likelihood of being effective when participants are overcome with emotions (e.g., when they want to yell, scream, catastrophize, or do something destructive instead of skillful). It can also be used as a teaching tool for how to figure out goals. Skip this worksheet if you also teach other handouts that have associated worksheets during this session.

If you are using a pros-and-cons worksheet for the first time with participants, begin by describing what is meant by "pros and cons." Then put the basic 2 × 2 grid up on the board, and work through several examples of pros and cons with participants. With drug addictions, for example, make a list of pros and cons of using drugs, and then a list of pros and cons of stopping the use of drugs. Stress the importance of filling out each of the four quadrants. Instruct participants to keep a copy of the completed worksheet, since it can be *very* hard for them to remember why not to engage in crisis behaviors when they are in emotion mind. For more detailed instructions in teaching pros and cons, see the teaching notes for Distress Tolerance Handout 5: Pros and Cons (Chapter 10, Section V).

✓ A. Guidelines for Skills Training

Discuss the guidelines on General Handout 3, and get each participant to agree to them. This is an important part of the treatment process, not a precursor to the process. Also discuss possible misconceptions about how to "get around" the guidelines. It can be useful after discussion of the guidelines to go around the room and ask each group member for an individual commitment to abide by them. In an open group, the guidelines should be discussed each time a new member enters the group. Often it is a good idea to have old members explain the guidelines to new members. Although the term "rules" is ordinarily not used, the expectation is that the guidelines will be followed as if they are rules. Note that presentation of the guidelines in an authoritarian way will probably alienate some clients, especially those for whom issues of control are important.

1. Participants Who Drop Out of Skills Training Are *Not* Out of Skills Training

There is only one way to drop out of skills training: missing four consecutive skills training sessions. Clients who miss 4 weeks of scheduled skills training sessions in a row have dropped out and cannot reenter for the duration of the time in their treatment contract. For example, if a client has contracted for 1 year, but misses 4 weeks in a row during the sixth month, then he or she is out for the next 6 months. At the end of the contracted time, the person can negotiate with the skills trainer(s) and the group about readmission (if he or she was in a group and it is continuing). There are no exceptions to this guideline. This guideline is the same as the rule for individual DBT psychotherapy. Mention that although it is technically possible to repeatedly miss three sessions in a row and come to the fourth session, it would be a violation of the spirit of the rule.

The message to communicate is that everyone is expected to come to skills training sessions each week. Presentation of this guideline offers an opportunity to discuss what constitutes an acceptable reason for missing a session. Not being in the mood, non-serious illness, social engagements, fear, beliefs that "No one in the group likes me," and so forth do not qualify. Serious illness, very important events, and unavoidable trips out of town do qualify as acceptable reasons.

2. Participants Who Join the Skills Training Group Support Each Other

There are many ways to be a supportive person when attending skills training sessions. As the group leaders, review with clients what is needed to be supportive.

a. Confidentiality

The importance of the confidentiality rule is self-evident. What may not be obvious is that the rule extends to "gossiping" outside sessions. The general notion here is that interpersonal problems between or among clients should be dealt with by the persons involved, either within or outside sessions. There are two exceptions to the confidentiality rule. First, clients can discuss what happens in skills training sessions with their individual therapists; this exception is important so that they can maximize the benefits of the therapy. But caution clients not to reveal other clients' last names unless absolutely necessary. The other exception has to do with the risk of suicide. If one client believes that another is likely to commit suicide, he or she can and should summon help.

b. Regular Attendance

Regular attendance—especially coming on time and staying for the entire session—is supportive. It is very hard to keep coming to a group when other people in the group do not treat it as important by coming to each session on time and staying until the end.

c. Practicing between Sessions

It is hard to keep practicing skills in a group when you are the only one who routinely practices between sessions. It can make the practicing member feel different or feel guilty that one person's practicing highlights others not practicing.

> **Note to Leaders:** Developing a group norm of coming on time and practicing skills between sessions is very important, but such a norm can be hard at times to develop. Discussing the importance of building norms at the start of each new module can be very helpful. My experience is that most skills training members want such norms to develop. See Chapter 4 for ideas on how to reinforce coming on time and doing homework that is assigned.

d. Validating Each Other and Avoiding Judgments

e. Giving Helpful, Noncritical Feedback When Asked

Members need to make every effort to validate each other and give helpful, noncritical feedback. This can set a tone of trust and support at the very beginning. Discuss this guideline, as well as how hard it may be for some members. In subsequent sessions when these guidelines are violated, you leaders can step in with guidance on how to replace judgments with nonjudgmental descriptions, critical feedback with helpful suggestions, and defensiveness with acceptance of other's comments.

f. Accepting Help from a Person Who Is Called for Help

It is not acceptable for a client to call someone; say, "I am going to kill myself," or "I am going to use drugs"; and then refuse to let that other person help. The inability to ask for help appropriately is a special problem for many individuals. Thus this rule begins the process in the skills training context of teaching how to reach out to peers for help when needed. Like the other rules, this rule is usually a relief to clients. The rule itself was suggested by one of our group clients.

Before this guideline was added, we occasionally had instances of a participant's calling another participant in desperate emotional pain, obliquely threatening suicide or other dysfunctional behavior, extracting a promise of confidentiality from the one called, and then hanging up after no apparent progress was made in the call. The helper was left with a very difficult dilemma: If the helper really cared about the caller, he or she would do something to help. Yet the helper clearly had not been able to do anything, and if he or she asked for outside help it would be violating a confidence. The resulting helplessness and anguish were enormous.

One of the strengths of group skills training is that members often build a strong supportive community among themselves. At times, they are the only ones who can really understand their mutual experiences. Since everyone's problems are public in the group, members need not be ashamed to ask one another for help. Not only is the opportunity for problem solving helpful to the caller, but the helper has a chance to practice generating problem solutions and reasons for living. In addition—and this point should be made to clients—such calls offer group members a structured chance to practice observing their own limits on how much help they are willing to give.

3. Participants Who Are Going to Be Late or Miss a Session Call Ahead of Time

This rule serves several purposes. First, it is a courtesy for clients to let you skills trainers know not to wait for latecomers before starting. Although we have a general rule in our groups of starting on time, it is difficult not to hold off on important material or announcements for the first few minutes, in the expectation that missing clients will show up any minute. This is a special problem in those weeks where only one or two clients are present at the beginning. Second, it introduces an added response cost for being late and communicates to clients that promptness is desirable. Finally, it gives information as to why a client is not present.

In a group context, when a person does not come to a session and gives no explanation ahead of time, group members (including the leaders) almost always start worrying about the welfare of the absent member. Sometimes, however, clients miss for reasons having nothing to do with problems. Thus not calling causes unnecessary worry for the group members. Just the fact that others will worry is often news to some group members; for others, the worry is a source of emotional support and may reinforce not calling. In any case, the rule offers a vehicle for addressing the behavior. Presentation of the rule is an opportunity to discuss the need for courtesy and empathy to the feelings of other group members, as well as the responsibility of each member to contribute to group cohesion.

4. Participants Do Not Tempt Others to Engage in Problem Behaviors

a. Participants Do Not Come to Sessions under the Influence of Alcohol or Drugs

The value of not using drugs or alcohol before coming to a skills group is reasonably self-evident; there is little need for extensive discussion of it. However, it does offer an opportunity to discuss the emotional pain that skills training attendance is likely to cause much of the time. Accurate expectations are essential here to head off demoralization. Once again, you can suggest that as clients learn emotion regulation skills, they will be better able to cope with the stress of skills training.

b. If Participants Have Already Used, They Should Come to Sessions Acting Clean and Sober

If a client has used drugs or alcohol, it may not be so clear why he or she should come to skills training anyway and act as if clean and sober. The reason is that for clients with substance use disorders, a rule saying not to come to skills sessions when using just gives these individuals with poor self-regulation a good excuse for not coming. Instead, my position is that skills learning is context-dependent, and thus, for individuals with substance problems, learning and practicing skills when under the influence of drugs or alcohol are particularly important. That is definitely the time when skills are needed.

c. Participants Do Not Discuss Problem Behaviors That Could Be Contagious to Others

Descriptions of dysfunctional behaviors can lead to behavioral contagion. In my experience, communications about self-injury, substance use, bingeing or purging, and similar behaviors elicit strong imitation effects among individuals with disordered emotion regulation. These urges to imitate can be very difficult to resist. Use the example of a person addicted to drugs listening to another person talking about drugs, and most participants will get the point immediately: The drug user trying to get off drugs will immediately have an urge to use drugs. Just as in individual DBT, clients in skills training must agree not to call or communicate with one another *after* a self-injurious act. Our group members usually welcome this rule. Before I instituted this rule, clients often complained that once they had given up dysfunctional behaviors themselves, it was very scary to listen to others describing their episodes of these behaviors.

5. *Participants Do Not Form Sexual or Confidential Relationships Outside Skills Training Sessions*

The key word in the fifth rule is "private." Clients may not form relationships outside the sessions that they then cannot discuss inside the sessions. DBT actually encourages friendships among group clients outside sessions. In fact, the support that members can give one another with daily problems in living is one of the strengths of group DBT. However, it also provides the possibility for interpersonal conflict that is inherent in any relationship. The key is whether interpersonal problems that arise can be discussed in the sessions (or, if that is too difficult or threatens to get out of hand, with you leaders privately). To the extent that such issues can be discussed and appropriate skills applied, a relationship can be advantageous. Troubles arise when a relationship cannot be discussed and problems increase to such an extent that one member finds it difficult or impossible to attend meetings, either physically or emotionally.

In presenting this rule, alert members that it is unacceptable for one member to demand complete confidentiality about problems from another member. This is especially crucial when it comes to plans for destructive behavior, important information that one person lies about in meetings, and other situations creating an untenable awkwardness for one member of the pair.

As discussed in Chapter 3, current sexual partners should be assigned to different groups at the onset. Thus this rule functions to alert group members that if they enter into a sexual relationship, one member of the pair will have to drop out of the group. To date, we have had several sexual relationships begin among group members; each created enormous difficulties for the partners involved. In one case, the initiating partner broke off the relationship against the wishes of the other, making it very hard for the rejected partner to come to group sessions. In the other, one member was seduced reluctantly, leading to trauma and tension in the group. Generally, this rule is clear to everyone involved. Without the rule, however, dealing with an emerging sexual relationship between clients is very tricky, since post hoc application of rules is unworkable with individuals who have disordered emotion regulation.

Note to Leaders: Exempted from the guideline above are skills training groups for friends and families, where couples, partners, and multiple family members often join. It is not reasonable or feasible to outlaw private relationships in these groups or in the multifamily skills groups commonly held with adolescents. In these situations, however, it is important to note that when relationship conflicts threaten the group, the leaders will approach the conflicts in a manner similar to that described above. That is, the topic will be discussed either in group (if it offers an opportunity to practice skills) or individually with one of the skills trainers (if the individuals having conflict do not have the requisite skills to address the conflict effectively within the group).

6. Additional Guidelines

Discuss any other guidelines you may wish to follow that are not on General Handout 3, and be sure that everyone writes them onto this handout.

7. Advanced Groups

In advanced groups, the DBT four-session-miss guideline may be modified. If so, discuss the criteria for determining whether an individual has or has not officially dropped out of skills training. For example, you may want to discussed what an "excused" session is (e.g., a session missed because of a physical illness, family emergency, vacation out of town, wedding, or funeral) and what an "unexcused" session is (e.g., a session missed because of fatigue, bad mood, psychiatric hospitalization, or a solvable problem).

✓ B. Skills Training Assumptions

An assumption is a belief that cannot be proved, but that all participants in skills training (clients and leaders alike) agree to abide by anyway.

1. People Are Doing the Best They Can

That is, given the multiplicity of causes in the universe (genetics, biological events, environmental events, consequences of previous behavior), each person at this one moment in time is what he or she is. Given who we each are and the fact that all behavior is caused, we are doing the best we can at this one moment, given the causes that have affected us.

2. People Want to Improve

This is similar to the Dalai Lama's statement that the common characteristic of all people is that they want to be happy.[2]

3. *People Need to Be Better, Try Harder, and Be More Motivated to Change

The fact that people are doing the best they can, and want to do even better, does not mean that their efforts and motivation are sufficient to the task.

The asterisk at the start of this assumption indicates that this is not always true. In particular, when progress is steady and at a realistic rate of improvement with no let-up or episodic drop in effort, doing better, trying harder and being more motivated is not needed.

4. *People May Not Have Caused All of Their Own Problems, but They Have to Solve Them Anyway

This assumption is true for adults, because the responsibility for their own lives rests with them.

The asterisk before this assumption indicates that this is not always true. With children and adolescents, as well as some disabled persons, parents and other caregivers must assist them with this task. For example, young children or disabled individuals cannot get themselves to treatment if parents or caregivers refuse to take them.

5. New Behaviors Must Be Learned in All Relevant Contexts

Behaviors learned in one context often do not generalize to different contexts, thus it is important to practice new behaviors in all the environments where they will be needed. (This is one of the main reasons it is important for participants to practice new skills in their daily environments.)

6. All Behaviors (Actions, Thoughts, Emotions) Are Caused

There is always a cause or set of causes for our actions, thoughts, and emotions, even if we don't know what these causes are.

7. Figuring Out and Changing the Causes of Behavior Works Better Than Judging and Blaming

This assumption is very much related to the previous one. When we agree that all behavior is caused, this leads to the understanding that blaming and being judgmental ("This should not be") are not effective in changing that situation or behavior.

> **Note to Leaders:** It is important to point out that our culture often encourages and models being judgmental, and so it's easy to respond in a judgmental manner. It is also important not to judge the judging. Letting go of judging is likely to get us to our goals of changing behavior more effectively.

C. Committing to Learning Skills

It is important to remember that you can never get too much commitment from clients to learning skills. Commitment in skills training is particularly important, because learning skills requires a fair amount of homework practice, and such practice not only takes time but can be difficult to do. Even if you have met individually with participants and worked on commitment, if time permits it can be very useful to review commitment in the group. The aim here is to focus attention on whether participants are still committed to coming to skills classes, doing the homework practice and generally putting substantial effort into learning new, skillful ways to solve problems and work toward their individual goals.

💬 Discussion Points:

1. Ask participants whether they are still committed to skills sessions and practice. Is there anyone who was never committed in the first place? If yes, ask, "Are you willing to commit to coming and practicing now?" Discuss.
2. Ask about difficulties participants may encounter with transportation, coming on time, and staying until the end of sessions. Troubleshoot difficulties with the group.
3. Ask about fears and concerns about coming to the group. Ask, "Who thinks it will be too difficult to share their homework with others? Who will be reluctant to ask questions when learning new skills?" Discuss.

✓ D. Diary Cards

1. What Is a Diary Card?

The DBT diary card is designed to track behaviors that clients are trying to decrease, as well as skills they are trying to increase. For the most part, the top half of the card tracks behaviors to be decreased, and the bottom half tracks skills to be practiced and increased. The top half is designed primarily for review in individual sessions. Because it is also important for individual therapists to track use of skills, clients rate the skills they use ("Used Skills") on a 7-point scale in one column on the top half. The bottom half, in contrast, lists the most important DBT skills taught. Participants are instructed to circle the skills they use each day. See Figure 4.1 in Chapter 4 for a sample diary card.

Only the bottom half of the card (pertaining to skills) is reviewed in skills training sessions. If you are conducting a skills-training-only program, and participants are either getting individual therapy elsewhere or are not in any individual therapy, give out only the bottom half of the card. In our friends-and-family skills program, we give out only the bottom half of the skills card. We do the same with parents in the adolescent multifamily skills program. The teens, however, have the complete card, which they review with their individual therapists. An exception here should be made if the skills trainers are also providing case management and/or crisis intervention to skills participants, in which case it makes sense to give them the complete card. Ask each participant to bring the diary card every week to the skills training session, but review only the bottom part of the card for even those who bring a complete card. My thinking on this issue (to block sharing of information on the top part of the card) is summarized in Chapter 3 in the discussion of the fourth skills training guideline: Participants do not tempt others to engage in problem behaviors.

2. Does the Diary Card Have to Be Printed on Card Stock?

The first diary cards were printed on card stock with a front and a back. It soon became clear, however, that card stock was very hard to fold up and keep somewhere inconspicuous when clients were homeless or when they were out in public (such as at work or at school). So we changed it to standard 8.5 × 11 paper. There are now many versions of our DBT diary cards online and also in computerized apps. Look up "DBT diary card" in your search engine and you will find them. As you will see, there are many variations.

3. How Is the Diary Card Used?

Go over the instructions in Chapter 4, Table 4.2, for filling out the diary card. In addition, do the following:

- **Tell clients to check each skill and circle it each day if they make any attempt to practice the skill.** Degree of skill practice (front of card) is rated according to the scale at the bottom of the card. Thus participants should rate their use of the skills they are learning. Note that maladaptive coping or problem solving (e.g., drinking, self-cutting) do not count as using skills.
- **Emphasize that clients need to practice skills already taught and learned, not just new ones.** This is crucially important in learning and change.
- **Troubleshoot problems in filling out the cards.** Engage in problem solving for difficulties.
- **Stress the confidentiality of cards.** Discuss ways to keep the cards confidential. Give out alternative cards with only acronyms if necessary. Suggest that participants not put their real names on cards, and that they use numbers or pseudonyms instead. Some participants do not want to use diary cards that can be understood by anyone else if they are found. In these instances, diary cards can be revised to use acronyms instead of the names of skills.

IV. BIOSOCIAL THEORY OF EMOTION DYSREGULATION (GENERAL HANDOUT 5)

> **Main Point:** Biosocial theory is an explanation of how and why some people have so much difficulty with emotion regulation and behavioral control.
>
> **General Handout 5: Biosocial Theory.** This handout covers both the biological and the social aspects of emotion regulation and behavioral control. In standard DBT, the information on this handout is ordinarily covered in individual therapy. In adolescent treatment it is discussed with both parents and teens. It is an optional handout for a skills-only program. For a more detailed review of the biosocial theory, see Chapter 1 and the references at the end of that chapter.
>
> **Worksheet:** None.

> **Note to Leaders:** As you will see, the biosocial theory puts a large emphasis on biology and on the behavior of others in the participants' social environment. Almost everyone will be comfortable with the emphasis on biology as an important factor in emotion dysregulation and behavioral dyscontrol. However, if not handled skillfully, the emphasis on the social environment can make many participants uncomfortable, and it can make those involved in their caregiving or others in their current environment particularly uncomfortable or defensive. Great care, empathy for others, and sensitivity are needed in

working with individuals who may not have been effective parents, or others who might fit into the invalidating category. That said, I have never watered down the theory to soothe parents or caregivers in a participant's social environment. Because I have not judged those in the social environment, I have generally found that parents, relatives, and others are grateful for the understanding and the guidance the theory gives them.

✓ **A. Biological Factors and Emotional Vulnerability: The "Bio" in Biosocial**

1. Characteristics of Emotionally Vulnerable Individuals

Individuals who are emotionally vulnerable:

- Are more sensitive to emotional stimuli.
- Experience emotions more often than others.
- May feel like emotions hit them for no reason, out of the blue.
- Have more intense emotions than others—emotions that feel like being hit by a ton of bricks.
- Have long-lasting emotions.

2. Biological Influences on Vulnerability

This vulnerability to high emotionality is highly influenced by biological factors:

- Genetics.
- Intrauterine factors during pregnancy.
- Brain damage or physical disorders after birth.

3. Individual Variation in Emotionality

Some people are just more emotional than others.

✓ **Discussion Point:** Ask participants to check off characteristics of emotional vulnerability that fit them. Discuss.

Discussion Point: Ask participants whether they have siblings or family members who have been markedly different in emotionality ever since (it seems) they were born. Discuss how this is probably due to biological differences.

Discussion Point: Individuals with serious brain disorders, traumatic brain injuries, and some other serious physical disorders that they acquired after birth will often have much more difficulty managing emotions than they had before the injury or disorder.

B. Biological Factors and Impulsivity

1. Characteristics of Impulsive Individuals

Individuals who are impulsive:

- Find it hard to inhibit behaviors.
- Are more likely to do things that get them in trouble.
- Have behaviors that often seem to come out of nowhere.
- Have moods that get in the way of organizing behavior to achieve goals.
- Have trouble controlling behaviors that are linked to their moods.

✓ **2. Biological Influences on Impulsivity**

Genetics and other biological factors also influence impulsivity.

✓   ### 3. Individual Variation in Impulsivity

Some people are just more impulsive than others.

✓   💬 **Discussion Point:** Ask participants to check off characteristics of impulsivity on General Handout 5 that fit them. Discuss.

💬 **Discussion Point:** Ask participants whether they have siblings or family members who have been markedly different in impulsivity ever since (it seems) they were born. Discuss how this is probably due to biological differences.

💬 **Discussion Point:** Individuals with serious brain disorders or traumatic brain injuries often will have much more difficulty managing impulses to act without thinking than before the injury or disorder. Discuss.

✓ ## C. The Invalidating Environment: The "Social" in Biosocial

1. Characteristics of the Invalidating Environment

The invalidating environment is characterized by:

✓
- Intolerance toward expressions of private emotional experiences, particularly those not supported by observable public events.

Example: Telling a child, "Nobody else feels like you do, so just stop being a crybaby."

- Intermittent reinforcement of extreme expressions of emotion, while simultaneously communicating that such emotions are unwarranted.

Example: Ignoring screams for help when a child falls off a tricycle until the screams get on the adult's nerves too much, and then responding in a cold and stern manner.

- Communications that specific emotions are invalid, weird, wrong, or bad.

Example: Telling a child, "That is such a dumb thing to say!"

- Communications that emotions should be coped with without support.

Example: Saying, "If you are going to keep crying, go to your room and come down when you get control of yourself."

✓
- Not responding to emotions that call for a response or action.

Example: Saying, "I can see you are upset about losing your textbook for tomorrow's exam," but not doing anything to help find the book.

- Confusing one's own emotions with the emotions of others.

Example: Saying, "I'm tired; let's all go to bed."

💬 **Discussion Point:** Elicit from participants other examples of invalidation in their own lives. Discuss.

✓ ## D. The Ineffective Environment: A Second "Social" in Biosocial

> **Note to Leaders:** I am using the term "parent" here, but it can mean "nonparental caregiver."

1. Reasons for Ineffective Parental Teaching

For several reasons, parents may be ineffective at teaching children emotion regulation and behavioral control.

a. **No Parent Is Perfect at Effective Parenting**

Most parents go through periods with their children where for a limited time it appears that they must be ineffective parents. This is normative in parenting. At these times, many parents get professional help in parenting.

b. **Many Parents Simply Do Not Know How to Be Effective Parents**

Many parents may not have had effective parenting themselves, and thus never learned what to do—how to discipline a child, and how to attend to and reinforce positive behaviors. These parents may not be aware that their parenting style does not fit what their children need.

✓ c. **Parents May Be Perfectionists**

Parents may be so perfectionistic or so highly concerned about appearances that they overemphasize internalizing all emotions and characterize impulsivity as a character flaw that can be remedied only if there is sufficient motivation. This is rarely sufficient alone.

✓ d. **Some Parents Have Serious Disorders**

Parents who have serious physical or mental disorders may not be able to attend to their children. They may themselves be highly emotionally dysregulated and impulsive.

✓ e. **Parents May Be Overstressed**

Some parents may be so overwhelmed that they cannot give their children the attention and coaching the children need. Severe illness in other family members, high-stress jobs, insufficient financial resources, multiple children, the absence of a second parent, and many other factors can interfere with the most caring parent's being able to give a child what is needed.

💬 **Discussion Point:** Ask participants if their parents have (or had) any of these characteristics. Ask parents if any of these descriptions fit them. Discuss.

2. *Reasons for Ineffective Adult Environments*

Sometimes adults get in environments that are ineffective and sometimes even destructive. Examples include:

a. **Work Environments**

Adults' work environments often excessively punish behaviors that don't meet the workplace standards, fail to reinforce effective behaviors, and fail to communicate respect. Any or all of these factors can lead to high emotionality in a vulnerable person. Although impulsive behaviors may not show up in the work setting, the stress of the workplace may lead to excess impulsivity outside work.

b. **Adult Relationships**

Many adult relationships can lead to high emotionality. This is particularly the case when partners or friends ignore effective behaviors and excessively punish unwanted behaviors. For many individuals who are vulnerable, an environment without nurturing and caring can lead to extreme sadness, loneliness, shame, and other extreme emotions. At times, sadness may spark high anger as well.

✓ c. **Insensitive Individuals**

Insensitive individuals who are very important to a person who is overly sensitive to invalidation can set off extreme emotional reactions when they invalidate the person's core beliefs, hopes, goals, accomplishments, or personal characteristics.

💬 **Discussion Point:** Ask participants whether they have been or are currently in any of the ineffective environments. Discuss.

✓ E. It's the Transaction That Counts

1. Escalation of Communication

A primary function of emotions is to communicate. When the communication is not received, the sender ordinarily escalates the communication. The more important the communication, the more the sender escalates it.

2. Escalation of Invalidation

At the same time, however, if the receiver does not believe the communication, each time the individual tries to communicate the same thing, the receiver will escalate invalidation.

3. Further Escalation of Both

As emotions escalate, invalidation escalates further—*and* as invalidation escalates further, emotions and their communication escalate further in turn.

4. What the Transaction Looks Like

A transaction looks like Figure 6.1, where A communicates to B and then B responds to A, who then communicates to B, and so on. In other words, each party in a transaction influences the other. A and B can represent two individuals, an individual and his or her environment, or two environments. The key idea is that over time, both sides influence each other.

> **Note to Leaders:** Describe the following scenario in as dramatic a fashion as possible. Act it out. It can also be helpful to put it on the board as you are acting it out.

✓   *Example:* Invalidation looks a lot like the following interchange.

SENDER: There's a fire.

RECEIVER: You're overreacting. What's wrong with you? There's no fire.

SENDER: Um, *there's a fire here!*

RECEIVER: You're crazy! *Just blow it out!*

[After many cycles of being invalidated for describing the situation, the sender responds in one of two ways:]

SENDER: OK, there's no fire. (What's wrong with me??)

RECEIVER: Good job!

[Or, when the sender is really desperate:]

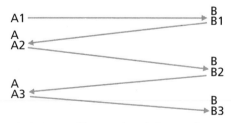

FIGURE 6.1. Transactional change diagram.

SENDER: FIRE!!! FIRE!!! HELP!!!

RECEIVER: Oh, no!! What can I do to help?

💬 **Discussion Point:** Ask participants to describe a transaction like this that has occurred in their lives. Probe for examples where participants were calling out "Fire!" when there was one, and situations where they themselves were invalidating someone else's cry of "Fire!" Discuss.

💬 **Discussion Point:** Often people who have been invalidated learn to exaggerate their communications to be sure the other person pays attention. Alas, once someone gets in this habit, the environment ordinarily gets in the habit of ignoring the person's communications. Elicit times when participants have exaggerated, and times when those they interact with have done so. Discuss ways to reduce the tendency to exaggerate.

5. Summary

In summary, highlight that each of us is influenced by our biological makeup, which then influences our behavior, which then influences our environment, which in turn reacts to and influences us in a never-ending transactional relationship over time. Such a transactional point of view is largely incompatible with blame, although it is not incompatible with identifying important causal factors in our own and others' behavior.

Caution: Remember that this biosocial theory fits individuals with very high emotion dysregulation. DBT skills, however, are effective for many other disorders, and it is important to provide a biosocial model that fits the disorder.

V. OVERVIEW: ANALYZING BEHAVIOR (GENERAL HANDOUT 6)

> **Main Point:** The ability to analyze our own behavior allows us to determine what causes it and what maintains it. Knowing this is important for any of us if we want to change our own behavior.
>
> **General Handout 6: Overview: Analyzing Behavior.** This overview handout can be reviewed briefly or skipped, depending on time. Do not teach the material while covering this page unless you are skipping the related handouts.
>
> **Worksheet:** None.

This section is aimed at helping clients develop the ability to analyze and understand ineffective, problematic behaviors and to identify missing effective behaviors that are needed.

A. Chain Analysis of Problem Behavior

A "chain analysis" is a series of questions to guide clients through figuring out what factors have led to problem behaviors and what factors might be making it difficult to change those behaviors.

B. Missing-Links Analysis

A "missing-links analysis" is a series of questions to guide clients through analyzing the factors associated with not engaging in effective behaviors that are needed or expected.

VI. CHAIN ANALYSIS OF PROBLEM BEHAVIOR (GENERAL HANDOUTS 7–7A)

> **Main Point:** Changing behavior requires us to understand the causes of the behavior we want to change. A behavioral chain analysis guides understanding of the chain of events leading to and following specific behaviors.

> **General Handout 7: Chain Analysis.** The ability to conduct a chain analysis of problem behaviors is a critical skill in DBT for both therapists and clients. The skill can be taught in a group setting as part of your standard curriculum, or it can be taught by individual therapists. Conducting chain analyses of problem behaviors by using General Worksheet 2 (see below) is a critical part of DBT. However, there are many ways to teach it, and there are many places and times to teach it in the course of therapy. In many treatment programs, individual therapists teach their clients how to do it in the course of individual therapy. It is ordinarily taught in residential and inpatient treatment programs.[3, 4] Inclusion of the chain analyses in skills training per se is optional. When participants are not in individual therapy, teaching chain analysis can be incorporated into skills training when there is time and it appears useful.
>
> **General Handout 7a: Chain Analysis, Step by Step.** This handout gives step-by-step instructions on how to do a chain analysis. It is important to review this handout in detail and link it closely with General Worksheet 2.
>
> **General Worksheet 2: Chain Analysis of Problem Behavior.** This is the worksheet for doing a chain analysis. Review this worksheet with participants, and link each item on it to the same item on Handout 7 or 7a. Note that two pages are given for listing behavioral links in the chain of events. Participants should use only as much space as needed and one page is often sufficient.
>
> **General Worksheet 2a: Example: Chain Analysis of Problem Behavior.** This is a sample, completed chain analysis worksheet.

✓ A. What Is Chain Analysis?

Any behavior can be understood as a series of linked components. These links are "chained" together, because they follow in succession one after the other; one link in the chain leads to another. For behaviors that are well rehearsed (practiced a lot), it may appear that the episode cannot be broken down into steps—that it "all happens at once." A "chain analysis" provides a series of questions (e.g., what happened before that, what happened next) for unlocking these links that sometimes feel stuck together.

The purpose of a chain analysis is to figure out what the problem is (e.g., being late for work, impulsively quitting a job); what prompts it; what its function is; what is interfering with the resolution of the problem; and what aids are available to help solve the problem.

✓ B. Why Conduct Chain Analyses?

A chain analysis is an invaluable tool for assessing a behavior to be changed. Although performing a chain analysis requires time and effort, it provides essential information for understanding the events that lead up to a particular problem behavior (i.e., behaviors participants want to change). Many attempts to solve a problem fail because the problem at hand is not fully understood and assessed.

By conducting repeated chain analyses, a person can identify the pattern linking different components of a behavior together. Figuring out what the links are is the first step in finding solutions to stopping the problem behavior. When any of the links of the chain can be broken, the problem behavior can be stopped.

✓ C. How to Do a Chain Analysis

> **Note to Leaders:** Following are two examples you can use to help participants see how to do a chain analysis. Chain analysis is better taught by example than by going over the steps below didactically.
>
> Ordinarily it is not a good idea in a group setting to demonstrate chain analysis by using a problem from the participants, as it may be very complicated and you may not have time to finish. You can use the

completed example on General Worksheet 2a. If you end before completing it, participants should read the example as a homework assignment. If doing chain analyses is an important part of your treatment, make reviewing and correcting them in sessions part of homework review.

✓   *Example 1:* Ask participants to go to General Worksheet 2a (the completed example of behavioral chain analysis). Review this example step by step, noting what information is being asked for, and highlighting how the information helps in understanding and ultimately changing the problem behavior. Point out that the questions on the worksheet correspond to the stepped descriptions in General Handout 7 and to the step-by-step instructions on General Handout 7a. Discuss the process and any difficulties participants have with the instructions and worksheet.

The chain analysis is structured to identify the critical pieces of information necessary to understand and solve a problem behavior. Steps 1–5 are about understanding the problem. Steps 6–8 are about changing the problem behavior. Going from the beginning of General Handout 7 to its end, ask participants to identify:

1. What exactly was the problem behavior?
2. What event in the environment started the chain of events (prompting event)?
3. What were the vulnerability factors for that particular day?
4. What was the chain of events, link by link, that led from the prompting event to the problem behavior?
5. What were the consequences of the behavior in the environment?

The next steps are these:

6. Identify skillful behaviors to replace problem links in the chain, and so to decrease the probability of this behavior's happening again.
7. Develop prevention plans to reduce vulnerability to prompting events and to starting down the chain.
8. Repair the negative consequences of the problem behavior for the environment and for oneself.

✓   *A special note on Step 8:* **When one is repairing negative consequences, it is extremely important to first figure out what has actually been harmed.** This is very hard for many individuals to do. For example, someone who betrays a person and says mean, untrue things about the person may try to repair by bringing flowers or candy, as if the damage done was to remove the person's flowers or candy. The repair that is necessary is to apologize, retract what was said, and also refrain from gossip in order to rebuild the person's trust.

A detailed description of each of these steps is given in General Handout 7a.

Note to Leaders: In the beginning, it may be very difficult for participants to identify separate steps that are part of a problem behavior. In other words, it is difficult for them to identify the steps that took place between Point A (when they were *not* engaging in the problem behavior) and Point B (when they were). With patience, a chain analysis can break this down into separate links.

Example 2: Give participants a clean copy of General Worksheet 2 (the blank worksheet for chain analysis). Go through the following example, and ask participants to track on the handout where they would put the information. At the end, discuss the value of the worksheet.

Step 1. The problem behavior: I yelled at my partner and stormed out of the room, slamming the door.

Step 2. The prompting event: I came home from work and my boyfriend was on the couch asleep [**beginning of the chain of events leading to yelling and slamming the door**].

Step 3. What made me vulnerable: The night before he had come home really late and was tired. He and I had not gone out together after work in a really long time and I got him to agree to go out the next night. I was really looking forward to going out when I got home.

Step 4. The specific behaviors and events that were links in the chain:

1st. When I saw him asleep I thought, "He is sleeping again. We're not going out."

2nd. I thought, "He does not love me."

3rd. I got furious right away.

4th. I wanted to hurt him like he hurt me.

Step 5. The consequences of the behavior—the harm my behavior caused:

a. In the environment: He was very hurt that I assumed he did not love me.

b. For myself: I felt guilty. I realized that I had ruined the evening for both of us.

Step 6. I can check the facts next time, since when I finally did in this situation, I found out he had taken a nap so that we would be able to have a really good time together.

Step 7. I can check the facts in my relationship with my partner when I start thinking he does not love me.

Step 8. Plans to repair, correct, and overcorrect the harm: I will make every effort to treat my partner as if he constantly loves me. I will also apologize to him and to make up our evening out that I ruined, I will plan an evening together for both of us that he will really like.

💬 **Discussion Point:** Discuss other ideas for some or all of the questions as you go through the example.

> **Note to Leaders:** Convey to participants the importance of not getting "hung up" by trying to do the analysis perfectly and identify all the parts of the chain exactly right. What is most important is that participants start using the chain analysis, as opposed to feeling overwhelmed by the complexity of doing it perfectly. Point out to participants that doing a chain analysis is a skill like any other, which means that practice matters and that people get better at doing the skill quickly. In our experience, conducting chain analyses over time leads participants to increased awareness of their thoughts and feelings.

> **Note to Leaders:** When completing a chain analysis, participants should focus on identifying the key dysfunctional links (thoughts, events, actions) that seem to contribute most to linking the prompting event with the problem behavior. One way to determine quickly whether a particular link is key is to imagine the probability of the problem behavior's occurring if that link had not been there. It is important to point out that links in a chain can be functional or dysfunctional, depending on whether the client responds to that link by moving farther away or closer to doing the problem behavior.

VII. ANALYZING MISSING LINKS (GENERAL HANDOUT 8)

> **Main Point:** Sometimes the problem is not the presence of problem behavior, but the absence of effective behavior. Analyzing missing links helps us identify what is interfering with effective behaviors that are expected or needed.

> **General Handout 8: Missing-Links Analysis.** This handout gives step-by-step instructions for how to do a missing-links analysis.

> **General Worksheet 3: Missing-Links Analysis.** This is the worksheet for analyzing missing links. It can also be used during sessions to analyze missing homework as a way to teach the skill. If it is not used as a teaching tool during a session, review the worksheet to be sure participants understand its use.

✓ **A. What Is Missing-Links Analysis?**

A "missing-links analysis" is a series of questions to help a person figure out what got in the way of behaving effectively. Its purpose is to show where in the chain of events something happened (or failed to happen) that interfered with effective behavior when it was needed or expected.

Two types of effective behaviors can be missing.

1. Expected Behaviors

Expected behaviors are ones you have agreed to do (e.g., get to work on time), have been instructed to do (e.g., skills training homework), have planned to do (e.g., clean your room), or have desperately hoped to do (e.g., exercise in the mornings).

2. Needed Behaviors

Needed behaviors are skillful behaviors that constitute effective responses in a specific situation (e.g., skillful interpersonal behavior to calm down a stressful interaction) or to address specific problems (e.g., getting up on time when your alarm clock is broken).

B. When Is Missing-Links Analysis Used?

Missing-links analysis and problem solving are likely to be sufficient when the problem is not knowing what was expected or needed, unwillingness to do what was expected or needed, or never having the thought enter your mind to do what was needed or expected.

Missing-links analyses together with chain analyses may be useful in figuring out the problem when you know what the effective behavior is but still do not do it. See below for an example.

C. Why Bother?

A missing-links analysis can be an invaluable tool for assessing situations when effective behaviors are repeatedly missing. As noted in discussing chain analysis, attempts to solve a problem often fail because the problem at hand is not fully understood and assessed.

An advantage of the missing-links analysis is that the questions can usually be asked and answered very rapidly.

✓ **D. How to Do It**

Tell clients: "Answer the questions on General Handout 8 until further questions would not be helpful or don't make sense. As soon as you get to that point, start problem solving."

For example, if a person did not know that an effective behavior was needed or expected, it is pointless to ask whether he or she was willing to do what was needed or expected. If a person is willful right from the start and decides not to engage in effective behavior, solving that problem is more important than asking whether the person thought about engaging in the behavior at a later point. If the thought of doing something effective never came to mind, asking what got in the way of effective behavior (other than never thinking of it) would not be very useful.

General Worksheet 3 (the missing-links analysis worksheet) is structured to identify the critical pieces of information necessary to understand and solve the missing behavior.

✓ **Practice Exercise:** Ask one participant to volunteer to have a missing behavior analyzed, and go through the questions and problem solving described on General Handout 8 and listed below. If time allows, do several examples.

> **1.** "Did you know what effective behavior was needed or expected?"
>
> If no, ask, "What got in the way of knowing?" Then stop questions and move to problem solving for what got in the way.
>
> If yes, move to Question 2.

2. "Were you willing to do the needed or expected effective behavior?"

If no, ask, "What got in the way of willingness to do an effective behavior?" Then stop questions and move to problem solving for lack of willingness.

If yes, move to Question 3.

3. "Did the thought of doing the needed or expected effective behavior ever enter your mind?"

If no, stop questions and move to problem solving for a way to get the thought to enter the participant's mind.

If yes, move to Question 4.

4. "What got in the way of doing the needed or expected effective behavior right away?"

Move to problem solving for what got in the way.

Make a concerted effort to generate a wide range of possible solutions. This can take more time than simply asking and answering questions. In a group setting, ask group members to help generate solutions. Refer to the problem-solving skill in the Emotion Regulation module if necessary (see Chapter 9, Section XI of this manual, and Emotion Regulation Handout 12: Problem Solving).

Discussion Point: Elicit from participants patterns of effective behaviors that are missing in their lives—or, if they cannot yet articulate a pattern, instances when they did not do something that was really important to do.

Practice Exercise: Ask one participant to volunteer to have a missing behavior analyzed, and ask another group member to volunteer to practice analyzing the missing behavior. Coach the person doing the analyzing. When doing so would not be disruptive to a group, encourage participants to analyze each other's missing homework behaviors.

Practice Exercise: When a person comes to skills training without doing all the homework assigned, hand out copies of General Worksheet 3 to each participant and have them fill it out as you ask the missing-links questions.

VIII. MISSING-LINKS ANALYSIS COMBINED WITH A CHAIN ANALYSIS (GENERAL HANDOUTS 7–8)

A complete analysis of missing behavior requires that you combine a missing-links analysis with aspects of a chain analysis of the same behavior. This should happen when the factors that contribute to you not doing something are complicated or are somehow preventing you from doing what is needed even when you know what that is. When this is the case, you start with a missing-links analysis and after question 4 switch to a chain analysis. Use the example below or one of your own to teach this.

Example 3: Missing behavior: I missed 45 minutes of a 1-hour weekly meeting at work that started at 8:30 A.M.

(Start with question 1 on General Handout 8 here.)

1. **Did I know what effective behavior was needed or expected?** Yes

2. **Was I willing to do what was needed?** Yes

3. **Did the thought of doing what was needed or expected ever enter my mind?** Yes

4. **What got in the way of doing what was needed or expected right away?** A chain of events.

(Start with question 2 on General Handout 7 or 7a here.)

Step 2. Describe the prompting event that started the chain of events: After I got up on time and made a cup of coffee, I brought in the morning newspaper. On the front page, there was an article about a scandal in our city that I was interested in and wanted to read [**beginning of the chain of events leading to being late**].

Step 3. **What made me vulnerable:** I had gone to bed late the night before. I had gotten little sleep, was very tired and moving slowly, and had little resistance to temptation.

Step 4. **The specific behaviors and events that were links in the chain:**

1st. As I was turning to the second page of the article, I glanced at the clock and saw that I did not have a lot of time.

2nd. I thought "Oh, well, I will dress really fast and get there on time."

3rd. The second page was really interesting, so I sat down for just a minute to read it.

4th. I was thinking I still had time.

5th. Just as I looked up at the clock and realized I really had to get a move on, . . .

6th. . . . the phone rang and it was my mother.

7th. I picked up the phone and started talking to her.

8th. Mom started chatting about something going on at home.

9th. I started worrying about getting off the phone to get to the meeting on time. (I still had time if I really put some energy into getting dressed, out of the house, and into the car to drive to work.)

10th. I felt guilty getting off the phone with Mom so fast.

11th. I stayed on the phone for 10 minutes (time I didn't have) listening to Mom.

12th. I finally did get off the phone.

13th. I saw the clock and realized I would be late by at least 10 minutes.

14th. I decided since I was going to be late anyway, I might as well not hurry.

15th. I finished reading the article.

16th. Then I dressed and left for work an hour after I usually leave.

Step 5. **The consequences of the behavior—the harm my behavior caused:**

a. **In the environment:** It took up the time of the people in the meeting who had to tell me what happened; it took time waiting to see whether I would be coming at the beginning; it made people feel less like I am a team player. People at the meeting were distressed that I was so late.

b. **For myself:** I felt guilty, and it also took a lot of my time to find out what had happened in the meeting.

Step 6. **Skills to replace problem links:**

2nd. Replace "Oh, well, I will dress really fast," with "I'd better dress now to be on the safe side; remind myself that when I read the paper before work, I am often late."

3rd. Don't sit down in the kitchen in the morning when I am tired.

7th. When I am running late, don't pick up the phone.

10th. Practice interpersonal skills to tell Mom I will call her later (and then call her!).

14th. Do pros and cons about giving up and giving in to being more late than necessary. Rush to get to work just a little bit late, rather than writing it off, relaxing, and being very late.

Step 7. **Ways to reduce my vulnerability in the future:**

■ Go to bed earlier to get more sleep (to reduce vulnerability).

■ Call Mom once a week, if only for a really brief chat (to reduce vulnerability).

Ways to prevent precipitating event from happening again:

- Stop taking the newspaper.
- Pick the paper up off the porch, but do not open it before work.

Step 8. Plans to repair, correct, and overcorrect the harm: I can apologize to my colleagues for being late, tell them I realize it is distressing when I come late, and let them know I will work harder at being on time in the future. I can be early for the weekly meetings of this group for the next 2 months, and I can offer to be the person who follows up on providing information to others who are late or miss a meeting. I can also offer to help other staff members out with tasks, and/or say yes when asked to help others out.

Discussion Point: Discuss other ideas for some or all of the questions as you go through the example.

References

1. Safer, D. L., Telch, C. F., & Chen, E. Y. (2009). *Dialectical behavior therapy for binge eating and bulimia.* New York: Guilford Press.
2. Dalai Lama. (2009, May 1–2). *Meditation and psychotherapy.* Conference held at Harvard University, Cambridge, MA.
3. Swenson, C. R., Witterholt, S., & Bohus, M. (2007). Dialectical behavior therapy on inpatient units. In L. A. Dimeff & K. Koerner (Eds.), *Dialectical behavior therapy in clinical practice: Applications across disorders and settings* (pp. 69–111). New York: Guilford Press.
4. Swenson, C. R., Sanderson, C., Dulit, R. A., & Linehan, M. M. (2001). The application of dialectical behavior therapy for patients with borderline personality disorder on inpatient units. *Psychiatric Quarterly, 72*(4), 307–324.

Mindfulness Skills

Mindfulness skills are central to DBT (hence the label "core" mindfulness skills for the first group of skills described below). The core skills are the first skills taught, and they underpin and support all of the other DBT skills. They are reviewed at the beginning of each of the other three skill modules and are the only skills highlighted throughout the entire treatment. DBT mindfulness skills are psychological and behavioral translations of meditation practices from Eastern spiritual training. Mindfulness skills are as essential for therapists and skills trainers to practice as they are for participants. Indeed, clinicians' practice of mindfulness has been found to be associated with a better therapeutic course and better outcomes.[1] Thus mindfulness practice is ordinarily the first agenda item in DBT treatment team meetings.

Mindfulness has to do with the quality of awareness or the quality of presence that a person brings to everyday living. It's a way of living awake, with eyes wide open. As a set of skills, mindfulness practice is the intentional process of observing, describing, and participating in reality nonjudgmentally, in the moment, and with effectiveness (i.e., using skillful means). In formulating these skills, I have drawn most heavily from the practice of Zen. But the skills are compatible with Western contemplative and other Eastern meditation practices, as well as with emerging scientific knowledge about the benefits of "allowing" experiences rather than suppressing, avoiding, or trying to change them. Both Eastern and Western psychologies, as well as spiritual practices, are converging on the same insights. Mindfulness practice per se was and is central to contemplative spiritual practices across denominations and beliefs, and the mindfulness practices included here may be incorporated into any individu-al's spiritual practices and beliefs. DBT, however, is specifically designed to be nondenominational (i.e., compatible with an array of beliefs and traditions), and thus practices are purposely provided in a secular format. No spiritual or religious convictions are expected or necessary for practicing and mastering these skills.

The mindfulness skills can also be thought of as the components that together make up the foundation for meditation practices taught in many psychological and stress reduction treatment packages (e.g., Mindfulness-Based Cognitive Therapy,[2] Mindfulness-Based Relapse Prevention,[3] Mindfulness-Based Stress Reduction[4]). In some ways, the mindfulness skills in DBT can be thought of as skills for beginners in mindfulness—that is, skills for individuals who cannot yet regulate themselves well enough to practice formal mindfulness meditation. They can also be thought of as skills for persons advanced in mindfulness—the skills such persons need to practice in everyday life. In this sense, these skills are the application of mindfulness meditation to everyday life.

What Is Mindfulness?

"Mindfulness" is the act of consciously focusing the mind in the present moment without judgment and without attachment to the moment. When mindful, we are aware in and of the present moment. We can contrast mindfulness with automatic, habitual, or rote behavior and activity. When mindful, we are alert and awake, like a sentry guarding a gate. We can contrast mindfulness with rigidly clinging to the present moment, as if we could keep a present moment from changing if we cling hard enough. When mindful, we are open to the fluidity of each moment as it arises and falls away. In "beginner's mind," each moment is a new beginning, a new and unique moment in time. We can contrast mindfulness with rejecting, suppressing, blocking, or avoiding the present moment, as if "out of mind" really did mean "out of existence" and "out of influence" upon us. When mindful, we enter into each moment.

"Mindfulness practice" is the repeated effort of bringing the mind back to awareness of the present moment, without judgment and without attachment; it includes, therefore, the repeated effort of letting go of judgments and letting go of attachment to current thoughts, emotions, sensations, activities, events, or life situations. In sum, mindfulness is a practice of entering into the current moment without reserve or grudge, entering into the cosmic process of existence with awareness that life is a process of constant change. Mindfulness practice teaches us to move into the moment and become aware of everything in it, functioning from there.

"Mindfulness everyday" is a way of living. It's a way of living with our eyes wide open. It is very difficult to accept reality with our eyes closed. If we want to accept what's happening to us, we have to know what's happening to us. We have to open up our eyes and look. Now a lot of people say, "I keep my eyes open all the time." But if we look at them, we'll see that they are not looking at the moment. They're looking to their past. They're looking to their future. They're looking to their worries. They're looking to their thoughts. They're looking to everybody else. They're looking absolutely everywhere else, except at the moment. Mindfulness as a practice is the practice of directing our attention to only one thing. And that one thing is the moment we are alive. The very moment we are in. The beauty of mindfulness is that if we look at the moment, just this moment, we will discover that we are looking at the universe. And if we can become one with the moment—just this moment—the moment cracks open, and we are shocked that joy is in the moment. Strength to bear the suffering of our lives is also in the moment. It's just about practice. It's not a type of practice where listening to it just once and going through it just once gets us there. Mindfulness is not a place we get to. Mindfulness is a place we are. It is the going from and coming back to mindfulness that is the practice. It's just this breath, just this step, just this struggle. Mindfulness is just where we are now, with our eyes wide open, aware, awake, attentive. It

can be extremely difficult. Things may come up that are difficult to bear. If that happens, we can step back, notice, let go. This moment will pass. Difficulty may come up again. It may be difficult again. We can look at it, let it go, let it pass. If it becomes too difficult at some moment, we can just gently stop. We can come another day, wait, and listen again.

"Meditation" is the practice of mindfulness while sitting or standing quietly for a period of time. Meditation is sometimes mistakenly thought to be the core of mindfulness. However, it is important not to confuse meditation and mindfulness. Although meditation implies mindfulness, the reverse is not necessarily so: Mindfulness does not require meditation. This distinction is very important. Although everyone can practice mindfulness, not everyone can practice meditation. Some cannot sit or stand still. Some are too terrified to look at their breath or watch their mind. Some cannot practice meditation now, but will be able to at a later point.

"Mindful meditation" is the activity of attending to, gazing, watching, or contemplating something. In Zen, for example, one is often given the instruction "Watch your mind." In other spiritual practices, one may be given words, texts, or objects to focus the mind on. In an art gallery, one stands or sits and gazes at artistic works. We attend to the chirp of the birds or the car engine sounding different than before. We watch the sun set and gaze at children frolicking in the park. Each of these is mindful activity. Although the term "meditation" is sometimes used to refer to thinking about something as in connection to the universe or the miracle of life, the more common understanding in secular circles is that of mindfulness. Just as common is the understanding that when one meditates, one is (usually) sitting quietly and is focusing on one's breath, one's bodily sensation, a word, or some other focus dictated by one's individual practice or tradition.

Meditation as a contemplative or mindfulness practice is both a secular practice, as in meditating on or contemplating art, and a religious or spiritual practice, as in contemplative prayer. Indeed, in all the major religions of the world, there is a tradition—however broad or narrow—of contemplative practice. This tradition within religions, often referred to as the "mystical" tradition, recommends mindfulness practices of various sorts and emphasizes spiritual experiences that may result from these practices. Whether mindful meditation and practice are secular or spiritual depends completely on the orientation and beliefs of the individual. For the spiritual person, mindfulness can be both a secular and a spiritual or religious practice.

In meditation and in mindfulness, there are two types of practices: "opening the mind" and "focusing the mind." Opening the mind is the practice of observing or watching whatever comes into awareness. In sitting meditation, it is simply noticing thoughts, emotions, and sensations that enter awareness without holding onto or pursuing them. It is like sitting and watching a conveyor belt going by—noticing what is going by on the conveyor belt, but not shutting off the belt to examine objects more closely. It is like sitting on a hill watching a harbor and noticing the boats entering and leaving without jumping onto one of the boats. For beginners or for persons with attention difficulties, opening the mind can be very difficult, because it is so easy to get caught up in a passing thought, emotion, or sensation and to lose the focus on awareness. For these individuals, focusing the mind is usually recommended.

When focusing the mind, one focuses attention on specific internal or external events. For example, when focusing on internal events, one might focus attention on a specific sensation succession (a series of sensations), emotions arising, thoughts going through the mind, or repeated words or phrases that have been decided before. For example, some schools of meditation give out mantras, or specific words to say with each breath. One instance of this is the "wise mind" practice (described below) of saying the word "wise" while breathing in and the word "mind" while breathing out. Another example is counting breaths (up to 10 and then starting over), which is a typical instruction in Zen. Guided mindfulness exercises given by clinicians or via meditation recordings give instructions of where and how to focus the mind. When focusing the mind externally one might focus on a leaf, a painting, a candle, another person or persons, or scenery, as in a walk in nature, a sunrise or sunset, and so forth.

There are also two stances one can take in practicing: either getting distance by pulling back and watching, or moving forward and becoming "what is" (by moving into what is being watched). Contrasts of these stances, stated in metaphorical language, are standing on a high mountain and picturing one's emotions as boulders far down below versus entering fully into the experience of one's emotions; sitting on the edge and watching the emptiness within oneself versus entering into and becoming the emptiness; noticing self-consciousness at a party versus throwing oneself completely into a party; and watching one's own sexual responses versus entering entirely into one's own sexual response.

Core Mindfulness Skills

States of Mind and the Mindfulness "Wise Mind" Skill

The core mindfulness skills are covered in Sections I–X of this module. In DBT, three primary states of mind are presented: "reasonable mind," "emotion mind," and "wise mind" (Section III). A person is in reasonable mind when he or she is approaching knowledge intellectually; is thinking rationally and logically; attends only to empirical facts; and ignores emotion, empathy, love, or hate in favor of being planful, practical, and "cool" in approaching problems. Decisions and actions are controlled by logic. The person is in emotion mind when thinking and behavior are controlled primarily by current emotional states. In emotion mind, cognitions are "hot"; reasonable, logical thinking is difficult; facts are amplified or distorted to be congruent with current affect; and the energy of behavior is also congruent with the current emotional state.

Wise mind is the synthesis of emotion mind and reasonable mind; it also goes beyond them: Wise mind adds intuitive knowing to emotional experiencing and logical analysis. In Mindfulness-Based Cognitive Therapy, two other states of mind are also discussed: "doing mind" or "doing mode" and "being mind" or "being mode."[5] Doing mind focuses on getting things done. It is multitasking, task-oriented, and driven. In contrast, being mind is "nothing-to-do" mind, where the focus is on experiencing rather than doing. These two states of mind are relevant to DBT mindfulness skills, because wise mind can also be considered as a synthesis of doing mind and being mind.

Mindfulness skills are the vehicles for balancing emotion mind and reasonable mind, being mind and doing mind, and other extreme sets of mind and action to achieve wise mind and wise action. There are three "what" skills (observing, describing, and participating). There are also three "how" skills (taking a nonjudgmental stance, focusing on one thing in the moment, and being effective).

Mindfulness "What" Skills

The mindfulness "what" skills are about what to do: "observe," "describe," and "participate" (Sections IV–VI). The ultimate goal of mindfulness skills practice is to develop a lifestyle of participating with awareness. Participation without awareness is a characteristic of impulsive and mood-dependent behaviors. Generally, paying special attention to observing and describing one's own behavioral responses is only necessary when one is learning new behaviors, when there is some sort of problem, or when a change is necessary or desirable. Learning to drive a stick-shift car, to dance, and to type are familiar examples of this principle. Consider beginning piano players, who pay close attention to the locations of their hands and fingers, and may either count beats out loud or name the keys and chords they are playing. As skill improves, however, such observing and describing cease. But if a habitual mistake is made after a piece is learned, a player may have to revert to observing and describing until a new pattern has been learned. This same deliberate reprogramming is necessary for changing impulsive or mood-dependent behavior patterns. Observing ourselves with curiosity and openness to what we will find can also, in time, lead to greater understanding and clarity about who we are. We find our "true selves" only by observing ourselves.

Observing

The first "what" skill (Section IV) is observing—that is, attending to events, emotions, and other behavioral responses, without *necessarily* trying to terminate them when they are painful or prolong them when they are pleasant. What the participants learn here is to allow themselves to experience with awareness, in the moment, whatever is happening—rather than leaving a situation or trying to terminate an emotion. Generally, the ability to attend to events requires a corresponding ability to step back from the event. Observing walking and walking are two different activities; observing thinking and thinking are two different activities; and observing one's own heartbeat and the heart's beating are two different activities. This focus on "experiencing the moment" is based on Eastern psychological approaches, as well as on Western notions of nonreinforced exposure as a method of extinguishing automatic avoidance and fear responses.

Describing

A second mindfulness "what" skill (Section V) is that of describing events and personal responses in words. The ability to apply verbal labels to behavioral and environmental events is essential for both communication and self-control. Learning to describe requires that a person learn not to take emotions and thoughts as accurate and exact reflections of environmental events. For example, feeling afraid does not necessarily mean that a situation is threatening to life or welfare. Many people confuse emotional responses with precipitating events. Physical components of fear ("I feel my stomach muscles tightening, my throat constricting") may be confused in the context of a particular event ("I am starting an exam in school") to produce a dysfunctional thought ("I am going to fail the exam"), which is then responded to as a fact. Thoughts ("I feel unloved" or "I don't believe anyone loves me") are often confused with facts ("I am unloved").

Participating

The third mindfulness "what" skill (Section VI) is the ability to participate without self-consciousness. A person who is participating is entering completely into the activities of the current moment, without separating him- or herself from ongoing events and interactions. The quality of action is spontaneous; the interaction between the individual and the environment is smooth and based in some part on habit. Participating can, of course, be mindless. We have all had the experience of driving a complicated route home as we concentrated on something else, and arriving home without any awareness of how we got there. But it can also be mindful. A good example of mindful participating is that of the skillful athlete who responds flexibly but smoothly to the demands of the task with alertness and awareness, but not with self-consciousness. Mindlessness is participating without attention to the task; mindfulness is participating with attention.

Mindfulness "How" Skills

The other three mindfulness skills are about *how* one observes, describes, and participates; they include taking a nonjudgmental stance ("nonjudgmentally"), focusing on one thing in the moment ("one-mindfully"), and doing what works ("effectively").

Nonjudgmentally

Taking a nonjudgmental stance (Section VII) means just that—taking a nonevaluative approach, not judging something as good or bad. It does not mean going from a negative judgment to a positive judgment. Although individuals often judge both themselves and others in either excessively positive terms (idealization) or excessively negative terms (devaluation), the position here is not that they should be more balanced in their judgments, but rather that judging should in most instances be dropped altogether. This is a very subtle point, but a very important one. The problem with judging is that, for instance, a person who can be "worthwhile" can always become "worthless." Instead of judging, DBT stresses the consequences of behavior and events. For example, a person's behavior may lead to painful consequences for self or others, or the outcome of events may be destructive. A nonjudgmental approach observes these consequences, and may suggest changing the behaviors or events, but would not necessarily add a label of "bad" to them. DBT also stresses accurate discrimination of one thing from another and description of what is observed. In discriminating, one determines whether a behavior meets a required definition or not. For example, a lawyer or judge can discriminate whether a certain behavior breaks the law or not. A diving judge can discriminate whether a diver's form matches the required form for the dive or not. Behavior may not be good or bad, but it can meet criteria for being against the law or for fitting the ideal model for a particular dive.

One-Mindfully

Mindfulness in its totality has to do with the quality of awareness that a person brings to activities. The second "how" skill (Section VIII) is to focus the mind and awareness in the current moment's activity, rather than splitting attention among several activities or between a current activity and thinking about something else. Achieving such a focus requires control of attention—a capability that many individuals lack. Often participants are distracted by thoughts and images of the past, worries about the future, ruminative thoughts about troubles, or current negative moods. They are sometimes unable to put their troubles away and focus attention on the task at hand. When they do become involved in a task, their attention is often divided. This problem is readily observable in their difficulties in attend-

ing to skills training sessions. The participants need to learn how to focus their attention on one task or activity at a time, engaging in it with alertness, awareness, and wakefulness.

Effectively

The third "how" skill (Section IX), being effective, is directed at reducing the participants' tendency to be more concerned with being "right" than with what is actually needed or called for in a particular situation. Effectiveness is the opposite of "cutting off your nose to spite your face." As our participants often say, it is "playing the game" or "doing what works." From an Eastern meditation perspective, focusing on effectiveness is "using skillful means." The inability to let go of "being right" in favor of achieving goals is often related to experiences with invalidating environments. A central issue for people who have been frequently invalidated is whether they can indeed trust their own perceptions, judgments, and decisions—that is, whether they can expect their own actions to be correct or "right." However, taken to an extreme, an emphasis on principle over outcome can often result in these individuals' being disappointed or alienating others. In the end, everyone has to "give in" some of the time. People often find it much easier to give up being right for being effective when it is viewed as a skillful response rather than as a "giving in."

Other Perspectives on Mindfulness

Three sets of supplementary mindfulness skills are included: mindfulness practice from a spiritual perspective; skillful means: integrating doing mind and being mind; and wise mind: walking the middle path (Sections XI–XVI). These skills add to and expand the core mindfulness skills described above, and each can be aligned with a spiritual perspective to a greater or lesser degree. They can be integrated into the teaching of the core skills, can be taught in an advanced skills course, or can be used in individual treatment settings as needed and as appropriate for the specific client.

Mindfulness Practice: A Spiritual Perspective

The focus on mindfulness from a spiritual perspective (Sections XI–XII) is included for a number of reasons. The practice of mindfulness itself has its origins in age-old spiritual practices. For many individuals, spirituality and religious practices are very important in their lives. Such practices can be important sources of strength and can also provide coping resources in difficult moments. Religious affiliation, in addition, can provide a community that often furnishes important spiritual and interpersonal support. Leaving out a recognition—and, indeed, a recruiting—of spirituality as a source of strength and sustenance when we discuss mindfulness practices, particularly mindful meditation, runs the risk of ignoring the spiritual diversity of the populations we treat. Including handouts on mindfulness from a spiritual perspective provides an avenue for helping clients strengthen their own spirituality and integrate it into their practices of mindfulness.

In contrast to the psychological goals of mindfulness, the goals of mindfulness from a spiritual perspective include experiencing ultimate reality as it is (something that is defined differently across cultures and religious practices), cultivating wisdom, letting go of attachments and radically accepting reality as it is, and increasing love and compassion toward self and others. For many, the practice of mindfulness also includes reflectiveness and the cultivation of ethical qualities. It is important here to keep in mind that spirituality and religion are two different things. Although there are many definitions of spirituality, a working definition is that it can be viewed as the "acknowledgment of a transcendent being, power, or reality greater than ourselves" (p. 14).[6] In particular, from this perspective, spirituality is a quality of the individual that has to do with regard for the spiritual, transcendent, or nonmaterial. As a practice, spirituality focuses on beliefs that in the universe "there is more than meets the eye"; that is, reality is not limited to what we can know via the material and sensory world. A spiritual perspective on mindfulness is designed to include every person. It is important here to recognize that spirituality can cover a vast terrain—from the community as a higher power (as is often said in 12-step groups), to humanistic views, mystical experience, religious practices, and (in DBT) wise mind.

Whereas spirituality is a quality of the individual, a religion is an organized community of individuals. Religions focus on beliefs, rituals, and practices oriented to bringing individuals within the community into closer relationship with the transcendent. Both spirituality and religion emphasize values and moral actions, and both can provide meaning, purpose, and hope to life. In particular, both can create meaning for those living lives of intense suffering. Purpose and hope can be extremely important in finding a way to build a life experienced as worth living.

Wise Mind from a Spiritual Perspective; Loving Kindness

Wise mind from a spiritual perspective (Section XIII) outlines different types of spiritual practices, as well as providing a list (see Mindfulness Handout 7a) of some of the many names and terms used with reference to the transcendent. It also provides a description of the experience of wise mind from this perspective. Many spiritual and religious practices share elements with mindfulness practices, including silence, quieting the mind, attentiveness, inwardness, and receptivity. These are characteristics of deep spiritual experiences. Many individuals have such experiences without any realization of their importance or validity. This handout helps both clients and clinicians understand such experiences. The emphasis across spiritual paths on love and compassion for even enemies is captured here in the mindfulness practice of loving kindness (Section XIV). Although written as a practice of wishing self and others well, it can also be practiced as brief prayers for the welfare of self and others.

How to Talk about Spirituality with Skills Training Participants

1. Do not be afraid to ask participants whether they are spiritual. If you need to define what you mean, you can say simply that it is the belief that "there is more to reality than what we can know through our senses." For those who are spiritual, you can ask whether they believe in God, a higher power, or the like.

2. Not only do you need to respect the spirituality (or its absence) of participants, but it is also important to set the tone in such a way that other group participants also act in a respectful manner.

3. Do no harm. Do not impose your own spirituality (or lack of it) on participants.

4. Find a path and a language that can be translated in multiple ways. Many of the notes provided in this chapter are aimed at giving you multiple ways to talk about various topics re-

lated to spirituality. You can also try to pick up on the language used by participants.

Notes for Agnostic Skills Trainers and Therapists

You do not need to be spiritual to teach mindfulness practice from a spiritual perspective. However, I suggest not teaching it if none of your participants are spiritual. A few clarifying points addressing common questions may make it easier for you to teach these skills.

1. *How do spirituality and therapy and skills go together?*

   The goal of psychotherapy and skills training is change. Change, however, requires acceptance of what is. The essential element across all spiritual and humanistic traditions is acceptance. Mindfulness emerged from spiritual contemplative practices. The common elements of contemplative practices are compassion, love, radical acceptance, and wisdom.

2. *Isn't this Buddhism or some other religion that I am not part of?*

   As noted in the earlier discussion of mindfulness, mindfulness is a practice that is nondenominational and transconfessional (i.e., it is compatible with an array of beliefs and traditions). Thus it is important to recognize that the "ultimate reality" that the spiritual person seeks to encounter can go by the name of God, Yahweh, the Great Spirit, Allah, Brahman, Atman, "no self," "emptiness," "essential essence," "essential nature," "the ground of being," "higher power," or a wide variety of other names. It is important for skills trainers to assist participants in linking the skills here to their own practices and terms.

3. *Isn't Zen a religion?*

   Zen is a practice, not a religion. Zen, Christian centering prayer, and many other contemplative and meditation practices across religions and cultures are similar in that they each focus on experiencing ultimate reality, however this is defined or understood. Although Zen was originally associated with Buddhism, as it has moved into Western culture it has expanded to embrace atheists, agnostics, and individuals across a wide variety of religious denominations and spiritual paths.

Skillful Means: Balancing Doing Mind and Being Mind

Among the growing number of treatments combining mindfulness meditation and yoga practices with behavioral interventions are Jon Kabat-Zinn's Mindfulness-Based Stress Reduction,[7] as well as Mindfulness-Based Cognitive Therapy[2] and Mindfulness-Based Relapse Prevention.[3] The latter two are also based on the work of Kabat-Zinn.[4] These treatments stress the differences between "doing mode" and "being mode." To bring these ideas into the fold of DBT, I have added the skill of skillful means (Section XV), and a handout focusing on the synthesis of these two concepts and titled Skillful Means: Balancing Doing Mind and Being Mind (Mindfulness Handout 9). Doing mind focuses on achieving goals; being mind focuses on present experiencing. Put another way, doing mind is "something-to-do" mind, and being mind is "nothing-to-do" mind. From a spiritual point of view, the difference between Martha and Mary in the Biblical story is that Martha was distracted by preparing what was needed for Jesus when he was visiting them, and Mary chose the "better part" by sitting at his feet and listening.[8] Being mind is the contemplative life path, and doing mind is the active life path. (For more on this topic, put the term "contemplative vs. active life" into your search engine.) The polarity between them is similar to that between reasonable and emotion mind. Wise mind brings the two into a synthesis. Without aspects of both being mind and doing mind, it is difficult if not impossible to lead a balanced life.

Wise Mind: Walking the Middle Path

"Walking the middle path" is living life between the extremes, or finding the synthesis between the extremes (Section XVI). This skill is, to a degree, a summary of previous skills with a few additions. The idea here is that mindfulness brings together opposites, finding the truth in alternate and opposite sides. As discussed previously, mindfulness skills focus on the synthesis of reasonable mind and emotion mind, as well as between doing mind and being mind. From a spiritual perspective, mindfulness skills bring together the material and the mystical—form and emptiness as one. (For a discussion of mysticism, see *Mysticism: Its History and Challenge* by Bruno Borchert.)[9] The two new oppositions have to do with finding the synthesis between acceptance on the one side and change on the other. In the first dichotomy, the main focus is on recognizing that one can give up attachments, as in radical acceptance of the moment, without at the same time suppressing the desire for change. The paradoxical point is that the very effort to reduce desire is itself a failure to radically accept desire. The supplementary skills in Chapter 8 include walking the middle path in the context of interpersonal relationships, with a particular emphasis on parent–teen relations. From a spiritual perspective, the middle path brings together the material and the mystical, form and emptiness, wise mind and the cloud of unknowing.[10, 28, 68] It is represented in the skills of replacing self-denial and asceticism with moderation, and replacing self-indulgence and hedonism with just enough satisfaction of the senses.

Managing Yourself Mindfully: Tips for Skills Trainers

What to Do When You Feel Judgmental

We skills trainers are often as likely to get judgmental as are our skills training participants. Like our participants, when we feel judgmental we often fail to take action or confront others and say what needs to be said, because we are afraid of coming across as judgmental to those we are working with. We start backing off and backing up, which lands us out of the moment and out of the flow. It is hard not to close up when we are afraid of something, and this is what usually happens when we will not confront another person for the fear of looking judgmental. As a skills trainer, what can you do to counteract this?

With colleagues, it can be helpful to start off by stating your fear of sounding judgmental and ask for help in reducing your judgmentalness. Practicing being nonjudgmental yourself is critical for the effectiveness of DBT in general, and for teaching mindfulness in particular. Consistent practice not only makes teaching nonjudgmentalness and confronting participants in a positive way much easier, but it also gives you support for getting back into the flow.

Although as a clinician you can speak about feeling judgmental with colleagues, you do not have the same luxury with skills training participants. Many individuals simply cannot tolerate the thought of their skills trainers' being judgmental, and they may blame themselves for the trainers' feelings of annoyance or irritation. What can you do to ease the situation at hand or prevent such a problem from unfolding?

■ *First, practice what you preach.* It is very difficult to engage in modeling nonjudgmentalness with participants if you are not consistently practicing the skill yourself. Practicing will help you quickly ease back into being nonjudgmental during a session if you start having difficulties.

■ *Second, practice opposite action when you feel judgmental.* The best way to do this is to start making validating statements in a situation that fills you with judgment (such as making comments about how the participants' behaviors are understandable, given current events or their history; how their behavior could not be otherwise, given the facts; etc.). Be sure to validate all the way, remembering to use a nonjudgmental voice tone. Keep talking until your judgmentalness goes down. Such comments constitute opposite action, and they are not unlike doing cognitive therapy on yourself. That is, as you speak to the participants, you are stating the nonjudgmental thinking that will ease you into nonjudgmental thinking yourself.

■ *Third, remember that acceptance is not a blank check for approval.* Although you may feel both the necessity and, simultaneously, the impossibility of acceptance when faced with extreme demands, egregious behavior, or untenable attacks, bear in mind that acceptance also entails accepting limits.

■ *Fourth, counteract the threat.* Judgmentalness and the anger that it breeds often have to do with your own fears, such as "If I cannot control this participant, he will commit suicide," "If I cannot get this point across, this participant will never get along with her daughter," or "I can't stand this one more second." In a skills training group, a very common threat is that one member's dysfunctional behaviors in the group will ruin skills training for other members. The function of judgmentalness here is often aimed at controlling these dysfunctional behaviors. In my experience, however, one of the fastest ways to lose control of another person is to try to control them. Although when a participant is highly suicidal, extremely aggressive, or passive, it can be *very* hard to control your own efforts to control the participant, nonetheless such self-control is often of paramount importance. How to do it? Use your skills! Check the facts (see Emotion Regulation Handout 8) and analyze clearly whether your feared outcomes are likely. Observe (see Mindfulness Handout 4) what is really going on, and ask wise mind (see Mindfulness Handout 3) whether your feared outcomes constitute a true catastrophe. Cope ahead (see Emotion Regulation Handout 19) can be useful for getting better at handling situations that you know precipitate judgmentalness in you. When you are with a participant or group, cheerlead yourself silently: In your mind, keep repeating cheerleading self-statements that counteract the threat (see Distress Tolerance Handout 9). I have used self-statements such as "Find the synthesis," "Therapy will work if I let it," "I can stand this," "I can manage this," "This is not a catastrophe," "My team will help me," and so on. At other times the threat is that you may be the cause of the problem you are trying to solve. This thought is such a threat that rather than try to solve the problem, you may immediately move to judgmental blaming of the participant. Opposite action for shame (see Emotion Regulation Handout 10) can be useful here. Talk with your participants and/or with your team about what you might have done to cause the immediate problem.

What to Do When You Slip Out of the Present

Often enough, we skills trainers respond not to a participant's action at the moment, but to a future action that could happen as a result of it. During a group session, for example, our thoughts about a participant may have the following trajectory: "What you are doing doesn't upset me, but it could get worse and upset the group; then other participants may drop out or not improve. My treatment will be a failure." When we are in a highly stressful moment with a participant who is angry at us or is attacking another group member, we have the option of throwing ourselves into the interaction of the moment matter-of-factly without malice, or we can sit there fuming and wait for the participant to come under control. Instead of treating the participants, we sometimes are waiting for them to quit being who they are. In a sense, we are washing dishes and thinking about having a cup of tea. As a skills trainer, what can you do to move yourself back into the present?

■ *Remind yourself that all you have to do in this moment is apply the treatment you are doing.* When you start thinking that you have to do therapy *and* control the participant, then you can get yourself into a mess. When you focus on thinking that all you have to do is apply the appropriate consequence to a functional or dysfunctional behavior when one appears, you will be in a much better place and shape. Ask yourself: What drives the need to hold up expectations and compare one reality to another? When your gauge inevitably misses the mark, you will get upset. To what extent is this going on with you?

■ *Take hold of the current moment.* If you find yourself slipping out of the moment and the nonjudgmental state, start observing physical sensations—the way you breathe, the way your body is positioned. Taking hold of the moment prevents venturing into the past or future. Being out of the moment may narrow your focus, reducing it to tunnel vision. It may also make getting distracted by other thoughts easier for you.

To Teach Mindfulness, Practice Mindfulness

Practice mindfulness both at home and at work. Ask yourself: Can a person who cannot play the piano teach piano? Can a person who has never done therapy teach therapy? Can a person who cannot hold a tennis racquet correctly teach tennis? Although there are types of behaviors you can teach even when you cannot do the behavior yourself (e.g., gymnastics), this is not the case with mindfulness. Thus it is extremely important that you, as a skills trainer, also have some type of mindfulness practice. Finding a mindfulness teacher can be very helpful, as can joining mindfulness practice groups, reading meditation/mindfulness/contemplative practice books (e.g., contemplative prayer books, Zen books), and attending mindfulness retreats led by teachers who have adequate credentials. Go to my website or blog to find Zen mindfulness retreats that I lead (*www.linehaninstitute. org/retreats.php*; *http://blogs.uw.edu/brtc/marsha-linehans-mindfulness-retreats*). There are many other teachers in the United States and internationally who also provide mindfulness and contemplative prayer retreats. Be sure to read the descriptions of the retreats, as schedules vary; in addition, some are primarily silent, and others have much more talking and discussion.

Selecting Material to Teach

There is a great deal of material for each skill in the mindfulness teaching notes on the following pages. You will not cover most of it the first time you teach specific skills. The notes are provided to give you a deeper understanding of each skill, so that you can both answer questions and add new teaching as you go. As in Chapter 6 (and throughout Part II of this manual), in this chapter I have put a checkmark (✓) next to material I almost always cover. On this manual's special website (*www.guilford.com/skills-training-manual*), I have put a star (★) on each handout that covers a standard DBT core skill not to be skipped. If I am in a huge rush, I may skip everything not checked (and on handouts without a star, I might skip them entirely or only review a few segments).

Also in this chapter (and in the rest of Part II), I have indicated information summarizing research in special features called "Research Points." The great value of research is that it can often be used to sell the skills you are teaching.

When you are teaching mindfulness skills (or any other DBT skills, for that matter), it is important that you have a basic understanding of the specific skills you are teaching. The first several times you teach, carefully study the notes, handouts, and worksheets for each skill you plan to teach. Highlight the points you want to make, and bring a copy of the relevant teaching note pages with you to teach from. Be sure to practice each skill yourself, to be sure you understand how to use it. Before long, you will solidify your knowledge of each skill. At that point, you will find your own favorite teaching points, examples, and stories and can ignore most of mine.

Teaching Notes

I. GOALS OF THIS MODULE (MINDFULNESS HANDOUTS 1–1A)

Main Point: The goal of practicing mindfulness skills for most people is to reduce suffering and increase happiness. For some, a goal of mindfulness is to experience reality *as it is.*

Mindfulness Handout 1: Goals of Mindfulness Practice. Briefly review the goals and benefits of mindfulness practice. Provide enough information to orient participants to the module, link the module to participant goals, and generate some enthusiasm and motivation for learning mindfulness skills. Summarizing one or two research findings can be very useful. It is common to cover the goals of practicing mindfulness and wise mind in one session. If you only have two sessions for mindfulness, start on some of the mindfulness "what" skills in the first session also. When time is short, you can skip this handout and teach the information orally and quickly.

Mindfulness Handout 1a: Mindfulness Definitions *(Optional).* This is an optional handout that you can give with or without review. The need for this handout depends on the sophistication level of the participants. If you do not give out this handout, it is important that you weave in at least some of its points as you teach.

Mindfulness Worksheet 1: Pros and Cons of Practicing Mindfulness *(Optional).* The worksheet is designed to help participants decide whether they have anything to gain from practicing mindfulness, particularly when they are feeling willful or apathetic and don't want to practice. It can be reviewed quickly if participants already know how to fill out a pros-and-cons worksheet. If not, instruct participants to fill out pros and cons both for practicing mindfulness skills and for not practicing. Also instruct them in how to rate intensity of emotions from 0 (the emotion is not there at all) to 100 (it would be impossible for the emotion to be more extreme). Explain that over time they will get better at rating their emotions, and the numbers will start to take on meaning. Numbers only mean something with reference to the person doing the rating. For example, an 80 for one person may be a 70 for another.

A. Goals of Mindfulness Practice

✓   💬 **Discussion Point:** Either before or after reviewing the handout, ask participants to check off each goal that is important to them in the boxes on the handout, and then share their choices. In what areas of their lives do they believe mindfulness might be of help?

Note to Leaders: With some participants, convincing them of the importance of mindfulness skills—which many have never heard of—can be a very hard sell. In these cases, it can be useful to let them know how widespread the teaching and practice of mindfulness are in many settings. For example, mindfulness practice is being taught in business schools, medical schools, and middle and high schools; it is also moving slowly into corporations.

✓   *1. Reduce Suffering and Increase Happiness*

- Reduce pain, tension, and stress.
- Increase joy and happiness.
- Improve physical health, relationships, and distress tolerance.
- Other goals that participants might have can also be discussed and written in the handout.

✓ **Research Point:** There is some evidence that the regular practice of mindfulness has beneficial effects. The major effects found for mindfulness alone include the following. Review several of these but not too many.

- Increased emotional regulation.[5]
- Decreased in both distractive and ruminative thoughts and behaviors.[11]
- Decreased dysphoric mood.[12]
- Increased activity of brain regions associated with positive emotion.[13]
- Enhanced immune response.[13]
- Decreased depression, anxiety.[14, 15]
- Decreased anger and emotional irritability, confusion and cognitive disorganization, and cardiopulmonary and gastrointestinal symptoms.[16]
- Reduction of pain symptoms, improvement of depressive symptoms in patients with chronic pain, and improvements in coping with pain.[17]
- Decreased psychological distress and increased sense of well-being.[18]
- Decreased risk of depression relapse or reoccurrence.[19]
- Increased healing of psoriasis.[20]
- Improved functioning of the immune system in patients with HIV.[21]

Most of these findings have been obtained with individuals who have practiced mindful meditation and yoga every day for eight or more weeks. Even very brief mindfulness practice, however, can be beneficial. In two of these studies, the mindfulness practice was very brief. More permanent and long-lasting gains, however, are likely to require a longer period of reasonably faithful practice.

✓ ## 2. Increase Control of Your Mind

Tell participants: "To a certain extent, being in control of your mind is being in control of your attention—that is, what you pay attention to and how long you pay attention to it."

■ *Increase your ability to focus your attention.* Say to participants: "In many ways, mindfulness practice is the practice of controlling your attention. With a lot of practice, you get better at it."[22] Explain that mindfulness reduces automaticity of attentional processes.[25]

■ *Improve your ability to detach from thoughts, images, and sensations.* Explain that often we react to thoughts and images as if they are facts. We get entangled in the events in the mind and cannot tell the difference between a fact in the world and thoughts or images of the world. Mindfulness, practiced often and diligently, can improve your skills of seeing the difference between facts and images and thoughts about facts.

Research Point: Acceptance and Commitment Therapy,[23] originally called Comprehensive Distancing Therapy,[24] focuses on just this: getting enough distance so that people can detach from their thoughts, images, and emotions. The central component of the therapy is teaching individuals how to step back and observe their minds—to see thoughts as thoughts, images as images, and emotions as emotions. Cognitive therapy also stresses the ability to differentiate thoughts, images, and emotions from facts.

■ *Decrease reactivity to mental events.* Say to clients: "Mindfulness is the practice of observing what is going on inside yourself as well as outside, without doing anything to change it. Thus, in some ways, you can consider it as a practice of observing things without reacting to or trying to change them. The ability to experience without reacting is essential in many situations. Mindfulness practice improves your ability to be less immediately reactive to everyday situations. It gives you a chance to take whatever time is needed before you react."

💬 **Discussion Point:** Draw from participants examples of how their inability to control their attention creates problems. Examples may include inability to stop thinking about things (e.g., the past, the future, current emotional pain or hurt, physical pain); inability to concentrate on a task when it is important to do so; and inability to focus on another person or to stay on a task because of distraction.

3. Experience Reality as It Is

✓   Ask participants: "If you walk across a dark room, is it better to see the furniture or not? Is it easier with the light on or with it off?" Explain that a fundamental goal of mind*fulness* is to reduce mind*lessness*—both of what is going on around us, and of what we ourselves are doing, thinking, and feeling.

The idea is that if we truly experience each present moment of our lives—if we let go of mental constructs, ideas, and judgments about what is—then we will ultimately see that our worst imaginings of reality are not true. We will at some point see that life itself is unceasing change, and also that clinging to any moment of reality is ultimately not in our best interests.

✓   **a. Be Present to Your Own Life**

Tell clients: "Mindfulness is the practice of being in the present. It is being present to your own life. Many people find at some point that their life is whizzing by and they are missing a lot of it. Children are growing up; friends that we care about are moving away; we are getting older. It is easy to be so focused on distractions, the past, or the future that we actually miss many positive things in our lives."

Example: "If you are walking in the forest, and you slightly change directions without knowing this, it may not take long before you are really far from where you were originally going."

✓   **Research Point:** Explain to clients that being present to our lives is the opposite of avoiding our lives and trying to avoid or suppress our experiences.

- Suppression increases the frequency of the very thoughts and emotions we are trying to suppress.[26, 27]
- Avoidance has no permanent effect on our well-being. When we avoid situations and events that prompt difficult emotions, this temporarily decreases the painful emotions, but it has no permanent effect on our response to these same situations and events in the future. When we avoid and escape painful emotions now, they will be painful in the future.
- Escape often causes more problems and rarely solves problems.

b. Be Present to Others

Mindfulness is focusing on the present moment and on the people we are with *now*. It is very easy to be around people but far away—thinking about something or someone else, looking for someone else to talk to, wishing we were somewhere else, planning what we will do next, dreaming about other things, focusing on our pain or our suffering. We are not present to the people around us. Others, of course, often notice this. They may eventually pull away from us; it is hard for them to be ignored in this way.

c. Experience Reality as It Is

■ *Connection to the universe.* Everyone and everything in the universe is connected. As physicists would point out, the universe is a network of interconnected atoms, cells, and particles that are constantly moving and changing. We touch the air around us that touches everything else around us, and on and on. Each move that we make interacts with the entire universe at some point. It is this point that we need to get across. However, knowing that we are interconnected is one thing; experiencing it is another.[28] Many people feel isolated and alone. Their experience of themselves is as outsiders. But once we see that the world and universe is an interconnected network, we can see that there is really no outside or inside. Thus our experience is built on the delusion of separation. Mindfulness is aimed at enhancing our experience of the universe as it is, without delusion or distortion.

■ *Essential "goodness."* Many individuals experience themselves as bad, unworthy, or somehow defective. Mindfulness is the practice of seeing ourselves as we are—ultimately simply ourselves and inherently neither good nor bad, but rather just as we are. From this perspective, all things in the universe, including ourselves, are good. (Although the use of the term "goodness" may seem to contradict the notion that "good" and "bad" are concepts in the mind of the observer, we cannot deny the use of "good" as an adjective and "goodness" as a term to denote a quality of something. Thus it is important not to move too far into a rigid notion that we can never use the term "good," as in my saying "Good boy" to my dog when he does something I have taught him, or "Good job" to a colleague at work. Once we have given up "good" and "bad" as judgments, we can revert to using them as shorthand comments about what is observed.)

■ *Essential validity.* "Validity" here means that each person has inherent significance which cannot be taken away or discounted. Each person's voice and needs warrant being heard and taken seriously. Each person's point of view is important.

💬 **Discussion Point:** Elicit from participants their own experiences of being connected to the universe, as well as experiences of being an outsider.

💬 **Discussion Point:** Elicit from participants their own experiences of being bad or unworthy, or of not being taken seriously. Discuss.

Note to Leaders: Sometimes individuals will be put off by references to Eastern meditation practice. You need to be very sensitive to this point. You can either divorce meditation from any religion or relate it to all religions.

1. The fact that meditation is now commonly used in the treatment of chronic physical pain and stress management programs, is increasingly being used in the treatment of emotional disorders, and is part of many wellness programs suggests that it can be practiced and be effective outside of any spiritual or religious context.

2. Eastern meditation practice is very similar to Christian contemplative prayer, Jewish mystical tradition, and forms of prayer taught in other religions.

Be alert to difficulties on this topic and discuss them. It is important not to push mindfulness onto religious participants if they start out by thinking of it as incompatible with their religion. Suggest that they practice what they can. Tell them to discuss it with others of the same religion. Give them time.

💬 **Discussion Point:** Ask participants how what you have said about mindfulness so far seems similar or different from their own spiritual practices.

B. Mindfulness Definitions

1. Universal Characteristics of Mindfulness

a. Intentionally Living with Awareness in the Present Moment

Explain that this means waking up from automatic or rote behaviors to participate and be present to our own lives.

b. **Without Judging or Rejecting the Moment**

Point out that this means noticing consequences, as well as discerning helpfulness and harmfulness—but letting go of evaluating, avoiding, suppressing, or blocking the present moment.

c. **Without Attachment to the Moment**

Emphasize that this means attending to the experience of each new moment, rather than ignoring the present by clinging to the past or grasping for the future.

> *Example:* "You can't be attached to having a newborn baby in the house, because quickly the baby will grow into a toddler."

2. *Mindfulness Skills*

"Mindfulness skills" are the specific behaviors that, put together, make up mindfulness.

3. *Mindfulness Practice*

a. **What It Is**

"Mindfulness practice" is the intentional practice of mindfulness and mindfulness skills. There are many methods of mindfulness practice.

b. **How It Can Be Practiced**

Mindfulness can be practiced at any time, anywhere, while doing anything. Intentionally paying attention to the moment, without judging it or holding on to it, is all that is needed.

c. **Meditation**

The similarities in meditation methods are much greater than the differences. Similarities are as follows:

- *Instructions to focus attention.* The focus is generally on either "opening the mind" to attend to all sensations and thoughts as they arise and fall away, or "focusing the mind" (which varies in what is attended to and may be a sacred word; a mantra given by a teacher; a word selected by the meditator; a story, event, phrase, or word; one's breath; sensations of the body and mind; or a large variety of other objects of focus).
- *Emphasis on observing nonjudgmentally,* without attachment or avoidance.
- *Emphasis on letting go of intellectual analyses* and logic, discursive thoughts, and distractions to gently bring oneself back to the practice, over and over again.
- *Letting the word or the practice do the work,* allowing oneself to go into the "cloud of unknowing"[29] and leave behind the "cloud of forgetting."
- *Carrying the practice into everyday life.*

d. **Contemplative or "Centering" Prayer**

Contemplative or "centering" prayer is a Christian mindfulness practice. Similar to meditation as described above, it emphasizes selecting a word to focus on. The difference is that contemplative prayer emphasizes a sacred word, interior silence, and the relationship with God within.[30] (See the work of Thomas Keating.[31])

e. **Mindfulness Movement**

Mindfulness movement has many forms:

- Dance (all religions; indigenous cultures)
- Martial arts (primarily Eastern religions)
- Walking or hiking with focused awareness on walking/moving and on the natural world
- Ritual music making (e.g., drumming)

C. The Importance of Practicing Mindfulness Skills

Emphasize to clients: "Mindfulness skills require practice, practice, practice. Mindfulness practice can be very difficult at first. Focusing the mind can take a lot of energy. Distractions may be frequent, and it is very easy to find that a few minutes after you started practicing your mindfulness skills, you have fallen out of it and are doing something else."

💬 **Discussion Point:** Discuss with participants the crucial importance of behavioral practice in learning any new skill. Behavioral practice includes practicing control of one's mind, attention, overt behavior, body, and emotions. Draw from participants their beliefs about the necessity of practice in learning: "Can you learn without practice?"

Example: "Mechanics have learned how to assess what is wrong with a car when it breaks down. It takes practice to be able to do that."

II. OVERVIEW: CORE MINDFULNESS SKILLS (MINDFULNESS HANDOUT 2)

> **Main Point:** Three sets of skills form the backbone of mindfulness practice: wise mind; the "what" skills of observing, describing, and participating; and the "how" skills of practicing nonjudgmentally, one-mindfully, and effectively.
>
> **Mindfulness Handout 2: Overview: Core Mindfulness Skills.** Use this handout for a quick overview of the skills. Do not teach the material from this handout unless you are skipping the related skill-specific handouts.
>
> **Mindfulness Worksheets 2, 2a, 2b: Mindfulness Skills Practice; Mindfulness Worksheet 2c: Mindfulness Core Skills Calendar.** These worksheets offer four variations for recording mindfulness skills practice. Each worksheet covers all of the mindfulness skills, and any one of them can be used with Mindfulness Handout 2 if you are using this handout as a review. Worksheet 2 provides space for recording practice of skills only twice between sessions; thus this worksheet can be a good starter worksheet with individuals you are trying to shape into more frequent skills practice. Worksheet 2a instructs participants to practice and gives multiple opportunities for each skill. Worksheet 2b calls for practicing each skill two times. Worksheet 2c is for those who like writing diaries and provides space for describing practice daily.
>
> These worksheets can be given again and again for each of the mindfulness skills if you do not want to use the worksheets specific to each skill. Either assign one worksheet to all participants (and bring copies of only one worksheet to the session), or allow participants to choose which worksheet they wish to fill out; giving them a choice increases their sense of control and may improve compliance. Bring new worksheets weekly to give to participants, so that they can incrementally mark the skills they practice.

✓ A. Wise Mind

Define "wise mind" for clients as "finding inside yourself the inherent wisdom that each person has within."

✓ B. "What" Skills

Tell clients that the "what" skills are "the skills that tell you *what* you should actually do when you practice mindfulness. There are three 'what' skills: observing, describing, and participating."

✓ C. "How" Skills

Explain to clients that the "how" skills are "the skills that teach you *how* to practice your mindfulness skills. Without the 'how' skills, you can veer far away from mindfulness itself. There are three 'how' skills: acting nonjudgmentally, one-mindfully, and effectively."

III. WISE MIND (MINDFULNESS HANDOUTS 3–3A)

> **Main Point:** Each person has inner wisdom. "Wise mind" is the mindfulness practice of accessing this inner wisdom. Entering the state of wise mind, we integrate opposites (including our reasonable and emotional states of mind), and we are open to experiencing reality as it is.
>
> **Mindfulness Handout 3: Wise Mind: States of Mind.** Because wise mind is a critical skill in DBT, this is not a handout that can be skipped. As you go through the concepts of "emotion mind," "reasonable mind," and "wise mind," it can be useful to draw the overlapping circles from the handout on the board and then fill them in. When trying to describe wise mind, it can be useful to draw a picture of a well in the ground (see Figure 7.1, p. 170) and use the drawing to explain the concept of "going within." You cannot ordinarily cover all the points about wise mind in one session; however, over several sessions you can cover most if not all points.
>
> **Mindfulness Handout 3a: Ideas for Practicing Wise Mind** *(Optional)*. It is useful to have this handout available, as it gives instructions for the various wise mind practice exercises.
>
> **Mindfulness Worksheet 3: Wise Mind Practice.** This worksheet lists several ways to practice wise mind, all described in more detail in Handout 3a. If you do not teach each type of wise mind practice, briefly describe them or tell participants that you will cover other ways of getting to wise mind in future classes. If you teach a different practice exercise, ask participants to write that exercise on their worksheet so that they will remember what it is. Next to each exercise on Worksheet 3, there are four boxes. Instruct participants to check off one box for every day they practice that exercise. If they practice more than four times in a week, put extra check marks outside the boxes. Review also how to rate wise mind practice. Note that the ratings are for how effective their practice was for getting into their own wise mind. These are not ratings of whether or not the practice calmed them or made them feel better. Also note at the bottom that the worksheet asks participants to list any and all wise things they did during the week. With some individuals, this may be an important worksheet or portion of a worksheet to give every week, even when you are not specifically teaching skills in the Mindfulness module.
>
> **Mindfulness Worksheets 2, 2a, 2b, 2c: Mindfulness Core Skills Practice.** These worksheets cover practice of all the core mindfulness skills, including the "what" and "how" skills. See the Section II overview for how to use these worksheets.

✓ **A. Wise Mind**

Wise mind is the inner wisdom that each person has. When we access our inner wisdom, we can say that we are in wise mind. Inner wisdom includes the ability to identify and use skillful means for attaining valued ends. It can also be defined as the ability to access and then apply knowledge, experience, and common sense to the situation at hand. For some people, accessing and applying their own inner wisdom are easy. For others, it is very hard. But everyone has the capacity for wisdom. Everyone has wise mind, even if they cannot access it at a particular point.

✓ **B. Reasonable Mind and Emotion Mind**

Reasonable mind and emotion mind are states of mind that get in the way of wise mind. Often what interferes with accessing our own wisdom is our state of mind at the time. We can be in different states of mind at different times. In one state of mind, we can feel, think, and act very differently than we do in another state of mind.

Example: A person might say, "I was out of my mind when I said that," meaning "I was not thinking clearly when I said that."

✓ **1. Emotion Mind**

Say to clients: "Emotion mind is your state of mind when your emotions are in control and are not balanced by reason. Emotions control your thinking and your behavior. When completely in emotion mind, you are ruled by your moods, feelings, and urges to do or say things. Facts, reason, and logic are not important."

✓ 💬 **Discussion Point:** Elicit from clients which emotions usually get in the way of their acting wisely.

a. Vulnerability Factors

Factors that make us all vulnerable to emotion mind include (1) illness; (2) sleep deprivation/tiredness; (3) drugs or alcohol; (4) hunger, bloating, overeating, or poor nutrition; (5) environmental stress (too many demands); and (6) environmental threats.

> *Example:* "You can wake up in emotion mind and be immediately worrying about work."

💬 **Discussion Point:** Elicit other vulnerability factors from participants.

b. Benefits of Emotions

Emotions, even when intense, can be very beneficial. Intense love fills history books as the motivation for relationships. Intense love (or intense hate) has fueled wars that in turn have transformed cultures (e.g., fighting to stop oppression and murders as in the battle against the Nazis). Intense devotion or desire motivates staying with very hard tasks or sacrificing oneself for others (e.g., mothers running through fires for their children). A certain amount of intense emotion is desirable. Many people, particularly those with emotional problems, have more intense emotions than most. Some people are the "dramatic" folks of the world and will always be so. People with intense emotions are often passionate about people, causes, beliefs, and the like. There are times when emotion mind is the cause of great feats of courage or compassion—when if reason were there at all, a person would not overcome great danger or act on great love.

c. Problems with Emotions

Problems occur when emotions are ineffective and control us. Emotions are ineffective when the results are positive in the short term but highly negative in the long term, or when the emotional experience itself does not fit the facts of our lives and is very painful, or when it leads to other painful states and events (e.g., anxiety and depression can be painful in themselves).

d. Different Effects of Emotions

Sometimes people become so emotional that they shut down and act like automatons. They may dissociate and appear very, very calm. Or they may isolate themselves, staying very quiet. They appear cool, deliberate, and reasonable, but their behavior is really under the control of overwhelming emotions that they would experience if they let go and relaxed. This is emotion mind; emotions are in control. At other times, of course, emotion mind looks, thinks, talks, and acts in very extreme ways.

✓ ### e. The Difference between Strong Emotion and Emotion Mind

Tell clients: "Don't confuse being highly emotional with emotion mind." Emotion mind is what occurs when *emotions are in control* at the expense of reason. People often have intense emotions *without* losing control. For example, holding one's newborn baby, walking up to receive an award, or finding out a loved one has died can each elicit intense emotions of love (for the baby), pride (at getting the award), or grief (over the loved one's dying). Each of these would be emotion mind only if the emotions crowded out reason and effectiveness.

✓   **2. Reasonable Mind**

Say to clients: "Reasonable mind is the extreme of reason. It is reason that is not balanced by emotions and values. It is the part of you that plans and evaluates things logically. When completely in reasonable mind, you are ruled by facts, reason, logic, and pragmatics. Emotions, such as love, guilt, or grief, are irrelevant."

a. Benefits of Reason

Reason can be very beneficial. Without it, people could not build homes, roads, or cities; they could not follow instructions; they could not solve logical problems, do science, or run meetings. Explain to clients: "Reason is the part of you that plans and evaluates things logically. It is your cool part. But, again, when you are completely in reasonable mind, you are ruled by facts, reason, logic, and pragmatics. Values and feelings are not important."

✓   **b. Problems with Reason**

Reasonable mind is cold and dismissive of emotions, needs, desires, and passion. This can often create problems.

Example: A hired assassin coolly and methodically planning the next murder is in reasonable mind.

Example: A task-focused person attending only to what must be done next, and ignoring even loved ones who want at least a nod hello, is in reasonable mind.

Say to clients: "It is hard to make and keep friends if you are only in reasonable mind. Relationships require emotional responses and sensitivity to others' emotions. When you ignore your own emotions and treat other people's emotions as unimportant, it is hard to maintain relationships. This is true about relationships in multiple settings—in families, with friends, and in work environments."

💬 **Discussion Point:** When other people say that "If you could just think straight, you would be all right," they mean "If you could be reasonable, you would do OK." Elicit from participants times other people have said or implied that if they would just not distort, exaggerate, or misperceive things, they would have far fewer problems. How many times have participants said the same thing to themselves?

💬 **Discussion Point:** Discuss pros and cons of emotion and reason. Draw from participants their experiences of being in reasonable mind and in emotion mind.

✓ **C. Wise Mind as the Synthesis of Opposites**

Explain to clients: "Wise mind is the integration of opposites: emotion mind and reasonable mind. You cannot overcome emotion mind with reasonable mind. Nor can you create emotions with reasonableness. You must go within and bring the two together."

> **Note to Leaders:** You do not need to cover each of the following points on wise mind every time through. Give just enough to get your point across. After making a few points, do one of the exercises described below before continuing with more information. You will be covering this section many times. Expand on your points a bit more each time through. (See Chapter 7 of the main DBT text for a fuller discussion of wise mind.)

✓   **1. Everyone Has Wise Mind**

Everyone has wise mind; some people simply have never experienced it. Also, no one is in wise mind all the time.

> **Note to Leaders:** Participants will sometimes say that they don't have wise mind. You must cheerlead here. Believe in participants' abilities to find wise mind. Use the metaphor that wise mind is like having a heart; everyone has one, whether they experience it or not. Use the "well" or "radio channel surfing" analogies below. Remind them that it takes practice to access and use wise mind.

2. Wise Mind Is Sometimes Experienced as a Particular Place in the Body

People sometimes experience wise mind as a particular point in the body. This can be the center of the body (the belly), or in the center of the head, or between the eyes. Sometimes a person can find it by following the breath in and out.

💬 **Discussion Point:** Elicit from participants where they think (or suspect) wise mind is within themselves.

3. It Is Not Always Easy to Find or Even Be Sure about Wise Mind

✓   �֎ **Story Point:** "Wise mind is like a deep well in the ground." (See Figure 7.1; show clients a copy of this figure, or draw it on the whiteboard or blackboard.) "The water at the bottom of the well, the entire underground ocean, is wise mind. But on the way down, there are often trap doors that impede progress. Sometimes the trap doors are so cleverly built that you actually believe there is no water at the bottom of the well. The trap door may look like the bottom of the well. Perhaps it is locked and you need a key. Perhaps it is nailed shut and you need a hammer, or it is glued shut and you need a chisel. When it rains emotion mind, it is easy to mistake the water on top of the trap door for wise mind."

Emotion mind and wise mind both have a quality of "feeling" something to be the case. The intensity of emotions can generate experiences of certainty that mimic the stable, cool certainty of wisdom. Continue the "well within" analogy above: "After a heavy rain, water can collect on a trap door within the well. You may then confuse the still water on the trap door with the deep ocean at the bottom of the well."

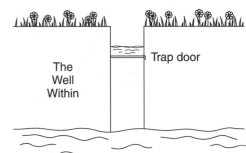

FIGURE 7.1. The well within: An illustration of wise mind.

💬 **Discussion Point:** Ask participants for other ideas on how to tell the difference between wise mind and emotion mind. There is no simple solution here. Suggest: "If intense emotion is obvious, suspect emotion mind. Give it time; if certainty remains, especially when you are feeling calm and secure, suspect wise mind."

✓   *Example:* Extreme anger often masquerades as wise mind. When really angry, we often think we are absolutely right in everything we think!

4. Wise Mind Is the Part of Each Person That Can Know and Experience Truth

It is where a person knows something to be true or valid. It is where the person knows something in a centered way.

5. Wise Mind Is Similar to Intuition

Wise mind is like intuition—or, perhaps, intuition is part of wise mind. It is a kind of knowing that is more than reasoning and more than what is observed directly. It has qualities of direct experience; immediate knowing; understanding the meaning, significance, or truth of an event without having to analyze it intellectually;[32] and "feelings of deepening coherence."[33]

6. Wise Mind Is Free of Conflict

✓   Tell clients: "In wise mind, you are free from conflict, making wise action almost effortless (even when it is difficult beyond words). Wise mind has a certain peace."

Example: "You are determined to pass a difficult college course or get a good evaluation at work. You have an assignment that will take up a lot of your time, and you would really like to just sit home and relax. But you think about the consequences of failing and know you will work on it."

✓   *Example:* "You are with your daughter in a boat on the river. You know how to swim, but your child does not, and she falls into the water. You immediately jump into the river to save her, even though the water is freezing."

Example: "You are deciding on a major for a program you're taking. One choice involves taking only classes you're likely to do well in without a lot of effort, but you don't like the job options afterward; the other choice involves taking more challenging classes, but getting specialized training for jobs you really like. In wise mind, you make the decision to go with what you like, even if it's harder."

> **Note to Leaders:** It is important here to point out that a goal of mindfulness and wise mind is not to make life all effort and work, work, work. Most people do not have to work all the time at keeping themselves regulated, doing things to keep their life on track, and moving toward their goals. The idea is to practice skills enough so that life gets easier and better. Wise mind is the road to that: In wise mind, it is easier to act in our own best interests instead of being controlled by our moods and emotions.

7. Wise Mind Depends on Integrating Ways of Knowing

Wisdom, wise mind, or wise knowing depends upon integration of all ways of knowing: knowing by *observing*, knowing by analyzing *logically*, knowing by what we *experience* in our bodies (kinetic and sensory experience), knowing by *what* we *do*, and knowing by *intuition*.[34]

8. Finding Wise Mind Consistently Can Take a Lot of Practice

� **Story Point:** "Learning to find wise mind is like searching for a new channel on the radio. First you hear a lot of static, and you can't make out the lyrics of the music—but over time, if you keep tuning in, the signal gets louder. You will learn to know right where the station is, and the lyrics become a part of you, so that you can access them automatically—just like you can finish the lyrics immediately if someone starts singing a song you know really, really well."

💬 **Discussion Point:** Elicit feedback from participants on their own experiences of wise mind.

💬 **Discussion Point:** Wise mind is getting to the heart of a matter. It is seeing or knowing something directly and clearly. It is grasping the whole picture when before only parts were understood. It is "feeling" the right choice in a dilemma, when the feeling comes from deep within rather than from a current emotional state. Elicit similar experiences and other examples from participants.

💬 **Discussion Point:** Wise mind may be the calm that follows the storm—an experience immediately following a crisis or enormous chaos. Sometimes a person may reach wisdom only when suddenly confronted by another person. Or someone else may say something insightful that unlocks an inner door. Elicit similar experiences and other examples from participants.

✓ D. Ideas for Practicing Wise Mind

1. About the Exercises

Conduct at least one or two practice exercises for going into wise mind, and be sure to describe several different methods of getting into wise mind. Of the exercises described below, I have found these to be most important: 1, 2, 4 (or 5), 6, and 8. Participants ordinarily have no idea what you are talking about until you do some practice exercises with them. Start with either Exercise 1 (stone flake on the lake) or 2 (walking down the spiral stairs) to give participants a sense of going within, or 3 (breathing "wise" in, "mind" out). Then select one or two more that you have tried yourself, or that you think your participants would like or find useful. You can give out Mindfulness Handout 3a: Ideas for Practicing Wise Mind. Although each exercise is also listed on Mindfulness Worksheet 3: Wise Mind Practice, having a handout can be useful, since participants often write all over, turn in, or throw away their worksheets. Briefly describe the exercises you do not do with them, so that, if they wish, they can practice these others by themselves.

Recommend that participants keep their eyes open when practicing mindfulness. The idea is to learn to be mindful and in wise mind in everyday life. Most of each day is lived with eyes open. Learning to be mindful with eyes closed may not generalize to everyday life with eyes wide open. That said, however, some teachers recommend closing eyes during many mindfulness and contemplative practices. Although it can be a matter of preference, it can also be a practice of willingness (distress tolerance) and mindfulness itself to keep eyes open and simply notice the discomfort (usually not too long lasting). At the beginning of mindfulness practice, this is definitely not a point worth arguing about. Encourage participants who are used to mindfulness or contemplative prayer with their eyes closed to try it for a while with eyes open. The first two exercises below (1 and 2) call for eyes closed.

2. General Steps for Leading Mindfulness Practice Exercises

- *Practice an exercise yourself* before you try to teach it.
- *Tell a story, present a problem, or describe a situation* that hits on a universal theme, to get the attention and interest of participants.
- *Relate the story, problem, or situation to yourself,* to highlight the importance of the skill or exercise being taught. This modeling can be particularly useful if participants are emotionally attached to you as the leader, since you are clearly asking them to try something that is important in your own life and you believe may be important in their lives also.

Example: "I was faced with a really big decision about where to send my child to kindergarten. Two schools were very good but had different strengths and weaknesses. I needed to be clear about what was really most important to me. In making my decision, it was important for me to access wise mind."

- *Orient participants to the reason for the exercise or practice.* People are less likely to try an exercise if they have no idea how it relates to themselves and their own personal goals. Make it clear that "this is an exercise that helps you get into wise mind," and explain how.
- *Remind participants to get in a "wide-awake" posture* (i.e., one where they will be likely to stay awake). Ordinarily, participants in a skills training group will be sitting in a chair. If so, it is best for them to keep both feet on the floor and sit in a posture that is likely to keep them both alert and comfortable.
- *Give clear and concise instructions* telling participants exactly what to do. See below for scripts. Demonstrate exercise if need be. Do not instruct participants to do more than one thing at the same time (e.g., count your breath and pay attention to sensations as they arise). If the instructions are brief and easily remembered, give instructions at the start of the practice. If the instructions are complicated and what participants do changes over time, give an overview before starting and then give instructions in sequence during the exercise. Even

for brief instructions, it can be helpful to make occasional guiding comments during the exercise to help individuals keep their focus. So that you don't distract participants during exercise, speak in a soft but steady voice, with brief instructions and pauses.

■ *Instruct participants on what to do if they get distracted.* Tell participants that if they get distracted, notice that they have stopped the exercise, or get lost, they should simply notice this and gently bring themselves back to the practice, starting over at the beginning. Remind participants to avoid judging themselves. The practice of noticing distractions and then coming back to the practice *is* the practice.

■ *Signal the start and end of the practice.* You can do this by using a mindfulness bell (e.g., "To start, I will ring the bell three times, and to stop, I will ring the bell once"), or you can signal verbally (e.g., "Start now," and at the end, "When you are ready, open your eyes," or "Bring yourself back to the room.").

■ *Invite participants to share and comment on their experiences.* This sharing is a critical part of the practice and should not be skipped. Going around the circle will usually be the quickest way, as it eliminates long waits between sharing. Allow individuals to say they don't want to share if they wish. In most groups, it is best to discourage cross-talk (i.e., responding to others' comments, discussing others' experiences). However, it can be useful to allow questions of fact or interpretation (e.g., "Did you say X?" or "I don't understand what you mean by XYZ; can you say more?").

■ *Give corrective feedback and troubleshoot.* This is a critical part of mindfulness teaching. It is particularly important to remind participants consistently that the goal of mindfulness practice is mindfulness practice.

3. Scripts for Exercises

> **Note to Leaders:** When reciting your script, your tone of voice and pace are of crucial importance. Try to use a low, gentle, semihypnotic tone; speak slowly; and leave pauses as you go. Bring people out of imagery gently.

✓ **a. Exercise 1: Imagining Being a Stone Flake on the Lake**

Start instructions with a soft voice, with pauses (. . .) as you go, using the following script (or something similar): "Sit in a comfortable but attentive position. Close your eyes. . . . As you sit there, focus your mind on your breath. . . . Attend to your breath coming in . . . and your breath going out . . . as you breathe naturally in and out. . . . " Then say something like this:

"Imagine you are by a lake on a warm sunny day. . . . It is a large, clear, very blue lake. . . . The sun is shining warmly on the lake. . . . Imagine that you are a small . . . stone . . . flake from a piece of stone near the lake, and imagine being gently tossed out onto the lake . . . out to the middle of the lake . . . skimming onto the cool, . . . clear, . . . blue . . . waters of the lake. . . . Imagine that you are slowly . . . very slowly floating down in the lake . . . noticing all that is in the lake as you gently float down . . . floating down in the cool, clear blue waters . . . gazing at what is around you . . . and now settling on the clear bottom of the lake, . . . at the center of the lake . . . gazing at the clear waters and what is nearby. . . . And when you are ready, open your eyes, come back to the room, trying to maintain your awareness of that clear center that is within you."

✓ **b. Exercise 2: Imagining Walking Down the Inner Spiral Stairs**

As with Exercise 1 above, start instructions with: "Sit in a comfortable but attentive position. Close your eyes. . . . As you sit there, focus your mind on your breath. . . . Attend to your breath coming in . . . and your breath going out . . . as you breathe naturally in and out. . . . " Then say something like this:

"Imagine there is an inner spiral staircase within you. . . . Imagine that you are walking down the staircase . . . going at your own pace . . . making the staircase as light or as dark as you wish . . . with as many windows as you wish . . . walking slowly down . . . and as you walk, noticing if you are tired or afraid . . . sitting down on the steps if you wish . . . walking down the stairs . . . as steep or as shallow as you wish . . . light or dark . . . noticing as you walk down moving toward your very center . . . toward your own wise mind . . . toward wisdom . . . simply walking down at your own pace . . . stopping and sitting when you arrive at a still point. . . . And when you are ready, open your eyes, come back to the room, trying to maintain your awareness of that clear center that is within you."

✓ **c. Exercise 3: Breathing "Wise" In, "Mind" Out**

Start instructions "Finding wise mind is like riding a bike; you can only learn it by experience. Keeping your eyes open, find a good place to rest your eyes . . . " as described above for Exercises 1 and 2. Then say:

"As you breathe in . . . say silently to yourself the word 'Wise' . . . and as you breathe out . . . say silently to yourself the word 'Mind.' . . . Continue saying 'Wise' as you breathe in . . . and 'Mind' as you breathe out."

Note to Leaders: You can substitute "Wise mind in" and "Wise mind out." You or participants may have other words that work better for various individuals, and that is fine.

d. Exercise 4: Asking Wise Mind a Question (Breathing In) and Listening for the Answer (Breathing Out)

Start instructions as described above for Exercise 3. Then say:

"As you inhale, ask yourself a question (e.g., What can I feel good about myself? Should I accept this job?). As you exhale, listen (don't talk, don't answer) for the answer. . . . Keep asking with each breath in and listening with each breath out. . . . See if an answer comes to you. . . . If not, perhaps there is no answer now."

Note to Leaders: The practice of asking wise mind a question and listening for the answer is in line with research showing that the impact of self-talk in interrogative form (questions) on future behavior may be different from the impact of declarative talk (assertions). Self-posed questions may lead to thoughts about intrinsic motivation to pursue a goal, leading the person to form intentions about that goal and increasing the likelihood of the person's performing behaviors linked to the goal.[35]

e. Exercise 5: Asking, "Is This Wise Mind?"

Start instructions as described above for Exercise 3. Then say:

"Bring to mind something you want to do or something you don't want to do, an opinion you have, or something you are doing right now. . . . Focus your mind on your breath . . . notice your breath coming in and your breath going out as you breathe naturally . . . in and out. As you inhale, . . . ask yourself, 'Is this wise mind?' . . . ('Is eating a second dessert wise mind?' 'Is not going to my therapy session wise mind?'). As you exhale, listen (don't talk, don't answer) for the answer. . . . Keep asking with each breath in and listening with each breath out. . . . See if an answer comes to you. . . . If not, perhaps there is no answer now, or perhaps you are too ambivalent to know the answer."

Note to Leaders: Exercise 5 is one you should definitely practice with participants. Accessing wise mind is one of the most important DBT skills. The questions can be anything: "What do I have to be proud of—

to help me feel good about myself?" "Should I continue to smoke pot?" "Do I really love him?" (While storming out of skills training early:) "Is this wise mind?" (When adamantly disagreeing with someone:) "Is this wise mind?"

f. Exercise 6: Attending to the Breath/Letting Attention Settle into the Center

Note to Leaders: Attending to one's breath is the most universal mindfulness practice. It can be woven into teaching about wise mind without a lot of orientation beforehand. It can be done with just a few breaths, while clients are sitting down, standing, or walking. It is very important to help participants let go of expectations about breathing. Expecting breaths to become slow or deep, expecting any other specific type of breath, or expecting to relax or feel differently while practicing can induce panic responses and actually interfere with experiencing wise mind. For some individuals, simple focusing on breathing for any extended length of time is not possible. As one participant once said, "I don't do breathing."

For many, a focus on breath alone allows their mind to generate trauma memories, ruminating thoughts, and traumatic and/or painful images. Extreme emotion and/or dissociation may be the result. Others get agitated immediately when they focus on their breathing. For these individuals, a shaping process is needed, and it may take a long time and/or exposure-based treatment before meditative breath focus becomes possible. For others, difficulties with attention or with sitting or standing still can make prolonged attention to breathing very difficult. The difficulties those with severe disorders often have with meditation practices are the principal reason why DBT does not require meditation (i.e., focus on breath) for individuals who cannot tolerate it.

Start instructions as described above for Exercise 3. Then say:

> "As you sit there, focus your mind on your breath . . . attend to your breath coming in and your breath going out . . . as you breathe naturally in and out. . . . Attending to your breath coming in and out, . . . letting your attention settle into your center . . . at the bottom of your breath when you inhale . . . just near your gut or in the center of your forehead. That very centered point is wise mind . . . as you breathe in and out . . . keeping your attention there at your very center . . . in your gut."

g. Exercise 7: Expanding Awareness

Note to Leaders: Begin this exercise by having participants attend to the breath for a few minutes and then expand their awareness. It is important that participants keep their eyes open during this exercise. You might add to the instructions, "Keeping your eyes focused where they are now, expand your awareness to the walls or to the floor or table." Most people will definitely notice the difference when taking this extra step.

Start instructions as described above for Exercise 3. Then say:

> "As you inhale and exhale normally, not changing your breathing . . . let your attention settle into your center . . . just near your gut. . . . As you breathe in and out . . . keeping your attention there at your very center . . . in your gut, gently expand your awareness to the greater space around you . . . not changing the focus or your eyes, but expanding the focus of your awareness . . . with widened awareness, keeping your primary awareness at your center."

Discussion Point: Ask participants to share their experience with expanding awareness, and to discuss how this is different from activities where they are so focused on a task, a game, or an interaction that they become oblivious to everything around them. The ability to be focused but aware of our surroundings is like that of a mother who, while working at home, is constantly aware of where her young child is. Contrast this with becoming lost in computer games, watching TV, or engaging in any other behavior patterns that can become addictive. Discuss the implications of this contrast with participants.

h. Exercise 8: Dropping into the Pauses between Inhaling and Exhaling

Start instructions as described above for Exercises 3. Then say:

"As you inhale, bring your attention up with your breath . . . notice the very top of your breath . . . at the top of your chest. Notice the very slight pause before your exhale. . . . As you reach this pause, drop yourself and your attention into the pause. . . . Notice as you exhale, letting your attention travel down with your breath. At the very bottom of your exhalation, before you inhale, drop yourself and your attention into that pause. . . . Continue breathing in and out, dropping yourself into the pauses, into wise mind."

> **Note to Leaders:** Some participants simply cannot do Exercise 8. It sounds incomprehensible and weird to them. Other participants, perhaps those with a poetic bent, love the exercise. Be prepared with another exercise when you plan to use this one.

✓ **E. Review of Between-Session Practice Exercises for Wise Mind**

Mindfulness Handout 3a lists all of the ideas described above for practicing wise mind. It is important to go over some of these if they are not practiced in the session.

IV. MINDFULNESS "WHAT" SKILLS: OBSERVE (MINDFULNESS HANDOUTS 4–4A)

Main Point: There are three mindfulness "what" skills and three mindfulness "how" skills. "What" skills are what we do when practicing mindfulness, and "how" skills are how we do it. The three "what" skills are observing, describing, and participating. Observing is paying attention on purpose to the present moment.

Mindfulness Handout 4: Taking Hold of Your Mind: "What" Skills. First, give a brief overview of each "what" skill. The key points are on this handout. Point out that a person can only do one thing at a time—observe, or describe, or participate—but not all three at once. If you are trying to teach all the core mindfulness skills in two sessions, cover wise mind and the "what" skills in their entirety in the first session. Observing, the first "what" skill, is fundamental to all mindfulness teaching and thus must be covered until participants understand what the practice is. Be sure to conduct practice exercises for observing before moving to the next skill. You will have a chance to do further teaching on these skills during the review of homework practice in the next session. These skills are best learned by practice, feedback, and coaching.

Mindfulness Handout 4a: Ideas for Practicing Observing *(Optional)*. This multipage handout gives instructions for three types of observing exercises: "coming back to your senses," "focusing the mind," and "opening the mind." It's useful to have this handout in the session. If you distribute the handout, be sure to describe (at least briefly) the differences between these three types of observing. For some groups of participants, these handouts may be overwhelming or confusing, and giving specific practice assignments may be more useful.

Mindfulness Worksheet 4: Mindfulness "What" Skills: Observing, Describing, Participating; Mindfulness Worksheet 4a: Observing, Describing, Participating Checklist; Mindfulness Worksheet 4b: Observing, Describing, Participating Calendar. These three worksheets offer three different formats for recording practice of mindfulness "what" skills. Worksheet 4 asks participants to practice mindfulness skills only twice between sessions. Worksheet 4a instructs participants to practice and gives multiple opportunities for each skill, as well as multiple check boxes for each skill. Worksheet 4b is aimed at participants who like to write. Assign one worksheet to all participants, or allow participants to choose; choosing may give them a greater sense of control and possibly improve adherence.

For participants new to mindfulness skills, asking them to practice all three "what" skills in a single week can be too much. It can be useful to ask which skill each participant has the most trouble with. For example, a person who has ADHD, or who ruminates a lot or gets completely lost in the moment, may want to practice observing first and then later practice the other skills. Observing is also a good first skill for a person who suppresses or avoids emotions or other experiences. A person who frequently distorts information or misinterprets what is going on may want to practice describing first. However, the skill of describing depends on accurate observation, so be sure the person has learned the skill of observing before you move to describing. The person who is usually an observer of others and does not jump in and participate in events may want to practice participating first. Although you ultimately want everyone practicing all the skills, it is often best to start with the skill a person wants to practice or believes is most needed.

Mindfulness Worksheets 2, 2a, 2b, 2c: Mindfulness Core Skills Practice. These worksheets cover practice of all the core mindfulness skills, including both the "what" and "how" skills. See Section II of this chapter for how to use these worksheets.

✓ A. The Mindfulness "What" and "How" Skills

There are three mindfulness "what" skills and three mindfulness "how" skills.

"What" skills are what we do when practicing mindfulness, and "how" skills are how we do it.

Each "what" skill is a distinct activity. Like walking, riding a bike, or swimming, the "what" skills are three separate activities. Thus "what" skills are practiced one at a time: We are either observing, or describing what has been observed, or participating in the moment. This is in contrast to the "how" skills (nonjudgmentally, one-mindfully, and effectively), which can be applied all at once.

Note to Leaders: You need not cover each of the points below every time through. Cover just enough to get your point across. You will be covering this section many times. Expand on your points a bit more each time through. Either before starting or after giving just a few points, do one or two exercises from the list at the end of this section. One of the brief introductory exercises followed by the lemon exercise can be very useful and engaging.

B. Why Observe?

✓ 1. We Observe to See What Is

Say to participants: "Observing is like walking across a room full of furniture with your eyes open instead of closed. You can walk across the room either way. However, you will be more effective with your eyes open. If you don't like the furniture in the room, you might want to close your eyes, but ultimately it's not very effective. You keep running into the furniture."

We all walk through life with our eyes closed sometimes, but opening our eyes and actually observing what's there can be very helpful. The good thing about observing is that it brings us into contact with the real, factual, present moment. That's where we all actually live—in the here and now. We can't experience the past; we can't experience the future; and if we're living in the past or the future, we're not really living. Observing is all about learning to feel fully alive in the here and now.

✓ 🗨 **Discussion Point:** Observing is the opposite of multitasking. As an example, discuss multitasking and driving, with an emphasis on how multitasking might interfere with seeing and responding to what is right in front of you—including other people.

2. We Observe to Get Information into Our Brains So That We Can Change

Research Point: Research shows that information coming into our senses will help us change in desired ways.

- Weighing ourselves consistently and seeing our weight regularly will often make our weight go down (if we feel too fat) or up (if we feel too thin).[36]
- Filling out diary cards is known to be reactive; that is, it can change the very behavior it is measuring.[37]

Discussion Point: Elicit from participants their own tendencies to avoid reality, particularly tendencies to avoid even noticing reality as it is. Discuss consequences of such avoidance.

Discussion Point: Elicit from participants, and discuss, any problems they have with attention.

✓ C. Observing: What to Do

✓ 1. Notice What You Are Experiencing through Your Senses

Say to clients: "Notice what you are experiencing through your eyes, ears, nose, skin, and tongue. You observe the world outside yourself through your five senses: seeing, hearing, smelling, tasting, and touching. You also observe the world inside yourself through sensing your thoughts, emotions, and internal bodily sensations."

a. Sense Objects or Events Outside or Inside Your Body

Tell participants: "What you sense depends on where you focus your attention. Ultimately, you will want to be able to observe events occurring within your mind and body (i.e., thoughts, sensations, emotions, images) and events occurring outside your body."

Note to Leaders: When you are helping clients begin a mindfulness practice, it is important to start with something somewhat difficult but also doable. When clients are first learning a skill, it is important for them to get reinforced for it. Shaping is important here as it is in learning any other new skill.

✓ D. Observing Practice Exercises

We all walk through life with our eyes closed. Opening our eyes and observing what's there can be very helpful—and practice in doing this is necessary.

1. Brief Introductory Exercises

✓   The following are very brief exercises that can be done as you first start teaching observing. You can do one exercise and then share the experience, or you can do several of these sequentially and then share. Ask participants to do these things:

✓
- "Attend to your hand on a cool surface (such as a table or chair) or a warm surface (such as your other hand)."
- "Attend to your thigh on the chair."
- "Attend to and try to sense your stomach, your shoulders."
- "Listen for sounds."
- "Follow your breath in and out; notice the sensation of your belly rising and falling."
- "Watch in your mind to see the first thought that comes in." (As a leader, you can facilitate this by yelling the word "Elephant!" first and then giving instruction.)

✓

■ "Stroke just above your upper lip; then stop stroking and notice how long it takes before you can't sense your upper lip any longer."

■ "Stand, arms relaxed at your sides, feet about a foot apart. Focus your attention on how your feet feel connecting with the floor. . . . Without moving your feet, find the spot where you feel most balanced over your feet."

💬 **Discussion Point:** Share experiences at end of exercises.

b. Sense Your Mind

Explain to clients: "Observing your thoughts can sometimes be very difficult. This is because your thoughts about events may often seem to you like facts instead of thoughts. Many people have never really tried to just sit back and watch their thoughts. When you observe your own mind, you will see that your thoughts (and also your emotions and bodily sensations) never stop following one another. From morning till night, there is an uninterrupted flow of events inside your mind; you might notice thoughts, emotions, and other bodily sensations. As you watch, these will come and go like clouds in the sky. This is what thoughts and feelings do inside the mind when just observed—they come and go."

👥 **Practice Exercise:** Instruct participants to sit with their eyes closed and listen as you say out loud a string of words (e.g., "up," "round," "salt," "tall"). Instruct them to observe what word comes into their minds following each word you say. Discuss the words that entered their minds.

■ *Some people are terrified to look at their own minds.* They've avoided it for years. For these individuals, it may be more effective to start observing things outside their bodies first—for example, sitting on a park bench and watching people walk by; or holding something in one hand, such as a leaf or a flower, and noticing the weight of the object, the texture, the smell, the shape.

■ *Some people can't stop analyzing their minds.* They're paying attention to their own experience all the time. For these individuals, it might be harder to start by observing their own minds, particularly if they are very used to analyzing themselves. In contrast, here it is important in observing the mind to adopt a curious attitude and simply watch what goes through the mind. That is, it is important not to try to understand the mind, figure out the mind, or analyze the mind. These are activities of "doing" mind. They are goal-directed. Observing is not goal-directed, other than toward noticing. Having a "Teflon mind"—a concept to which I return later—is essential here.

> **Note to Leaders:** Some people dissociate or sense themselves leaving their bodies when observing. For people having trouble staying "inside themselves," it can be useful to suggest that they imagine that the place they go outside themselves is a flower. The flower is connected to their center by a long stem. Their center is the root of the flower. Instruct them to imagine coming down the stem to the root. Have them do this each time and then observe at the root.

2. Pay Attention on Purpose to Right Now—As It Happens

Mindful observing can be thought of as paying attention to present experiences on purpose. Instruct clients: "To observe, you simply step back, be alert, and notice. When you observe, it is the only thing you are doing, nothing else. Don't react, don't label, don't describe; just notice the experience. When you observe, you pay attention to direct physical sensation."

3. Observe by Controlling Attention

Explain to clients: "When you can control your attention, you can control your mind. There are two types of attending: focusing the mind and opening the mind."

a. Focusing the Mind

"Focusing the mind" is the practice of concentrating attention on specific activities, objects, or events. Many things can be used for focusing the mind. Give clients these examples:

- "The most common mindfulness practice is observing your breath. Your breath is the only thing that you can be certain you will always have for as long as you live. You can lose your arm; you can lose your leg; you can lose many things. But as long as you are alive, you have breath. Focusing attention on your breath is a central part of all mindfulness meditation and contemplative prayer practices."
- "Some schools of meditation give mantras or specific words to say with each breath."
- "Guided mindfulness exercises given by therapists, or meditation recordings, give intermittent instructions on where and how to focus the mind."
- "Counting breaths in and breaths out up to 10 and then starting over is a typical instruction in Zen."
- "Saying the word 'wise' when breathing in and the word 'mind' when breathing out is a way to focus your mind. Some people practice using a word such as 'calm.'"

Mindfulness of current emotions (see Emotion Regulation Handout 22), mindfulness of current thoughts (Distress Tolerance Handout 15), and mindfulness of others (Interpersonal Effectiveness Handout 12) are other examples of focusing the mind, as are the exercises described in the "Focusing the Mind" portion of Mindfulness Handout 4a.

b. Opening the Mind

In "opening the mind," instead of focusing on specific activities, objects, or events, we focus our attention on observing or watching whatever comes into awareness as it comes in and as it goes out of awareness. It is noticing thoughts, emotions, and sensations that enter awareness, without holding onto or pursuing the topics coming into mind. When opening the mind, we attempt at each moment to expand awareness to moment-to-moment experiencing. Thus the object in opening the mind is to observe the flow of moment-to-moment experience. This is like sitting and watching an operating conveyor belt, noticing the objects that go by on the belt, but without shutting down the belt to look at the objects more closely. Another metaphor for this is sitting on the shore of a stream in autumn and watching the leaves go by on the water without following any of the leaves to pay closer attention.

In Zen this practice is called *shikentaza,* which is mindfulness practice without the support of focusing on the breath or other techniques for concentrating the mind. This is also called "choiceless awareness"[38] to indicate that an individual notices anything that comes into awareness, not choosing one thing to pay attention to.

> **Note to Leaders:** For participants who have attention difficulties (or sometimes even high anxiety), the practice of opening the mind can be very difficult, because they keep getting caught up in thoughts, emotions, or sensations that come into awareness. Focusing the mind is recommended for these participants.

✓   ### 4. *Practice Wordless Watching: Observe without Describing What Is Observed*

Observing without describing can be very hard, and for many people this takes a lot of practice. Our minds may be in the habit of immediately adding labels to anything we observe. We hear "chirp, chirp" and think "bird"; we hear "vroom, vroom" and say "car"; we sense our breath and say "breath"; we see a picture of a bird on the wall and say "bird." We often trade observations for concepts, such as hearing "chirp, chirp" and thinking, "I know what that is: a bird." But when hearing "chirp, chirp," we aren't actually seeing any birds. For all we know, somebody out there could be practicing bird calls. It could in fact be a bird, but we didn't observe a bird. It was only an observed sound. All we can know for sure is the sound we hear. Observing is noticing the sound "chirp, chirp." That's it. That's all. In fact, jumping to label the sound as "bird" gets in the way of paying attention to the sound. This is like trying to text and drive, or talk on a cell phone and engage in an in-person conversation at the same time: No one can observe well while describing (the second "what" skill) at the same time. Grasping this idea may be difficult for many participants. They might even think it is not possible actually to observe something without the mind's saying anything. For many people, the mind is a constantly chattering set of thoughts.

💬 **Discussion Point:** Elicit from participants their own tendencies to label observations.

✓ **5. Observe with a "Teflon (or Nonstick) Mind"**

Allowing emotions, thoughts, images, and sensations to come and go is central to mindful observing. A "Teflon/nonstick mind" is important in practicing opening the mind, and also in practicing focusing the mind. In both practices, thoughts, emotions, and images will come up in the mind. The idea is to let all experiences—feelings, thoughts, and images—flow out of the mind, rather than either grabbing experiences or holding onto them, or pushing experiences away.

Say to clients: "Observing inside your mind can be like sitting on a hill looking down on a train that's going by. Some of the train cars are thoughts, strung together. They come into view. They go out of view. Some of the train cars are emotions, feelings. Each thought and feeling arises, comes closer, then passes, and goes away down the tracks and around the hill out of sight. The trick is not to get caught in the content of the thought or feeling. Watch, observe, but do not get on the train."

✓ **a. Avoid Pushing Away Experiences**

"Experiential avoidance"[39] is trying to suppress or avoid experiencing what is happening in the present, in the moment. Some individuals may be afraid to observe their thoughts. Some thoughts are scary, and others may be thoughts a person would like to not have. If worried about any particular thought, a person may try to get rid of it, to shut it out of the mind.

Research Point: However, there is scientific evidence[27, 40] that trying to shut out thoughts is the best way to keep having them. The harder a person tries to shut them out, the more they will pop back into the mind. The best way to get rid of unwanted thoughts is to step back and simply observe them. They will go away by themselves. The attempt to avoid or suppress our own experiences is associated with higher, not lower, emotion dysregulation.[41, 42]

---

b. Avoid Holding on to Experiences

"Experiential hunger" is trying to hold on to positive experiences. We try to create positive experiences at the expense of noticing what is currently in our lives. People often overindulge in drugs, alcohol, sex, fast driving, and other exciting activities, seeking an emotional high or a thrill. Everyday life seems boring.

We may try to hold on to a sense of security or a sense of being loved. Holding on to damaging relationships, or being overly demanding of those we love, are often efforts to hold on to a false sense of safety and security. Life is too scary otherwise.

It is even possible to become overly "addicted" to spiritual experiences. Mindfulness meditation and/or prayer can become efforts to have "spiritual highs." Individuals constantly seeking reassurance or frequently demanding proof of unwavering love fall into the same category. When this happens, the individuals can become like ocean fish swimming around and around, constantly searching for the water.

Note to Leaders: It is essential to help participants observe in a nonattached way. Thus whatever happens in their minds is "grist for the mill," so to speak. No matter what they do, they can just "step back" and observe. Get feedback. Work with participants until they get the idea of observing. Check how long each person can observe. It is common to have to start and restart many times in the course of 1 or 2 minutes.

6. *Observe with a "Beginner's Mind"*

Each moment in the universe is completely new. This one moment, right now, has never occurred before. In "beginner's mind," we focus our minds on noticing the experience of each moment, noticing that each moment is new and unique. It is easy to forget this. We forget to observe and notice the moment. A new moment may be very much like a previous moment. We may find ourselves saying "same old, same old," but actually everything is changing, is constantly new. In reality, we are always in "beginner's mind"; that is, every moment is indeed new and unique. In observing, we take the stance of an impartial observer, investigating whatever appears in our conscious minds or strikes our attention.

Say to clients: "Nothing has ever been in your mind that has not gone away. If you just watch your mind, thoughts, images, emotions, and sensations all eventually go away. It is a fascinating thing. If you just sit there and look at them, they go away. When you try to get rid of thoughts they keep coming back."

7. *Practice, Practice, Practice to Train the Mind to Pay Attention*

Emphasize to clients: "Learning to observe your own mind takes patience and practice. It means training your mind to pay attention. It may seem impossible to ever get your attention under control, but it is possible. It just takes practice, practice, and more practice."

Story Point: An untrained mind is like a TV that gets 100,000 different channels, but the person watching the TV doesn't have a remote control. The mind keeps turning to the same stations over and over and over again—most of which are painful for participants.

Story Point: A Zen metaphor compares an untrained mind to a puppy. The untrained mind causes problems just like a puppy that pees where it's not supposed to, chews up its owner's favorite shoes, eats garbage, and throws up. Likewise, the untrained mind wanders all over, gets itself (and the person) in trouble, and ruminates about things that make the person feel worse.

✓ 8. *Keep Bringing the Mind Back to Observing*

Say to clients: "Observe by *bringing your mind back to observing* over and over, each time that you notice being distracted. Most people, when they practice observing, find that their minds frequently and sometimes very quickly start thinking about something—and before they know it, they become lost in their thoughts, unaware of the present moment, no longer observing. Whenever your attention is drawn away from observing and awareness, gently but resolutely push distractions to the side as if you are dividing the clouds in the sky, and return, single-mindedly, to the object of attention. The idea here is to observe being distracted—that is, to observe yourself as you become aware that you were distracted. Notice, if you can, when you start to become distracted. Practice noticing distractions."

9. *Observing Requires Controlling Action*

The first rule of observing is to notice the urge to quit observing. One of the first things that happens when people start practicing observing is that they want to quit. They get bored; they get tired; they experience painful emotions; their bodies start hurting; they remember something else important they need to do; something else catches their interest; and on and on and on.

Tell participants: "You don't have to act on whatever comes into your mind. When you're observing, you might notice you feel sleepy. Notice it, but don't fall asleep. Instead, bring your attention back to whatever you are observing. You might notice you're hungry. But don't get something to eat right now. Instead, notice that you're hungry; notice that your attention has been pulled into thinking about food. Notice that, and then bring your attention back to whatever you were observing."

💬 **Discussion Point:** Elicit from participants estimates of their own ability to stay focused on observing for any length of time. Discuss strategies for increasing the ability to continue observing in the face of temptations to quit.

Note to Leaders: A common problem for many participants is that they forget why they are observing in the first place. They see no benefit. They may feel worse—certainly not better or calmer. They want to quit. At these times it can be helpful to do a quick review of the pros and cons (see Mindfulness Worksheet 1: Pros and Cons of Practicing Mindfulness), and to remind them (and have them remind themselves) that very little can be accomplished in this life without the ability to observe. Ultimately, this ability will depend somewhat on the ability to tolerate distress and to inhibit impulsive urges. This may be quite a task for some participants, requiring much practice before they can comfortably stay quiet and stay still long enough to fully observe something within or without.

---

10. Observing Is Very Simple, but It Can Also Be Surprisingly Hard

To make the point to participants about the surprising difficulty of observing, try one of the following exercises; the first focuses on not seeing what is there, and the second on seeing what is not there.

👥 **Practice Exercise 1:** Hold up a page or poster, or put up a PowerPoint slide, with the sentence below written in the form shown. Instruct participants to observe the sentence, and then ask them, "What do you see?"

The yellow bird flew through
through orange curtains
into blue sky.

Take the display down and discuss. People ordinarily do not notice that the word "through" is repeated. (It's at the end of the first line and the beginning of the second line.) Put the display up again, and ask whether participants now see the word "through" two times. Discuss participants' experiences. Because people know how to read and write, they have expectations about words and sentences. If people saw the extra word the first time they read the sentence, they probably ignored it; they knew from past experience that it probably wasn't supposed to be there. If they weren't giving it their full attention, they may not have noticed the extra word. Their minds automatically "saw" the words as they should be. It's good to practice observing, because it's very easy not to see things that are there like the extra word above.

👥 **Practice Exercise 2:** Hold up a page or poster, or put up a PowerPoint slide, with the image in Figure 7.2. Ask participants what shapes they see inside the box. It's clear that there are three black circles and that each has a notch, like a missing pie piece. In addition, many people see a triangle when they look at the shapes in Figure 7.2. But in fact, there is no triangle in the box. The notches in the three circles happen to line up with each other. If there

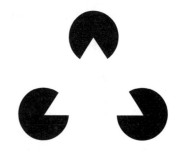

FIGURE 7.2. Three notched black circles with a "missing" triangle: An illustration of how surprisingly difficult observing can be.

were lines that connected the three notches, then there would be a triangle. But there are no connecting lines, and so there is no triangle shape. Our minds, however, can provide these "missing" lines, so we "see" a triangle even though it isn't really there. Discuss participants' experiences. The mind has the ability to fill in blanks, so we "see" something we expect even when it's missing. When the mind isn't fully paying attention, it can also erase something unexpected, even though it's there. In fact, most people stop paying attention when they think they know what something is. This can be useful and save us a lot of time. But it can cause lots of problems when what we think we see doesn't line up with what's really out there.

11. Observing Can Be Very Painful at Times

The trouble with observing is that people may wind up seeing things they do not want to see. This can be hard. In particular, those with histories of trauma may find observing very scary. They are afraid to watch what goes through their minds. Some are worried that thoughts and images that ordinarily cause enormous anxiety will race through their minds. Others are afraid of thoughts and images of the past, particularly when these set off intense emotions of sadness or anger. However, there is research showing that control of attention can reduce rumination.[43]

> **Note to Leaders:** Remind participants to step back within themselves, not outside of themselves, to observe. Observing is not dissociating. As described in an earlier Note to Leaders, if some individuals have difficulty staying inside instead of going outside themselves, suggest that they try imagining that the place they go outside themselves is a flower.

12. Practice Exercises for Observing That Require Preparation*

The following exercises need supplies and require some advance preparation. They are fairly active, most people find them fun, and they are very good for younger groups or people who are somewhat resistant to practice. They are also very good for people who have difficulty sitting still or focusing without much to do, thereby opening the door to traumatic images or thoughts.

✓   **a. Finding Your Lemon**

Hand one lemon to each person. Instruct participants to examine the lemon (by touching it, holding it, smelling it, etc.), but not to eat the lemon. After a period of time, collect all the lemons in one place. Mix up the lemons. Ask participants to come and find their own lemons. This can be done with other things (e.g., pennies), but be sure that the objects you choose look reasonably similar and will require examination to tell the difference.

b. Holding Chocolate on Your Tongue

Hand out a small piece of chocolate to each person. Have each person unwrap the chocolate. Before starting, give these instructions: "Put the piece of chocolate on your tongues. Hold it in your mouth, noticing the taste, the texture, the sensations in your mouth. Do not swallow. Notice the urge to swallow." Start by ringing a bell, and end in 3–5 minutes by ringing the bell. (Substitute some other sound for the bell if necessary.)

c. Eating or Drinking with Awareness

Give something to eat or to drink to each participant (or have participants select something from an array of food or drinks). Then instruct participants to eat (or drink) what they have selected very slowly, focusing on the feel of the food (or drink) in their hands; the smell, the

---

*All exercises in this section (and later in this chapter) marked with note number 44 are adapted from Miller, A. L., Rathus, J. H., & Linehan, M. M. (2007). *Dialectical behavior therapy with suicidal adolescents*. New York: Guilford Press. Copyright 2007 by The Guilford Press. Adapted by permission.

texture, the temperature, the sound, and the taste of the food (or liquid) in their mouths; the sensations of swallowing; and urges to eat or drink more slowly, faster, or not at all.

d. What's Different about Me?[44]

Two group members pair off and mindfully observe each other. Then they turn their backs, change three things (e.g., glasses, watch, and hair), and turn back toward each other. Can they notice the changes?

e. Observation of Music[44]

Play a piece of music and ask group members to listen quietly and to observe nonjudgmentally, while fully letting the experience surround them (their thoughts, emotions, physiological changes, urges). Variations include playing segments of two or three very different pieces (in terms of style, tempo, etc.) and having group members observe changes in the music and their internal reactions.

f. Mindfully Unwrapping a Hershey's Kiss[44]

Have each group member sit in a comfortable position with a Hershey's Kiss in front of him or her. Then say: "After I ring the bell the third time, observe and describe the outside of the Hershey's Kiss to yourself. Feel the differences in the texture between the paper tag and the foil. As you begin to unwrap the chocolate, note how the shape and texture of the foil change in comparison to the paper tag, as well as the chocolate. Feel the chocolate and how it changes in your hand. If your mind wanders from the exercise, note the distraction without judgment, and then return your attention to the chocolate."

g. Repeating an Activity[44]

Instruct participants: "When the bell rings, sit at the table with your arms resting on the table. Very slowly, reach several inches to pick up a pen. Raise it a few inches, and then set it down. Move your hand back to its original position of rest. While you repeat this action throughout the time period, experience each repetition with freshness, as though you have never done it before. You can allow your attention to wander toward different aspects of the movement: watching your hand or feeling the muscles contracting. You can even notice your sense of touch, being aware of the different textures and pressures. Let go of any distractions or judgments you may have. This activity will help you to become mindful of a simple activity that you perform often throughout the day."

h. Focusing on Scent

Bring in and distribute scented candles. Then instruct group members: "Choose a candle. When the bell rings, sit back in your chair and find a comfortable and relaxed position. Close your eyes, and begin to focus on the smell of the candle. Let go of any distractions or judgments. Notice how the smell makes you feel and what images it evokes." Afterward, discuss observations, emotions, thoughts, feelings, and sensations with participants: "How did the scent make you feel? What images came to your mind? Did the smell remind you of anything in particular?"

i. Mindfully Eating a Raisin

Bring in and distribute raisins. Then ask group members to hold a raisin; observe its appearance, texture, and scent; then put it in their mouths and slowly, with awareness, begin eating—noticing the tastes, sensations, and even the sounds of eating. This can also be done with candies (sweet tarts, caramels, fruit chews, fireballs, etc.). Eating a raisin (or other small food) is a very well-known exercise that is typically done in mindfulness-based treatments.

j. Observing Emotions

Say to participants: "Notice the emotions you are experiencing, and try to note how you know you are having those emotions. That is, what labels do you have in mind? What thoughts, what body sensations, and so on give you information about the emotions?"

k. What's My Experience?

Tell participants: "Focus your mind on your experience this very moment. Be mindful of any thoughts, feelings, body sensations, urges, or anything else you become aware of. Don't judge your experience, or try to push it away or hold onto it. Just let experiences come and go like clouds moving across the sky."

l. Noticing Urges[44]

Instruct participants: "Sit very straight in your chair. Throughout this exercise, notice any urges—whether to move, shift positions, scratch an itch, or do something else. Instead of acting on the urge, simply notice it." Then discuss the experience with participants. Was it possible to have an urge and not act on it?

m. Mindfulness of the Five Senses

The exercises for observing through the five senses are limited only by your imagination and creativity.

- *Sight.* Have participants pick a picture on a wall or an object in the room to look at, or ask them to pass around pictures or postcards. Or light a candle in the middle of the room, or go for a walk in an area with flowers or other sights to see. Instruct participants to contemplate or gaze at the sight.
- *Touch.* Bring things with various textures to pass around. Instruct participants to close their eyes and hold and examine the object(s) with their hands, and/or rub the object(s) on their skin. Find a nearby grassy place to walk barefoot, and ask participants to notice the feel of the ground on bare feet.
- *Smell.* Bring in aromatic things, such as spices, herbs, perfumes, perfumed soaps or candles, gourmet jelly beans, or other foods or aromatic oils. Instruct participants to close their eyes and focus on their sense of smell.
- *Taste.* Bring various small but tasty bites to eat. Try to make some tastes very different and some very similar. Have participants sample each bite to eat separately. Instruct them to focus on the taste and, if they are good cooks themselves, to try to inhibit analyzing the taste for what elements make up the taste.
- *Sound.* Instruct participants to close their eyes and listen to sounds in the room. Or bring a large mindfulness bell and ring the bell very slowly (but completely each time). Or put on a musical recording, instruct participants to listen, and have them make an effort to keep their attention on the sound only.

13. Practice Exercises for Awareness

Ordinarily, have participants practice the following exercises with eyes open. Speak in a low and gentle voice tone. You can give all the instructions at once or you can follow the script, with pauses (. . .). You can do one exercise and then share the experience, or you can do several of these sequentially and then share. As described earlier with the scripts for wise mind exercises, set up the practice as follows, and then continue with one of the scripts below:

"Sit in a comfortable but attentive position. Keeping your eyes open, find a good place to rest your eyes . . . looking down with only slightly open eyes, or keeping your eyes more open. You might want to clear the space in front of you so as to not be too distracted."

a. **Expanding Awareness While Staying Aware of Your Center**

"See if you can let your attention settle into your center . . . at the bottom of your breath when you inhale . . . just near your gut. That very centered point is wise mind . . . as you breathe in and out . . . keeping your attention there at your very center . . . in your gut. . . . Now, as you keep your center of attention in your gut, expand your awareness outside . . . noticing in the periphery of your vision the colors of the walls or floor or table, objects in the room, people nearby . . . maintaining all the while awareness of your gut . . . your center point . . . your wise mind."

b. **Awareness of Threes**

"Stay focused on your breathing . . . in and out, for three breaths . . . and, maintaining your awareness of your breath, expand your awareness to your hands . . . just holding both in your awareness for three breaths. . . . Now, expand your awareness even further . . . maintaining awareness of your breath and of your hands, include in your awareness sounds . . . staying aware of all three for three breaths . . . letting go of perfection if you lose awareness of one . . . starting over again."

> **Note to Leaders:** The two exercises above are very good for working on the ability to focus attention. Many people who have problems with emotion regulation or impulse control have great difficulties in controlling attention. With much practice of these exercises, their control of attention will gradually improve.

c. **Watching Train Cars**

"Imagine you are sitting on a hill near train tracks, watching train cars go by. . . . Imagine that thoughts, images, sensations, and feelings are cars on the train. . . . Just watch the train cars go by. . . . Don't jump on the train. . . . Just watch the train cars go by. . . . If you find yourself riding the train, jump off and start observing again. . . . Just noticing that you got on the train . . . watching the train cars . . . watching your mind again."

> **Note to Leaders:** There are many variations on the "train cars" image. For the train cars, you can substitute boats on a lake, sheep walking by, and so forth.

d. **Watching Clouds in the Sky**

"Imagine that your mind is the sky, and that your thoughts, sensations, and feelings are clouds. . . . Gently notice each cloud as it drifts . . . or scurries . . . by."

✓ E. Review of Between-Session Practice Exercises for Observing

It is important to go over some of these exercises with participants if they are not practiced in the session. If time is short, leaf through the pages of Mindfulness Handout 5a with participants, just so they see how many ways there are for practicing observing. If you have time, ask participants to review some of the ideas and check off in the boxes practices they think would be useful for them.

V. MINDFULNESS "WHAT" SKILLS: DESCRIBE (MINDFULNESS HANDOUTS 4–4B)

> **Main Point:** Describing is the second of the three mindfulness "what" skills; it is putting into words what is observed.

Mindfulness Handout 4: Taking Hold of Your Mind: "What" Skills. This is the same handout used to teach the skill of observing. Review the "Describe" section of the handout with participants.

Mindfulness Handout 4b: Ideas for Practicing Describing *(Optional)*. As with previous practice handouts, this list may be overwhelming; if so, it should be skipped. Most of the describing practice takes place in writing on the worksheets, but this handout can be used to find specific exercises to assign in areas where a participant is having trouble describing accurately.

Mindfulness Worksheets 2, 2a, 2b, 2c: Mindfulness Core Skills Practice. These worksheets provide for practice of wise mind skills, "what" skills, and "how" skills. For instructions on how to use them, see Section II of this chapter.

Mindfulness Worksheet 4: Mindfulness "What" Skills: Observing, Describing, Participating; Mindfulness Worksheet 4a: Observing, Describing, Participating Checklist; Mindfulness Worksheets 4b: Observing, Describing, Participating Calendar. These worksheets are the same as those used in teaching the skill of observing. Choose one to distribute, or let the participants choose. The focus in teaching describing is on examining what is written to be sure that it was actually observed, nothing more, nothing less. The skill of describing permeates all of the worksheets in DBT. Each asks participants to describe something they have observed. To coach participants in describing, it is important to review these worksheets throughout all the modules, not just in the Mindfulness module.

A. Why Describe?

Note to Leaders: You can jump-start teaching this skill by using exercises to make the teaching points below before you go on to explain what you mean by the skill of describing.

✓   **Practice Exercise:** Looking right at one of the participants, ask him or her to tell you what you are thinking. Insist upon it. When the person cannot, turn to another person and ask him or her to describe what you are thinking. Keep at it. Insist, saying, "Other people tell you what you are thinking; why can't you tell me what I am thinking?" When they cannot, discuss how often we think we know what another person is thinking. Elicit times when others have insisted they know what participants are thinking but really do not.

✓   **Practice Exercise:** Turn to one of the participants and say, "I'm really tired, it's late." Then ask the participant to describe your intent or motive for saying that. Insist upon it. When a participant cannot do it or gets it wrong, ask another participant. Discuss how often we think we know other people's motives. Elicit times when others have insisted they know participants' minds but really do not. How does that make the participants feel?

✓   **Practice Exercise:** Ask one of the participants to describe what you are doing tomorrow. Insist upon it. When this person can't do it, turn to another person and ask him or her. Act as if you expect participants to be able to do this. When they cannot, discuss how often we say something about the future, like "I can't do this" or "I'll never make this," as if we are describing facts. Elicit times when others have acted as if they can describe what participants are going to do or not do—as if they know the facts. Ask, "Which is worse: describing your own future as facts, or having others describe it for you?"

1. Describing Distinguishes What Is Observed from What Is Not Observed

Describing develops the ability to sort out and discriminate observations from mental concepts and thoughts about what we observe. Confusing mental concepts of events with events themselves (e.g., responding to thoughts and concepts as if they are facts) can lead to unnecessary emotional distress and confusion.

Example: "When you find out that your child stole money, your mind might immediately describe that as 'My child is going to end up going to jail,' and that description causes emotional distress."

Responding to thoughts about events as if they were facts can lead to ineffective actions when the thoughts do not match the actual event.

Example: "Describing your boyfriend's not being dressed yet when you come home before going out to your birthday dinner as not loving you may ruin your chances of having a nice dinner together."

2. Describing Allows Feedback from the Larger Community

Those around us can correct or validate our perceptions and descriptions of events.

Example: Think of how children learn: They say words, and parents and others correct them until they become very proficient at accurately describing what they observe.

Example: In Zen, the interview with the teacher, called *dokusan*, gives students an opportunity to describe their experiences during their mindfulness practice. An important component of these interviews is the teacher's helping the students drop concepts and analyses of the world and instead respond to what is observed.

Example: After a party, one person often describes events to another and asks whether the other person saw it the same way. This can also be very important when getting consultation about interpersonal problems at work or in other settings.

3. Describing Observations by Writing Them Down Allows Observation of the Information

Observing, as discussed above, can change behavior in desired directions. Describing can also, at times, provide a means of processing the information we have observed. Many people, for example, find writing diaries very helpful in organizing the events they observe throughout their days.

> **Research Point:** Describing and labeling emotions regulates emotions.[45] Brain imaging research has shown that when individuals describe their emotional responses, the very act of labeling the emotions changes brain responding in the direction of emotion regulation.[46]

✓ **B. Describing: What to Do**

✓ ### 1. To Describe Is to Add Words to an Observation

Describing is putting words on experiences. Describing follows observing; it is labeling what is observed. True describing involves just sticking with the facts.

Example: If I am looking at a painting, the words "landscape," "green," "yellow," and "brush strokes" might come to mind. That would be an example of describing. It's simply applying basic descriptors to what's there.

Example: Describing internal experience, I could say, "I observe a feeling of sadness arising."

💬 **Discussion Point:** Discuss the difference between describing and observing. Again, observing is like sensing without words. Describing is using words or thoughts to label what is observed.

✓ 👥 **Practice Exercise:** Draw the image in Figure 7.3 on a board, or move the features of your face to mimic an emotional expression similar to that of a person experiencing sadness, anger, or fear. Exaggerate your expression somewhat. Then ask participants to describe your face. Almost always, they will use emotional terms ("sad," "angry," "afraid"). Give a number of people the opportunity to speak; then point out that no one observed an emotion. They observed features of your face (e.g., eyebrows together, creases in the forehead, lips tight together, etc.). Tell them: "A hint about how to describe things is to imagine that you are instructing someone in how to draw something, or instructing a designer on how to put together a setting for a movie."

FIGURE 7.3. A facial expression for giving participants practice in describing.

✓ **2. If It Wasn't Observed, It Can't Be Described**

No one has ever observed the thoughts, intentions, or emotions of another person.

✓ **a. No One Can Observe the Thoughts of Others**

Although we can observe thoughts that go through our own minds, we can only infer or guess what another person is thinking. Assumptions of what others are thinking are just that: assumptions in our own minds.

Example: "You think I'm lying" is not a description of an observation. "I keep thinking that you think I am lying" is a description.

Example: "You are just thinking up ways to get out of going to the party with me" is not a description of an observation. "I think [or believe] that you are trying to come up with ways to get out of going to the party with me" is a description. Tell participants: "Note also that when the sentence is framed this way, you clarify that you are describing your own thoughts."

Example: "You disapprove" is not a description. "I think you disapprove" is a description.

"When you do X, I feel [or think] Y" is a good way to describe personal reactions to what others do or say.

Example: Saying, "When you raise your eyebrows and purse your lips like that [X], I start thinking you think I'm lying [Y]" is also a form of describing. Say to participants: "Putting it this way shows that you are describing your own thoughts, which you can observe."

💬 **Discussion Point:** Discuss how describing a thought as a thought requires one to notice that it is a thought instead of a fact. Give examples of the differences between thinking, "You don't want me," and the other person's actually not wanting you; or thinking, "I am a jerk," and being a jerk. Get feedback. Get lots of examples. It is crucial that participants understand this distinction.

💬 **Discussion Point:** Elicit from participants times when others have misinterpreted their thoughts. Discuss how this feels.

👥 **Practice Exercise:** Have participants practice observing thoughts and labeling them as thoughts. Suggest labeling them into categories (e.g., "thoughts about myself," "thoughts about others," etc.). Use the conveyor belt exercise described earlier in this chapter, but this time as thoughts and feelings come down the belt, have participants sort them into categories: "For example, you could have one box for thoughts of any sort, one box for sensations in your body, and one box for urges to do something (such as to stop describing)."

✓ **b. No One Can Observe the Intentions of Others**

Speaking about the inferred intentions of others is not describing and can cause trouble. This is so because (1) it is extremely difficult to read other people's intentions correctly; and (2) incorrectly characterizing others' intentions can be exceptionally painful, particularly when they are socially unacceptable intentions. People often pay attention to the effects of what other people do and then assume that these effects were intentional.

Example: "I feel manipulated" translates into "You are manipulating me."

Example: "I am feeling hurt" translates into "You did that to hurt me."

Example: "When you tell me that you are going to quit school if I don't give you a better grade, I feel manipulated" is a more accurate example of describing.

✓ **c. No One Can Observe the Feelings or Emotions of Another Individual**

We cannot see the internal experiential components of emotions. We can, however, observe many components of emotions, such as facial expressions, postures, verbal expressions of emotions, and emotion-linked actions. But expressive behaviors can be misleading. The expressions associated with various emotions may be very similar, and because of this, we may often be wrong in our beliefs about the emotions of others.

Example: Many people sound as if they are angry or irritated when they are very anxious.

Example: People often withdraw from others when they are ashamed, leading others to say they are angry.

We may also often incorrectly assume that someone who does something must have wanted to do it, when the person may instead have felt coerced or afraid to say no. The same is true when thinking about things a person does not do: We may assume, "If you wanted to, you would have done it."

Example: To someone with an alcohol problem who has fallen off the wagon again, we may say incorrectly, "You just don't want to stay sober."

Example: If we call a person very late at night and he answers the phone, we may assume incorrectly that "He wants to talk to me."

💬 **Discussion Point:** It is sometimes easiest to get this point across by asking participants to think of times people have "described" their thoughts or feelings incorrectly. Also ask for times when they have "described" others' emotions, thoughts, or intentions incorrectly. Highlight here the difference between inferences and descriptions based on observation.

Note to Leaders: Describing is similar to checking the facts, an emotion regulation skill. See Emotion Regulation Handout 8.

✓ **d. No One Has Ever Observed a Concept, a Meaning, a Cause, or a Change in Things**

Concepts and meanings are the results of our putting together in our minds a number of observations to make sense out of them. Causes and changes are inferred from observing the world and making logical deductions from our observations.

Example: Say to participants, "I see you hit a ball with a cue, and the ball moves; I infer that hitting the ball caused the movement. But I did not observe the 'cause,' because this is a concept, not something I can observe."

Conclusions and comparisons such as "more" or "less," or any differences between things, are also the results of mental calculations that occur in our minds.

Example: We see a person acting very irritable one day, and very calm the next day. We may say, "I see you are calmer than you were yesterday." Actually, the statement is based on comparing in our minds what we observed on one day with what we are observing today, and then forming a conclusion. But conclusions about things and how they have changed are concepts, not things we can observe. We can, of course, observe the conclusions we draw in our own minds.

C. Describing Practice Exercises

Like the introductory exercises for observing practice described earlier, these are very brief exercises that can be done as you first start teaching describing. You can do one exercise and then share the experience, or you can do several of these sequentially and then share. You can weave the instructions and questions in as you cover the teaching points. These exercises do not need a setup.

- ■ "Observe and then describe the first thought running through your mind."
- ■ "Observe and then describe a picture on the wall or an object on the table."
- ■ "Observe sounds in the room for a few minutes, and then describe the sounds you heard."
- ■ "Observe sensations in your body, and then describe one or more of your sensations."
- ■ "Observe your thoughts as if they were on a conveyor belt. As they come by, sort them by descriptive category into boxes—for instance, planning thoughts, worry thoughts."

✓ D. Review of Between-Session Practice Exercises for Describing

Mindfulness Handout 4b lists a number of ideas for practicing describing. It is important to go over some of these with the participants.

VI. MINDFULNESS "WHAT" SKILLS: PARTICIPATE (MINDFULNESS HANDOUTS 4–4C)

Main Point: Participating, the third mindfulness "what" skill, is entering wholly into an activity.

Mindfulness Handout 4: Taking Hold of Your Mind: "What" Skills. This is the same handout as used in teaching the skills of observing and describing. Review the "Participate" section of the handout with participants.

Mindfulness Handout 4c: Ideas for Practicing Participating. Participants frequently have difficulty finding ways to practice participating. This is particularly true for socially shy individuals. This handout is brief and can be a useful source of ideas.

Mindfulness Worksheet 2, 2a, 2b: Mindfulness Core Skills Practice; Mindfulness Worksheet 2c: Mindfulness Core Skills Calendar; Mindfulness Worksheet 4: Mindfulness "What" Skills: Observing, Describing, Participating; Mindfulness Worksheet 4a: Observing, Describing, Participating Checklist; Mindfulness Worksheet 4b: Observing, Describing, Participating Calendar. These worksheets are the same as those used in teaching the skills of observing and describing. Each asks participants to describe their participation practice. It is important to point out to participants in homework review that practicing skills during the week is the homework, not writing their descriptions of their homework experience.

✓ A. Participating: What Is It?

Participating is entering wholly and with awareness into life itself, nonjudgmentally, in the present moment. Participating is the ultimate goal of mindfulness.

Note to Leaders: Do not feel you have to go over all these points each time. Remember that you will be reviewing this skill multiple times and can review new points at later times.

B. Why Participate?

✓ ### 1. The Experience of "Flow" Is Associated with Participating

The state of "flow" is widely considered an optimal experience—incompatible with boredom, and associated with intense enjoyment and a sense of control. It is a critical characteristic of "peak experience."[47]

Example: Being fully immersed in an activity like skiing or running can give one a sense of maximum well-being or a sense of ecstasy.

2. Participating Is Incompatible with Self-Consciousness

When we "become what we are doing," there is a merging of action and awareness, so that we are no longer aware of ourselves as separate from what we are doing.

3. Participating Is Incompatible with a Sense of Exclusion

When we become what we are doing, we are no longer aware of ourselves as separate from what we are doing or from our environment. We lose awareness of the separation of ourselves and everything else. We forget ourselves, and thus forget ourselves as outside or inside.

4. In Participating, Effort Seems Effortless

In a state of flow, there is an effortlessness of action. We are absorbed in what we are doing, in what is happening. We are aware of a sense of movement, speed, and ease. Life and what we are doing become like a dance. Even great effort seems effortless.

5. In Participating, We Are Present to Our Own Lives and the Lives of Loved Ones

When we become what we are doing, we do not miss our own lives. We also do not miss being part of the lives of others. Compassion and love, toward ourselves or others, requires our presence.

6. Participating Is a Fundamental Characteristic of Skillful Behavior

To be experts in any task, we must practice and "overlearn" that task. Expertise in any activity requires mindful awareness of the task without the distractions of thinking about ourselves, others, or even the task. A person who thinks about running while running loses the race. In great acting, an actor becomes the role. A great dancer becomes the dance. In the Olympics, gymnasts let their bodies do the work.

✓ ## C. Participating: What to Do

Make one or more of these suggestions to participants:

- "Enter into present experiences. Immerse yourself in the present."
- "Throw yourself completely into activities."
- "Don't separate yourself from ongoing events and interactions. Engage completely; immerse yourself in the moment; become involved; join with; opt in."
- "Become one with what you are doing."
- "Let go of self-consciousness by acting opposite to it. Abandon yourself to the moment. Concentrate in the moment such that you and what you are doing become "merged" as if there is only now, only what you are doing."
- "Act intuitively from wise mind, doing just what is needed in each situation."
- "Go with the flow; respond with spontaneity."

Example: Observing and describing are like "stop, look, and listen." Participating is like walking across the street.

Example: Tell clients, "If it is raining, just play in the puddles like a kid would; enjoy the rain."

✓ **D. Choosing When to Observe, When to Describe, and When to Participate**

1. Observing and Describing When Something Is New or Difficult

Instruct participants: "Step back from participating in an activity when you are making errors or don't know how to do something. When you are participating, you are very aware, but you are not actively focusing your attention on yourself and analyzing the details of what you are doing. At times you must step back, slow down, and pay attention to what you are doing. In particular, when you notice there's a problem in your life, you need to step back and actively observe and describe both the problem situation and your responses to it. You can then figure out what's wrong, learn the skills needed to solve the problem, and return to participating."

Example: "You can only play the piano really well if you participate in the act of piano playing—that is, if you play fully. But if you've learned an incorrect technique, you may want to learn the correct version. To do so, you have to step back and observe and describe what you're doing wrong, then practice the correct way over and over until you're skilled. You can then stop observing and participate again."

💬 **Discussion Point:** We step back from participating to understand and improve things. Share examples of participating (e.g., driving a car): "When you switch cars to one with a different way of driving, or if you go to England and have to drive on the left side of the road, you suddenly need to stop, observe, and describe." Elicit other examples from participants.

2. Doing the Most Practice of the Most Difficult Skill

Tell clients: "Practice most the mindfulness skill you find most difficult. Different people have trouble with different skills." Give these illustrations:

✓ *Example:* Some people participate all the time, and that's their problem. They don't notice that they're participating in a way that's driving others crazy. Other people have a lot of trouble with participating, especially people who are shy, socially anxious, or afraid of failing. All they do is stay on the sidelines and observe. Still others have busy, analytical minds. They also stay back from living in the moment, but instead of just observing, they are analyzing, thinking, and ruminating about each event as it occurs. Life is like a running commentary on the universe. Describing is in overdrive.

💬 **Discussion Point:** It's important to emphasize practicing the skill that's hardest or most needed for each participant. Discuss with participants which "what" skill (observing, describing, participating) is their strength and which is their weakness. The one they find most needed is the one they should practice the most.

💬 **Discussion Point:** Discuss the relationships among the three mindfulness skills. Remind participants: "When you are observing, observe; when you're describing, describe; when you're participating, participate."

E. Participating Practice Exercises

1. Laugh Club

Explain to participants that laughing can have very positive effects on health and happiness. Instruct all to start laughing with you and continue until you stop. Then start laughing, keeping it up for several minutes. (Do not worry if some refuse; it can be very difficult *not* to laugh when others are laughing.)

2. Sound Ball[44]

The game here is throwing and catching sounds. To throw a sound, a person brings his or her hands up, bends toward another person, and mimics throwing a basketball to the other person, while at the same time making a sound ("uuuggggg," "zoopitydo," "luloulee," or any other nonsense sound). Generally, the sound is "thrown" in a drawn-out, sing-song voice. The person "catching the song" brings his or her hands up near the ears, bends back, and imitates the sound. That person then throws a different sound to someone else, and so on. Have everyone stand in a circle and practice the concept until everyone gets how the game is played. Then start the game. The idea is to throw and catch sounds as fast as everyone can.

3. Rain Dance

Ask everyone to stand in a circle. Instruct everyone that their task is to do whatever the person on their left is doing, changing what they are doing when the person to their left changes. Remind them not to look at you, just focus on what the person on their left is doing. Start by rubbing your hands up and down together. Once everyone, including the person on your left, is rubbing hands, you stop rubbing your hands together and start snapping your fingers. Follow this with the following moves: patting your thighs; stepping up and down; patting your thighs again; snapping your fingers again; rubbing hands together again; and standing still. This is called the "rain dance" because it sounds like rain in a forest.

✓   ### 4. Improvisation

Improvisation can be a lot of fun and involves the practice of mindful participating with spontaneity. It also involves letting go of being separate from others and throwing oneself into the story plot that is unfolding as each person takes a turn. If you have an improv teacher who can come to teach a group class, or if one of your group leaders has experience with improv (or is willing to read up and experiment with it), this can be a very good way to increase participants' (and your own) mindful participation skills.

a. Improvisation 1

To begin this exercise, have group members sit or stand in a circle. Instruct participants that the idea of the mindfulness practice is for each person to become part of the community that is the circle of persons. The idea is to become part of the circle, advancing the community's story. The first person begins by saying a word to start a story. Each person says only one word as the story goes around the circle. Each person tries to respond as quickly as possible with a word that advances the story line that has been told by the time it gets to him or her. The idea is for participants to give up thinking ahead and let go of clinging to their own story lines when necessary. (Example: "A . . . boy . . . once . . . fell . . . from . . . the . . . sky . . . ")

b. Improvisation 2

Have participants stand in a circle. Use the same instructions as above, except instead of having each person say only one word, ask each person to say a phrase. (Example: "Once upon a time . . . there was a big bear. . . . The bear was ferocious . . . but the bear was also kind. . . . A little boy nearby . . . saw the bear . . . ")

5. Row, Row Your Boat in Rounds

Divide the participants into two, three, or four groups, and then sing "Row, Row, Row Your Boat" in rounds. Here are the words: (a) "Row, row, row your boat," (b) "Gently down the stream," (c) "Merrily, merrily, merrily, merrily," (d) "Life is but a dream." While singing, the participants are to throw themselves into pantomiming the song: (a) rowing, (b) hands waving slightly up and down to signify moving down the stream, (c) hands up and head going from side to side, (d) hands together and head laid down on hands.

6. Dances

There are many circle folk dances that a group can do to music. Two easy dances are as follows.[48]

a. Shepherd's Dance

Standing in a circle, each person puts both arms out to his or her neighbors, right hand palm up and left hand palm down on the neighbor's palm. The dance is done to a count of 4, starting with (1) the left foot out and pointed straight forward, (2) left foot out pointed to the left, (3) then pointed out to the back, and then (4) back down on the floor next to the right foot. Then repeat with the right foot: (1) pointed to the front, (2) to the right, (3) to the back, and (4) back down next to the left foot. Then step (1) left foot to left, then right foot left and down next to the left foot; and repeat the same steps three more times for (2), (3), and (4). Repeat the two sequences over, and keep repeating until the music stops. This can be done to any music with a four-count beat. The music we use is the "Shepherd's Dance."[49] When we don't have this music available we have danced while we sang "We Shall Overcome."

b. Invitation Dance

What makes this next dance special is the instruction at the beginning. Before you start, suggest to participants: "Invite a person in your life (living or dead) to dance with you." Then, standing in a circle, have each person put both arms out in front of him or her, palms up in an inviting and willing posture. The dance involves two steps to the right and one step to the left: (1) right foot to right, left foot moves right and down next to right foot; and (2) repeat. Then (3) left foot to left, then right foot left and down next to the left foot. Tell participants: "When you are moving to the right, turn the hips and body toward the right. Then, when you are moving to the left, turn the left foot toward the left and bring the right foot down next to it, with hips and body toward the left. Repeat the sequence, and keep repeating until the music stops." This can be danced to "Red Rain" by Maria Farantouri (*www.youtube.com/watch?v=BVsHTWLYu9g*). (Start first step going right with beat at approximately 48 seconds in.) This dance can also be done with "Nada Te Turbe," a hymn that originated in the Taizé religious community in Spain, and that has a much easier beat to dance to. It is a Christian song in Spanish, but an English translation can be found on YouTube (*www.youtube.com/watch?v=fvfTVxgkWpo*). Any other music with a similar beat would work. I usually teach the dance first with "Nada Te Turbe" and then go to "Red Rain."

> **Note to Leaders:** The idea of "inviting others to dance with you in your mind" came from my experience with this dance, where I always invite all the psychiatric unit inpatients in the world to dance with me. When I suggested this to my graduate students, they found it extremely moving, with many in tears. So be prepared for an emotional response to this. Be sure to have participants share their experiences after the dances.

7. Walking

Have everyone stand in a single-file line and then walk for some minutes at the pace of the leader. Instruct participants to space themselves approximately an arm's length from each other.

8. Backward Writing[50]

Give each participant a piece of paper and a pencil. Instruct them to hold the pencil in the non-dominant hand, and then to write the alphabet backward from Z to A. A variation is writing with a different hand: Ask participants to describe their favorite vacation or memory by writing it down, using the hand they do not normally write with. Then ask them to discuss what they observed about their experience.

9. Origami

Bring in a simple set of origami instructions (the instructions for making a box are easy enough to follow). Hand out the flat pieces of paper, and ask the group to follow your lead with the folds. Walk the group through the steps. When the origami creations are complete, you can discuss a couple of things with participants. First, you can discuss participants' ability to stay mindful, noticing of being judgmental or nonjudgmental, and so on. Second, you can discuss how the piece of paper that started as a square or rectangle has now changed form (different function, shape, etc.).

10. Changing Seats

In our groups (and treatment teams!), people tend to want to sit in the same place they always sit. Before beginning this exercise, wait until all group members are seated and settled. Give a general instruction to observe and be mindful of reactions to what is to come. Then ask everyone to get up and move to a seat on the opposite side of the room. Share in terms of awareness of willfulness, as well as resistance to change. Ask participants to share observations of what they see/experience differently in their new seats.

11. Balancing Eggs

This is an exercise learned from a Chinese psychiatrist who visited my clinic. Bring in a set of raw eggs at room temperature. Clear a space on a table (don't use a tablecloth). Give each person an egg. Instruct each person to hold the egg lightly with his or her fingers with the large end on the table, and then try to balance the egg in such a way that when the participant takes the fingers away, the egg stays balanced on its end. Continue until most participants get their eggs balanced.

> **Note to Leaders:** It is important for you to practice this exercise before you try to teach it to participants. It takes more concentration and mindfulness than you might be expecting.

12. Calligraphy

Calligraphy is an expressive and harmonious form of writing. If you have a calligraphy teacher who can come to a group to teach a class (or calligraphy books to work from), practicing calligraphy can be a wonderful mindfulness practice, as it requires mindful concentration on the moment. To work with this in class, you will need supplies, such as paper, pens or brushes, and ink.

13. Ikebana

Ikebana is a disciplined form of Japanese flower arranging. As with calligraphy, doing it well requires mindful concentration and presence to the moment. If you have an ikebana teacher who can come to a group to teach a class (or ikebana books to work from), this is for many a mindfulness practice. You will also need a few flowers and leaves or branches.

14. Becoming the Count

Instruct participants: "Become the count of your breath. Become only 'one' when you count 1, become only 'two' when you count 2, and so on."

15. Tai Chi, Qigong, Hatha Yoga, Spiritual Dance

There are very many forms of mindful movement, including martial arts, yoga, and dance. Practiced with concentration and awareness of present movement of the body, each is a long-standing form of mindfulness practice.

16. Hand Exercise[44]

Have the group members stand around an oval or rectangular table. Each member is instructed to place his or her left hand on the table. Then each member places his or her right hand underneath the left hand of the person to the right. One person starts the sequence by picking the right hand off the table and quickly placing it back down. The person to the right quickly lifts up his or her right hand. The hand movements continue around the circle in sequence, until someone does a double tap. This move reverses the direction of the hand movements, and these continue in the reverse direction until someone does a double tap again. Anyone who picks up a hand too early or too late removes that one hand and leaves the other hand on the table (if the other hand was doing what it was supposed to do). The exercise continues until only a couple of hands are left.

17. Snap, Crackle, and Pop[44]

All group members are instructed to say "snap" when they cross their chests with their left or right arms and point either immediately left or right; to say "crackle" when they raise their left or right arms over their heads and point immediately left or right; and to say "pop" when they point at anyone around the circle (who need not be immediately left or right). Any one person starts by saying "snap" while simultaneously pointing either immediately left or right. Whoever receives the point says "crackle" while simultaneously pointing immediately left or right. Whoever receives the point says "pop" while pointing at anyone in the circle. That person then starts with "snap" and begins the sequence again. Anyone who misspeaks or misgestures, while trying to maintain a reasonably fast pace, is out of this portion of the exercise. These people then become "distracters" and stand outside the circle trying to distract their peers (verbally, without physical contact). The "snap–crackle–pop" sequence continues until there are only two people remaining in the circle.

18. Last Letter, First Letter[44]

To begin this exercise, have group members sit in a circle. The first person begins by saying a word. Then the individual to the right must say a word that starts with the last letter of the word the first person says. (Sample sequence: "bus," "steak," "key," "yellow," etc.) Tell participants: "As you continue around the circle, let go of any distractions. Notice any judgments you may have regarding your ability to think of a word quickly." Afterward, discuss observations with the participants.

✓ ### 19. Acceptance by the Chair

Remind participants that the focus of participating is to experience one's unity with the universe. With all participants seated, ask them to close their eyes and then listen to you saying:

> "Focus your attention on your body touching the chair you sit in. . . . Consider how the chair accepts you totally, holds you up, supports your back, and keeps you from falling down on the floor. . . . Notice how the chair does not throw you off, saying you are too fat or too thin or not just right. . . . Notice how accepting the chair is of you. . . . Focus your attention on your floor holding up the chair. . . . Consider the kindness of the floor holding you up, keeping your feet out of the dirt, providing a path for you to get to other things. . . . Notice the walls enclosing you in a room, so everyone going by does not hear everything you say. . . . Consider the kindness of the walls. . . . Notice the ceiling keeping the rain and winter cold and hot summer sun from beating down on you. . . . Consider the kindness of the ceiling. . . . Allow yourself to be held by the chair, held by the floor, and held by the walls and ceiling. . . . Notice the kindness."

You might want to read the following poem by Pat Schneider.[51] It highlights the idea that love and acceptance are all around us. The point here is to let go of rigid ideas about where we can find love, acceptance, respect, and generosity.

The Patience of Ordinary Things*

It is a kind of love, is it not?
How the cup holds the tea,
How the chair stands sturdy and foursquare,
How the floor receives the bottoms of shoes
Or toes. How soles of feet know
Where they're supposed to be.
I've been thinking about the patience
Of ordinary things, how clothes
Wait respectfully in closets
And soap dries quietly in the dish,
And towels drink the wet
From the skin of the back.
And the lovely repetition of stairs.
And what is more generous than a window?

✓ F. Review of Between-Session Practice Exercises for Participating

Mindfulness Handout 4c lists a number of ideas for practicing participating. It is important to go over some of these with participants.

VII. MINDFULNESS "HOW" SKILLS: NONJUDGMENTALLY (MINDFULNESS HANDOUTS 5–5A)

Main Point: "How" skills are *how* we observe, describe, and participate. There are three "how" skills: acting nonjudgmentally, one-mindfully, and effectively. Nonjudgmentalness is letting go of evaluating and judging reality.

Mindfulness Handout 5: Taking Hold of Your Mind: "How" Skills. The "how" skills can be taught in one session. First give a brief overview of each skill: nonjudgmentally, one-mindfully, and effectively. The key points are on the handout. You will need to spend more time on nonjudgmentalness the first time through the skills, as the concepts are difficult for most participants to grasp. They can also be difficult for skills trainers to grasp clearly, so be sure to review them carefully before you teach them. Nonjudgmentalness is fundamental to all mindfulness teaching and thus must be covered until participants understand what the practice is. It is important to pay attention to the nuances of this skill. Be sure to conduct practice exercises for nonjudgmentalness before moving to the next skill. You will have a chance to do further teaching on these skills during the review of homework practice. These skills are best learned through practice, feedback, and coaching.

Mindfulness Handout 5a: Ideas for Practicing Nonjudgmentalness. The first five practice ideas for nonjudgmentalness are organized in order from easiest to hardest. For individuals who are having difficulties reducing judgmentalness, these practice exercises can be assigned in order, one exercise per week.

Mindfulness Worksheets 2, 2a, 2b: Mindfulness Core Skills Practice; Mindfulness Worksheet 2c: Mindfulness Core Skills Calendar. These worksheets are the same as those used in teaching the "what" skills of observing, describing, and participating. Each asks participants to describe their mindfulness practice. When the worksheets are used for this skill, ask participants to practice the skills of observing, describing, and participating *nonjudgmentally*.

---

*From Schneider, P. (2005). The patience of ordinary things. In *Another river: New and selected poems*. Amherst, MA: Amherst Writers and Artists Press. Copyright 2005 by Pat Schneider. Reprinted by permission.

> **Mindfulness Worksheet 5: Mindfulness "How" Skills: Nonjudgmentalness, One-Mindfulness, Effectiveness.** This worksheet provides space for recording only two practices of a "how" skill for the week.
>
> **Mindfulness Worksheet 5a: Nonjudgmentalness, One-Mindfulness, Effectiveness Checklist; Mindfulness Worksheet 5b: Nonjudgmentalness, One-Mindfulness, Effectiveness Calendar; Mindfulness Worksheet 5c: Nonjudgmentalness Calendar.** Worksheets 5a and 5b offer different formats for recording how skills practice. Worksheet 5c is an advanced worksheet for the single skill of nonjudgmentalness. It is most useful when you are working with someone on replacing judgmental thoughts, statements, assumptions, and/or expressions with nonjudgmental ones. This worksheet can also be very useful for DBT treatment teams in working with typical judgmental thoughts and assumptions about individual therapists, skills training leaders, and/or individual therapy/skills training participants.

✓ **A. Two Types of Judgments**

There are two types of judgments: judgments that *discriminate* and judgments that *evaluate*.

✓ **1. Judgments That Discriminate**

To "discriminate" is to discern or analyze whether two things are the same or different, whether something meets some type of standard, or whether something fits the facts.

Some people are paid to compare things to standards or to predict consequences—that is, to judge. Teachers give grades; grocers put out "good" food or produce and discard "bad" food. The word "good" is also used to give children and adults feedback about their behavior, so they will know what to keep doing and what to stop.

Example: An expert jeweler discriminates whether a stone purported to be a diamond is really a diamond or not.

✓ *Example:* A U.S. Supreme Court judge discriminates whether an action or law violates the Constitution.

Example: A criminal court judge discriminates whether an action is against the law or not.

✓ *Example:* Judges in a spelling contest discriminate whether contestants' spelling is the same as or different from that in the dictionary.

Discriminations are necessary. Discriminating between a swimming pool with water in it and one without water is essential before a swimmer dives into it. A person who can discriminate is often called a person with a "good eye" (e.g., a butcher who can select the piece of meat that will be most tender when cooked). Discriminating the effects of angry versus conciliatory behavior toward other people is essential to building lasting relationships.

✓ **2. Judgments That Evaluate**

To "evaluate" is to judge someone or something as good or bad, worthwhile or not, valuable or not.

Evaluations are something we add to the facts. They are based on opinions, personal values, and ideas in our minds. They are not part of factual reality.

✓ **3. Letting Go of Evaluations, Keeping Discriminations**

Our aim in nonjudgmentalness is to let go of judgments that evaluate as good and bad, and to keep judgments that discriminate and see consequences.

"Good" and "bad," however, are sometimes used as shorthand for describing consequences.

✓ *Example:* When fish is slimy and old, and won't taste good if it's eaten, we say it is "bad." If it is rotten and will make us sick, we say it is "bad." If it is fresh and not contaminated, we say it is "good."

Example: When people hurt others or are destructive, we call them "bad." When they help others, we call them "good."

Example: If it rains on a parade and people are distressed, we call it "bad." If it is sunny and people are happy, we call it "good."

Example: We say that people have "good judgment" when they are skilled at seeing the consequences of their own behaviors or decisions.

But it is easy to leave out stating consequences and simply call other people or events "good" and "bad." When we use "good" and "bad," we often forget that we are adding something to reality. We forget that we are predicting consequences. We treat our judgments as facts. People also treat their judgments of us as facts.

✓ Discriminations can easily become judgmental as well. Discriminations can turn into judgments when we exaggerate differences between two things. That is, we describe what we believe to be factual rather than what we observe to be factual. Discrimination against various people or ideas is based on judging certain characteristics of the people or certain ideas as "good" or "bad." When we feel threatened by differences, it is easier to become judgmental.

Example: Black people are inferior to whites.

Example: Women are less worthwhile than men.

Example: Homosexuals are evil people.

4. *The Nature of Evaluations*

✓ Judgments that evaluate as good or bad are in the mind of the observer. They are not qualities of what the observer is judging.

We are judgmental when we add an evaluation of worth or value to what we have observed. "Good" and "bad" are never observed. They are qualities put on things by the person observing. If something can be worthwhile, valuable, or good in the eyes of one person or group, it can always be viewed as worthless, of no value, or bad by another person or group. An important mindfulness skill is *not* judging things in this manner.

✓ *Example:* Different cultures see different things as good and different things as bad. Different families have different values. Different schools have different rules for what is good behavior and what is bad behavior. The same is true in different companies.

✓ ⚽ **Story Point:** Imagine that a tiger chases a man for dinner. What does the man think? "No, no! This is bad!" If the tiger catches the man and eats him, his family members might say, "This is terrible! This is bad!!" Or they might say, "He should not have been out there alone," "They [the guides on his safari] should have protected him and not let him out there by himself," or the like. What does the tiger say, however? The tiger says, "Yum, yum."

5. *The Nature of Nonjudgmentalness*

✓ Nonjudgmentalness is describing reality as "what is," without adding evaluations of "good" and "bad" or the like to it.

💬 **Discussion Point:** Discuss the difference between discriminating and being judgmental. Elicit examples of when people have been judged as good or bad, and when something they have done has been judged as meeting a standard or not. For example, a person may get a B on a math test, but may not feel that the teacher is judging the person or the performance as "bad."

💬 **Discussion Point:** Discuss when discrimination between characteristics of people leads to unjust behaviors—as, for example, in discrimination based on race, gender, sexual orientation, age, or disability. Knowing that two things are different may be an important discrimination, but it may be far more important to be an accurate judge of whether the observed difference makes a difference. Refusing to hire a man without hands as a pianist does not mean he cannot be hired as a tap dancer, for instance.

B. Why Be Nonjudgmental?

1. Judgments Can Have Damaging Effects on Relationships

Negative judgmentalness creates conflict and can damage relationships with people we care for. Very few of us like people who are judgmental of us. Judging others might get people to change temporarily, but more often it leads people to avoid or retaliate against those who judge them badly.

2. Judgments Can Have Negative Effects on Emotions

Adding judgments can have a huge impact on our emotions. When we add evaluations of "good" and "bad" to people or things around us, it can have a strong effect on our emotional responses to the persons or things we are judging. It is then often difficult to recognize that we have created the judgments, and thus have created the very events that can dysregulate our emotions.

✓ 💬 **Discussion Point:** Elicit from participants whether they have more difficulty judging themselves or judging others. Do they often feel judged by others? What about judgments they hear around them, or on radio, TV, or the Internet? (Notice if they are judging those who judge.)

✓ ### 3. Changing the Causes of Things Works Better Than Judging

Everything that has happened in the universe has been caused. Changing the causes of things works better than judging things we don't like.

In other words, saying that things "should" not have happened, or saying that they are "bad" and "should" be different, is ineffective and does not change things. If we want drunk drivers off the road, we need to develop circumstances that cause them to stop drinking and driving. We may need stronger laws against drunk driving or more police patrols to enforce the law. We may also need to provide effective treatment for people with alcohol problems, and to persuade other people not to drive with people who are drinking.

Similarly, if we want people to vote for something we believe in, we have to give them a cause to vote our way. We will need to provide persuasive arguments that they will believe, or arguments against voting against our position. Or if we want a new dog to urinate outside instead of on our new carpets, we have to cause a new behavior to develop by training the dog.

✓ *Example:* Standing near a table, ask participants to imagine that on the table is a priceless heirloom—a white lace tablecloth that is 300 years old and has been in your family all that time. Then, holding a small object in your hand, ask them to imagine that what you are holding is a glass of fine red wine. As you continue dropping the object on the table, picking it up, and dropping it again, keep asking, "Should this glass of red wine spill on the table?" If they or you say yes, then put your other hand out and catch the object before it hits the table. Comment that if you don't want the glass of wine to spill on the table, you have to do something to cause it not to hit the table when it is dropped. If you or they then comment that the glass of wine would not drop on the table if you did not open your hands, comment that you would have to change the neural firing of your brain for that not to happen.

💬 **Discussion Point:** If making demands does not change reality, why do we keep making them? The answer: Sometimes expressing our demands really does change reality. Getting angry, pouting, or crying out about the unfairness of what someone has done does sometimes make people change, just to get us to stop acting so angry, stop pouting, or stop crying. Elicit from participants times this has been true for them. What are the positive consequences of this? What are the negative consequences? Discuss.

4. Nonjudgmentalness Is Fundamental to Mindfulness

Nonjudgmentalness is stressed in all mindfulness-based treatments (including Mindfulness-Based Cognitive Therapy, Mindfulness-Based Stress Reduction, and Mindfulness-Based Relapse Prevention), as well as in all treatments that emphasize acceptance of others and of oneself and one's own behavior. It is central to all spiritual traditions of mindfulness.

✓ C. Nonjudgmentally: How to Do It

1. Let Go of Good and Bad

View and describe reality as "what is." Let go of evaluating people, their behavior, and events as good or bad.

Example: Let go of saying that a person or the person's behavior is either "bad" or "good."

Example: Let go of saying that a person or characteristic is "worthless" or "worthwhile."

Example: Let go of calling oneself a "bad person" or a "good person."

The goal here is to take a nonjudgmental stance when observing, describing, and participating. Judging is any labeling or evaluating of something as good or bad, as valuable or not, as worthwhile or worthless. Letting go of such labeling is being nonjudgmental.

✓ 2. Replace Evaluations with Simple Statements of "It Is," or with Descriptions of What Is

The goal is not to replace "bad" with "good," to switch "worthless" for "worthwhile," or to make other similar replacements. If you are good, you can always be bad; if you are worthwhile, you can always be worthless. Second, changing a negative judgment into a positive judgment can obscure the negative consequences of an event. For example, saying that a rotten piece of meat is good instead of bad could cause someone to eat it and then get sick. The idea is to eliminate evaluations entirely.

Example: When buying a new house, rather than asking, "Is it a good house?", we might ask, "Is it a house I will like?" or "Is it a house that will last a long time without a lot of repairs?" or "Will I be able to sell it for more than I bought it for?"

Example: If we call a pillow a "good pillow," we are using judgmental language instead of saying, "I like this pillow."

But does this mean that we cannot say "Good job" to someone or use positive words to praise others? *No*, it does not! Positive judgments have far fewer negative consequences than do negative judgments. In general, once we reduce our internal judgmentalness, we can go back to using the phrase "Good job" and the like to mean specific things. For example, if I say, "Good job!" to one of my students after hearing her present her handling of a very difficult problem in therapy, I would usually mean "You responded to that very effectively." Saying, "Good job!" to a 3-year-old boy who has mastered a new task may mean "I am proud of you."

✓ 3. Let Go of "Should"

Nonjudgmentalness involves letting go of the word "should." That is, it means letting go of being persons who define how the world should be, and letting go of demands on reality to be what we want it to be simply because we want it to be that way. When being nonjudgmental, we let go of saying and thinking that things should be different than they are. We also let go of saying that we ourselves should be different than we are.

✓   ### 4. Replace "Should" with Descriptions of Feelings or Desires

Nonjudgmentalness involves replacing "should" with describing how we feel or what we desire: "I want things to be different," "I want to be different than I am," or "I hope you will do this for me." An alternative is to replace "should" with "This is caused": "Everything is as it should be, given the causes of the universe."

✓   ## D. Getting the Concept of Nonjudgmentalness Across
✓   ### 1. Nonjudgmentalness Does Not Mean Approval

Being nonjudgmental means that everything *is* what it is, and that everything is *caused*. Rather than judging something as good or bad, it is more useful to describe the facts and then try to understand the causes. When things happen that are destructive, that we do not like, or that do not fit our values, we have a better chance of stopping or changing them if we try to understand and then change the causes. Yelling "Bad!" doesn't stop that many things. Even if we believe that there is an "evil force" or a "devil" in the world, understanding how it works and why it does what it does when it acts is a more effective strategy for getting change.

💬 **Discussion Point:** Participants may believe that by saying something is not "bad," then they must be saying it is "good," and vice versa. This is true only if people have the dichotomy "good–bad" in their minds in the first place and use that to describe things. Elicit from participants all the times others have applied judgments to them when they felt their doing, thinking, or feeling was neither good nor bad.

💬 **Discussion Point:** Elicit from participants times when others have called them "bad" and expected immediate change, versus times when others have tried to help them understand the causes of their own behaviors and help them change. What are the differences?

✓   ### 2. Nonjudgmentalness Does Not Mean Denying Consequences

A person who stops judging can still observe or predict consequences. It is often very important to observe and remember consequences of behaviors and events, particularly when consequences are either destructive to things we value or highly rewarding to us. And it can be very important to communicate these consequences to other people. Saying, "This piece of meat is bad," is a shorthand way of saying, "It is filled with bacteria and may make you sick if you eat it." Saying, "This paint will look really good in my house," means "I will really like this color if we use it in my house." Behavior that is destructive to others or to ourselves can still be labeled "bad." Behavior that is constructive or helpful to others or ourselves can still be labeled "good."

Judgments are often easier than describing consequences of things. People often use judgmental statements as a shorthand for consequences all the time, and eventually forget what consequences they are referring to. When there are a lot of negative consequences to a behavior, it can be easier to use "good" and "bad" as shorthand all the time.

✓   *Example:* Saying a person has "good judgment" means that when the person makes decisions, the outcomes are ordinarily beneficial to the person and/or to others.

✓   *Example:* All societies judge murder as "bad," because the consequences of allowing people to kill others whenever they want to harms the community as a whole.

Example: In politics, one side says, "This is good, good, good," while the other side says, "This is bad, bad, bad." However, these are only personal evaluations.

It is easy to simplify "good" and "bad" events or behaviors to "good" and "bad" people.

💬 **Discussion Point:** Discuss the difference between describing and judging. Judging is labeling something in an evaluative way as "good" or "bad." Describing is "just the facts." The facts may be that something is destructive or harmful, constructive or helpful.

💬 **Discussion Point:** Get examples of the difference between judging and noticing consequences: "Your behavior is terrible," versus "Your behavior is hurting me" or "What you are doing is going to result in my getting hurt"; "I am stupid and bad," versus "I missed my appointment for the third time, and this is going to get me in trouble with my friends if I don't change."

3. Nonjudgmentalness Does Not Mean Keeping Quiet about Preferences or Desires

✓ Asking for change is not judgmental.

But preferences and desires often become judgments on reality as it is.

- Saying that things "should" change (simply on our say-so) is judgmental.
- Saying that things "should" be different puts a demand on reality.
- Saying that things "should" be different implies that there is something wrong or bad about reality as it is.
- Saying that things "should" be different implies that a consequence that is caused should somehow not occur. This would, of course, require changing the rules of the universe.

✓ The important point here is this: Who says so? If each person gets to determine what "should" be at any given moment, we could say that each person has the power to be "God" of the universe. This would, of course, be a mighty responsibility, as changing one thing to fit our preferences on a particular day might have unintended consequences for the entire universe.

✓ 👥 **Practice Exercise:** The following exercise is a good way to make the point that "shoulds" are indeed based on preferences. Ask a participant to tell you something that he or she thinks "should" be different than it is. Then ask, "Why?" Once the person answers, ask why that should be so. For example, if a person says, "People should love others more," you would ask, "Why should people love others more?" Then when the person gives an answer, you ask again, "Why?" For example, if the person then responds, "Because when people are more loving, there is less war," you would ask, "And why should there be less war?" For each answer the person gives, you continue to ask, "And why should that be so?" You do this even if the person says, "Because it is God's will." In that case, you ask, "And why should God's will be carried out?" Ultimately, you will get to a final answer: "Because I want it to be that way." At that point, you can point out that the person is turning his or her own wishes into a demand on reality. Even if the person's wish is shared by most people on earth, even if it would be valued by most people, even if it is praiseworthy and wonderful, it is still a preference turned into a command. Alas, reality as a whole does not work by our commands. Changing reality requires changing causes.

✓ Saying that one thing *should* (or *must*) occur in order for a second thing to occur is *not* judgmental.

✓ *Example:* Saying, "I should turn the car key if I want the car to start," "I should study if I want to make good grades," or "I should look for a job if I want to find a job" is not judgmental. The trick here is to avoid the implication that "to be a good person, I should turn the car key, study, or look for a job." It is also important to avoid the implication that "to be a good person, I should want to start the car, make good grades, or find a job."

✓ 4. Values and Emotional Responses to Events Are Not Themselves Judgmental

A person can like something without also saying that it is good or bad. For example, many people dislike certain foods without judging those foods "bad." Values are principles, standards, or qualities that are considered desirable and admirable. Things that we value are things we believe are important for our welfare or the welfare of society at large. Generally, we have an attachment to our values (i.e., positive emotional feelings about our values). This is why it can be so difficult when someone disagrees with our values. We feel threatened. It is easy to view such people as "bad." Wanting, desiring, or admiring something, however, is not itself judging. Hating or feeling disgusted by something is not necessarily judgmental.

Judgments are often shorthand for describing preferences.

Example: Saying that a room looks "bad" or a book was "terrible" is based on a personal preference in decorating or in reading material (or sometimes on a personal or community standard for how rooms should look or how books should be written).

Example: Saying, "I should get the job because I am more experienced," is really just my preference that they give me the job, or my value that more experienced people should get jobs over less experienced people.

We often forget that such judgments are shorthand and take them as statements of fact. When values and preferences are very important, we feel threatened by people who disagree with us. Being threatened can easily lead to our calling others "bad."

💬 **Discussion Point:** Judging is often a way of getting out of responsibility. Explain: "If I don't like what other people are doing and want them to stop it, I can say, 'That is bad,' and I don't have to own up to the fact that the real reason they should stop is that I (and maybe others) don't like it, don't believe in it, or don't want the consequences." Elicit from participants times when others have tried to control their behavior by stating judgments as facts. Get examples of when they have tried that with someone else. Give your own examples here.

✓ **5. *Statements of Fact Are Not Judgmental, but Judgments Often Go Along with the Statements of Fact***

Many words have literal meanings that are not judgmental, but are almost always used as judgmental statements. A statement of fact may be a judgment because the fact is simultaneously being judged. For instance, "I am fat" may simply be a statement of fact. But if one adds (in thoughts, implication, or tone of voice) that being fat is bad or unattractive, then a judgment is added. A favorite judgmental word of participants I work with is "stupid," as in "I did a stupid thing," "I am stupid," or "What a stupid thing to say." Judgments often masquerade as statements of fact, so they can be hard to catch. Mental health professionals are very good at this sometimes. I once had a therapist try to convince me that calling a client "narcissistic" (for saying she felt more "real" when she was around me) was not a judgmental statement.

💬 **Discussion Point:** Discuss the difference between a judgment and a statement of facts. Get examples of judgmental statements masquerading as descriptions of facts.

> **Note to Leaders:** Some participants will believe that there really is an absolute "good" and an absolute "bad." You need to be dialectical here and search for a synthesis of different points of view. Do not expect participants to throw out judgments without a fight! Expect participants to bring up Hitler (or, more rarely, sexual abuse) as an example of "bad" with a capital B. Thus the next teaching point is important: Judgments have their place. Letting go of judging is an idea that will grow over time. Don't force it at the beginning. You can usually get more mileage out of focusing first on reducing self-judgments. (See Chapter 7 of the main DBT text for a more extensive discussion of these points.)

✓ **6. *Don't Judge Judging***

Emphasize to participants: "It is important to remember that you cannot change judging by judging judging."

E. Nonjudgmentalness Practice Exercises

As it is for developing the "what" skills (observing, describing, participating), practice is important for developing the "how" skills. You can do one exercise and then ask participants to share their experiences of it, or you can do several of these sequentially and then ask them to share.

p194

1. Any Participating Exercise

When asked to participate in a task such as those described for participating (see Section VI, E), most people have judgmental thoughts either about themselves or others. Using participating exercises to practice nonjudgmentalness works best if you first start the exercise and then, after a few minutes, stop and ask people whether they are judging themselves. For example, are they thinking, "I look silly," or "I'm really stupid, I can't do this"? Almost always, when the exercise restarts, people find it easier to let go of judgments.

2. Walking Slowly in a Line

Ask participants to walk slowly in a line, either around in a circle indoors or single file outdoors. What almost always happens in this exercise is that people start judging the person in front of them or behind them, or they judge the person giving the instructions. As above, it is useful to stop in the middle and review who is already judging. Then start again.

3. Describing Something That Is Disliked

Ask each person to describe a disliked interaction with someone or a disliked characteristic of another person or of herself. Have participants practice describing these things without using judgmental words or tone of voice.

4. Starting Over without Judgments

During the session, stop anyone who uses a judgmental voice tone or judgmental words. Ask the person to start the sentence over and to drop judgmental words and voice tone. Do this every session, even when other skills are being taught, and individuals will ultimately get in the habit of being nonjudgmental.

F. Nonjudgmentalness Practice Exercises for Between Sessions

The following are individual practice ideas for participants who are having lots of trouble with judgmental thoughts. The practice exercises are listed in order from easiest to hardest. Check up on each assignment each week, and give the next assignment once the current exercise is mastered. Each suggestion is a daily practice that starts over on the next day. These exercises are also included in Mindfulness Handout 5a, along with other ways to practice nonjudgmentalness; it is important to go over this handout with participants. Ask participants to do the following:

- "Practice observing judgmental thoughts going through the mind. Remember, do not judge judging."
- "Count up judgmental thoughts each day. You can do this in one of several ways. You can tear up pieces of paper, put them in a pocket on one side, and move them to a pocket on the other side each time you notice a judgment. Or buy a golf or sports counter, and each time a judgment goes through, push the counter. Or record judgments on a cell smartphone each time one comes by. At the end of each day, write down the count, and start over the next day. Remember that observing and recording behavior can be an effective way of changing behavior."
- "Replace judgmental thoughts, statements, or assumptions with nonjudgmental ones." (See below for tips on how to do this.)
- "Observe your judgmental facial expressions, posture, and voice tones (both internal and external). It can sometimes be helpful to ask caring others to point these out."
- "Change judgmental voice tones and expressions to nonjudgmental expressions (and, if necessary, apologies)."

G. Tips for Replacing Judgmental Thoughts

See also the list under item 3 on Mindfulness Handout 5a.

■ "Describe the facts of the event or situation—*only* what is observed with your senses." (For example, "The white fish is not fresh and has a fishy smell.")

■ "Describe the consequences; keep to the facts." (For example, "This fish may taste rancid when cooked.")

■ "Describe your own feelings in response to the facts. Emotions are not judgments." (For example, "I don't want to serve this fish for dinner.")

VIII. MINDFULNESS "HOW" SKILLS: ONE-MINDFULLY (MINDFULNESS HANDOUTS 5–5B)

> **Main Point:** Acting one-mindfully, the second of the three mindfulness "how" skills, consists of focusing attention on the present moment and bringing the whole person to bear on one task or activity.
>
> **Mindfulness Handout 5: Taking Hold of Your Mind: "How" Skills.** This is the same handout used in teaching the skill of nonjudgmentalness. Review the "One-Mindfully" section of the handout with participants. It is important to note that this skill encompasses two ideas: being completely present to the moment, and doing one thing at a time. Both have to do with focusing the mind.
>
> **Mindfulness Handout 5b: Ideas for Practicing One-Mindfulness** (Optional). It is useful to have this handout available, as it gives a number of practice exercises for one-mindfulness.
>
> **Mindfulness Worksheets 2, 2a, 2b: Mindfulness Core Skills Practice; Mindfulness Worksheet 2c: Mindfulness Core Skills Calendar; Mindfulness Worksheet 5: Mindfulness "How" Skills: Nonjudgmentalness, One-Mindfulness, Effectiveness; Mindfulness Worksheet 5a: Nonjudgmentalness, One-Mindfulness, Effectiveness Checklist; Mindfulness Worksheet 5b: Nonjudgmentalness, One-Mindfulness, Effectiveness Calendar.** These worksheets are the same as those used in teaching the skills of observing, describing, and participating, as well as nonjudgmentalness. Each asks participants to describe their mindfulness practice. For this skill, ask participants to practice one-mindfulness and then record their experience.

✓ **A. One-Mindfully: What Is It?**

✓ *1. One-Mindfully Means Being Completely Present in This One Moment*

One-mindfulness means, for "just this moment," being present to our lives and what we are doing. Like nonjudgmentalness, living one-mindfully is central to all mindfulness teaching and contemplative practices. It is central to both psychological and spiritual traditions of mindfulness.

a. The Past Is Over

The past is over; it does not exist in the present. We may have thoughts and images of the past. Intense emotions may arise within us when we think about the past, or when images of the past go through our minds. We may worry about things we did in the past or things others did. We may wish that our pasts were different, or wish that we were still in the past. But it is crucial to recognize that these thoughts, images, feelings, and wishes are occurring in the present.

Trouble starts when, instead of being aware of thinking about the past, we become lost in the past or in past thinking and imagining. We stop paying attention to what is happening right here and now, and instead focus our minds inadvertently on thoughts and images about the past. Our emotions now may be identical to the emotions we felt in the past, making us think that we are actually living in the past or that the past is living in us.

b. The Future Has Not Come into Existence

The same points can be made with respect to the future. It does not exist. We may have many thoughts about and plans for the future. Intense emotions may arise within us when we think about the future. We may have many worries about the future. Indeed, we may spend many hours and endless nights worrying about the future. But, as with worries about the past, it is very important to remember that our worries about the future are occurring in the present. Just as we can get lost in our thoughts and images of the past, we can get lost in ruminating about the future.

Living in the present can include planning for the future. It simply means that when we plan, we plan with awareness that we are doing it (i.e., we plan as a present-moment activity).

✓ ### 2. One-Mindfully Means Doing One Thing at a Time

One-mindfulness also means doing one thing at a time, with awareness. It is focusing attention on only *one* activity or thing at a time, bringing the whole person to bear on this thing or activity.

> **Research Point:** This notion is very similar to an effective therapy for chronic worriers developed by Thomas Borkovec.[52] The essence of the therapy is "Worry when you are worrying." It involves setting aside 30 minutes each day to worry. Explain: "You go to the same place each day, and try to spend the whole time worrying. During the rest of the day, you banish worries from your mind, reminding yourself that you will attend to that particular worry during your worry time. There is a similar technique for fighting insomnia: writing down all the things you need to remember for the next day before you go to sleep, so you won't have to wake up to think about them."

B. One-Mindfully: Why Do It?

✓ ### 1. The Pain of the Present Moment Is Enough Pain for Anyone

Adding to a painful present moment all the pain from the past and all the pain from the future is too much. It is too much suffering.

> **Research Point:** One of the reasons mindfulness is an effective treatment for physical pain is that it keeps us in the present. Ruminating about suffering in the past, and dreading suffering in the future, both increase the pain in the moment. The road to less pain is letting go of past and future pain, and suffering only the pain of the present moment.

✓ ### 2. Multitasking Is Inefficient

There is now quite a bit of research on multitasking (doing more than one thing at a time). Contrary to what most people believe, trying to juggle two things at once does not save time. In fact, it cuts down on the ability to do things quickly.[53–59]

3. Life, Relationships, and Beauty Pass You By

When life is led in mindlessness of the present, the present whizzes by. We do not experience many of the things we care about. We do not smell the roses.

C. One-Mindfully: How to Do It

✓ ### 1. Be Present to Your Own Experiences

Being present to our own experiences is the opposite of avoiding or trying to suppress our present experiences. It is allowing ourselves to be aware of our current experiences—our feelings, our sensations, our thoughts, our movements and actions.

2. Rivet Yourself to Now

The next step is to actively focus and maintain awareness of what we are experiencing now, what is happening now, and what we are doing now. This involves letting go of thoughts of both the past and the future. We spend much of our time living in the past (which is over), living in the future (which is not here yet), or responding to our concepts and ideas of what reality is rather than what it actually is. Thus a primary aim of one-mindfulness is to maintain awareness of the moment we are in.

✓   *Example:* "You are in a meeting and very bored. Rather than sitting and thinking about all the things you would rather be doing, throw yourself into listening. Focus on the present. This can stop you from being miserable."

    Example: "When you are driving, drive. When you're walking, walk. When you are eating, eat."

3. Do Only One Thing at a Time

✓

Doing only one thing at a time is the opposite of how people usually like to operate. Most of us think that if we do several things at once, we will accomplish more; this is not true. The trick is to have our minds completely on what we are doing at the moment. This refers to both mental and physical activities.

✓   *Example:* "You have five dishes to wash, but you can only wash one at a time."

However, this does not mean that we cannot switch from one thing to another and back. Focusing on one thing in the moment does not mean that we cannot do complex tasks requiring many sequential activities. But it does mean that whatever we do, we should attend fully to it. Thus the essence of the idea is acting with undivided attention. The opposites are mindlessness (i.e., automatic behaviors without awareness) and distracted behavior (i.e., doing one thing while thinking about or attending to another).

💬 **Discussion Point:** Discuss an example of doing two things at once, such as sitting in skills training and thinking about the past or worrying about the future. Explain: "A mindfulness perspective would suggest that if you are going to think about the past, you should devote your full attention to it. If you are going to worry about the future, devote your full attention to it. If you are going to attend class, devote your full attention to it." Get participants to come up with other examples (e.g., watching TV or reading while eating dinner).

D. One-Mindfulness Practice Exercises

Mindfulness Handout 5b lists a number of ideas for practicing being one-mindful. It is important to go over some of these with participants.

IX. MINDFULNESS "HOW" SKILLS: EFFECTIVELY (MINDFULNESS HANDOUTS 5–5C)

> **Main Point:** Acting effectively, the third of the three mindfulness "how" skills, is doing what works and using skillful means.
>
> **Mindfulness Handout 5: Taking Hold of Your Mind: "How" Skills.** This is the same handout used in teaching the skills of acting nonjudgmentally and one-mindfully. Review the "Effectively" section of the handout with participants. The key point here is that to reach one's goals, to reduce suffering, and to increase happiness, using effective means is critical. Willfulness (the opposite of the skill of willingness; see Distress Tolerance Handout 13: Willingness) and pride, however, often get in the way. The best way to teach this skill is to find a way to appeal to each participant's ultimate self-interest.

Mindfulness Handout 5c: Ideas for Practicing Effectiveness. Practicing effectiveness can be difficult if you do not have a situation where effectiveness is needed. This handout gives some ideas on how to practice.

Mindfulness Worksheets 2, 2a, 2b: Mindfulness Core Skills Practice; Mindfulness Worksheet 2c: Mindfulness Core Skills Calendar; Mindfulness Worksheet 5: Mindfulness "How" Skills: Non-judgmentalness, One-Mindfulness, Effectiveness; Mindfulness Worksheet 5a: Nonjudgmentalness, One-Mindfulness, Effectiveness Checklist; Mindfulness Worksheet 5b: Nonjudgmentalness, One-Mindfulness, Effectiveness Calendar. These worksheets are the same as those used in teaching the "what" skills, as well as nonjudgmentalness and one-mindfulness. Each asks participants to describe their mindfulness practice. For this skill, ask participants to practice the skills of effectiveness. To do this, participants need to be vigilant for situations where they are tempted to do something dysfunctional or ineffective. These are the situations where effectiveness is needed. Also encourage participants to write down times when they easily or even automatically act in an effective manner.

✓ A. Effectively: What Is It?

Acting effectively is doing what works to achieve our goals. The goal here is to focus on doing what works, rather than what is "right" versus "wrong" or "fair" versus "unfair." Generally, it is the opposite of "cutting off your nose to spite your face." Acting effectively means using skillful means to achieve our goals.

✓ B. Why Act Effectively?

Without the skill to use effective means, it is difficult to reach our goals, reduce suffering, or increase happiness. Being right or proving a point may feel good for the moment, but in the long term, getting what we want in life is more satisfying.

Example: "Yelling at the reservation clerk who says you do not have a reservation for a hotel room (when you know you called and made one) may make you feel good in the moment, but actually getting a hotel room (which may require skillful means) would be likely to make you feel even better."

C. Effectively: How to Do It

1. Know the Goal or Objective

Doing what works (what is effective) requires, first, knowing what our goal or objective in a particular situation is.

✓ 💬 **Discussion Point:** Not knowing what we want makes effectiveness hard. It can be very hard to know what we want when emotions get in the way. We can mistake being afraid of something with not wanting something, being angry at someone with not wanting to be close to the person, being ashamed of our own actions with not wanting to be around certain people. Discuss with participants when confusion over goals and objectives interferes with effectiveness. Elicit examples of when emotions have interfered.

2. Know and React to the Actual Situation

Being effective requires knowing and reacting to the actual situation, not to what we think the situation *should* be.

Example: Signs on the freeway tell people to drive in the right lane except to pass. People who tailgate slower drivers in the left lane, switch their lights off and on, or keep honking (instead of just passing from the right lane) are acting as if all people are willing to follow highway directions. All are not!

Example: A person wants to get a raise at work, but thinks the supervisor should know without being told that a raise is deserved, and so the person refuses to ask for it. In this case, the person is putting being right over achieving the goal of getting a raise.

💬 **Discussion Point:** Get examples of participants' "cutting off their noses" to make a point. Share examples of your own here as well—the more outrageous or humorous, the better.

3. *Know What Will and Won't Work to Achieve Goals*

Effectiveness requires knowing what will and what won't work to achieve our goals. Much of the time, we know what is and is not effective if we are calm and can think about our options. At other times, however, being effective means asking for help or asking for instructions in what to do. To be more effective, some participants may need to improve their problem-solving skills (see Emotion Regulation Handout 12). An openness to experimenting, to staying aware of the consequences of what we do, and sufficient humility to learn from our mistakes are essential to effectiveness.

Example: "If you want people to remember your birthday, you can call to remind them beforehand, rather than letting them forget."

Example: "When the goal is to make someone happy, it is more effective to do what you know will make them happy than to take a stand and be 'right.' "

✓ *Example:* "When things are going wrong at the airport, it is more effective to talk calmly to the people who can help you than to yell at them. Yelling and making a scene can cause the reservations person to put you on a flight far in the future!"

✓ ### 4. *"Play by the Rules" When Necessary*

Effectiveness also involves "playing by the rules" when this is needed to achieve a goal. Playing by the rules is most important in situations where we are in a low-power position and what we want is important.

Example: Being an involuntary patient in a state hospital is a situation in which playing by the rules is vitally necessary. Staff members make the rules about when a patient gets privileges. Right or wrong, they have the power, not the patients.

Example: Other examples of situations that call for playing by the rules include being a prisoner in jail, an applicant for a bank loan, or a person going through security at an airport. In each situation, other people make the rules and can enforce them.

5. *Be Savvy about People*

Effectiveness often means being "political" or savvy about people. It is taking people where they are (rather than where they "should" be) and going from there. Different people are like different cultures. What works in one culture may not work in another. Focusing on what's "right" instead of what works is like trying to impose our own culture on another country when visiting.

💬 **Discussion Point:** Get examples of when participants have imposed their own cultures or views on others. Also, when have others imposed in this way on participants?

6. *Sacrifice a Principle to Achieve a Goal When Necessary*

Effectiveness sometimes requires sacrificing principles to achieve a goal. In extreme situations (e.g., a concentration camp, where not playing by the rules would mean death), most people are willing to sacrifice their principles even if the rules are not fair. In real life, this is sometimes very hard. It can be especially hard just when it is needed most, with people in authority positions.

💬 **Discussion Point:** Discuss with participants which "how" skill (taking a nonjudgmental stance, focusing on one thing in the moment, being effective) is their strength and which is their weakness. The one they have most difficulty with is the one to practice the most.

✓ **D. Effectiveness Practice Exercises**

Mindfulness Handout 5c lists a number of ideas for practicing effectiveness. It is important to go over some of these with participants.

X. SUMMARY OF THE MODULE

At the end of the Mindfulness module, summarize states of mind, the mindfulness "what" skills (observing, describing, participating), and the mindfulness "how" skills (taking a nonjudgmental stance, focusing on one thing in the moment, being effective). If you have used supplemental skills (see Sections XI–XVI, below), they should also be summarized. Remind participants that they need to continue practicing mindfulness skills throughout all of the skills training modules (and beyond).

XI. OVERVIEW: OTHER PERSPECTIVES ON MINDFULNESS (MINDFULNESS HANDOUT 6)

> **Main Point:** There are many possible approaches to mindfulness, and many possible outcomes that can be obtained from the practice of mindfulness. This set of handouts can be taught in their entirety, or you can select specific skills to fit the individuals you are working with. Mindfulness Handout 7a highlights the role of spirituality in mindfulness practices for both leaders and participants. The handout is meant to promote discussion; there is no worksheet for it.
>
> **Mindfulness Handout 6: Overview: Other Perspectives on Mindfulness Skills.** Review this handout quickly unless you plan on skipping the handouts associated with each topic (Mindfulness Handouts 7–10).
>
> **Worksheet:** There is no worksheet associated with this handout.

✓ **A. Mindfulness: A Spiritual Perspective**

Mindfulness as a psychological practice is a derivative of mindfulness as a spiritual practice.

B. Skillful Means: Balancing Doing Mind and Being Mind

"Skillful means" is a set of skills for balancing being present to the moment with doing what is needed in the moment, and for working toward goals while at the same time letting go of attachment to achieving goals.

C. Wise Mind: Walking the Middle Path

"Walking the middle path" is a set of skills highlighting the importance of finding the synthesis between opposites, rather than condemning one side or the other.

> **Note to Leaders:** The content of these mindfulness skills from another perspective and of Mindfulness Handouts 6–10 can be woven into your teaching of the core mindfulness skills (Mindfulness Handouts 1–5) or can be covered separately. These skills can be taught in any order. The content easiest to integrate into core mindfulness skills is that of Mindfulness Handout 7. It does not necessarily add new content to Mindfulness Handout 1; it simply extends the list of goals. These goals, taken together, can be presented as psychological goals and spiritual goals. The concepts of being mind and doing mind are prominent in

Mindfulness-Based Stress Reduction therapy and similar treatments. If you are treating individuals who have family members in adolescent DBT, then teaching Mindfulness Handout 10 makes sense, since walking the middle path (finding the synthesis between opposites) is an important skill in adolescent DBT.

XII. MINDFULNESS PRACTICE: A SPIRITUAL PERSPECTIVE (MINDFULNESS HANDOUT 7)

Main Point: Mindfulness can be practiced for spiritual, psychological, medical, and/or humanistic reasons. The practice of mindfulness is very old, arising initially from spiritual practices across many cultures and spiritual practices. Its modern-day presence is found in the contemplative prayer and meditation practices common across the wide array of spiritualities in our times.

Mindfulness Handout 7: Goals of Mindfulness Practice: A Spiritual Perspective *(Optional).* This is an optional handout. Depending on the group you are teaching, it can be added after Handout 1: Goals of Mindfulness Practice (and reviewed *very* quickly), or it can be taught after participants have been through mindfulness teaching one or more times. If added to Handout 1, mention the list of outcomes here as outcomes many mindfulness practitioners speak about. Pay just enough attention so that participants have a good idea of what many believe the benefits of mindfulness practice may be, particularly for spiritual individuals. *Do not* let this handout interfere with teaching the "what" and "how" mindfulness skills.

Worksheet: There is not a new worksheet for this handout. Assign Mindfulness Worksheet 1 if needed.

Note to Leaders: Be sure to read my rationale for inclusion of a spiritual perspective at the beginning of this chapter. You do not need to be spiritual yourself to teach this skill. However, I suggest not teaching it if none of your skills training participants are spiritual or have an interest in spirituality. Find out by asking. Your task in teaching this skill is to assist participants in grounding their mindfulness practice firmly within their own spiritual practices. Remember not to confuse spirituality with religion. See discussion at the beginning of the chapter on this topic.

✓ **A. The Goals of Mindfulness Practice from a Spiritual Perspective**

- To experience ultimate reality—the transcendence of boundaries and the ground of our being, which leads to an awareness of our intimate wholeness with the entire universe.
- To grow in wisdom of the heart and of action.
- To experience freedom by letting go of attachments.
- To increase love and compassion toward ourselves and others.

Each of these goals is discussed in detail below.

✓ 💬 **Discussion Point:** Ask participants to read Mindfulness Handout 7 and check off on the handout each goal that is important to themselves. Discuss participants' goals. Use the teaching notes below to address questions that arise about goals or to make teaching points.

B. Experience Ultimate Reality

1. Our Minds Are Spacious

Our minds are spacious; that is, there is no boundary enclosing our minds.

- *Spacious mind is the opposite of rigidity and inflexibility.* Flexibility[60] is one of the hallmarks of emotional well-being.[61–66] Emotion regulation, problem solving, and coping with stressful life events require a flexible repertoire of responses that a person can use as the situation requires.

■ *Spacious mind is empty mind.* This type of emptiness is experienced as liberating and joyful rather than painful and constricted. "Empty" in this sense does not mean being empty-headed. It is an acceptance of the fact that everything in the universe is in a state of continual change. Thus nothing is permanent (although we experience much in the universe as permanent). Even the self is continuously changing. "Emptiness" also means being empty of "self" or "ego." It is the process of emptying ourselves of attachments and of letting go of clinging.

> **Note to Leaders:** "Emptiness" is a concept that can be difficult to understand. It is best left to more advanced teaching, after you have worked with wise mind for some time. Although the term "emptiness" is used extensively by Buddhist writers, particularly in Zen, it is also an important concept in Christian and other religious writings.

Practice Exercise: Instruct participants to close their eyes, and then to examine what is going on in their minds and ask themselves, "Where are the boundaries of my mind?" or "Can I see the walls around my mind?" Afterward, ask them to share and discuss observations.

Practice Exercise: Following the exercise above, ask participants to walk around the room for a few steps and then stop. Ask, "Where did walking go?" Discuss how thinking, desiring, wanting, and so forth are behaviors of the mind (and of the body also). "Where does walking go? Where do my thoughts, desires, urges, and so on go?" These questions have the same answer.

■ *In spacious mind, everything comes and goes.* If we watch our minds for a while, we can see this. What was in our minds 5 seconds, 5 minutes, or a year ago is not in our minds now. Thoughts, feelings, and desires may come into our minds over and over and over. But they also go out of our minds over and over and over.

Practice Exercise: Instruct participants to close their eyes and then to observe their minds for a few minutes. Ask them to observe thoughts coming and going, feelings and sensations coming and going. Then ask: "Where do thoughts go? Where are thoughts coming from?"

■ *Spacious mind is still.* If we practice mindfulness long enough, uncluttered by our constant inner chatter, ruminations, thoughts, and images, we will gradually develop a clarity within which our thoughts and emotions come and go. We will experience the stillness of our minds.

■ *Under high emotional arousal, our minds become constricted and inflexible.* Feeling constricted and mentally inflexible can be extremely painful and scary. We cannot change this experience through willpower or by mental command. Trying to suppress, deny, or avoid this experience makes it worse. In wise mind, all of us are sometimes constricted and inflexible. Because everything in our mind comes and goes, this sense of being constricted and inflexible also comes and goes.

✓ **C. We Are Each Intimately Connected with the Entire Universe**

We cannot be separate from the universe even if we try to be. We are connected to even the farthest star in the universe. Mindfulness is a path to experiencing this connection. *Everything in the universe is interconnected.* This is a major finding of modern physics. It is also a tenet of all major religions and spiritual paths. Given this reality, each of us is also interconnected with the entire universe.

✓ ■ *There are no outsiders in the universe.* If everything is interconnected, then it logically follows that the universe is *one* with many parts. Therefore, although we can feel like outsiders and we can be treated as outsiders, in reality there are no outsiders and no insiders.

✓ ■ *We are connected even if we don't experience the connection.* The floor touches the door to outside; the door touches the porch or sidewalk; the sidewalk touches the street; the street goes so many places; and so on and so on. If we close our eyes and do not experience something right in front of us, does that mean it has disappeared from the universe and is no longer connected to us? Opening our eyes, we see that it is still there.

■ *It is very easy to experience ourselves as isolated, alone, and unconnected when troubles arise.* If we have not experienced being loved or cherished by others, it can be extremely difficult to experience our connections to others. This is particularly true if others have not stayed connected to us. We lose the reality that we are intimately connected to the entire universe.

■ *The experience of being unconnected, of being an outsider, or of not fitting in can be extremely painful.* Fear and shame are common emotions here. We cannot change this experience at will; trying to suppress it is also not effective. Mindfulness practices of mindfulness of current emotions and mindfulness of current thoughts can be very helpful here.

■ *The absence of a sense of connection can also be due to beliefs that life must go the way we want it to if we are to be content.* Practicing radical acceptance and willingness (distress tolerance skills) can be very helpful here.

■ *All of us sometimes feel alone and unconnected.* Some people, however, feel unconnected, like outsiders, and alone almost all the time. They may be physically alone and treated as outsiders much of the time. In contrast to others who have been chosen as life partners or best friends, they may be unchosen. They may have no family or friends to love and cherish them. Thus their experience may fit the facts of their everyday experience, and these facts should not be denied or downplayed. However, it is still true that in reality no one is unconnected, outside, or alone in the universe.

■ *Some people are quite content being alone and feeling like outsiders, and don't care if they fit in or not.* (Of course, these people as well are really not alone and are not outsiders.) More than likely, this feeling of contentment is due to these people's having not been judged and not judging themselves as inadequate or unacceptable for being the way they are.

■ *The absence of a sense of connection may be due to inadequate awareness of the present moment.* Sometimes people are very connected but just don't experience or see it. This may be due to being too busy to notice (i.e., "not taking time to smell the flowers") or to having a habit of inattentiveness to everyday life.

■ *Finding connection and building a sense of inclusion take much more work for some people than for others.* Say to participants: "The fact that you are not an outsider in the universe does not mean that you are not an outsider in the community that you are in or that you want to be in. You may not be alone in the universe, but you may be alone in your home. The universe as a whole may love and cherish you, but there may be no person who loves and cherishes you enough to call you on the phone or want to live with you."

■ *The absence of a sense of connection may be due to having a very rigid idea of what it means to be connected, loved, or included.* This tendency is quite common in situations where one person makes up the rules, so to speak, for what counts as being connected, loved, or included.

Example: A person may be loved by a very forgetful person, but feel unloved if the person forgets his or her birthday.

Example: A person may be loved by a significant other with very different taste. This person may feel misunderstood or unloved upon receiving a gift from the significant other that he or she does not like.

Example: A person may have expectations about how a friend should express affection. This person may expect to be always picked up from the airport, or to be able to borrow money indefinitely, and may feel rejected when these events don't happen.

✓ 💬 **Discussion Point:** Ask participants about their own feelings of being unconnected, being outsiders, being alone, or not fitting in. Ask each person whether such experiences set off emotions of shame or of fear or other emotions. Ask what is most likely: that these feelings of being unconnected are due primarily to (1) life experiences of being judged; (2) life experiences of being physically alone, not included, or ignored much of the time; (3) being unaware of present-moment connections; and/or (4) something else entirely.

Note to Leaders: It may be critical to help participants develop a sense of lovability, inherent acceptability, and connection. The goal here is to transform their experience of being outsiders to an experience of insider status. Although many are treated as outsiders by their families or communities, no one really is an outsider—since if we are actually "one," there are no outsiders and no insiders.

It can also be very important to connect participants' own spiritual or religious beliefs to this view of our connection to the universe. Quotations that might help follow.

Many authors have written about our intimate connection to the entire universe. Here are just a few examples:

Lord Byron, the poet, wrote: "Are not the mountains, waves and skies a part of me and of my soul, as I of them?" (p. 530).[67]

Henry Miller, the novelist, wrote: "We invent nothing, truly. We borrow and re-create. We uncover and discover. All has been given, as the mystics say. We have only to open our eyes and hearts, to become one with that which is" (p. 57).[68]

Charlene Spretnak, a writer on women and spirituality, has noted: "There are sacred moments in life when we experience in rational and very direct ways that separation, the boundary between ourselves and other people and between ourselves and Nature, is illusion. Oneness is reality. We can experience that stasis is illusory and that reality is continual flux and change on very subtle and also on gross levels of perception."[69]

✓ D. Grow in Wisdom

When we are in wise mind, we gain access to our inner wisdom. The practice of mindfulness over time leads to increases in wisdom and wise action.

1. Wisdom Is Practical

Wisdom is practical; that is, it is concretely beneficial to life and well-being. Wise mind is a way to access good judgment and skillful means. Good judgment is figuring out what is needed in any given moment, and skillful means is doing what is needed.

2. A Wise Person Is Balanced

A mark of wise mind practice is a growing sense of greater integration. In the stillness of wise mind, we can find harmony, balance, and quieting of extreme emotions.

3. Wisdom Involves Both the Heart and the Brain

In wise mind, there is wisdom of the heart as well as of the brain. Thus, in wise mind, we access our capacity for intuitive knowing, and develop sensitivity and a capacity to "read hearts." In wise mind, we have depth of understanding, in addition to good judgment and application of existing knowledge (as noted above).

✓ E. Experience Freedom

Mindfulness practice enables us to free ourselves from the demands of our own desires, cravings, and intense emotions.

1. Freedom Is the Ability to Want Something We Lack and to Find a Life Worth Living without It

We need the ability to have a tragic and sad past, or a present that is not what we would want, and still have a sense of liberation and freedom. The idea is not to suppress feeling, wishes, and desires, but to live with them as friends.

2. The Drive to Stop Pain No Matter What Is the Opposite of Freedom

Much of life involves managing situations that are painful but cannot be solved immediately. Although it is easy to think that we can just get rid of pain through positive thinking, ignoring pain, or suppressing pain, the fact is that these strategies often do not work. Our use of these strategies is usually based on the delusion that we cannot stand the pain. We feel compelled to do something to stop the pain. We are slaves to our incessant urges to escape from the present moment.

3. When We Are Free, We Have a Sense of Liberation and Absence of Constraints

We are free to be who and what we are. We are free to change. Freedom is the falling away of desperation and limits.

✓ F. Increase Love and Compassion

Finally, mindfulness practice enables us to increase love and compassion toward ourselves and others. Compassion is one of the hallmarks of being in wise mind. It is difficult to find any discussion of wise mind or of experiencing reality as it is, of religious or spiritual awakening, or of wisdom or enlightenment without a corresponding discussion of love and compassion.

1. Wise Mind Lets Go of Judgmental Thinking

Tell participants: "As you settle more often in wise mind, you will find that you become more tolerant and more likely to radically accept yourself and others, as well as less likely to judge, criticize, and reject yourself and others."

2. Wise Mind Is Loving

The outcome of wise mind is a greater capacity for love—love of others and love of oneself.

3. Wise Mind Is Compassionate

Say to participants: "Compassion makes much more sense once you realize that you and the universe are one. Cutting off your arm is cutting off your friend's or your neighbor's arm. Hurting others is hurting yourself."

💬 **Discussion Point:** Elicit participants' reactions to these points and discuss. The last point in particular can be difficult for participants to understand; the interconnectedness of the entire universe is a conceptual idea but not an experienced reality for many.

XIII. WISE MIND: A SPIRITUAL PERSPECTIVE (MINDFULNESS HANDOUT 7A)

Main Point: Spiritual words and concepts are often universal beliefs that, depending on one's own religion, are stated in vastly different words. It is important to see the commonalities across various practices and cultures. It is also important to be able to select the part of a practice that conforms to one's own beliefs and practices.

Mindfulness Handout 7a: Wise Mind from a Spiritual Perspective *(Optional)*. Depending on the group you are teaching, this optional handout can be added after Mindfulness Handout 8: Practicing Loving Kindness to Increase Love and Compassion (and reviewed *very* quickly), or it can be brought out if the topics covered come up in a discussion of mindfulness at some other point. Similar to Mindfulness Handout 7, this handout can be useful for spiritual and/or religious participants and their families, particularly those who are uncomfortable with mindfulness or the term "mindfulness" due to its association with Buddhism.

Worksheet: There is no worksheet for this handout.

A. Wise Mind as Contemplative Practice

In the widest meaning, the experience of wise mind can be viewed as a contemplative experience. Contemplative practices are associated with all of the major religions, as well as with naturalist/humanistic contemplative practices.

✓ *1. Wise Mind as Unity with the Sacred*

The experience of wise mind, from these perspectives, is the experience of unity with the sacred when entered into wholly and completely. "The sacred" here is referred to in various traditions as "the divine within," God, the Great Spirit, Yahweh, Brahma, Allah, Parvardigar, "ultimate reality," "the totality," "the source," "our essential nature," "no self," "emptiness," "the core of our being," "the ground of being," "our true self," and countless other names.

2. Wise Mind Experiences as Spiritual Experiences

Such experiences are often termed "spiritual" or "enlightenment" experiences. "The well within" as a metaphor for wise mind (see Figure 7.1) intentionally opens into an underground ocean so as to accommodate these beliefs.

✓ ### B. Wise Mind as "Going Home"

Wise mind can be considered "going home" or "going to our true home." When we are out of wise mind, we can feel lost. The loneliness we feel is homesickness.

1. Wise Mind as True Self

Wise mind is sometimes considered to be our true self. From this perspective, we are each one with ultimate reality. Just as wise mind is our true home, it is our true self as well.

2. Seven Characteristics of Spiritual Experiences

Seven characteristics of deep spiritual or mystical experiences are as follows:

- *Experiential.* The experience involves direct, unmediated experience of reality.
- *Unitary or nondual.* The experience is characterized by awareness of nonduality and non-separation—of no distance between oneself, the ultimate reality, and all other beings.
- *Ineffable or nonconceptual.* What is experienced is ungraspable and incomprehensible. It can only be communicated with metaphors. It is compared with going into the "cloud of unknowing."[10, 29, 70]
- *Giving certitude.* In the midst of the experience, certainty is total, undeniable, and clear.
- *Practical.* The experience is concretely beneficial to one's life and well-being.
- *Integrative.* The experience is psychologically integrative, establishing harmony of love, compassion, mercy, kindness, and quieting of extreme emotions.
- *Sapiential.* The experience leads to wisdom, enhanced capacity for intuitive knowledge, the capacity to "read hearts," and the ability to discern the motives of others.[71]

✓ *3. "The Dark Night of the Soul"*

The inability to access wise mind can be experienced as "the dark night of the soul," described by St. John of the Cross in his book of the same name.[72] The dark night of the soul is a metaphor for a depth of loneliness and desolation.

XIV. PRACTICING LOVING KINDNESS (MINDFULNESS HANDOUT 8)

> **Main Point:** Anger, hate, hostility, and ill will toward ourselves and others can be very painful. The practice of loving kindness is a form of meditation that involves reciting specific positive words and phrases repeatedly, to cultivate compassion and loving feelings as an antidote to negativity.

Mindfulness Handout 8: Practicing Loving Kindness to Increase Love and Compassion *(Option-al).* Although this is an optional handout, it can be very useful in a number of ways. As presented here, loving kindness is a meditation aimed at increasing love and compassion for others. As such, it would also fit well with a number of skills in the Interpersonal Effectiveness module (e.g., see Interpersonal Effectiveness Handout 6). It can also be used as an an opposite action for anger and hate as well as disgust aimed at self and others (see Emotion Regulation Handout 10). Because loving kindness involves some imagery, it can also be used as a skill to improve the moment (see Distress Tolerance Handout 9).

Mindfulness Worksheet 6: Loving Kindness. Review this worksheet with participants. The worksheet gives participants an option to describe two incidents of practicing loving kindness. Remind them that they can describe other times on the back of the page. Instruct participants to check off which individual(s) they send loving kindness to. If they send loving kindness to more than one person while practicing, then they should check more than one person for the practice episode. Remind them to practice on people, including themselves, toward whom they want to increase or continue a sense of loving kindness. The series of warm wishes the participant used should be listed next. Remind participants that they can use the script in Mindfulness Handout 8, or they can make up their own. Review also how to rate loving kindness practice. Note that the ratings are for how effective the participants' practice was in increasing love, compassion, and connection, as well as increasing wisdom and a sense of happiness and personal validity.

A. Loving Kindness: What Is It?

✓ ### 1. A Practice of Mentally Sending Warm Wishes

Say to participants: "Loving kindness is the practice of mentally sending warm wishes to yourself and to others. Loving kindness is very similar to praying for people, except that rather than praying for their welfare, you are wishing for their welfare. Warm wishes can be sent to yourself, to others you know, to people you don't know, and to all beings everywhere. The wishes can be for any positive outcome, such as for happiness, safety, health, contentment, love, and so on."

2. An Ancient Spiritual Meditation Practice

Loving kindness is an ancient spiritual meditation practice developed originally as a Buddhist practice (*metta* meditation), but it is compatible with all spiritual traditions. The aim of the practice is to increase love and compassion for self and others.

3. A Form of Visualization

Tell participants: "Loving kindness can also include visualizing the persons you are sending wishes to—that is, calling up images of them in your mind."

B. Loving Kindness: Why Do It?

1. Ill Will, Hate, and Anger toward Self and Others Can Be Wearing

Strong negative emotions can be corrosive psychologically; they can also have negative physical effects, such as raising blood pressure and increasing risk of heart attacks.[73–75]

2. Loving Kindness Reduces Self-Hate

Hating oneself is extremely painful. Loving kindness focuses on reducing self-hate. Tell participants: "Besides being painful all by themselves, hate, anger, and disgust directed at yourself make it much more difficult to take good care of yourself. Self-hate can lead to an attitude that you don't deserve positive events, soothing, or even your rights to be upheld. In turn, this attitude can complicate depression, increase feelings of inadequacy, and decrease feelings of worth and efficacy."

3. Ill Will, Hate, and Anger Interfere with Interpersonal Effectiveness

Say to participants: "It is much more difficult to live, work, and negotiate with persons you have difficult relationships with. Loving kindness can help you improve these relationships."

✓ ### 4. Daily Loving Kindness Practice Increases Positive Emotions

> **Research Point:** Data suggest that a daily practice of loving kindness works to increase daily experiences of positive emotions (including love, joy, gratitude, contentment, hope, pride, interest, amusement, and awe), and to decrease negative emotions.[76] The practice of loving kindness increases social connectedness,[77] and mounting research suggests that it has potential as an effective psychological intervention. Neuroimaging studies suggest also that loving kindness practice is associated with increased activation of brain areas involved with emotional processing and empathy. Over time, these positive emotions predict both increased satisfaction with life and reduced depressive symptoms.[78] In addition, daily practice of loving kindness can also increase self-acceptance and improve relationships over time.[79]

> **Note to Leaders:** There is preliminary but potentially significant research indicating that loving kindness meditation may not be as useful for individuals with a high tendency to brooding rumination.[80] These individuals may do better with a mindful focus on breathing.[81] I would suggest encouraging participants to try both and letting them decide which practice is best for them.

✓ ## C. Loving Kindness: How to Do It

✓ ### 1. The Core Component: Sending Loving Kindness toward Ourselves and Others

The content of loving wishes can vary. The script provided in Mindfulness Handout 8 is a common one, but there are also many other versions—for example, "May I live with ease" ("May John live with ease"), "May I be safe and protected" ("May John be safe and protected"), "May I be healthy and whole" ("May all beings be healthy and whole"), "May I be filled with joy" ("May all beings be filled with joy"), and so on. Generally, however, only four or five wishes for each person should be made, as it is hard to remember many others.

✓ ### 2. Select Wishes That Are Sincere

Sincerity is a key point. Tell participants: "If your wish is not sincere, from your heart, then it can become like saying a mantra where the words themselves mean very little. Once the words lose meaning, your mind can repeat the words even while you think of other things. So it is important that the wishes have real meaning for you. Don't repeat only one wish over and over. Instead, go through a brief list of meaningful wishes, and then start over."

💬 **Discussion Point:** Ask participants what positive wishes they would like to make to themselves and others.

✓ ### 3. Start with Wishes for Self or a Loved One

Suggest to participants: "Start by practicing only on yourself or only on someone you already love until you understand how to do the practice. The standard way is to start with wishes for yourself, because it is hard to love others when you don't love yourself. Generally, it is easier to go next to a person you love or a friend. Practice repeatedly with one person until you feel a sense of loving kindness and/or compassion, and then move to the next person. Then it can be useful to send wishes to a person you are having difficulties with or are angry at. End with all living beings." Positive results have been found with very brief loving mindfulness practices; lasting changes, however, are more than likely to require a consistent regimen of practice.

> **Note to Leaders:** It is important to remind participants to practice only on people they want to increase love and compassion for.

4. Try to Let Go of Tension or Tightness

Say to participants: "Try to let go of any tension or tightness after each round of wishes, but do not worry if you find it hard to relax. Simply let go as much as possible."

✓ ### 5. If Thoughts or Distractions Intrude, Just Notice Them and Gently Return to the Practice

Tell participants: "When thoughts take you away from loving kindness, notice it and make a wish for your own happiness, and then continue. Remember that mindfulness practice is not about forcing your mind to stay focused, but rather about noticing when your mind is distracted by thoughts, emotions, sounds, or other sensations, and then gently bringing your mind back. You can say, 'My mind has taken a walk. I think I will come back home to loving kindness.' Let go of judgmental and critical thoughts. Let go of perfectionism."

> **Note to Leaders:** Note that the instructions here are almost identical to previous instructions for observing mindfulness practice.

XV. SKILLFUL MEANS: BALANCING DOING MIND AND BEING MIND (MINDFULNESS HANDOUTS 9–9A)

> **Main Point:** In everyday life, wise living requires us to balance working to achieve goals (on the one hand) with, *at the very same time*, letting go of attachment to achieving goals (on the other hand).
>
> **Mindfulness Handout 9: Skillful Means: Balancing Doing Mind and Being Mind** *(Optional)*; **Mindfulness Handout 9a: Ideas for Practicing Balancing Doing Mind and Being Mind** *(Optional)*. Both of these optional handouts can be particularly useful for participants who have read about or participated in one of the mindfulness-based forms of CBT.[4, 82] The concepts of doing mind and being mind were taken from these approaches. Handout 9 integrates these concepts with that of wise mind. Handout 9a lists practice exercises. The handouts may be particularly useful for individuals who tend toward overdoing. Generally, these handouts are useful with individuals who have already gone through mindfulness training several times.
>
> **Mindfulness Worksheet 7: Balancing Being Mind with Doing Mind.** Review this worksheet with participants. It is almost identical to Mindfulness Worksheet 3: Wise Mind Practice, but it also lists the practice exercises given in Handout 9a. If you have taught a different practice exercise, ask participants to write that exercise on their worksheet so that they will remember what it is. Review where participants have questions. As on Worksheet 3, for each exercise there are four boxes. Instruct participants to check off one box for every day they practice the indicated exercise. If they practice more than four times in a week, tell them to put extra checkmarks outside the boxes. Review also how to rate wise mind practice, if you have not done so already. Note that the ratings are for how effective their practice was in getting into their own wise mind. These are not ratings of whether or not the practice calmed them down or made them feel better. Also note that at the bottom, the worksheet asks participants to list any and all *wise* things they did during the week.
>
> **Mindfulness Worksheet 7a: Mindfulness of Being and Doing Calendar; Mindfulness Worksheet 8: Mindfulness of Pleasant Events Calendar; Mindfulness Worksheet 9: Mindfulness of Unpleasant Events Calendar.** Each of these worksheets is a calendar that asks participants to record their mindfulness practice each day. Review the worksheets you plan to assign to participants. Each worksheet asks participants to attend to the present moment, noticing their sensations, moods, feelings, and

thoughts during their mindfulness practice and also as they are writing their practice down. The calendars focus on mindfulness during frazzled moments (7a), pleasant events (8), and unpleasant events (9).

✓ **A. Skillful Means**

Each person has the capacity for skillful means. "Skillful means" is a term in Zen; it refers to any effective method that aids a person to experience reality as it is, or, in DBT terms, to enter fully into wise mind.

✓ **B. Doing Mind and Being Mind**

"Doing mind" and "being mind" are states of mind that in their extremes can get in the way of skillful means and of wise mind. Doing mind focuses on achieving goals; being mind focuses on experiencing. The polarity between them is similar to that between reasonable mind and emotion mind.

✓ **C. The Need for Both Doing Mind and Being Mind**

Without aspects of both being mind and doing mind, it is difficult if not impossible to lead a balanced life. Once we let go of balance and, instead, live at one extreme or the other, we start seeing reality from that extreme perspective. We become biased, and experiencing reality as it is becomes elusive.

Note to Leaders: The concepts of doing mind and being mind are drawn from the mindfulness-based treatment manuals. For those in skills training who have experienced multiple episodes of major depression, it may be useful to give them information on Mindfulness-Based Cognitive Therapy as an evidence-based treatment for depression and the self-help book based on it.[82] For those with addictions, Mindfulness-Based Relapse Prevention may be useful, and for those with chronic physical pain, Mindfulness-Based Stress Reduction may be of value.[3, 4]

✓ **D. Doing Mind**

✓ **1. Doing Mind Focuses on Achieving Goals and Doing What Is Needed**

Say to clients: "When you are in doing mind, similar to reasonable mind, you view thoughts as facts about the world. You are comparing where you are now to where you want to be in the future. You compare your own behavior and that of others now and in the past to what you want it to be. In its extreme form, doing mind is relentlessly task focused, climbing to the top with ambition. At this extreme, doing mind is driven mind."

Doing mind is necessary for getting work done, for meeting goals, for planning, and for evaluating whether we are living our lives according to our values. Processing incoming information and using the information to help us achieve both immediate and long-range goals is clearly important.

✓ **2. Too Little Doing Mind Can Interfere with Achieving Important Goals**

Deficits in doing activities can be destructive. This is particularly true for those individuals who spend many of their waking moments "zoning out," sleeping, or living lives of leisure or lethargy that ignore their very real needs. Many individuals resort to drugs in order to mobilize themselves to work toward goals. Cocaine, amphetamines, and high levels of caffeine, for example, are used by many to produce an artificial state of doing mind.

✓ **Discussion Point:** Elicit from participants their own experiences of doing mind. Ask how many always feel the need to be doing something; feel guilty if they are not productive; and/or fill their time with activities, activities, activities to keep from having nothing to do.

💬 **Discussion Point:** Elicit from participants addictive behaviors that they cannot stop—that they spend far too much time planning for or doing.

💬 **Discussion Point:** Ask what artificial means participants have used to produce doing mind. What helps them to produce short-term doing mind naturally when they need it?

3. Too Much Doing Mind Can Become an Automatic Mode of Being

When we spend too much time in doing mind, we start living our lives on automatic pilot. We act out of habit and do not notice when the situation or context has changed and something else is needed. It can be very easy to make both little and big mistakes.

▪ *Problems with doing occur when we become addicted to "doing."* Workaholics are caught in doing mind. They work excessively, caught in always doing something. They feel an intense drive to always be doing something productive and, alas, they do not enjoy work. We could call them "doing-aholics." Perfectionists are also caught in doing mind.

▪ *People with any types of addiction are caught in doing mind.* The addictive activity is so compelling that although the persons may be in the present (forgetting about the long-term harm their addiction is causing), their awareness of the present is rigidly focused on just the one addictive activity. Out of awareness are the wider universe; the people whom they love and who love them; and the responsibilities and promises they are forgetting.

✓ ▪ *In doing mind, we lose sight of the value of the present moment,* because we look at the present and the past in terms of how close or far we are from some future goal. We are immersed in activity, losing sight of all else happening around us, like a workaholic who never stops to smell the roses.

✓ E. Being Mind

1. Being Mind Is "Beginners' Mind"

✓ Say to participants: "In being mind, you are open and curious about the moment you are in. Thoughts are viewed as sensations of the mind, arising and falling, coming and going. You are focused on immediate, moment-to-moment experiencing with an open mind; you accept that each moment is as it is. You let go of evaluating the past and the present. There is only 'just this moment.' In its extreme form, being mind focuses on immediate, moment-to-moment experiencing, with no thought of goals or of consequences of current action or absence of action."

2. Too Little Being Mind Can Interfere with Living Life to Its Fullest

✓ ▪ *Being mind is "nothing-to-do, nowhere-to-go" mind.* Tell participants: "When there is nothing to do and nowhere to go, being mind is the place to be. Being mind is the path to spacious mind, to awareness or our connection to the entire universe—the floor that touches our feet and the furthest star in the universe. Being mind is like lying in the grass on a warm sunny day, head in your arms, lotion on your body, just feeling the warm sun beating down. Or it is like lying on your back on a cool summer evening, gazing at the sky and watching the stars. It is watching the clouds going by. Or it is simply attending to a touch on the arm or a smile from someone you know."

✓ ▪ *Being mind is being present to one's life.* Many people find at some point that they have missed a lot of their own lives. Almost always, this is a very sad realization. It is like having a garden full of beautiful roses but never stopping to smell them. Appreciating life requires experiencing life.

▪ *Deficits in being mind can be as destructive as deficits in doing mind.*

Generally, a deficit in being shows up as an excess of doing: Individuals spend many of their waking moments comparing themselves to others, or comparing their progress in life now to what they expected it to be or wanted it to be. Many individuals find these incessant comparisons so difficult that they try to escape with drugs. Opiates in particular bring about a state of artificial being mind that provides an escape from the anxiety and shame that doing mind run amuck can sometimes create.

💬 **Discussion Point:** Elicit from participants their own experiences of being mind. What artificial means have they used to produce being mind? What helps them to produce being mind naturally when they need it?

💬 **Discussion Point:** Discuss the pros and cons of both types of mind. Draw from participants their experiences of doing mind and of being mind.

✓ **3. Too Much Being Mind Can Be Indulgent and Self-Centered**

An excess of being mind can be focused on personal experience at the expense of others and their needs, and of what needs to be done in the moment. Say to participants: "When this happens, being mind can be destructive if there is something that needs to be done or somewhere you need to go. Sitting in meditation, lying around on the beach, or watching the clouds go by is all well and good. But it won't do when you are driving somewhere and need to follow a map; when you have a weekly budget and need to plan, buy, and cook meals for the week; when homework needs to be done; or when e-mail needs to be answered."

Example: "Someone who just sits on the couch meditating all day never gets any work done and is stuck in being mind. 'Now, now, now' can interfere with planning for the future for yourself and for those you love and/or are responsible for."

F. Review of Practice Exercises for Balancing Doing Mind and Being Mind

Mindfulness Handout 9a lists a number of ideas for bringing being mind into everyday doing mind life. There are also exercises for increasing doing mind when needed. It is important to go over some of these with participants.

XVI. WISE MIND: WALKING THE MIDDLE PATH (MINDFULNESS HANDOUT 10)

Main Point: The "middle path" is a synthesis of extremes. Ordinarily, when we are at an extreme on any continuum, we are in danger of distorting reality.

Mindfulness Handout 10: Walking the Middle Path: Finding the Synthesis between Opposites. This handout can be useful for participants who need to work on balancing the priorities in their lives. It is also compatible with an adolescent skills training module, Walking the Middle Path. Generally, like the previous handout, this handout is useful with individuals who have already gone through mindfulness training one or more times. With individuals for whom the main focus of treatment is on interpersonal relationships, however, Handout 10 can be important in its own right, independent of other mindfulness handouts.

Mindfulness Worksheet 10: Walking the Middle Path to Wise Mind. Note that the worksheet lists several polarities that could be out of balance. The first polarity is emotion mind versus reasonable mind. If you have not reviewed Handout 10, you can still use this worksheet if you wish; you can simply tell participants to work on the first polarity only, or you can very briefly describe what is meant by each polarity without going into too much detail.

Mindfulness Worksheet 10a: Analyzing Yourself on the Middle Path. Review the instructions for each step. At Step 1, instruct participants to think through whether they are out of balance on each of the three polarities. They should put an X in the middle if they are not out of balance, or put an X toward the end where they are most of the time. At Step 2, remind participants that they need to be very specific in describing what they do that is too much (i.e., too extreme) or too little. This may take a fair amount of coaching and review if you have not already taught the mindfulness skill of describing. Step 3 is very important: What is out of balance for one person may not be out of balance for another. Remind participants that being out of balance means living in a way that knocks them off their center, out of wise mind. At Step 4, be sure participants know how to be very specific when they commit to making changes in the next week. Remind them to be realistic in what they write down. Review also how to rate their practice.

Mindfulness Worksheet 10b: Walking the Middle Path Calendar. This worksheet offers opportunities for recording daily practice in a different format from that of Worksheet 10. It can also be used in conjunction with Worksheet 10a.

✓ A. Wise Mind: The Middle Path between Extremes

In wise mind, we replace "either–or" with "both–and" thinking, in an effort to find a synthesis between positions. Wise mind is all of the following things.

✓ 1. A Synthesis of Reasonable Mind and Emotion Mind

A person who uses facts and reason alone ignores values and the feelings of others; in essence, this person lets go of empathy in making a decision. This is the person who insists on taking the shortest route on the highway because it is more efficient, ignoring everyone else's desire to enjoy the scenery even if it is not as efficient. A person who is ruled by emotions is mood-dependent, ruled by the current mood. This is the person who refuses to take the scenic route because he or she is angry at everyone else and is not in the mood for being civil.

✓ 2. A Synthesis of Doing Mind and Being Mind

The middle path combines doing with being. The key here is to do what is needed with awareness. Skillful means is doing what is needed to be effective, while at the same time experiencing fully the uniqueness of each moment in the moment.

The middle path between doing and being has been written about for thousands of years and across many cultures. In 2400 B.C., the Egyptian sage Ptahhotep wrote: "One that reckons accounts all the day passes not a happy moment. One that gladdens his heart all the day provides not for his house. The bowman hits the mark, as the steersman reaches land, by diversity of aim. He that obeys his heart shall command."[83]

This is similar to the proverb "All work and no play makes Jack a dull boy." Some writers have added a second part to this proverb: "All work and no play makes Jack a dull boy; all play and no work makes Jack a mere toy."

✓ 3. A Synthesis of Intense Desire for Change and Radical Acceptance

The middle path also involves radically accepting the present without suppressing an intense desire for something else. The middle path from this perspective includes simultaneously passionately throwing your entire self into working toward goals, while at the same time letting go of having to achieve your goals.

✓ 4. A Synthesis of Self-Denial and Self-Indulgence

All of us at times need to deny ourselves something we want. At times, however, indulging ourselves can be good for the soul. The middle path here combines moderation with satisfying the senses, self-care, and pleasant events. The point is that either extreme—self-denial or self-indulgence—can interfere with finding wise mind.

> **Note to Leaders:** When you are making the points above, it can be very useful to draw a balance beam on a whiteboard with each of the polarities written at either end. See Mindfulness Handout 10 for examples. If a whiteboard is not available, give out Handout 10.

✓ 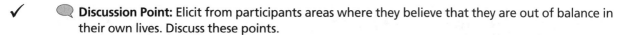 **Discussion Point:** Elicit from participants areas where they believe that they are out of balance in their own lives. Discuss these points.

    Discussion Point: Balance is not always a 50–50 split. What is out of balance for one person may not be out of balance for another. As noted earlier, being out of balance means a living style that knocks each person off his or her own center, out of his or her own wise mind. Elicit from participants times when something was out of balance for them but not for others. How did that feel?

B. Dialectical Abstinence

In working with people with addictions (to use of alcohol/drugs or to other behavioral patterns), the synthesis of opposites is referred to as "dialectical abstinence." In dialectical abstinence, the person strategically shifts between 100% absolute abstinence "in the moment" (so long as the person refrains from addictive behaviors) and relapse management (should the individual lapse or relapse).

- *In every moment that the individual is abstinent* (from drugs or dysfunctional behaviors), every cell in the individual's body is committed fully to absolute abstinence from the addictive behavior. Each move is intended to get the individual further and further down the road away from a life with the addictive behavior, and closer to a life worth living without the behavior.
- *In every moment after a person has relapsed*, the individual radically accepts the relapse and focuses on getting back up, so to speak; he or she applies all the skills necessary to get back into abstinence.

See Distress Tolerance Handout 17 for more information on dialectical abstinence.

C. Summary of Other Perspectives on Mindfulness Skills

Summarize both core and supplemental mindfulness skills that have been covered.

References

1. Grepmair, L., Mitterlehner, F., Loew, T., Bachler, E., Rother, W., & Nickel, M. (2007). Promoting mindfulness in psychotherapists in training influences the treatment results of their patients: A randomized, double-blind, controlled study. *Psychotherapy and Psychosomatics, 76*(6), 332–338.
2. Segal, Z. V., Williams, J. M. G., & Teasdale, J. D. (2013). *Mindfulness-based cognitive therapy for depression* (2nd ed.). New York: Guilford Press.
3. Bowen, S., Chawla, N., & Marlatt, G. A. (2011). *Mindfulness-based relapse prevention for addictive behaviors: A clinician's guide.* New York: Guilford Press.
4. Kabat-Zinn, J. (1990). *Full catastrophe living: Using the wisdom of your body and mind to face stress, pain, and illness.* New York: Delacorte.
5. Williams, J. M. G. (2008). Mindfulness, depression and modes of mind. *Cognitive Therapy and Research, 32*(6), 721–733.
6. Miller, W. R., & Martin, J. E. (1988). Spirituality and behavioral psychology: Toward integration. In W. R. Miller & J. E. Martin (Eds.), *Behavior therapy and religion* (pp. 13–24). Newbury Park, CA: Sage.
7. Kabat-Zinn, J., Lipworth, L., & Burney, R. (1985). The clinical use of mindfulness meditation for the self-regulation of chronic pain. *Journal of Behavioral Medicine, 8*(2), 163–190.
8. Luke 10:38–42. (Any version of the Bible; see, e.g., *www.devotions.net/bible/00bible.htm*)
9. Borchert, B. (1994). *Mysticism: Its history and challenge.* York Beach, ME: Samuel Weiser.
10. Johnston, W. (2005). *The cloud of unknowing* and *The book of privy counseling.* New York: Doubleday.
11. Jain, S., Shapiro, S. L., Swanick, S., Roesch, S. C., Mills, P. J., Bell, I., et al. (2007). A randomized controlled trial of mindfulness meditation versus relaxation training: Effects on distress, positive states of mind, rumination, and distraction. *Annals of Behavioral Medicine, 33*(1), 11–21.
12. Broderick, P. C. (2005). Mindfulness and coping with dysphoric mood: Contrasts with rumination

and distraction. *Cognitive Therapy and Research, 29*(5), 501–510.

13. Davidson, R. J. (2003). Alterations in brain and immune function produced by mindfulness meditation. *Psychosomatic Medicine, 65*(4), 564–570.

14. Gross, C. R., Kreitzer, M. J., Reilly-Spong, M., Winbush, N. Y., Schomaker, E. K., & Thomas, W. (2009). Mindfulness meditation training to reduce symptom distress in transplant patients: Rationale, design, and experience with a recycled waitlist. *Clinical Trials, 6*(1), 76–89.

15. Kabat-Zinn, J., Massion, A. O., Kristeller, J., Peterson, L. G., Fletcher, K. E., Pbert, L., et al. (1992). Effectiveness of a meditation-based stress reduction program in the treatment of anxiety disorders. *American Journal of Psychiatry, 149*, 936–943.

16. Speca, M., Carlson, L. E., Goodey, E., & Angen, M. (2000). A randomized, wait-list controlled clinical trial: The effect of a mindfulness meditation-based stress reduction program on mood and symptoms of stress in cancer outpatients. *Psychosomatic Medicine, 62*(5), 613–622.

17. Chiesa, A., & Serretti, A. (2011). Mindfulness-based interventions for chronic pain: A systematic review of the evidence. *Journal of Alternative and Complementary Medicine, 17*(1), 83–93.

18. Pradhan, E. K., Baumgarten, M., Langenberg, P., Handwerger, B., Gilpin, A. K., Magyari, T., et al. (2007). Effect of mindfulness-based stress reduction in rheumatoid arthritis patients. *Arthritis and Rheumatism, 57*(7), 1134–1142.

19. Sephton, S. E., Salmon, P., Weissbecker, I., Ulmer, C., Floyd, A., Hoover, K., et al. (2007). Mindfulness meditation alleviates depressive symptoms in women with fibromyalgia: Results of a randomized clinical trial. *Arthritis and Rheumatism, 57*(1), 77–85.

20. Kabat-Zinn, J., Wheeler, E., Light, T., Skillings, A., Scharf, M. J., Cropley, T. G., et al. (1998). Influence of a mindfulness meditation-based stress reduction intervention on rates of skin clearing in patients with moderate to severe psoriasis undergoing phototherapy (UVB) and photochemotherapy (PUVA). *Psychosomatic Medicine, 60*(5), 625–632.

21. Creswell, J. D., Myers, H. F., Cole, S. W., & Irwin, M. R. (2009). Mindfulness meditation training effects on CD4+ T lymphocytes in HIV-1 infected adults: A small randomized controlled trial. *Brain, Behavior, and Immunity, 23*(2), 184–188.

22. Tang, Y. Y., Ma, Y., Wang, J., Fan, Y., Feng, S., Lu, Q., et al. (2007). Short-term meditation training improves attention and self-regulation. *Proceedings of the National Academy of Sciences USA, 104*, 17152–17156.

23. Hayes, S. C., Strosahl, K. D., & Wilson, K. G. (2012). *Acceptance and commitment therapy: The process and practice of mindful change* (2nd ed.). New York: Guilford Press.

24. Hayes, S. C., & Melancon, S. M. (1989). Comprehensive distancing, paradox, and the treatment of emotional avoidance. In L. M. Ascher (Ed.), *Therapeutic paradox* (pp. 184–218). New York: Guilford Press.

25. Fischer, N. (2008). *Mindfulness.* Lecture presented at the Benedicktushof, Holzkirchen, Germany.

26. Giuliano, R. J., & Wicha, N. Y. Y. (2010). Why the white bear is still there: Electrophysiological evidence for ironic semantic activation during thought suppression. *Brain Research, 1316*, 62–74.

27. Wegner, D. M., Schneider, D. J., Carter, S. R., & White, T. L. (1987). Paradoxical effects of thought suppression. *Journal of Personality and Social Psychology, 53*(1), 5–13.

28. Stapp, H. P. (2007). *Mindful universe: Quantum mechanics and the participating observer.* New York: Springer.

29. Walsh, J. (Ed.). (1981). *The cloud of unknowing.* New York: Paulist Press.

30. Jager, W. (1994). *Contemplation: A Christian path.* Ligori, MO: Triumph Books.

31. Keating, T. (n.d.). *The method of centering prayer.* Available from *www.cpt.org/files/WS-Centering Prayer.pdf*

32. Deikman, A. J. (1982). *The observing self: Mysticism and psychotherapy.* Boston: Beacon Press.

33. Polanyi, M. (1958). *Personal knowledge.* Chicago: University of Chicago Press.

34. May, G. G. (1982). *Will and spirit: A contemplative psychology.* San Francisco: Harper & Row.

35. Senay, I., Albarracin, D., & Noguchi, K. (2010). Motivating goal-directed behavior through introspective self-talk: The role of the interrogative form of simple future tense. *Psychological Science, 21*(4), 499–504.

36. Butryn, M. L., Phelan, S., Hill, J. O., & Wing, R. R. (2007). Consistent self-monitoring of weight: A key component of successful weight loss maintenance. *Obesity, 15*(12), 3091–3096.

37. Nelson, R. O., & Hayes, S. C. (1981). Theoretical explanations for reactivity in self-monitoring. *Behavior Modification, 5*(1), 3–14.

38. Krishnamurti, J. (1991). *The collected works of J. Krishnamurti: Vol. 5. 1948–1949, Choiceless awareness.* Dubuque, IA: Kendall/Hunt.

39. Hayes, S. C., Wilson, K. G., Gifford, E. V., Follette, V. M., & Strosahl, K. (1996). Experiential avoidance and behavioral disorders: A functional dimensional approach to diagnosis and treatment. *Journal of Consulting and Clinical Psychology, 64*(6), 1152–1168.

40. Wegner, D. M., & Erber, R. (1992). The hyperaccessibility of suppressed thoughts. *Journal of Personality and Social Psychology, 63*(6), 903–912.

41. Levitt, J. T., Brown, T. A., Orsillo, S. M., & Barlow, D. H. (2004). The effects of acceptance versus suppression of emotion on subjective and psychophysiological response to carbon dioxide challenge in patients with panic disorder. *Behavior Therapy*, 35(4), 747–766.

42. Roemer, L., & Borkovec, T. D. (1994). Effects of suppressing thoughts about emotional material. *Journal of Abnormal Psychology*, 103(3), 467–474.

43. Teasdale, J. D., Segal, Z., & Williams, J. M. G. (1995). How does cognitive therapy prevent depressive relapse and why should attentional control (mindfulness) training help? *Behaviour Research and Therapy*, 33(1), 25–39.

44. Miller, A. L., Rathus, J. H., & Linehan, M. M. (2007). *Dialectical behavior therapy with suicidal adolescents*. New York: Guilford Press.

45. Cioffi, D. (1993). Sensate body, directive mind: Physical sensations and mental control. In D. Wegner & J. W. Pennebaker (Eds.), *Handbook of mental control* (pp. 410–442). Englewood Cliffs, NJ: Prentice-Hall.

46. Lieberman, M. D., Eisenberger, N. I., Crockett, M. J., Tom, S. M., Pfeifer, J. H., & Way, B. M. (2007). Putting feelings into words: Affect labeling disrupts amygdala activity in response to affective stimuli. *Psychological Science*, 18(5), 421–428.

47. Csikszentmihalyi, M. (1997). *Finding flow: The psychology of engagement with everyday life*. New York: Basic Books.

48. Beatrice Grimm taught me these dances at Benedicktushof in Germany.

49. Besser, B. (n.d.). Shepherd's dance. On *More beginner's dances* [CD]. (Available from Barbara Besser, Nienberger Kirchplatz 1, D-4861 Munster, Germany)

50. Based on Bays, J. C. (2011). *How to train a wild elephant and other adventures in mindfulness*. Boston: Shambhala.

51. Schneider, P. (2005). The patience of ordinary things. In *Another river: New and selected poems*. Amherst, MA: Amherst Writers and Artists Press.

52. Borkovec, T. D., & Inz, J. (1990). The nature of worry in generalized anxiety disorder: A predominance of thought activity. *Behaviour Research and Therapy*, 28(2), 153–158.

53. Rubinstein, J. S., Meyer, D. E., & Evans, J. E. (2001). Executive control of cognitive processes in task switching. *Journal of Experimental Psychology: Human Perception and Performance, 27*(4), 763–797.

54. Jackson, M. (2004). Pressured to multitask, workers juggle a fragmented existence. *Health*, 10, 26.

55. Healy, M. (2004). We're all multitasking, but what's the cost? *Los Angeles Times*. Retrieved from *www.umich.edu/~bcalab/articles/LATimesMultitasking2004.pdf*

56. Henig, R. M. (2005). Driving? Maybe you shouldn't be reading this. *The New York Times*. Retrieved from *www.umich.edu/~bcalab/articles/NYTimesMultitasking2004.pdf*

57. Rubinstein, J., Meyer, D., & Evans, J. E. (2001). Is multitasking more efficient?: Shifting mental gears costs time, especially when shifting to less familiar tasks. Retrieved from *www.apa.org/news/press/releases/2001/08/multitasking.aspx*

58. Cable News Network. (2001, August 5). CNN Tonight: Multitasking has problems, study finds. Retrieved from *www.umich.edu/~bcalab/articles/CNNTranscript2001.html*

59. Anderson, P. (2001, December 6). Study: Multitasking is counterproductive. Retrieved from *www.umich.edu/~bcalab/articles/CNNArticle2001.pdf*

60. McClure, E. B., Treland, J. E., Snow, J., Schmajuk, M., Dickstein, D. P., Towbin, K. E., et al. (2005). Deficits in social cognition and response flexibility in pediatric bipolar disorder. *American Journal of Psychiatry*, 162(9), 1644–1651.

61. Bonanno, G. A., Papa, A., Lalande, K., Westphal, M., & Coifman, K. (2004). The importance of being flexible. *Psychological Science*, 15(7), 482–487.

62. Gross, J. J. (1998). Antecedent- and response-focused emotion regulation: Divergent consequences for experience, expression, and physiology. *Journal of Personality and Social Psychology*, 74(1), 224–237.

63. Gross, J. J. (1998). The emerging field of emotion regulation: An integrative review. *Review of General Psychology*, 2(3), 271–299.

64. Pennebaker, J. W., & Seagal, J. D. (1999). Forming a story: The health benefits of narrative. *Journal of Clinical Psychology*, 55(10), 1243–1254.

65. Lester, N., Smart, L., & Baum, A. (1994). Measuring coping flexibility. *Psychology and Health*, 9(6), 409–424.

66. Cheng, C. (2001). Assessing coping flexibility in real-life and laboratory settings: A multimethod approach. *Journal of Personality and Social Psychology*, 80(5), 814–833.

67. Byron, G. G. (1979). Childe Harold's pilgrimage. In M. H. Abrams (General Ed.), *The Norton anthology of English literature* (4th ed., Vol. 2, pp. 518–541). New York: Norton. (Original work published 1812–1818)

68. Miller, H. (1958). *The smile at the foot of the ladder*. New York: New Directions.

69. Spretnak, C. (n.d.). Retrieved from *www.famousquotes.com/author/spretnak*

70. Butcher, C. A. (Trans.). (2009). *The cloud of unknowing with the book of privy counsel: A new translation*. Boston: Shambhala.

71. Teasdale, W. (1999). *The mystic heart: Discovering a universal spirituality in the world's religions.* Novato, CA: New World Library.

72. St. John of the Cross. (1990). *Dark night of the soul* (E. A. Peers, Ed. & Trans.). New York: Image Books.

73. Williams, J. E., Paton, C. C., Siegler, I. C., Eigenbrodt, M. L., Nieto, F. J., & Tyroler, H. A. (2000). Anger proneness predicts coronary heart disease risk: Prospective analysis from the Atherosclerosis Risk In Communities (ARIC) Study. *Journal of the American Heart Association, 101*(17), 2034–2039.

74. Markowitz, J. H., Matthews, K. A., Wing, R. R., Kuller, L. H., & Meilahn, E. N. (1991). Psychological, biological and health behavior predictors of blood pressure changes in middle-aged women. *Journal of Hypertension, 9,* 399–406.

75. Shapiro, D., Goldstein, I. B., & Jamner, L. D. (1996). Effects of cynical hostility, anger out, anxiety, and defensiveness on ambulatory blood pressure in black and white college students. *Psychosomatic Medicine, 58*(4), 354–364.

76. Fredrickson, B. L., Cohn, M. A., Coffey, K. A., Pek, J., & Finkel, S. M. (2008). Open hearts build lives: Positive emotions, induced through loving-kindness meditation, build consequential personal resources. *Journal of Personality and Social Psychology, 95*(5), 1045–1062.

77. Hutcherson, C. A., Seppala, E. M., & Gross, J. J. (2008). Loving-kindness meditation increases social connectedness. *Emotion, 8*(5), 720–724.

78. Hofmann, S. G., Grossman, P., & Hinton, D. E. (2011). Loving-kindness and compassion meditation: Potential for psychological interventions. *Clinical Psychology Review, 31*(7), 1126–1132.

79. Carson, J. W., Keefe, F. J., Lynch, T. R., Carson, K. M., Goli, V., Fras, A. M., et al. (2005). Loving-kindness meditation for chronic low back pain: Results from a pilot trial. *Journal of Holistic Nursing, 23,* 287–304.

80. Barnhofer, T., Chittka, T., Nightengale, H., Fisser, C., & Crane, C. (2010). State effects of two forms of meditation on prefrontal EEG asymmetry in previously depressed individuals. *Mindfulness, 1,* 21–27.

81. Feldman, G., Greeson, J., & Senville, J. (2010). Differential effects of mindful breathing, progressive muscle relaxation, and loving kindness meditation on decentering and negative reactions to repetitive thoughts. *Behaviour Research and Therapy, 48*(10), 1002–1011.

82. Williams, J. M. G., Teasdale, J. D., Kabat-Zinn, J., & Segal, Z. V. (2007). *The mindful way through depression: Freeing yourself from chronic unhappiness.* New York: Guilford Press.

83. Geary, J. (2007). *Geary's guide to the world's great aphorists.* New York: Bloomsbury USA.

CHAPTER 8

Interpersonal Effectiveness Skills

Goals of the Module

Interpersonal response patterns taught in DBT skills training are divided into three sections. The first section focuses on the core interpersonal skills of obtaining objectives while maintaining relationships and self-respect. These skills are very similar to those taught in many assertiveness and interpersonal problem-solving classes. The second section is designed for individuals who want help in developing and maintaining relationships. It focuses on decreasing interpersonal isolation by addressing how to find friends, get them to like you, and then build the sensitivity and communication skills necessary for maintaining friendships. How to end destructive relationships is also covered. The third section covers skills for walking the middle path, which have to do with balancing acceptance and change in relationships. These skills were developed for working with adolescents' families,[1]* but they can be useful for individuals, as well as for any group members who wish to develop better communication and collaboration skills.

Core Interpersonal Effectiveness Skills: Obtaining Objectives While Maintaining Relationships and Self-Respect

The core interpersonal effectiveness skills include effective strategies for asking for what one needs,

for saying no, and for managing interpersonal conflicts skillfully. "Effectiveness" here has to do with "doing what works" in these areas.

Many individuals possess reasonably effective interpersonal skills in a general sense. Problems arise in the application of these skills to specific situations. People may be able to describe effective behavioral sequences when discussing how another person encounters a problematic situation, but they may be completely incapable of generating or carrying out a similar behavioral sequence for their own situation. It is important to remember here what is meant by the term "skill": "the ability to use one's knowledge effectively and readily in execution or performance."[2] Thus having a skill means not only having a specific response in one's behavioral repertoire (e.g., saying "no"), but also having the ability to respond in a way likely to have the intended effect. The ability to hold a flute in your hands, blow out air, and move your fingers over the flute's finger holes, for example, does *not* mean that you are a skillful flute player. Mastering any skill of consequence ordinarily takes practice and feedback, often repeated many times over.

Even if people have a very strong knowledge of interpersonal skills, any number of factors can interfere with their use of those skills. For example, an interpersonal mistake that many individuals make is premature termination of relationships. Such termination can be due to difficulties in several skill areas. Problems in distress tolerance can make it difficult to tolerate fears, anxieties, or frustrations that are typical in conflictual situations. Problems in emotion regulation can lead to difficulties with decreasing anger, with frustration, or with fear of another's reaction. Inadequate problem-solving skills can make it difficult to turn potential relationship conflicts into positive encounters. Problems

---

*Sections XIV–XVII of this chapter, as well as other material marked with note number 1, are adapted from Miller, A. L., Rathus, J. H., & Linehan, M. M. (2007). *Dialectical behavior therapy with suicidal adolescents*. New York: Guilford Press. Copyright 2007 by The Guilford Press. Adapted by permission.

with attending to the moment in a nonjudgmental fashion (i.e., problems with mindfulness) can make it difficult either to assess personal wishes and goals or to assess what is needed to improve the situation.

Obtaining Objectives Skillfully

The core interpersonal effectiveness skills (Sections I–IX of this chapter) teach participants how to apply specific interpersonal problem-solving, social, and assertiveness skills to modify aversive environments and to obtain their goals in interpersonal encounters. The module focuses on situations where the objective is to change something (e.g., requesting someone to do something or take a point of view seriously) or to resist changes someone else is trying to make (e.g., saying no). Thus it is most properly considered a course in assertion, where the goal is for persons to assert their own wishes, goals, and opinions in a manner that leads other people to respond favorably. The skills taught in this part of the module maximize the chances that a person's goals in a specific situation will be met, while at the same time not damaging (and, ideally, even enhancing) the interpersonal relationship and/or the person's self-respect. The instructional content is divided into several segments.

Factors That Reduce Effectiveness and Goal Identification

Sections I–IV deal with identifying factors that contribute to interpersonal effectiveness, as well as things that interfere with being effective. The particular behavioral patterns needed for social effectiveness are almost totally a function of a person's goals in a particular situation. Thus the ability to analyze a situation and to determine goals is crucial for interpersonal effectiveness. Section IV of the module in particular addresses this challenge.

Objectives Effectiveness: DEAR MAN

Section V focuses on objectives effectiveness—specific skills for getting what one wants, summarized with the mnemonic DEAR MAN: Describe, Express feelings, Assert wishes, Reinforce, (stay) Mindful, Appear confident, and Negotiate.

Relationship Effectiveness: GIVE

Section VI covers relationship effectiveness—skills for keeping a relationship, summarized with the mnemonic GIVE: (be) Gentle, (act) Interested, Validate, (use an) Easy manner.

Self-Respect Effectiveness: FAST

Section VII describes skills for self-respect effectiveness—keeping one's self-respect; the mnemonic here is FAST: (be) Fair, (no) Apologies, Stick to values, (be) Truthful.

Section VIII focuses on guidelines for modulating how intensely to ask for what one wants or say no. Section IX, the last section of core skills, focuses on troubleshooting—how to figure out why interpersonal skills may not be working.

In this part of the module, it is especially easy to spend too little time on teaching the skills of asking or saying no in an effort to have time for everything else. At least half of this part should be devoted to the objectives, relationship, and self-respect effectiveness skills (Sections V, VI, and VII). In-session practice and role plays of these new behaviors are essential; these activities constitute an important part of all interpersonal skills training programs. However, integrating behavioral practice of new behaviors within sessions can be one of the most difficult aspects of skills training for new therapists and for those not trained in behavior therapy. Thus it can be very easy to just let it slip by in this module.

Skills for Building Relationships and Ending Destructive Ones

The skills in this part of the module (Sections X–XIII) are designed specifically to teach individuals how to meet new people and interact in a way that facilitates the development of trust and friendship, and that reduces the likelihood of conflict. It also covers how to end relationships that are damaging.

Finding Potential Friends

In Section XI, the skills are aimed at getting individuals started at actively finding people who might become their friends. This is particularly important for those individuals who are isolated and feel lonely much of the time.

Mindfulness of Others

Mindfulness of others and sensitivity to others' needs are critical components of developing and maintaining relationships and are covered in Section XII. Notice as you teach these skills that the mindfulness skill of describing is referred to often. Describing one's own or another's reactions, thoughts, or feelings is the opposite of making judgmental comments about oneself or others. This is a critical interpersonal skill, because judgmentalness is often poisonous in both new and ongoing relationships.

How to End Relationships

Staying in destructive relationships too long can, of course, be just as problematic as not having relationships. Skills for those who have difficulty ending relationships are covered in Section XIII. These individuals often have enormous difficulties in saying no, as well as difficulties in observing their own limits. Emotion dysregulation is often the culprit here—fear of what might happen to oneself or the other if the person leaves the relationship, out-of-control grief at another's current or potential suffering, excessive guilt at causing another pain, and compassion for another while failing to have compassion for oneself. In these cases, people often vacillate between avoidance of conflict and intense confrontation. Unfortunately, the choice of avoidance versus confrontation is often based on an individual's current emotional state (i.e., mood dependency) rather than on the needs of the situation. Interpersonal effectiveness skills are difficult to develop in a vacuum; perhaps more than any other set of skills, they depend on simultaneous improvement across all skill areas.

The skills in this part of this module do not cover the finer points of finding love or a life partner, or of developing intimate relationships and deep and lasting friendships. Nor are the skills directed at how to make time alone more palatable. The skills, however, are essential basic skills for anyone who wants to meet new people, find and keep love or a partner, form and maintain lasting intimate friendships, and build a life where time spent alone is filled with satisfying activities.

Walking the Middle Path

As noted above, the skills for walking the middle path (Sections XIV–XVII) were originally designed for family skills training with adolescents and their caregivers. The skills, however, are also important for adults and can be helpful in any relationship. They are also essential for DBT skills trainers. There are three skill sets in walking the middle path: dialectics, validation, and behavior change strategies. Taken together, the skills in this part of the module focus on balancing acceptance and change in interpersonal relationships.

Dialectics

The skill of dialectics is covered in Section XV. As discussed in Chapter 1, dialectics as a world view forms the basis of DBT. It has three primary characteristics. The first stresses the wholeness of reality and directs our attention to the immediate and larger contexts of behavior, as well as to the interrelatedness of individual behavior patterns. Second, from a dialectical perspective, reality is comprised of internal opposing forces (thesis and antithesis), and out of their synthesis evolves a new set of opposing forces. Dichotomous, extreme thinking, behavior, and emotions are viewed as dialectical failures; the individual has become stuck in polarities unable to move to synthesis. Third, dialectics assumes that the nature of reality is change. Both the individual and the environment are undergoing continuous transition. In essence, every relationship is one of continuous transition and change.

Validation

Although validation as a skill is covered as one of the relationship effectiveness GIVE skills (see above and Section VI), it is retaught in Section XVI in more depth, because it is so essential to developing and maintaining close and intimate relationships. Validation has to do with communicating clearly to others that you are paying attention to them, that you understand them, that you are nonjudgmental, that you have empathy, and that you can see the facts or the truth of their situation. The key to teaching validation is for participants already to have a firm foundation in mindfulness. Validation requires the ability to observe and describe without necessarily adding to what is observed, and to listen and interact nonjudgmentally. As you teach the validation skills, you may need to review the mindfulness skills. How to recover from invalidation is also included in this section. This skill teaches participants how to validate themselves effectively when necessary. For a thorough discussion of validation and how to use it see Linehan (1997).[3]

Strategies for Changing Behavior

Finally, the middle path skills include basic behavioral contingency management skills. The basic idea is that systematic and contingent application of consequences following others' behaviors can have an enormous impact on their behavior in the future. Although telegraphing consequences of behavior is part of the core DEAR MAN skills taught in Section V (Reinforce), in this section specific contingency management skills are taught—including positive and negative reinforcement, shaping, extinction, satiation, and punishment. These are the very same skills that therapists also use in DBT. (See Chapter 5 in this manual, and also see Chapter 10 of the main DBT text.)

Selecting Material to Teach

As noted above, there is a great deal of material for each skill in the interpersonal teaching notes that follow. Most of it you will not cover the first time you teach specific skills. The notes are provided to give you a deeper understanding of each skill so that you can answer questions and add new teaching as you go. As in Chapters 6 and 7, I have put a checkmark (✓) next to material I almost always cover. If I am in a huge rush, I may skip everything but checkmarked points. Similarly, on this manual's special website (*www.guilford.com/skills-training-manual*), I use stars (★) for core handouts I almost always use.

And as in Chapter 7, I have indicated information summarizing research in special "Research Point" features. The great value of research is that it can often be used to sell the skills you are teaching.

Moreover, as when you are teaching any skills module, it is important that you have a basic understanding of the specific interpersonal effectiveness skills you are teaching. Decide what skills you are going to teach first. Carefully study the teach-

ing notes, handouts, and worksheets for each skill you have selected to teach. Highlight the points you want to make, and bring a copy of the relevant pages with you to teach from. Practice each skill, and make sure you understand how to use it yourself. Before long you will solidify your knowledge of each skill. At that point, you will find your own favorite teaching points, examples, and stories, and can ignore mine.

Finally, a number of handouts in this module offer brief, optional, multiple-choice quizzes of skills taught. They can be used within group sessions and discussed, or can be assigned as homework. An answer key for all of these handouts is provided below, and the key for each handout is provided at the end of the sections in which the handout might be used.

Answer Key for Multiple-Choice Handouts

Interpersonal Effectiveness Handout 11a: Identifying Skills to Find People and Get Them to Like You
- Effective answers: 1A, 2B, 3A, 4A, 5A, 6B, 7B, 8B, 9B, 10B, 11B, 12A

Interpersonal Effectiveness Handout 12a: Identifying Mindfulness of Others
- Effective answers: 1B, 2B, 3A, 4A, 5A, 6A, 7B, 8B, 9B, 10A, 11B, 12B

Interpersonal Effectiveness Handout 13a: Identifying How to End Relationships
- Effective answers: 1B, 2B, 3B, 4A, 5B, 6B, 7B, 8B

Interpersonal Effectiveness Handout 16c: Identifying Dialectics
- Effective answers: 1A, 2B, 3B, 4B, 5A, 6C, 7B, 8B

Interpersonal Effectiveness Handout 18a: Identifying Validation
- Effective answers: 1B, 2A, 3A, 4B, 5A, 6B, 7B, 8B

Interpersonal Effectiveness Handout 19a: Identifying Self-Validation
- Effective answers: 1A, 2B, 3A, 4B, 5A, 6B

Interpersonal Effectiveness Handout 22a: Identifying Effective Behavior Change Strategies
- Effective answers: 1B, 2B, 3A, 4A, 5B, 6B, 7B, 8A

Teaching Notes

I.   GOALS OF THIS MODULE (INTERPERSONAL EFFECTIVENESS HANDOUT 1)

Main Point: The basic goal of this module is for participants to learn how to be effective in interpersonal interactions, so that their interactions with others will have outcomes they want. These skills teach participants how to be effective at achieving their own goals without alienating the other person or losing their self-respect. Interpersonal effectiveness skills are also necessary for strengthening current relationships and for finding and building new relationships.

Interpersonal Effectiveness Handout 1: Goals of Interpersonal Effectiveness Skills. This handout is intended to orient participants to interpersonal goals for which the skills taught in this module might be very useful. Go over it briefly, link the module to participants' goals, and generate some enthusiasm for learning the interpersonal effectiveness skills. Then move to the next handout. If time permits, have participants checkmark the goals that are most important to them. Spend more time on the handout later, if necessary.

Interpersonal Effectiveness Worksheet 1: Pros and Cons of Using Interpersonal Effectiveness Skills *(Optional).* This worksheet is designed to help participants (1) decide whether they want to use interpersonal skills instead of power tactics to get what they want, and (2) decide whether to go after what they want instead of giving up on getting it. Its major use is to communicate that the goal is to be *effective* in getting what they want (i.e., in reaching their own goals). It is not about being nice, following rules, giving in, or doing what other people want. This worksheet can also be used as an exercise to improve the likelihood of being effective when a person is overcome with emotions (e.g., when the person just wants to yell and scream, or to avoid an interpersonal situation completely). It can also be used as a teaching tool for how to figure out goals. For instructions in teaching pros and cons, see the teaching notes for the Distress Tolerance module (Chapter 10, Section V) on reviewing pros and cons as a way to make behavioral decisions. Assign this worksheet as optional if you teach other handouts in the session that have associated worksheets.

✓   💬 **Discussion Point:** Either before or after reviewing Interpersonal Effectiveness Handout 1, ask participants to check off each goal that is important to them in the boxes on the handout, and then to share choices.

The goals of interpersonal effectiveness skills include the following:

✓   A. Be Skillful in Achieving Objectives with Others

The skills in this section are a variation on assertiveness skills. They have to do with being interpersonally effective in two sets of situations.

1. Asking Others to Do Things

✓   Skills for asking others to do things we would like them to do include making requests, initiating discussions, solving problems in relationships/repairing relationships, and getting others to take our opinions seriously.

2. Saying No to Unwanted Requests Effectively

Skills for saying no to unwanted requests include resisting pressure from others and maintaining a position or point of view.

✓   💬 **Discussion Point:** Ask participants whether they have more trouble asking for what they want or saying no to unwanted requests from others. Ask who has trouble getting others to take their opinions seriously. Are there some people with whom, or some times when, being assertive is harder? How about easier?

💬 **Discussion Point:** Discuss with participants how they view their own interpersonal skills. Some individuals will be skillful at asking for things but not skillful at saying no, whereas others can say no but cannot ask for anything. Still others are deficient across the board. Sometimes individuals are able to apply skills in some situational contexts but not in others. For example, some people may be quite comfortable at saying no to strangers but not to friends; others may be able to ask for help from friends but not from their bosses. Elicit from each person the situations and skills he or she feels are strong (enough) and those that need further work.

> **Note to Leaders:** The major goal here is for participants to see the relevance of interpersonal effectiveness skills training to their own lives by seeing areas in which they need improvement. Keep in mind that participants' descriptions of their strengths and weaknesses in these skills may not correspond with their actual skill levels. Some will report having no skills, but are able to apply skills in role plays; others may report strong skills, but then demonstrate clear deficits in role plays. Both sorts of participants will benefit from support and encouragement in their process of building mastery and a fact-based sense of self-efficacy.
>
> Feel free to share with participants your own areas of strength and weakness. This can serve to normalize the notion of skill deficits by highlighting that we all have areas in which we can improve our skills. In my experience, some individuals are exceptionally skilled in many interpersonal situations and may present as if they do not need interpersonal effectiveness skills training. However, a closer discussion, especially of various situational contexts, will reveal that almost everyone can use some skills training. Therefore, even with a very skilled person, make every effort to identify areas where that person can use improvement.

✓ **B. Build Relationships, Strengthen Current Relationships, and End Destructive Ones**

Skills for relationships include skills for doing these things:

- Not letting hurts and problems build up.
- Heading off problems.
- Repairing relationships (or ending them if necessary).
- Resolving conflicts before they get overwhelming.

Unattended relationships can develop cracks that create enormous stress. This stress then increases emotional vulnerability, and life can go downhill. Unattended relationships often blow up, and can end even when people want them to continue. Having the ability to repair relationships is much more important than keeping them from "tearing" in the first place. However, the longer relationships remain unattended to, the harder they are to repair. Relationships that are ignored can weaken and disappear. Once a relationship disappears, it can be difficult to resurrect it. Sometimes, rather than disappearing, relationships become intolerably difficult; thus learning how to end an intolerably painful and hopeless relationship is also an important skill.

> **Note to Leaders:** If you plan on teaching the skills for building relationships and ending destructive ones (Sections X–XIII of this module), then stress these skills as a way to both find and build new relationships, as well as to end hopeless relationships.

✓ **C. Walk the Middle Path**

A final set of interpersonal effectiveness skills involves "walking the middle path" (a concept covered in Chapter 7 among the supplementary mindfulness skills). If you are teaching these skills, emphasize these points to participants:

▪ Keeping relationships requires balancing our own priorities with the demands of others.
▪ Relationships require balancing change with acceptance without letting go of either.

Maintaining relationships also require us to remember that relationships are transactional. For relationships to work, it is important to practice looking at all sides of situations, finding the kernel of truth in other people's views. Although we need to have skills that can get others to change their behavior, we must also balance that with accepting others as they are.

II. FACTORS REDUCING INTERPERSONAL EFFECTIVENESS (INTERPERSONAL EFFECTIVENESS HANDOUTS 2–2A)

Main Point: Lack of skill, indecision, interference from emotions, prioritizing short-term goals over long-term goals, interference from the environment, and interpersonal myths can each make interpersonal effectiveness very difficult.

Interpersonal Effectiveness Handout 2: Factors in the Way of Interpersonal Effectiveness. This handout can be reviewed quickly. If time is short, skip the discussion and lecture points provided below. You can revisit this handout later to troubleshoot difficulties in using interpersonal effectiveness skills successfully.

Interpersonal Effectiveness Handout 2a: Myths in the Way of Interpersonal Effectiveness (Optional). This handout can be used as part of an exercise on identifying and challenging worry thoughts and myths. See Section F below for a detailed description. If time is short, skip this handout and instead describe several myths when introducing the factors that interfere with interpersonal effectiveness.

Interpersonal Effectiveness Worksheet 2: Challenging Myths in the Way of Interpersonal Effectiveness (Optional). Listing the same myths as on Handout 2a, this worksheet helps participants develop new challenges or rewrite the challenges discussed in group sessions in more personal language. The important point is for the participants to "own" a challenge, not to necessarily think up one on their own. There are also spaces for participants to write in and challenge their own myths. Be careful about assigning too much homework, but if you assign this worksheet, be sure to review it with participants. If necessary, instruct them in how to rate intensity of emotions. (For instructions, see Chapter 10, Section VI.)

Interpersonal Effectiveness Worksheet 7: Troubleshooting Interpersonal Effectiveness Skills. If participants have already gone through the Interpersonal Effectiveness skills module once and this is their second time, encourage them to use this worksheet. It covers the same topics, organized in the same sequence as in Handout 2 above. However, it is overwhelming and hard to use when participants are going through the module for the first time. It works much better when given at the module's end or when these skills are repeated.

(Interpersonal Effectiveness Handout 9: Troubleshooting: When What You Are Doing Isn't Working. This handout may also be appropriate when the module is repeated. It also covers the same topics in the same sequence as Handout 2 and Worksheet 7.)

✓ **Being interpersonally skillful is hard.** There are many reasons why interactions may not be effective.

✓ **A. Lack of Needed Skills**

Say to participants: "When you lack skills, you don't know what to say or how to act. You don't know how to behave in order to obtain your interpersonal goals."

1. Lack of Ability versus Lack of Motivation

Lack of ability to behave in a certain way is very different from lack of motivation. Emphasize that people learn social behaviors by observing someone else do them first, practicing them, and refining them until they can be used to obtain good results. People sometimes don't have enough opportunities to observe; therefore, they don't learn the behaviors. Or they may not have the chance to practice the behaviors they do observe.

2. Ability, Observation, and Modification

Tell participants: "Having a skill means that you not only have a specific ability (for instance, to say no), but that you can do two other things."

- "You have the ability to observe the effect of what you do and how you do it on others."
- "And you can then modify what you do, based on this feedback, in order to have an intended effect. Becoming interpersonally effective usually requires that critical skills are overlearned, so that they are automatic when needed. Any skill of consequence, however, ordinarily takes practice and feedback many times over to master."

Practice Exercise: Hold up your hands as if you are holding a flute, and ask participants to do the same. Then ask participants to pucker their lips and blow air as they move their fingers over the imaginary holes in the flute. Ask them: "Does this mean that all of you can now play the flute?" The same can be said for sports, public speaking, solving problems, and—most importantly—interpersonal skills. Elicit examples of skills participants have learned that took lots of practice to get proficient at.

> **Note to Leaders:** When I teach this, I do the practice exercise above first. Then, using the information below, I explain why the ability to blow air and move my fingers does not mean that I can play a flute.

✓ **B. Indecision**

Say to participants: "Even if you have the ability to be effective, you may not know or can't decide what you want. There are several ways that indecision can hinder you."

- "Not knowing what you really want can be confusing and get in the way of being clear about what you are asking for or saying no to."
- "Indecision on how to balance your needs with those of others can lead to ambivalence and make it hard for you to know how insistent to be in asking or saying no to things."
- "Vacillating between asking for too much and not asking for anything, or between the equal extremes of saying no to everything and giving in to everything, can keep you in an extreme position and make you unlikely to be effective."

Discussion Point: Discuss the tendency to go to extremes of asking (or saying no) versus not asking (or giving in). Also discuss tendencies to go to extremes: complete neediness (asking in a clinging, begging, grasping, or hysterical manner) versus complete self-sufficiency (never asking, saying yes to everything); complete worthiness (asking in an inappropriately demanding manner or refusing belligerently) versus complete unworthiness (never asking or saying no). Elicit examples.

✓ C. Interference from Emotions

Tell participants: "Emotions may get in the way of your ability to behave effectively. You may have the capability to use interpersonal skills, but your skills are mood-dependent and are interfered with by your emotions."

- Emotions can inhibit skillful actions or overwhelm known skills. In fact, emotions can be so strong that emotional actions, words, and facial and body expressions become automatic.
- Automatic emotional reactions can be based on previous conditioning. Or they can be a result of believing myths (discussed below).
- A person can have skills in one set of situations but not in another, or in one mood but not in another, or in one frame of mind but not in another.

💬 **Discussion Point:** Elicit examples of strong emotions interfering with skillful behavior.

💬 **Discussion Point:** Elicit examples of having variable skills, depending on current emotions or mood.

✓ D. Prioritizing Short-Term Goals over Long-Term Goals

Several factors can cause us to give priority to short-term over long-term goals. Two major ones are low distress tolerance and failure to think about consequences.

1. Low Tolerance for Distress

Low distress tolerance often leads us to jump into a situation and demand what we want, even when it is not in our long-term interest or is inconsistent with our long-term goals, values, and/or self-respect.

Example: If our tolerance for conflict is low, we might end a relationship that we really want, or give in to another person's wishes when we know we don't really want to.

2. Failure to Consider Consequences

Sometimes we don't think about the consequences of our actions for ourselves and the people we are interacting with. When angry, we may make threats and demand our way right this minute; in a calmer moment later, we realize that getting what we want is less important than the relationship.

💬 **Discussion Point:** Elicit examples of putting short-term over long-term goals and regretting it later.

✓ E. Interference from the Environment

Environmental factors, including other people, may preclude effectiveness. At times even the most skilled individuals cannot be effective at getting what they want, keeping others liking them, or behaving in ways that they respect.

- When the environment is powerful, other people may simply refuse to give us what we want, or they may have the authority to make us do what they want. Saying no or insisting on our rights under these circumstances may have very negative consequences.
- Sometimes there is no way to keep the other person liking us and also get what we want or say no. People may be threatened, jealous, or envious, or may have any number of other reasons for not liking someone.
- When we are faced with a conflict, and achieving an objective is very important (e.g., food or medical care for ourselves or our children), we may have to act in ways that damage our pride or otherwise hurt our self-respect.
- Fully applying ourselves to being interpersonally effective is the only way to know whether the environment is preventing effectiveness. This includes preparing for assertiveness ahead

of time, and getting feedback on the plan from trusted individuals, such as getting DBT skills coaching.

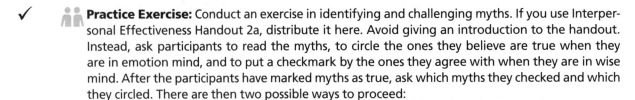 **Discussion Point:** Some people believe that all failures to get what they want from someone else are failures in skills. They have difficulty seeing that sometimes the environment is simply impervious to even the most skilled individuals. Thus, when they fail to get what they want by using interpersonal effectiveness skills, they may fall back into hopelessness, try an aggressive response, or threaten (e.g., blackmail) other people. Although increased interpersonal skills should increase the probability of getting objectives met, they are not a guarantee. Elicit times when participants have been very skillful (or seen someone else be skillful) but not successful at getting what was wanted.

> **Note to Leaders:** Some individuals have a very unrealistic view of the world and of what skilled people can do. The idea that people often don't get what they want or need isn't clear to them. The belief that people can always get what they want and need precludes the necessity of developing distress tolerance skills. Without such skills, frustration often turns into anger. Be very careful on this point, especially during homework discussions.

✓ ## F. Interpersonal Myths

All people have some worries about standing up for themselves, expressing opinions, saying no, and so on. Sometimes worries are based on myths about interpersonal behavior.

Tell participants that they can counteract worries and myths in several ways:

- Arguing against them logically.
- Checking the facts (see Emotion Regulation Handout 8).
- Practicing opposite action (see Emotion Regulation Handout 10).
- Practicing cope ahead with imagined negative consequences (see Emotion Regulation Handout 19).

Counteracting worry thoughts and myths is an example of cognitive modification or cognitive therapy. It can sometimes be useful in getting people to do things they really want to do but are afraid to do. Challenges to myths can be used to challenge worries that crop up about trying interpersonal skills.

✓ 🧍🧍 **Practice Exercise:** Conduct an exercise in identifying and challenging myths. If you use Interpersonal Effectiveness Handout 2a, distribute it here. Avoid giving an introduction to the handout. Instead, ask participants to read the myths, to circle the ones they believe are true when they are in emotion mind, and to put a checkmark by the ones they agree with when they are in wise mind. After the participants have marked myths as true, ask which myths they checked and which they circled. There are then two possible ways to proceed:

1. Ask those who checked or circled a myth to offer challenges to one or both.

2. Use the devil's advocate technique to discuss myths. In this strategy, you present a myth and then make an extreme statement in favor of the myth, thus getting participants to argue the case for the counterstatements. As the participants argue against the myth, you continue to make extreme and universal (i.e., applying to all people) arguments to the myth. After several arguments, you give in and agree with the participants. (See Chapter 7 of the main DBT text for further discussion of this strategy.) The discussion on each statement should be resolved by transcending the extremes to find a synthesis or balancing point of view.

Not every myth has to be discussed in this exercise; the participants should be included in choosing which ones to go over. Whichever strategy you use, the task of participants is to develop personalized challenges or counterarguments against the myths. Ask everyone to write challenges down as participants think them up. Be sure that each challenge on the one hand contradicts the myth in some way, and on the other hand is at least somewhat believable to individual participants. For example, one participant might be able to challenge the myth "I don't deserve to get what I want or need," with "I do deserve to get what I want and need," but this might be too strong for (and therefore rejected by) another participant. However, the second participant might be able to practice the challenge "Sometimes it's OK for me to get things I want or need." These challenges can be used as cheerleading statements later, to help participants get themselves to act effectively.

Note to Leaders: A homework assignment might be to have participants complete the challenges not covered during the exercise above. Another assignment might be to have them observe themselves over the week and write down any other myths that they operate by. They should also think up challenges to these other myths.

It is important to have participants practice reviewing their personalized challenges, in order to develop a strong habit of overcoming their myths. It can be very effective to have participants develop a plan for reviewing their challenges, such as placing them on their refrigerators or bathroom mirrors for daily review.

Discussion Point: If you don't use Handout 2a, ask participants what worry thoughts, assumptions, beliefs, and myths have gotten in the way of their asking for what they want or need and saying no to unwanted requests. Then generate challenges as noted in the exercise above for some or all of the myths.

Discussion Point: Unmanaged worries can interfere with effectiveness even if they are not based on myths (e.g., "This person might get upset with me for asking," or "I hope my anger doesn't get out of control," or "This person might say no to my request, and I won't get what I want"). Elicit from participants worries that get in the way of effectiveness.

G. Interplay of Factors

Say to participants: "Very often, a combination of various factors may be keeping you from being effective. For example, the less you know, the more you worry, the worse you feel, the more you can't decide what to do, the more ineffective you are, the more you worry, and so on. Or the more you experience nongiving and authoritarian environments, the more you worry, the less you practice skillfulness, the less you know, the worse you feel, the more you can't decide what to do, and so on."

III. OVERVIEW: CORE INTERPERSONAL EFFECTIVENESS SKILLS (INTERPERSONAL EFFECTIVENESS HANDOUT 3)

Main Point: Introduce the core DBT interpersonal effectiveness skills. These are the basic assertiveness skills necessary to achieve objectives, maintain relationships, and enhance self-respect. These three sets of skills are referred to by the mnemonics DEAR MAN, GIVE, and FAST. The effectiveness of these skills depends in part on two additional skills: clarifying priorities and determining how intensely to ask or say no.

Interpersonal Handout 3: Overview: Obtaining Objectives Skillfully. This overview handout can be reviewed briefly or skipped, depending on time. Do not actually teach the material while going over the points below unless you are skipping the related handouts, all of which are ordinarily taught.

Worksheet: None.

Say to participants: "The skills in this section of the module are aimed at being effective when you ask someone for something or respond to a request, while at the same time maintaining or even improving both the relationship and your self-respect."

✓ A. Clarifying Priorities

Tell participants: "Clarifying your priorities is the first and most important interpersonal skill. It is the essential task of figuring out (1) what you actually want and how important it is, compared to (2) keeping a positive relationship and (3) keeping your own self-respect.

✓ B. Objectives Effectiveness Skills: DEAR MAN

Say to participants: "DEAR MAN is DBT shorthand for the set of skills enabling you to effectively obtain your objective or goal."

✓ C. Relationship Effectiveness Skills: GIVE

Continue: "GIVE is DBT shorthand for the set of skills enabling you to create or maintain a positive relationship while you also try to obtain your objective."

✓ D. Self-Respect Effectiveness Skills: FAST

Continue: "FAST is DBT shorthand for the set of skills enabling you to maintain or increase your sense of self-respect while at the same time trying to obtain your objective."

✓ E. Skills for Evaluating Your Options

Conclude the overview by telling participants: "Every situation is different. Sometimes it is very important to push hard to obtain your objective; at other times it can be equally important to give up your personal goals in favor of someone else's. These skills help you figure out how hard to push for what you want and how strong to hold to saying no to someone else."

IV. CLARIFYING GOALS IN INTERPERSONAL SITUATIONS (INTERPERSONAL EFFECTIVENESS HANDOUT 4)

> **Main Point:** To use interpersonal skills effectively, we have to decide the relative importance of (1) achieving our objective, (2) maintaining our relationship with the person(s) we are interacting with, and (3) maintaining our self-respect. The skills we use depend on the relative importance of these three goals.
>
> **Interpersonal Effectiveness Handout 4: Clarifying Goals in Interpersonal Situations.** This handout reviews the goals and priorities an individual might have in any interpersonal situation. Be sure that participants understand this handout before moving on, as it is an important underpinning of subsequent handouts. Generally, what is most difficult for participants to understand is that all three of these priorities must be considered in every goal-directed interpersonal situation.
>
> **Interpersonal Effectiveness Worksheet 3: Clarifying Priorities in Interpersonal Situations.** Review this worksheet with participants. In describing the prompting event, remind them to use the mindfulness "what" skill of describing (see Mindfulness Handout 4). This is very important, because when it comes to interpersonal conflict or fears about an interpersonal situation, individuals often fail to notice that much of what they describe as happening in a situation is actually their interpretations or assumptions.

✓ A. Why Clarify Goals?

To be effective in interpersonal interactions, it is important for us to know what we actually want—in other words, what our goal is. This is no easy task, however. Many interactions get off track because we are not clear about what we really want. Interactions also get off track when emotions interfere with knowing what we want.

Example: "If you are afraid of asking for what you want or of saying no to a request, you may be too afraid even to think about what you want."

Example: "Shame and thinking you don't deserve to get what you want can interfere with believing it is OK to have goals and objectives."

✓   💬 **Discussion Point:** Elicit from participants times when they have had trouble figuring out what their actual goal was in an interpersonal interaction. Discuss how these interactions turned out.

✓ **B. Three Potential Goals in Interpersonal Situations**

✓ **1. Objectives Effectiveness**

Say to participants: "Objectives effectiveness refers to attaining your objective or goal in a particular situation. Generally, the objective is the reason for the interaction in the first place."

Emphasize: "The key question to ask yourself here is '**What specific result or change do I want from this interaction?**' This is the specific change or outcome you want from the other person by the end of the interaction. It may be what the other person is to do, to stop doing, to commit to, to agree to, or to understand. It is important for the objective to be as specific as possible. The clearer you are about what you want, the easier it will be to apply objectives effectiveness skills, and the clearer you will be as to whether or not you succeed in reaching your goal."

✓   *Examples:*

- "Standing up for your rights in such a way that they are taken seriously."
- "Requesting others to do something in such a way that they do what you ask."
- "Refusing an unwanted or unreasonable request and making the refusal stick."
- "Resolving interpersonal conflict."
- "Getting your opinion or point of view taken seriously."

💬 **Discussion Point:** Elicit from participants which goals they find important (standing up for rights, making requests, refusing requests, etc.). Which are hardest and require the most skills?

✓ **2. Relationship Effectiveness**

Tell participants: "Relationship effectiveness refers to keeping or improving the relationship, while at the same time trying to achieve your goal in the interaction."

Emphasize: "The key question to ask yourself here is '**How do I want the other person to feel about me after the interaction is over (whether or not I get the results or changes I want)?**' At its best, you will get what you want, and the person may like or respect you even more than before. This likelihood is increased by using relationship effectiveness skills."

Examples:

- "Acting in a way that makes the other person actually want to give you what you are asking for or feel good about your saying no to a request."
- "Balancing immediate goals with the good of the long-term relationship."

a. Improving a Relationship Can Be a Main Objective

Explain to participants: "If the main goal of the interaction is to get the other person to notice, like, or approve of you, or to stop criticizing or rejecting you, then enhancing the relationship is the objective and should be considered under objectives effectiveness. In that case, relationship effectiveness refers to choosing a way to go about developing, improving, or keeping the relationship that does not at the same time damage the relationship over the long run."

> *Example:* "You understand the other person's perspective, while at the same time you ask this person to change how he or she treats you. You avoid threats, judgments, or attacks."

✓ **b. Always Making the Relationship the Main Objective Doesn't Work**

Many individuals, of course, are highly concerned with maintaining relationships, approval, and liking. Some are willing to sacrifice personal objectives for the sake of interpersonal relationship goals. They may operate under the myth that if they sacrifice their own needs and wants to other people, their relationships will go more smoothly, approval will be ever forthcoming, and no problems will arise.

💬 **Discussion Point:** Elicit examples of when participants have made relationships overly important, at the expense of their own objectives and self-respect—or even the relationships themselves.

✓ **c. Subverting Personal Needs in a Relationship Doesn't Work**

Draw a time line on the blackboard like that in Figure 8.1. At the left end of the time line, mark the beginning of a relationship. Then move the chalk toward the right as if time were marching on, and discuss how a relationship goes if a person constantly subverts his or her own needs for the sake of a relationship. Although a person can survive in such a relationship for some time, frustrations will build up and will have to be dealt with. Usually at the point where frustrations are long-standing, the unmet needs are large, and the sense of inequity is extreme, one of two things will happen: The frustrated individual will (1) blow up and thereby risk losing the relationship through the other person's rejection; or (2) in frustration, leave the relationship on his or her own. Either way, the relationship comes to an end or is in serious jeopardy.

💬 **Discussion Point:** Discuss the ways in which constantly subverting personal needs for the sake of a relationship has worked in participants' lives. Usually someone can give examples of how he or she has blown up and ruined a relationship. Behaviors that may show up at the far end of the continuum include violent acts or threats, screaming or yelling, saying very hurtful things, and suicide attempts. (Other dysfunctional behaviors can also be used as examples.) Such behaviors often function to get someone else to take a person's feelings and opinions seriously, or they may function to get other people to change their behavior. It is important to elicit from participants how blowing up or walking out of relationships inadvertently jeopardizes their own goals.

d. Extreme Behaviors May Be Effective in the Short Term but Not over the Long Term

Say to clients: "Extreme, unskillful behaviors early in a relationship may get you what you want in the moment, but they can also jeopardize a relationship's very existence in the long run. Employing interpersonal skills will not only enhance your relationships, but improve your chances of obtaining interpersonal and social approval rather than the opposite."

💬 **Discussion Point:** A strategy that is sometimes useful at this point and at many other points is to ask participants to imagine another person behaving toward them in extreme ways, such as using violence, threats of suicide or other terrible acts, or blowing up. Ask, "How would it feel?"

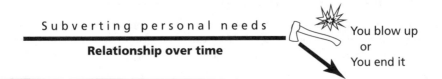

FIGURE 8.1. Over time, subverting personal needs in a relationship usually ends the relationship.

From that perspective, individuals often find it easier to see the dysfunctional nature of these behaviors. The main goal here is to elicit participants' commitment to the value of learning and practicing interpersonal skills. Of course, commitments often waver in the actual situations where employing the skills is necessary; nonetheless, obtaining commitment is the first step in the process of shaping interpersonal skills.

> **Note to Leaders:** Participants may have great difficulty seeing this point. In my experience, some individuals believe that extreme behaviors are not only effective but are the only behaviors possible, given the circumstances of their lives or of the group or culture in which they are living. It is essential at this point to help them develop some insight into how these strategies are self-defeating in the long run. Other individuals confuse the idea that a behavior can have a consequence (e.g., can be inconveniencing or hurtful) with the idea that the person *intends* the consequence. It is important to discuss the difference.

✓ ### 3. Self-Respect Effectiveness

Instruct participants: "Self-respect effectiveness is maintaining or improving your respect for yourself, and respecting your own values and beliefs, while you try to attain your objectives. Self-respect effectiveness means acting in ways that fit your sense of morality, and that make you feel a sense of competence and mastery."

Emphasize: "The key question to ask yourself here is '**How do I want to feel about myself after the interaction is over (whether or not I get the results or changes I want)?**'"

a. Improving Self-Respect Can Be a Main Objective

Say to participants: "If the main goal of the interaction is to do something that will enhance your self-respect, then enhancing self-respect is the objective and should be considered under objectives effectiveness. This is particularly the case when the simple act of standing up and speaking is most important—in other words, when actually getting what you want is not as important as asserting what you want (such as asking for something, saying no, or expressing an opinion). In these cases, self-respect effectiveness refers to how you go about improving or keeping your self-respect. Relationship effectiveness refers to choosing a way to improve your self-respect that does not at the same time inadvertently damage your self-respect either short term or long term."

Examples: Again, give a number of examples:

- "Standing up for yourself."
- "Defending a friend."
- "Stepping forward to do or say something courageous."
- "Voting for what you really believe in (even if you are in the minority or will lose friends over your vote)."

✓ #### b. Always Making Self-Respect the Main Objective Doesn't Work

Some individuals make maintaining their self-respect the major issue in almost all interactions. Always wanting to be "on top" or to have control or power, never letting another person win in an interaction, wanting to prove a point or defend a position no matter what— each of these positions can compromise long-term effectiveness.

✓ #### c. Violating Our Own Moral Values Diminishes Self-Respect in the Long Term

Giving in on important things just for the sake of approval, lying to please others or to get what we want, or any activity that is experienced as "selling out" or "selling our souls" diminishes self-respect over time.

✓   **d. Acting Helpless Also Diminishes Self-Respect in the Long Term**

Even if acting helpless is strategic—that is, deliberately calculated to get someone to do something—the strategy will inevitably lead to reduced mastery and self-respect if it is overused.

💬 **Discussion Point:** Elicit from participants times when they have done things in relationships that reduced their sense of self-respect. When have they acted in ways that enhanced their sense of self-respect? Where do they need to improve their skills?

C. Deciding on the Relative Importance of the Three Effectiveness Types

1. All Three Types Must Always Be Considered

Emphasize that participants need to consider all three types of effectiveness in every situation with a specific interpersonal objective or goal.

✓   ### 2. Each Type of Effectiveness May Be More or Less Important in a Given Situation

Note that, generally, one type of effectiveness may lose importance when pursuing it will interfere with a more highly valued type of effectiveness.

✓   ### 3. The Effectiveness of a Behavior in a Particular Situation Depends on a Person's Priorities

Discuss the following examples of situations, goals, and priorities.

Example:

Situation: Diego's landlord keeps his damage deposit unfairly.

Objective: Get the damage deposit back (most important to Diego).

Relationship: Keep the landlord's good will and liking, or at least keeping good reference (second most important).

Self-respect: Not lose self-respect by getting too emotional, "fighting dirty," threatening.

Example:

Situation: Carla's best friend wants to come over and discuss a problem; Carla wants to go to bed.

Objective: Go to bed.

Relationship: Keep a good relationship with the friend (most important to Carla).

Self-respect: Balance caring for the friend with caring for herself (second most important).

Example:

Situation: Tiffany wants a raise; her boss wants sex in return.

Objective: Get the raise; stay out of bed with the boss.

Relationship: Keep the boss's respect and good will (second most important).

Self-respect: Not violate her own moral code by sleeping with the boss (most important to Tiffany).

💬 **Discussion Point:** Elicit from participants times they have risked losing what they want, a relationship, or their self-respect for a short-term relationship gain.

Examples may include attempting or threatening suicide or violence to get what they want or keep someone from leaving; attacking another person for voicing criticism; lying (and being found out) to get something; demanding to get their way; laying a "guilt trip" on another person to get that person to do something; and so on.

✓　👥 **Practice Exercise:** Have participants generate other situations and identify the objective(s) in the situation, the relationship issue, and the self-respect issue for each situation. Discuss priorities for each situation. Continue generating situations until it is clear that the participants have grasped the essential points. The following examples can be used; however, be sure to ask participants what would be most important to them before suggesting the priority given in boldface at the end of each example.

Example:

Situation: Yvonne is in a very difficult financial situation and has overdrawn her bank account. There is now a big overdraft fee on the account. Yvonne goes to the bank to ask a clerk to remove the fee.

Objective: Get the overdraft fee removed from the account.

Relationship: Keep the clerk's good will.

Self-respect: Not lie about what happened; not get too emotional and cry in front of the clerk.

In a very serious financial situation, getting the objective may be most important.

Example:

Situation: A friend asks Tony to engage in an illegal activity with him or her.

Objective: Not do anything illegal.

Relationship: Keep a good relationship with the friend.

Self-respect: Not go against Tony's values.

If engaging in activity could lead to legal trouble, getting the objective may be most important.

Example:

Situation: Sharon's boss asks her to stay overtime and finish a project.

Objective: Go home and relax.

Relationship: Keep a good relationship with the boss.

Self-respect: Balance self-care with doing the job well.

If the boss does not overdo these types of requests, keeping the relationship may be most important.

Example:

Situation: Sharon's boss asks her to stay overtime and finish a project.

Objective: Go to her child's piano recital right after work.

Relationship: Keep a good relationship with the boss.

Self-respect: Balance self-care with doing the job well.

Even if the boss does not overdo these types of requests, going to the piano recital may be most important.

Example:

Situation: Jim's younger sister asks him to cover for her and tell their parents she spent the night at Jim's place, which is not true.

Objective: Keep his sister out of trouble.

Relationship: Maintain a good relationship with his sister.

Self-respect: Not violate his moral code of not lying.

If lying is not a large violation of Jim's moral code, the objective may be most important. If it is, self-respect may be most important.

Example:

Situation: Juanita gets into a controversy with her partner about a political issue.

Objective: Voice her opinion and have it taken seriously.

Relationship: Maintain a good relationship with her partner.

Self-respect: Stand up for what she believes.

Self-respect may be most important.

Practice Exercises: Ask participants to generate areas where they need to ask for something or say no to something. Work with participants in describing objectives, relationship issues, and self-respect issues. Discuss variations of which would be most important.

V. OBJECTIVES EFFECTIVENESS SKILLS: DEAR MAN (INTERPERSONAL EFFECTIVENESS HANDOUTS 5–5A)

Main Point: Objectives effectiveness skills help us to be as effective as possible in achieving our objectives or goals. The term DEAR MAN is a way to remember these skills.

Interpersonal Effectiveness Handout 5: Guidelines for Objectives Effectiveness: Getting What You Want (DEAR MAN). This handout describes the skills to use when a person wants to ask for something, say no, maintain a position or point of view, or achieve some other interpersonal objective. The skills are Describe, Express, Assert, Reinforce, (stay) Mindful, Appear confident, and Negotiate. Teach these didactically rather quickly, and then move to doing role plays.

Interpersonal Effectiveness Handout 5a: Applying DEAR MAN Skills to a Difficult Current Interaction *(Optional).* This handout gives examples of how to handle situations where the other person also has very good interpersonal skills and keeps refusing legitimate requests or keeps asking for what he or she wants even when the first person keeps saying no. Material here can be woven into your teaching or can be given to participants as a take-home to read. Skills described can be practiced if there is time or can be covered in advanced classes.

Interpersonal Effectiveness Worksheet 4: Writing Out Interpersonal Effectiveness Scripts. This is a worksheet for participants who want to figure out what they are going to do and say *before* they practice their interpersonal skills. Review the worksheet with participants and remind them to use the mindfulness "what" skill of describing (Mindfulness Handout 4) when describing the prompting event. Notice that this sheet requires participants to write down their goals for objectives, relationship, and self-respect effectiveness. You might want to review these definitions, as well as one or two examples, when you review this sheet. For this lesson on DEAR MAN skills, tell participants to fill out the worksheet through Step 6 (or as far as you have taught).

Interpersonal Effectiveness Worksheet 5: Tracking Interpersonal Effectiveness Skills Use. This is a general worksheet for tracking use of interpersonal effectiveness skills. Like Worksheet 3, it requires describing the prompting event and figuring out and writing down interpersonal priorities. It also asks about conflicts in priorities. (This part does not need to be filled out if there were no conflicts.) Next, participants describe what they actually said and did in the situation. The check lines are included on the sheet as a reminder of what the skills actually are, and to cue the participants both in practice and in writing down. Finally, the worksheet asks how the interaction went. Here you want the participants to say

> whether they actually got their objectives met and what effects the interaction had on the relationship and their own self-respect.

A. What Is Objectives Effectiveness?

Say to participants: "Objectives effectiveness refers to attaining your objective or specific goal in a particular situation. The objective is ordinarily the reason for the interaction in the first place. These skills are really the same thing as assertiveness skills. Several types of situations call for objectives effectiveness or assertiveness."

- ■ "Getting others to do what you ask them to do."
- ■ "Saying no to unwanted requests and making it stick."
- ■ "Resolving interpersonal conflict or making changes in relationships."
- ■ "Getting your rights respected."
- ■ "Getting your opinion or point of view taken seriously."

✓ ## B. The DEAR MAN Skills

Tell participants: "You can remember these skills with the term DEAR MAN.[4] This stands for <u>De</u>scribe, <u>E</u>xpress, <u>A</u>ssert, <u>R</u>einforce, (stay) <u>M</u>indful, <u>A</u>ppear confident, <u>N</u>egotiate."

✓ ### 1. *Describe the Situation*

Instruct clients: "When necessary, begin by briefly describing the situation you are reacting to. Stick to the facts. No judgmental statements. Be objective."

Why describe? Beginning an assertion by reviewing facts can be useful for a number of reasons. First, it ensures that the other person is oriented to the events leading to the request, refusal, opinion, or point of view. Also, sticking to objective facts helps the two parties get on the same page and begin a pattern of agreeing. Finally, if the other person is not in agreement on the basic facts of the situation, it gives the participant a fair warning that the assertion might not be well received or successful.

Remind participants that describing here is just like using the mindfulness skill of describing. When there is conflict or fear that the other person will disagree with a participant's version of events, describing accurately can be very difficult. To help participants get the idea of describing observable facts, have them consider what a third party could have observed, or would agree had occurred. Or participants might consider what could be submitted for evidence in a court.

Example: "I've been working here for 2 years and have not gotten a raise, even though my performance reviews have been very positive."

Example: "This is the third time you've asked this week for a ride home from work."

Example: "I have gone over our budget and our outstanding debts very carefully, to see whether we do or do not have enough money for a vacation."

Example: "I bought this shirt 2 weeks ago, and the receipt says I can return it within 90 days. The clerk refused to take it back, saying it was on sale. But, I have my receipt right here, and it says I can return it."

✓ 👥 **Practice Exercises:** Role-play some of these examples, and elicit feedback from group members on the experience of describing events. Suggest that participants try describing really difficult interpersonal situations (briefly, giving just the facts) or times when they were angry with someone. Be sure to give feedback when participants drift from describing events to describing interpretations as if they were the events. For example, they should only say, "This is the third time you have left the front door unlocked," as a prelude to asking someone to stop leaving the door unlocked if it is indeed the third time.

Note to Leaders: Practice Exercises are essential in teaching interpersonal skills. Once a chunk of material is presented and discussed, move to rehearsal, where the material just learned can be practiced. To get a good situation to practice, elicit examples from participants, dream them up yourself, or use one or more of the examples given below. Rehearsal techniques are as follows:

• *Rapid rehearsal.* Go around the room and have each person briefly rehearse a particular skill. For example, ask participants to describe a problem situation where they want to ask for something. For example, "There are a lot of dishes to wash," as a prelude to asking someone to help wash the dishes. Next, have participants practice going around and expressing feelings or opinions about a situation (either the one practiced for describing or a new one), and likewise for asserting (by asking for something or refusing directly) and for reinforcing. You can have everyone practice on the same situation (which either you or the participants make up), or have each person use a situation from his or her own life. Practicing on the same situation is usually quicker if time is of the essence. Use this procedure at least once for each individual skill.

• *Role playing with a leader.* One person can rehearse (role-play) a situation with you, the leader, during the session. Usually, this is done when the participant is describing homework and it seems useful to try acting differently in the situation right away. It can also be used when a participant wants (or needs) help with particular types of situations.

• *Role playing with other participants.* Participants can role-play a situation, taking turns playing the person who is asking or saying no and the other person in the situation. Taking the part of the other person can be very important, because it gives participants an idea of what it feels like when someone else uses behavioral skills on them.

• *Dialogue rehearsal.* If a participant simply cannot role-play or refuses to do so, present the situation in story fashion: Ask, "Then what would you say?" Wait for a response, and then say, "OK, then the other person says _____. What would you say next?"

• *Covert rehearsal.* If a participant refuses even dialogue rehearsal, ask him or her to role-play the situation mentally and imagine giving a skilled response. Do a fair amount of prompting to guide the participant's attention and focus.

Do not sacrifice rehearsal in order to present more material. Role playing is often the most difficult procedure for therapists with little experience in behavior therapy; nonetheless, it is essential. (You might try the role-play procedures with your DBT consultation team, or even with a friend, to get some practice.) Role playing can also be hard for participants at first, but with experience it gets easier. At the beginning, you sometimes have to pull or drag them through the practice. The most important thing with a reluctant role player is that you not fall out of role, even if he or she does. Just keep responding to the person as if you are actually in the situation you are rehearsing. Usually this will do the trick, and the person will get back into the role play.

2. <u>E</u>xpress Clearly

Say to participants: "Next, express clearly how you feel or what you believe about the situation. Don't expect the other person to read your mind or know how you feel. For instance, give a brief rationale for a request or for saying no."

Why express? Explain to participants: "By sharing your personal reactions to the situation, you are making it easier for the other person to figure out what you really want from the interaction. This can help alert the other individual to what makes the situation important to you, and can potentially draw personal interest to your situation. This can make you feel vulnerable at times, but it also has the advantage of providing important information to the other person."

Example: "I believe that I deserve a raise."

Example: "I'm getting home so late that it is really hard for me and my family."

Example: "I am very worried about our current finances."

Example: "I believe that I have a right to return this, and I am distressed that your clerk would refuse to take it back, particularly because there is no damage to it and I have the receipt."

✓ **Practice Exercises:** Role-play some examples, and elicit feedback from group members on the experience of hearing expressions of feelings. This can help clarify the value of expressing genuine thoughts and feelings.

✓ Note that the <u>D</u>escribe and <u>E</u>xpress skills are not always necessary. For example, a person might simply ask a family member going to the grocery store to get some orange juice (without saying, "We're out and I'd like some"). In a hot, stuffy room, the person could ask someone else to open a window (without necessarily saying, "The room is stuffy and I'm feeling hot"). In saying no to a request, the person might simply say, "No, I can't do it." Every participant, however, should learn and practice each of the skills, even if not all of them are always needed.

3. *Assert Wishes*

Tell participants, "The third DEAR MAN skill is to ask for what you want. Say no clearly. Don't expect people to know what you want them to do if you don't tell them. Don't beat around the bush, never really asking or saying no. Don't tell them what they *should* do. Be clear, concise, and assertive. Bite the bullet and ask or say no."

Example: "I would like a raise. Can you give it to me?"

Example: "I have to say no tonight. I just can't give you a ride home so often."

Example: "We simply do not have the money for the vacation we planned for this year."

✓ *Example:* "Will you accept a return on the shirt?"

✓ #### a. **Expressing Is Not Asserting**

Many individuals feel very uncomfortable with asking an assertive question, and will need practice and simple feedback on whether or not they are actually asking a question (often confusing <u>E</u>xpress with <u>A</u>ssert).

b. **Asking versus Demanding**

Some individuals feel very strongly that asking for things is weak, and that in many instances they should not have to ask for what they want, as others should be told or know what to do and do it. There are two points to make here.

- First, orient them to the difference between assertiveness and aggressiveness. When people get their way by demanding and not giving the other person any say in the outcome, this is controlling, is potentially hostile, and tends to damage relationships. The group might give feedback on who wishes to be spoken to that way.
- Second, if a person tells someone what to do (rather than asking the person to do something), but does not request feedback on whether or not he or she will do it (i.e., with a question such as "Will you do that for me?"), then by the end of the interaction the person will not be certain whether or not the goal has been reached. Has the other person committed to, agreed upon, or accepted anything?

✓ **Practice Exercise:** Role-play the "demanding/telling" versus the "asking" strategies with participants, asking for feedback on strength of assertiveness (such as on a scale from 0 to 10).

✓ **Practice Exercise:** Role-play some examples, and ask each group member to role-play making one request to the person sitting next to him or her. Go all around the circle. Afterward, have participants discuss how it felt to be assertive, as well as how it felt to be asked. Give feedback to participants if they ask in a harsh or demanding way.

4. _Reinforce_

Say to participants: "The fourth DEAR MAN skill is to reinforce the other person. That is, identify something positive or rewarding that would happen for the other person if he or she gives the response you want. This can involve taking time to consider the other person's perspective and motivation, and drawing connections between what you're asking for and what the person wants or needs. Alternatively, you could offer to do something for the other person, if the other does this thing for you. At a minimum, express appreciation after anyone does something consistent with your request."

The basic idea here is that people are motivated by gaining positive consequences (and by avoiding negative consequences). Explain to participants: "Linking your request to consequences that other people desire will make them more likely to agree. Also, if other people do not gain at least some of the time from complying with a request, taking no for an answer, or listening to your opinions, then they may stop responding in a positive way."

Example: "I will be a lot happier and probably more productive if I get a salary that reflects my value to the company."

Example: "I would really appreciate it if you would accept that I can't always give you rides home."

Example: "I think we will both sleep better if we stay within our budget."

Example: "My hope is that we can work this out, so that I can continue shopping in this store and encouraging my friends to do likewise."

💭 **Discussion Point:** The notion of behaviors' being controlled by consequences, instead of by concepts of "good" and "bad" or "right" and "wrong," can be particularly difficult for some participants to grasp. Discuss this idea with participants.

Emphasize to clients that "carrots" are more effective than "sticks." That is, motivating with positive consequences (carrots) tends to be more effective than punishments (sticks) not only for maintaining positive relationships, but also for getting people actually to follow through with desired behaviors once the punishment is past. Although identifying positive consequences often takes more effort, it tends to pay off in effectiveness. However, when a request is extremely important and there are either no options for positive consequences or they have not worked, it may be necessary to motivate by introducing a negative consequence.

> **Note to Leaders:** If you plan to teach the behavior change strategies of reinforcement, punishment, and extinction (see Section XVII of this chapter and Interpersonal Effectiveness Handouts 20–22), or have already taught them, you can reference the first two here. Extinction can be referenced later when you review the broken record and ignoring attacks (see below).

5. _(Stay) Mindful_

Tell participants: "The next DEAR MAN skill is to stay mindful of your objectives in the situation. Maintain your position and avoid being distracted onto another topic. There are two useful techniques here."

a. The "Broken Record"

Instruct clients: "The first technique is to act like a skipping record on a turntable. That is, keep asking, saying no, or expressing your opinion over and over and over. This can include starting the DEAR script again from the top, or from any part that seems to make the most sense. Keep saying the exact same thing. The idea is that you don't have to think up something different to say each time. The key is to keep a mellow voice tone—'kill them with kindness,' so to speak. The strength is in the persistence of maintaining the position."

Go around and practice this with each person. This is perhaps one of the most important objectives effectiveness skills. Participants can usually learn it without much trouble, because it is easy to do and remember.

b. Ignoring Attacks and Diversions

Tell participants: "The second technique is that if another person attacks, threatens, or tries to change the subject, ignore their threats, comments, or attempts to divert you. Just keep making your point and don't take the bait."

If participants object to this (and many will), continue: "Paying attention to attacks gives the other person control. When you respond to an attack, you often lose track of your objective—and when that happens, the other person has taken control of the conversation. Also, if you pay attention to attacks, respond to them in any way, or let them divert you in the slightest, then you are reinforcing the attacks and diversions—which means that they are likely to occur more often. If you want to respond to the attacks, that is another issue and can be dealt with at another time or after this discussion is finished."

Example: Here is an instance of giving the other person control:

REQUESTER: Would you give me the money you owe me?

OTHER: You are such a jerk for bringing up the fact that I owe you money when you know I don't have much money.

REQUESTER: I'm not a jerk for wanting my money back.

OTHER: Yes, you are. You went and told my wife that I owe you money and that I am 3 months late in paying you back.

REQUESTER: No, I did not tell her that. Who told you that? [And on and on and on.]

Check to be sure that participants see that this is an example of getting off track.

💬 **Discussion Point:** Once participants get the hang of this skill, it can be quite fun to use. Elicit feedback on this point from participants, paying special attention to their belief that they have to respond to every criticism or attack made by another.

Note to Leaders: Be sure to practice both ignoring attacks and the "broken record" with all participants. Used together, these two strategies constitute a very effective skill for maintaining a refusal or putting pressure on someone to comply with a request. When the other person attacks, a participant should simply replay the "broken record." It is extremely difficult to keep attacking or criticizing a person who doesn't respond or "play the game." But being a broken record and ignoring diversions are a lot harder than they look. The only way for participants to get the hang of these skills is to practice. Also, it can be a nice idea to have participants practice with each other, to see what having their own attacks and diversion strategies ignored or having another person keep repeating a request, opinion, or refusal feels like. The key to both the "broken record" and ignoring attacks is to keep hostility out of the voice while keeping on track.

✓ ### 6. *Appear Confident*

Encourage clients: "Use a confident voice tone, and display a confident physical manner and posture, with appropriate eye contact. Such a manner conveys to both the other person and yourself that you are efficacious and deserve respect for what you want. No stammering, whispering, staring at the floor, retreating, saying you're not sure, or the like."

✓ 💬 **Discussion Point:** Note that the skill is "<u>A</u>ppear confident," not "<u>B</u>e confident." Note that it is perfectly reasonable to be nervous or scared during a difficult conversation; however, acting nervous or scared will interfere with effectiveness. Elicit examples from participants about situations where it may be important to appear confident even when they are not.

💬 **Discussion Point:** How confident to act in a given situation is a judgment call. A person needs to walk a fine line between appearing arrogant and appearing too apologetic. Elicit examples from participants.

✓ *7. Negotiate*

Say to participants: "The final DEAR MAN skill is negotiation. Be willing to give to get. Offer and ask for alternative solutions to the problem. Reduce your request. Maintain your no, but offer to do something else or solve the problem another way."

Continue: "An alternative technique is to 'turn the tables'—that is, to turn the problem over to the other person. Ask for alternative solutions."

Example: "What do you think we should do? I'm not able to say yes, and you really seem to want me to. What can we do here? How can we solve this problem?"

💬 **Discussion Point:** Negotiating or turning the tables is useful when ordinary requesting or refusing is going nowhere. There are many variations on the negotiating strategy. Get participants to discuss any time they have negotiated or turned the tables.

C. Applying DEAR MAN Skills to a Difficult Current Interaction

To turn around a really difficult situation, a person can focus the skills on the other person's behavior right now. See Interpersonal Effectiveness Handout 5a for examples of effective and ineffective scripts for the following four steps.

1. Describe the Current Interaction

Tell participants: "If the 'broken record' and ignoring don't work, make a statement about what is happening between you and the other person now, but without imputing the person's motives."

2. Express Feelings or Opinions about the Interaction

Say: "For instance, in the middle of an interaction that is not going well, you can express your feelings of discomfort in the situation."

3. Assert Wishes in the Situation

Say: "When a person is refusing your request, you can suggest that you put the conversation off until another time. Give the other person a chance to think about it. When another person is pestering you, you ask him or her politely to stop it."

4. Reinforce

Say: "When you are saying no to someone who keeps asking, or when someone won't take your opinion seriously, suggest ending the conversation, since you aren't going to change your mind anyway."

👥 **Practice Exercise:** Using Interpersonal Effectiveness Handout 5a, go around the room and have one person read an example of an effective statement, and the next person read one of the ineffective statements. Keep going until everyone has had a chance to read a statement. Discuss the difference in emotional responses to both types of statements.

✓ **D. Elicit and Review Ideas for Practicing DEAR MAN Skills**

An essential component of interpersonal skills training is behavioral rehearsal, both in sessions and between sessions as homework. It is important to discuss situations where DEAR MAN skills can be used.

1. Use the Skills If a Situation Arises

Emphasize that participants are to try to use their skills when a situation occurs between sessions where they can ask for something or say no.

2. Actively Search for Practice Situations

Say to participants: "If nothing arises in daily life to provide an opportunity to practice, it is important to dream up situations where you can practice. That is, do not just wait for a situation to arise where you can practice. Actively search out situations." If no situations arise naturally, suggest creating opportunities to practice. The practice ideas listed below are examples of ones participants can create for practice.

💬 **Discussion Point:** Elicit from participants what DEAR MAN skills they are willing to practice during the week. Describe items below if participants have difficulty coming up with something. Discuss any objections to doing DEAR MAN. Be flexible here. Remember your principles of shaping. (See Chapter 10 of the main DBT text.)

3. Practice Ideas

- "Go to a library and ask for assistance in finding a book." (Variation: "Go to a store and ask the salesperson to help you find something.")
- "While you are talking with someone, change the subject."
- "Invite a friend to dinner (at your house or at a restaurant)."
- "Ask a waiter/waitress at a restaurant a question about your bill."
- "Take old books to a used-book store and ask how much they are worth."
- "Pay for something costing less than $1.00 with a $5.00 bill, and ask for change."
- "Ask for special 'fixings' on a sandwich at a fast-food restaurant." (A variation of this is to ask for a substitution on the menu when ordering a meal.)
- "Ask a store manager to order something you would like to buy that is not usually carried by the store."
- "Ask coworkers or classmates to do a favor for you (such as fix you a cup of coffee while they are fixing their own, let you look at their notes, or lend you their textbook)."
- "Ask someone you know for a ride home."
- "Disagree with someone's opinion."
- "Ask a parent, spouse, partner, or child to accept more responsibility in a specific area."
- "Ask a friend for help in fixing something."
- "Ask a person to stop doing something that bothers you."
- "Ask somebody you don't know well what time it is."

VI. RELATIONSHIP EFFECTIVENESS SKILLS: GIVE (INTERPERSONAL EFFECTIVENESS HANDOUTS 6–6A)

> **Main Point:** Relationship effectiveness skills are aimed at maintaining or improving our relationship with another person while we try to get what we want in the interaction. The term GIVE is a way to remember these skills.
>
> **Interpersonal Effectiveness Handout 6: Guidelines for Relationship Effectiveness: Keeping the Relationship.** This handout describes the GIVE skills: (be) Gentle, (act) Interested, Validate, (use an) Easy

manner. Quickly teach these skills didactically, and then, as with the objectives effectiveness skills, move to doing role plays.

Interpersonal Effectiveness Handout 6a: Expanding the V in GIVE: Levels of Validation *(Optional)*. This material lists six different ways to validate (the V in GIVE). It can be covered with or without using the handout. A fuller description of these steps in validation is provided in the later discussion of walking the middle path for interpersonal effectiveness (see Section XVI of this chapter, and Interpersonal Effectiveness Handouts 17 and 18).

Interpersonal Effectiveness Worksheet 4: Writing Out Interpersonal Effectiveness Scripts; Interpersonal Effectiveness Worksheet 5: Tracking Interpersonal Effectiveness Skills Use. These worksheets are the same as those used for the DEAR MAN skills. Instructions for their use can be found at the start of Section V, above.

✓ **A. What Is Relationship Effectiveness?**

Tell participants: "Relationship effectiveness refers to improving or maintaining a good relationship with the other person in an interaction, while at the same time trying to obtain your objective."

✓ "When improving a relationship is the main objective, interpersonal effectiveness focuses on *how* you go about trying to improve the relationship. For instance, is your voice gentle and respectful, or are you angry and yelling? Do you ask, or do you demand? Do you listen to the other person, or do you cut this person off?"

Example: "If you cry and throw a tantrum every time your best friends forget your birthday, you will surely get them to remember your birthday in the future, but they may remember it with bitterness instead of love and affection. A more effective approach might be gently reminding them a few days ahead of time, or asking them with an easy manner to put your birthday in their calendar so they remember it."

Emphasize that relationship effectiveness is always needed in any interaction. Participants will sometimes insist that they have no relationship goal in certain interactions—for example, when dealing with a store clerk they never intend to see again, or when breaking up with a significant other. You can generally dispel this idea by asking them to imagine two scenarios. In the first one, the objective goal is met (e.g., a participant's significant other understands that the relationship is over), but the interaction is not relationship-effective (e.g., the significant other leaves wishing that the participant would drop dead). In the second scenario, the objective goal is met, and this time the interaction is relationship-effective (e.g., the significant other leaves thinking that the participant has handled this very respectfully, and wishing the best for the participant). Ask: All things being equal, which scenario would group members prefer? The presence of a relationship goal becomes obvious. It is simply a lower priority.

✓ **B. The GIVE Skills**

Say to participants: "You can remember these skills with the term GIVE. This stands for (be) Gentle, (act) Interested, Validate, and (use an) Easy manner."

✓ **1. (Be) Gentle**

Tell clients: "Being gentle means being nice and respectful in your approach. People tend to respond to gentleness more than they do to harshness." Clarify that gentleness specifically means four things: no attacks, no threats, no judging, and no disrespect.

a. **No Attacks**

Begin by saying: "People won't like you if you threaten them, attack them, or express much anger directly."

b. **No Threats**

Continue: "Don't make 'manipulative' statements or hidden threats. Don't say, 'I'll kill myself if you . . . ' Tolerate a 'no' to requests. Stay in the discussion even if it gets painful. Exit gracefully."

Emphasize that attacks and threats have limited effectiveness: "When you use punishment, threats, or aggression to get what you want, people may do what you want while you are around them. But when you are not around them, or when you cannot see or monitor what they are doing, they will be unlikely to do what you want."

Example: A customer service agent at an airport may be very courteous to a person yelling and screaming about a missed flight. But the same agent may surreptitiously keep this person off the next flight to his or her destination.

> **Note to Leaders:** This point concerning threats may be very sensitive with some participants. I usually present it as if it is not sensitive, and then ask whether anyone has made threats or been accused of making threats. The idea is to normalize the interpersonal behavior (making threats, "manipulating") that some may have been accused of by others. Acknowledge how hard it is to stop such behavior.

Usually this question will come up: "What does and doesn't sound like a threat?" More specifically, participants may ask how a person can communicate a desire to leave a relationship or situation, to quit something because it is too hard (e.g., a job or school), or to express an extreme wish (e.g., to commit suicide, beat up a child, or get a divorce) in such a way that others do not take it as a threat. This is a good question. Generally, the best way is for the person to couple the communication with a statement of wanting to work on the relationship or job, or not wanting to commit suicide or file for a divorce.

Say to participants: "The idea is to make it sound as if you are taking responsibility for the situation, even if you did not cause it, rather than making it the other person's responsibility. When others feel you are making them responsible, they usually say that you are threatening or manipulating them. In general, if you say that you are going to kill or harm yourself, use drugs, hit the children, start smoking again, or go off your diet, but at the same time say that you want help or that you know you can control yourself, it is not a threat. But it is a threat to say you are going to do these things if others do not change what they are doing. It is a threat to say or even imply that you are going to commit suicide, harm yourself, or use drugs if someone else doesn't come through for you, do what you want, cure you, or make things better."

Another option is for participants to share dysfunctional desires by *mindfully describing* the urges, as opposed to voicing the urges directly. For example, the statement "My urges for suicide are getting high," or "I'm noticing a strong urge to use alcohol," will generally sound less threatening than "I want to kill myself," or "I'm going to a liquor store."

✓ c. **No Judging**

Continue: "The third part of gentleness is no judging. That means no name calling, 'shoulds,' or implied put-downs in voice or manner. No guilt trips."

💬 **Discussion Point:** The injunction not to judge is woven throughout all of the skills. But it is so important that it is emphasized here as a separate skill. Elicit from participants times when they have felt judged by others. Try a role play to help them see what it feels like to be judged.

✓   **d. No Disrespect**

Say: "The last part of gentleness is no disrespect. That means no sneering, expressing contempt or scorn, or walking out on conversations. Also, again, it means no put-downs."

💬 **Discussion Point:** Elicit times when participants have used skillful words, but have communicated nonverbally that they have no respect for the other's opinion or request. What does it feel like? Remember, people almost always pay attention to nonverbal communication over the words used. When have you done the same thing? Discuss.

✓   **2. (Act) Interested**

Say to participants: "The second GIVE skill is to be interested in the other person. Listen to the other person's point of view, opinion, reasons for saying no, or reasons for making a request of you. Don't interrupt or try to talk over the other person. Don't mind-read thoughts or intentions without checking them out. Don't assume that your ideas about what is going on inside the other's mind are correct, especially if you think the other person is being intentionally hostile, hurtful, rejecting, or simply uncaring. If you have a concern about what the other person is thinking or is motivated by, gently ask, and listen to the answer. Be sensitive to the other person's desire to have the discussion at a later time, if that's what the person wants. Be patient." (Note that this is Level 1 validation on Interpersonal Effectiveness Handout 6a.)

    a. People Respond Well to Interest

Tell participants: "People will feel better about you if you seem interested in them and you give them time and space to respond to you."

    b. The Skill Is "Act" Interested, Not "Be" Interested

Continue: "There are times when you may want for someone to have a positive experience interacting with you, and you are not actually interested in what they want to talk about. Choosing to listen means deliberately choosing to be effective in achieving your goal of helping them have a positive experience interacting with you."

💬 **Discussion Point:** Elicit examples from participants.

✓ 👥 **Practice Exercise:** Divide participants into pairs. (If necessary, pair one client with one of your leaders.) Instruct participants that when you indicate "Start," one person should start talking to his or her partner about any topic, and the partner should listen intently, nod occasionally, and in general appear very interested. After several minutes when you indicate "Switch," the talker should continue talking on the topic, but the partner should look as uninterested as possible (e.g., file nails, look around, pick up things to read, go through his or her wallet or purse). After several minutes, stop and then do it again, this time with the listening partner now doing the talking. Discuss how difficult it was to keep talking or even stay organized on the topic once no one was listening.

> **Note to Leaders:** This exercise is a very effective way to demonstrate the negative effects of discounting or invalidating another person. Many participants also want to discuss how often this happened, or is still happening, to them in their lives. The main point is that no matter what has happened to them, it is not effective to turn around and do the same to others. You can also note that when they feel ignored, participants can apply objectives effectiveness skills to get others to change such behaviors.

💬 **Discussion Point:** Some people find it very easy to be quiet and listen to others. But other people find it very hard. Such a participant may have a racing mind and may always be a step or two ahead of the person talking, or may have an impulsive tongue that just seems to start talking on its own. Discuss.

3. *Validate*

Say to participants: "The third GIVE skill is validation. This means communicating that the other person's feelings, thoughts, and actions are understandable to you, given his or her past or current situation." (Note that this is actually an example of Level 2 validation on Interpersonal Effectiveness Handout 6a.)

a. Validate the *Why* Even While Disagreeing with the What

Note that we can validate a reason why a person is feeling, thinking, or doing something, without agreeing with what they are actually thinking or doing.

Example: We can say, "I know that you feel you have to yell at me, because if you don't you will keep things inside of yourself and never get what you want. At the same time, I don't like it at all, and I really want you to stop yelling and try just telling me what you want me to do."

✓

b. Validate with Words

Continue: "Acknowledge with words the other person's feelings, wants, difficulties, and opinions about the situation, without judgmental words, voice tone, facial expression or posture."

Story Point: Tell the following story or one like it.

"Johnny is sitting in class, trying to pay attention, and he accidentally knocks his notebook off his desk, making a loud noise on the floor. The peers next to him chuckle. The teacher stops in her tracks and says, 'There you go again, John, disrupting the class, trying to get attention. . . . I am really getting tired of this behavior!' Johnny feels extremely embarrassed, hurt, and angry, since he'd been making a true effort to focus and behave more skillfully. He later goes home and recounts the story to his mother, who replies, 'Why do you keep doing this to yourself? You're never going to get into college at this rate. You'd better shape up!'"[1]

Discussion Point: Ask participants what they think Johnny must have felt after his teacher's and mother's responses. Why were these responses so hurtful? What was missing from their responses?[1]

c. Read and Validate the Other's Nonverbal Signals

Say to participants: "Validating often requires you to read and interpret the other person's nonverbal signals, such as facial expression and body language. These are clues to figuring out what problems the person might be having with your request or your saying no. Acknowledge those feelings or problems. For example, you can say, 'I know that you are very busy,' 'I can see that this is really important to you,' 'I know this will take you out of your way a bit,' or something like that." (Note that this is an example of Level 3 validation on Interpersonal Effectiveness Handout 6a.)

Continue: "In addition, notice and validate when other people are right about what they are saying, when their behavior fits the facts of the situation, or when they are making a lot of sense given the current facts." (Note that this is an example of Level 5 validation on Interpersonal Effectiveness Handout 6a.)

Example: "You are demanding that a person return something you loaned him or her. The person reminds you that he or she already gave it back. Drop your defensiveness and admit you were wrong when you remember that the other person is correct."

d. Actions Speak Louder Than Words

Explain to participants: "Validating with words can sometimes be invalidating. This is true when the situation calls for action but we only validate with words. It is important to validate with action when the situation calls for it and you believe another's request is indeed valid." (Note that this is an example of Level 5 validation on Interpersonal Effectiveness Handout 6a.) You can give these two examples of ineffective validation with words only:

Example: "You are returning a shirt you bought, but you don't have your receipt. The store clerk asks you to follow him to go and talk with his supervisor. You say, 'I understand that we will need to talk with the supervisor,' but you don't make a move to follow the clerk."

Example: "You are screaming out the window in a fire, 'Help me, help me, it's hot in here,' and the firefighter yells up, 'I see that you are hot,' instead of climbing up right away to get you out."

Practice Exercise: Ask a participant to come stand near you. Then put your foot on the participant's foot. Ask the participant to tell you when it starts to hurt. As soon as he or she says something, keep your foot pressure at that level and say, "I can see that this hurts your foot." Repeat several times. Discuss.

Emphasize that **validating others is effective for improving relationships any time**: "A conflict situation does not have to arise; you don't need to make a request of someone or want to say no to validate another's feelings, thoughts, or actions."

> **Note to Leaders:** For a fuller understanding of validation see notes associated with handouts 17–18. You can also read a chapter I wrote that describes validation in great detail.[3]

4. (Use an) Easy Manner

Tell participants: "The final GIVE skill is an easy manner. That is, try to be lighthearted. Use a little humor. Smile. Ease the other person along. Wheedle. Soothe. This is the difference between the 'soft sell' and the 'hard sell.' Be political."

Discussion Point: Elicit from participants conversations they have had where the tension was so thick it could be cut with a knife; the moments seemed to drag on and on; or it felt like walking near a land mine, where any wrong step could lead to an explosion. Using an easy manner helps create a comfortable atmosphere in such situations. It helps to convey the message that the conversation is safe and that the other person can be relaxed, without worrying too much. Discuss.

Emphasize to participants: "Get people to like giving you what you want. People don't like to be bullied, pushed, or made to feel guilty." Although some participants may have been called manipulators by others, a really good manipulator makes other people like giving in. The premise in DBT is that individuals need to learn to be better at inducing others to do what they want them to do, while at the same time getting the others to like doing it.

VII. SELF-RESPECT EFFECTIVENESS SKILLS: FAST (INTERPERSONAL EFFECTIVENESS HANDOUT 7)

> **Main Point:** Self-respect effectiveness skills help us to keep or improve our self-respect, while at the same time we try to get what we want in an interaction. The term FAST is a way to remember these skills.
>
> **Interpersonal Effectiveness Handout 7: Guidelines for Self-Respect Effectiveness: Keeping Respect for Yourself.** This handout describes the self-respect effectiveness skills: (be) Fair, (no) Apologies, Stick to values, (be) Truthful. As with the DEAR MAN and GIVE skills, teach these didactically rather quickly, and then move to doing role plays.

> **Interpersonal Effectiveness Worksheet 4: Writing Out Interpersonal Effectiveness Scripts; Interpersonal Effectiveness Worksheet 5: Tracking Interpersonal Effectiveness Skills.** These worksheets are the same as those used for the DEAR MAN and GIVE skills. Instructions for their use can be found at the start of Section V, above.
>
> **Interpersonal Effectiveness Worksheet 13: Self-Validation and Self-Respect** *(Optional)*. This might be a good worksheet to use when interpersonal effectiveness skills fail and self-validation is needed. The worksheet can be used in conjunction with Handout 7 (see above), as well as with Interpersonal Effectiveness Handout 17: Validation.

✓ A. What Is Self-Respect Effectiveness?

Say to participants: "Self-respect effectiveness refers to acting in a manner that maintains or increases your self-respect after an interpersonal interaction. *How* you go about attempting to obtain your objectives requires self-respect effectiveness skills. The key question here is how to ask for what you want or say no to a request in such a way that you will still respect yourself afterward."

Example: Some people lose respect for themselves if they cry and/or get extremely emotional during an interpersonal interaction. Others lose self-respect if they give in and act passively, rather than sticking up for themselves. Still others lose respect for themselves if they get extremely angry, mean, or threatening.

Ask: "Do you stand up for your peer group's values or your own values? Do you put on a tough attitude to avoid humiliating yourself, but at the same time lose self-respect by being mean and tough? Do you lie or tell the truth? Do you act competent or incompetent?"

Emphasize that **self-respect effectiveness is always needed in any interaction**. The usual problem here is that on the one hand, participants have not considered how to keep their own self-respect, or, on the other hand, they have focused on it to the extreme. The goal here is to identify the skills needed to keep self-respect while not forgetting the mindfulness "how" skill of effectiveness (see Mindfulness Handout 5). Tell participants: "Giving up getting your objective in favor of doing what you believe is necessary to keep your self-respect is not always the best decision."

✓ B. The FAST Skills

Say to participants: "You can remember these skills with the term FAST. This stands for (be) Fair, (no) Apologies, Stick to values, (be) Truthful."

✓ 1. (Be) Fair

Tell participants: "The first FAST skill is to be fair to yourself and the other person in your attempts to get what you want. It is hard to like yourself over the long haul if you consistently take advantage of other people. You may get what you want, but at the risk of your ability to respect yourself."

Continue: "Validate your own feelings and wishes as well as the other person's. It is also hard to respect yourself if you are always giving in to others' wishes and never sticking up for your own wishes or beliefs."

💬 **Discussion Point:** Some individuals always prioritize others' needs ahead of their own. What impact does this have on self-respect? Discuss with participants.

✓ 2. (No) Apologies

Say to participants: "The next FAST skill is not to overapologize. When apologies are warranted, of course, they are appropriate. But no apologizing for being alive, for making a request, for having an opinion, or for disagreeing. Apologies imply that you are wrong—that you are the one making a mistake. This can reduce your sense of mastery over time."

Explain that **excessive apologies can hurt relationships**. Making an apology can at times enhance a relationship. Excessive apologies, however, often get on other people's nerves and usually reduce both relationship and self-respect effectiveness.

✓ ### 3. _Stick to Values_

Continue: "The third FAST skill is to stick to your own values. Avoid selling out your values or integrity to get your objective or to keep a person liking you. Be clear on what, in your opinion, is the moral or valued way of thinking and acting, and hold on to your position."

💬 **Discussion Point:** When a situation is dire, or lives are at stake, people might choose to give up their values. The problem is that many individuals have black-and-white views on this issue: Either they are willing to sell out everything to get approval and liking (to give up their entire "selves," it seems), or they interpret everything as an issue of values and view flexibility of any sort as giving up their integrity. Elicit examples.

Note to Leaders: This Discussion Point assumes that participants know their own values and are clear about what they believe is moral and immoral. Many individuals, however, have difficulties with one or both of these. For these individuals, it can be helpful to review Emotion Regulation Handout 18: Values and Priorities List.

Note that **values can be at issue in relationships**: "A conflict between what others want you to do and what your own moral code or personal values tell you to do is not uncommon. It is difficult to maintain your self-respect when you give in to others and do or say things you believe to be wrong. It can also be very difficult to stand up for yourself, particularly when your values are not the values of the other people in the relationship. Losing your self-respect in a relationship can lead over time to a corrosion of the relationship. This corrosion, or falling apart, can sometimes be very subtle, but in the end it can destroy a relationship."

💬 **Discussion Point:** Elicit and discuss times when participants have been in a situation where a person or group wants them to do or say something that conflicts with their own moral values. Discuss the difficulties of standing up for oneself. Discuss the consequences of giving in and violating one's own values.

✓ ### 4. _(Be) Truthful_

Tell participants: "The final FAST skill is to be truthful. Don't lie, act helpless when you are not, or exaggerate. A pattern of dishonesty over time erodes your self-respect. Even though one instance may not hurt, or may even occasionally be necessary, dishonesty as your usual mode of getting what you want will be harmful over the long run. Acting helpless is the opposite of building mastery."

💬 **Discussion Point:** At times, being honest may actually reduce relationship effectiveness. The "little white lie" was invented for just this reason. Any attempt to convince participants that honesty is always the best policy will probably fail. Discuss this point with participants. The crucial idea is that if one is going to lie, it should be done mindfully rather than habitually.

Stress that **mastery is the opposite of passivity**. Building mastery requires doing things that are difficult, that involve a challenge. Helplessness is the enemy of mastery. Overcoming obstacles is one route to mastery. Most successful people in this world do not have fewer obstacles; they just get up after falling down more often than unsuccessful people do. Getting up after falling down is mastery. Falling down is irrelevant. The drive to mastery seems to be innate.[5] Small children learning how to walk keep falling down and getting up, falling down and getting up.

Note to Leaders: The concept of mastery here is very similar to the skill of building mastery in emotion regulation (see Emotion Regulation Handouts 14 and 19).

💬 **Discussion Point:** Elicit from participants times when they have done things that reduce their own sense of self-respect. When have they enhanced their sense of self-respect? Where do they need to improve their skills?

✓ **C. Balancing Self-Respect Effectiveness and Objectives Effectiveness**

Make these points to participants in regard to balancing self-respect and objectives effectiveness:

- ◾ "No one can take away your self-respect unless you give it up."
- ◾ "Using DEAR MAN skills can improve your self-respect by increasing your sense of mastery. But using DEAR MAN ineffectively sometimes leads to a loss of self-respect for the other person."
- ◾ "You can also enhance self-respect by giving up things you want for the welfare of the other person."
- ◾ "Balancing what you want and what the other person wants and needs might be the best path to self-respect."

✓ **D. Balancing Self-Respect Effectiveness and Relationship Effectiveness**

Make these points to participants in regard to balancing self-respect and relationship effectiveness:

- ◾ "Using GIVE skills well will probably enhance your sense of self-respect, because most people's sense of self-respect is somewhat dependent on the quality of their relationships."
- ◾ "However, if you frequently use GIVE skills with a person who abuses you or doesn't care about you, your self-respect is likely to erode over time."
- ◾ "Using GIVE skills when they are needed, and putting them away when harshness and boldness are necessary, might be the best path to self-respect."

✓ **VIII. EVALUATING YOUR OPTIONS: HOW INTENSELY TO ASK OR SAY NO (INTERPERSONAL EFFECTIVENESS HANDOUT 8)**

Main Point: It is important to consider whether to ask for something or say no, and how strongly to ask or say no.

Interpersonal Effectiveness Handout 8: Evaluating Options for Whether or How Intensely to Ask or Say No. The first page of this handout can be reviewed rather quickly. "Factors to Consider" should be discussed to be sure that participants understand each point. Getting and giving examples are both important here. Interpersonal Effectiveness Worksheet 6 can also be used to teach this skill either before or after going over the factors to consider in Handout 8.

Interpersonal Effectiveness Worksheet 6: The Dime Game: Figuring Out How Strongly to Ask or Say No. Use this worksheet with participants in class as a way to teach this skill. Bring 10 dimes with you to the class, and extra copies of the worksheet for participants to use as homework practice.

✓ **A. Range of Intensities for Asking and for Saying No**

💬 **Discussion Point:** Draw a vertical line on the board with "Low intensity" at the top (number it 1) and "High intensity" at the bottom (number it 10), like Figure 8.2. Identify low-intensity behaviors (not asking, hinting, asking tentatively, giving in to other's requests, etc.), and high-intensity behaviors (speaking firmly, insisting, resisting, refusing to negotiate, etc.). Go around the room and ask each participant to identify where he or she tends to fall on this continuum, and what the pros and cons are of that approach.

Alternative Discussion Point: Instead of having the discussion described above, review levels of intensity on the first page of Interpersonal Effectiveness Handout 8, and then ask participants to put a checkmark where they usually fall when asking for something and another checkmark when saying no. Then ask participants to put an X where they wish they could be for both. Discuss.

1. Interpersonal Effectiveness Changes as Situations and Timing Change

What works in one situation at one point in time may not work in another situation or in the same situation at another point in time.

Example: "Being pushy may get your 16-year-old child to pick you up from work when you are too tired to take a bus, but may not work when you ask your husband or wife."

Example: "Asking your mother to make you a special meal that she always makes you when you go home may be very effective at one point in your life, but when your mother is in bed dying of cancer, asking may damage your self-respect and sense of morality."

Emphasize that appropriateness is not black or white; **there are levels for asking and saying no.** Being interpersonally effective requires thinking through whether it is appropriate to ask for something or to say no to a request. Contrary to what many people think, the answer is not usually as clear-cut as it is for the example of the mother in bed with cancer. Instead, there are levels of asking and levels of saying no.

2. Analyze Each Situation to Determine How Intensely to Ask or Say No

Tell participants: "Asking and saying no can be very intense and firm, where you try every skill you know to change the situation and get the outcome you want. Asking and saying no can also

Low intensity (let go, give in)

Asking	Saying no
Don't ask; don't hint.	1. Do what the other wants without being asked.
Hint indirectly; take no.	2. Don't complain; do it cheerfully.
Hint openly; take no.	3. Do it, even if you're not cheerful about it.
Ask tentatively; take no.	4. Do it, but show that you'd rather not.
Ask gracefully; but take no.	5. Say you'd rather not, but do it gracefully.
Ask confidently; take no.	6. Say no confidently, but reconsider.
Ask confidently; resist no.	7. Say no confidently; resist saying yes.
Ask firmly; resist no.	8. Say no firmly; resist saying yes.
Ask firmly; insist; negotiate; keep trying.	9. Say no firmly; resist; negotiate; keep trying.
Ask and don't take no for an answer.	10. Don't do it.

High intensity (stay firm)

FIGURE 8.2. Options for whether or how intensely to ask or say no.

be of very low intensity, where you either don't ask or say no, or are very flexible and willing to accept the situation as it is."

✓ B. Factors to Consider

Go over the "Factors to Consider" from Interpersonal Effectiveness Handout 8 with participants.

1. Capability (Your Own or the Other Person's)

Encourage participants: "Increase the intensity of asking if the other person has what you want. Increase the intensity of saying no if you do *not* have (and therefore cannot give or do) what the other person wants."

2. Your Priorities

When an objective is very important, the intensity of asking or saying no should be higher. When getting an objective interferes with a relationship and/or with self-respect, then intensity should be lowered to the degree that the relationship and self-respect are important. Say to participants: "Often relationship issues are such that you may be willing to trade an objective for keeping the other person happy. If so, lower the intensity of the response. If getting an objective requires sacrificing your self-respect, then intensity might need to be lowered."

3. Self-Respect

Say: "Increase the intensity of asking if you usually do things for yourself and are careful to avoid acting helpless. Increase the intensity of saying no if saying no will *not* result in feeling bad about yourself, and if wise mind says no."

4. Rights

Say: "Increase the intensity of asking if the other person is required by law or moral code to give you what you want. Increase the intensity of saying no if you are *not* required by law or morals to give the other person what he or she wants (in other words, saying no would *not* violate the other person's rights)."

5. Authority

Continue: "Increase the intensity of asking if you are responsible for directing the other person or telling him or her what to do. Increase the intensity of saying no if the other person does *not* have authority over you, or if what the person is asking is not within his or her authority."

6. Relationship

Go on: "Increase the intensity of asking if what you want is appropriate to the current relationship. Increase the intensity of saying no if what the other person wants from you is *not* appropriate to the current relationship."

7. Long-Term versus Short-Term Goals

Continue: "Increase the intensity of asking if being submissive will result in peace now but create problems in the long run. Increase the intensity of saying no if giving in will get you short-term peace but *not* a long-term relationship you wish to have."

8. Reciprocity

Say: "Increase the intensity of asking if you have done at least as much for the other person as you are requesting, and you are willing to give if the other person says yes. Increase the intensity of saying no if you do *not* owe the other person a favor, or the other person does *not* usually reciprocate."

9. Homework

Say: "Increase the intensity of asking if you know all the facts necessary to support a request, and both the goal and the request are clear. Increase the intensity of saying no if the other person's request is *not* clear or you are *not* sure of what you would be saying yes to."

10. Timeliness

Tell participants: "Increase the intensity of asking if this is a good time to ask (the other person is in the mood for listening and paying attention; he or she is likely to say yes to a request). Increase the intensity of saying no if this is *not* a bad time for you to say no."

Point out here that **wise mind** can be used as an additional factor in deciding whether to ask or say no and how intensely to push for what one wants. Tell participants to use wise mind to calibrate the importance of other factors described above, and to attend to any factors not included in the list. The more important a factor, the more it should be weighted in the final tally of pros and cons for levels of intensity. In using wise mind as a factor, however, it is important actually to be in wise mind (and not in emotion mind).

✓ **C. Figuring Out How Strongly to Ask or Say No: The Dime Game**

Practice Exercise: Use Interpersonal Effectiveness Worksheet 6 to give participants practice in deciding whether or how strongly to ask for something or say no to a request.

✓　　1. *Ask a participant to give an example of a situation where he or she is trying to decide whether to ask for something or say no to someone.* Be sure to use a real situation, not one made up. Give the participant the 10 dimes you brought to the session. Using that situation, go over the worksheet. Ask each question on the left side if the person is trying to decide whether to ask someone for something. Ask questions on the right side if the person is trying to decide whether to say yes or no to a request. On the left side, have the participant put a dime in the bank for each "yes" answer. On the right side, have him or her put a dime in the bank for each "no" answer.

✓　　2. *On the left side, count the number of "yes" responses.* The participant should then go into wise mind and decide whether one or more "yes" responses should be added or subtracted. If after this adjustment there are more "yes" than "no" responses, then participants should make the request. The more "yes" responses, the stronger the request should be.

✓　　3. *On the right side, count up the number of "no" responses.* The participant should then go into wise mind and decide whether one or more "no" responses should be added or subtracted, and also whether other factors should be considered. If there are more "no" than "yes" responses, then the participants should say no to a request made of him or her. The more "no" responses, the more it makes sense to increase the intensity of saying no to the other person.

　　4. *Ask participants for another situation* where they are having difficulty asking for something or saying no to something. Put the 10 dimes back on the table, and then go through the questions on Worksheet 6 with another participant, following the instructions above. Continue doing this with several participants.

IX. TROUBLESHOOTING INTERPERSONAL EFFECTIVENESS SKILLS (INTERPERSONAL EFFECTIVENESS HANDOUT 9)

> **Main Point:** Difficulty in obtaining an objective can be due to many possible factors. When we can identify the problem, we can often solve it and be more effective at getting what we want.

Interpersonal Effectiveness Handout 9: Troubleshooting: When What You Are Doing Isn't Working. This handout gives questions for diagnosing which factors are reducing interpersonal effectiveness. These are the same factors briefly described on Interpersonal Effectiveness Handout 2. Troubleshooting is best taught by reviewing Worksheet 7 (see below).

Interpersonal Effectiveness Worksheet 7: Troubleshooting Interpersonal Effectiveness Skills. Have participants follow along with the worksheet as you review the material. It may be useful to have participants mark on the worksheet their most common problems as you go through. If you do this, give them extra copies of the worksheet to use as homework.

✓ Tell participants: "When what you are doing isn't working, you can troubleshoot by asking yourself the questions on Interpersonal Effectiveness Handout 9 and Worksheet 7."

✓ A. Lack of Skill

Say to participants: "When you lack the skills, you don't know how to act or speak effectively to obtain your objectives, maintain the relationship, and keep your self-respect."

Many people have simply not been taught the interpersonal skills they need to be interpersonally effective. In this module, the skills are taught, but only a limited amount of time is spent on each skill. A participant may have missed some of the important skills classes, or may have been too shy to do role plays. To be interpersonally effective takes much practice and much role playing. Practice also takes discipline and the overcoming of fear. Some participants may not have practiced enough to get a skill down.

✓ Have participants ask themselves: **"Do I have the skills I need?"** The first step in answering this question is to carefully read over the instructions for each skill tried. If this does not help, the next step is to write out a script and then practice the script with a friend or in front of a mirror. Participants should get some coaching if needed in how to use the skills or in how to select the skill likely to be the most effective.

💬 **Discussion Point:** Elicit from participants interpersonal effectiveness skills they believe they have not learned sufficiently to use in daily life. Discuss whether their problems are due to not learning them in the first place or not practicing them enough to feel confident in using them. Discuss possible solutions to such problems.

Note to Leaders: This is a good time for you to share with participants times you have misused interpersonal skills and how you revised what you were doing to get a better outcome. It is important to encourage both participants and their individual therapists (if they have such therapists) to review and practice skills often, to be sure that the participants are using the skills correctly. It is very easy just to assume this, but the assumption is often incorrect.

✓ B. Unclear Objectives

Tell participants: "Not knowing your objectives in a situation can make it almost impossible to be effective. When you don't know what you want, getting what you want is mostly based on chance."

✓ Have participants ask themselves: ASK: **"Do I know what I want in the interaction?"** If they are not sure, they should fill out a pros-and-cons worksheet (Interpersonal Effectiveness Worksheet 1) comparing different objectives; they can also use emotion regulation skills, including opposite action, to reduce fear and/or shame about asking or saying no.

💬 **Discussion Point:** Elicit from participants times when they were ambivalent about what they really wanted, could not decide on an objective, or did not know what their priorities were in a situation. Discuss the role of fear of conflict or of potential guilt or shame in these situations.

💬 **Discussion Point:** Elicit from participants times when fear and shame have gotten in the way of knowing what they want. When this is the case, it may be very hard to reduce indecision and ambivalence without first reducing anxiety and fear. Similarly, a person may feel ashamed of asking for something or feel too ashamed to say no. As with anxiety and fear, reducing shame may be an essential first step in clarifying goals. Discuss ways of figuring out what is wanted.

✓ **C. Short-Term Goals Interfering with Long-Term Goals**

Explain to participants that at times, impulsively going for short-term goals can interfere with getting what we really want in the long term. This is true when we sacrifice a relationship or our self-respect to get an immediate goal or reduce distress. It can also happen when we consistently give up getting what we want or need in order to avoid conflict and keep others happy in the short term.

✓   Have participants ask themselves: **"Are my short-term goals getting in the way of my long-term goals?"** If they are not sure, they should fill out another copy of Interpersonal Effectiveness Worksheet 1, comparing short-term with long-term goals. Advise them, "Wait until you are not in emotion mind to do this. Try to get in wise mind."

💬 **Discussion Point:** Elicit from participants times when they have let short-term goals trump long-term goals. Discuss the consequences of doing that for themselves, as well as the consequences for the long-term relationship with the other person.

✓ **D. Emotions Getting in the Way of Skills**

Say to participants: "At times, your emotions may be so extreme that you simply cannot get into wise mind in order to figure out what to do and say. Instead of saying something skillful, you make emotional statements that are extreme and ineffective—or you retreat into silence, pout, or leave the interaction, which are also ineffective strategies. Out-of-control sobbing and crying may make it all but impossible to communicate what you want to say. Although tears can often be an effective communication, at other times they can become a vortex of catastrophizing: The more you cry, the more distressed you become; the more you cry, the less you can control what you say and do during interactions. This can also happen with extreme anger or other intense emotions. In these situations, you can be said to fall into a sea of dyscontrol. Reasonable mind does not have a chance to surface and moderate the influence of emotion mind. You may have the skills, but emotions interfere with using your skills."

✓   Have participants ask themselves: **"Am I too upset to use my interpersonal skills?"** Explain to them: "Trying complicated skills when you are at your skills breakdown point can be intensely frustrating and eventually lead you to give up on skills. The problem is that you may be so far into emotion mind that you don't even know you have hit your skills breakdown point. One solution is to practice your most important interpersonal skills over and over when you are *not* in emotion mind. However, even when you have practiced the skills, you are sometimes too overwhelmed with emotion to use them. When this happens, use crisis survival and emotion regulation skills to stop out-of-control unskillful responses and to reduce emotional arousal."

Give participants this list of skills to use when they are upset:

- *The STOP skill* (see Distress Tolerance Handout 4) to keep from saying things they will regret.
- *Opposite action* (see Emotion Regulation Handout 10) to get themselves to use skills they know they need to do but don't want to use.
- *Self-soothing skills* (see Distress Tolerance Handout 8) before an interaction, to get themselves calm enough for the interaction.
- *TIP skills* (see Distress Tolerance Handout 6) to regulate their emotions rapidly. If they can get their emotions regulated, taking a short break before the interpersonal interaction to do so will be well worth it.
- *Mindfulness of current emotions* (see Emotion Regulation Handout 22) to become aware

of their emotions—particularly those that may be interfering with their skills—and then to refocus completely on the present objective.

💬 **Discussion Point:** Elicit from participants emotions that get in their way interpersonally. Make a list on the board. Then elicit skills that could be used both to regulate emotions and to help participants use interpersonal skills more effectively.

✓ E. Worries, Assumptions, and Myths Interfering

Tell participants: "Worries about negative outcomes, and assumptions and myths about the value of expressing your opinions or thoughts, can cause much trouble when you are trying to improve your interpersonal skills. Some beliefs invalidate ever asking for what you want, such as believing that asking for things or saying no is always selfish. Other myths interfere with maintaining relationships, such as believing that people should know what you want without having to ask."

✓   Have participants ask themselves: **"Are worries, assumptions, and myths getting in the way of using interpersonal skills?"** Then advise them: "Try challenging myths and checking the facts when you are worrying and making assumptions. Practicing opposite action *all the way* is a good way to test assumptions and myths about feared negative consequences. It is important when practicing to focus both on your current objectives and on the other person."

💬 **Discussion Point:** Elicit worries, assumptions, and myths that get in the way of skillful behavior. Write some on the board. Get participants to counter myths for each other, and write their revisions on the board. Be sure all participants also write down the revisions in their notes.

💬 **Discussion Point:** Even when worries are true (e.g., maybe the other person *does* become annoyed by the request or says no), they can distract participants from being fully present when asserting themselves, and therefore can decrease effectiveness. Discuss options for managing worries, such as pushing away, turning the mind, and (if necessary) pros and cons of worrying.

✓ F. Environment More Powerful Than Skills

Say to participants: "When you don't reach your objectives, it is helpful to search for ways in which you were not skillful. It is also important to consider the power of the environment, compared to your own power as a person making a request or saying no. For example, in a company beset by financial losses, requests for raises may be denied no matter how skillful you are in asking. If the police arrive at your home with a warrant for your arrest, your refusing to be arrested will probably be met with force. Refusing to pay a bill that you owe may mean dealing with a bill collector. Getting a stubborn spouse or partner to empty the garbage every night may be met with a resistance that no use of skills can overcome."

✓   Have participants ask themselves: **"Are the other people in the interaction so powerful that they don't have to do anything I ask? Do they have the authority to make me do what they want?"** Advise them: "Try problem solving just to be sure. If the objective is important, try to find an ally who is as powerful as or more powerful than the person you are interacting with. If all else fails, practice radical acceptance of not getting what you want, or of having to do what someone else asks you to do."

💬 **Discussion Point:** Discuss how and why some people might resist a request or refuse to accept no from another person, simply because they feel personally threatened by the request or the refusal. Ask participants to discuss possible solutions to such a problem.

💬 **Discussion Point:** Elicit situations where skills didn't work and couldn't be made to work because the other person in an interaction was so powerful that a participant had almost no influence or leverage. Discuss what it would be like to practice radical acceptance in these situations.

💬 **Discussion Point:** Elicit situations where participants were powerful and someone else did something outrageous to get them to do what the other person wanted. What did that feel like?

> **Note to Leaders:** When done intentionally as a means of influence, the use of outrageous behavior (including threats of dire consequences such as suicide, being unable to cope, losing everything, etc.) is rightfully called "manipulation." This can, and at times should, be discussed. However, it must be done carefully. See an extensive discussion of this topic in Chapter 1 of the main DBT text.

X. OVERVIEW: BUILDING RELATIONSHIPS AND ENDING DESTRUCTIVE ONES (INTERPERSONAL EFFECTIVENESS HANDOUT 10)

> **Main Point:** This section of the module teaches supplementary DBT skills for building relationships and trust with other people, as well as for ending relationships that are destructive, hopeless, or unwanted.
>
> **Interpersonal Effectiveness Handout 10: Overview: Building Relationships and Ending Destructive Ones.** This is an overview handout to be reviewed briefly. Stay on it longer if you are using it to review skills already taught. If you are teaching only some of the skills on this handout, consider skipping the overview entirely. Do not teach the material while covering this handout, unless you are skipping the related handouts (Interpersonal Effectiveness Handouts 11 through 13a).
>
> **Worksheet:** None.

✓ A. Finding Friends and Getting Them to Like You

Forming friendships is the first step in reducing interpersonal isolation and loneliness. Covered here are basic principles of finding people and developing friendships—including the principles of proximity and similarity, as well as very basic skills of starting and maintaining a conversation, expressing liking, and joining groups.[6]

✓ B. Mindfulness of Others

Friendships last longer when we are mindful of others. This skill includes observing and paying attention to others, describing what is observed rather than judging it, and participating in the flow of interactions. The skill of mindfulness of others is an extension of the relationship effectiveness skills (GIVE) taught earlier in this module.

✓ C. Ending Destructive, Hopeless, or Unwanted Relationships

Sometimes relationships must be ended. This can be the case when there is little hope of improving a relationship, the relationship is abusive, or it interferes with very important lifetime priorities. These skills focus on how to end such relationships effectively.

XI. SKILLS FOR FINDING POTENTIAL FRIENDS (INTERPERSONAL EFFECTIVENESS HANDOUTS 11–11A)*

> **Main Point:** Finding people and getting them to like us often requires an active effort. It usually does not happen by itself. To be successful, we have to know where and how to look.
>
> **Interpersonal Effectiveness Handout 11: Finding and Getting People to Like You.** This handout reviews skills for how to search for friends, as well as some ideas on how to be effective at finding them.

---

*The skills in this section are adapted from Linehan, M. M., & Egan, K. J. (1985). *Asserting yourself.* New York: Facts on File. Copyright 1985 by Facts on File Publications. Adapted by permission of the authors.

Review each section, and then discuss it before moving to the next section. This handout can be taught didactically or very interactively, depending on time.

Interpersonal Effectiveness Handout 11a: Identifying Skills to Find People and Get Them to Like You (*Optional*). Skip this handout if you do not have extra time, or give it out as homework and then discuss it at the next session. The correct responses are listed below in the teaching notes, as well as at the end of the introduction to this chapter.

Interpersonal Effectiveness Worksheet 8: Finding and Getting People to Like You. Review this worksheet with participants. Remember to remind participants to use the mindfulness "what" skills of describing (see Mindfulness Handout 4) when describing events and what they or others have said or done. This is "practicing mindfulness" when participants are writing down homework practice. The first section of the worksheet asks participants to describe any opportunities they have had to make contact with people, to mix with people like them, to ask questions or give answers, or to join in a group conversation. It is essential here to get participants to think flexibly and "outside the box."

✓ A. Why Find Friends?

Say to participants: "Finding people and getting them to like you is the first step in decreasing isolation and loneliness. It is also important whenever you move to a new location, take a new job, or join a new group."

💬 **Discussion Point:** For some people, making friends is very easy and seemingly effortless. For others, it can take a lot of work and a long time. Some people have lots of friends to do things with; others have only one or two very good friends. Some people have lots of acquaintances but few good friends; others have a few good friends but very few acquaintances. Elicit from participants what types of friends they have and what types of friends would they like to have.

1. Friends Are Essential for Happiness

Many people believe that "needing" friends and relationships means being emotionally dependent, and that they should be able to be happy alone. This belief flies in the face of almost everything we know about human happiness. Although there are indeed some people who are happy with lives of solitude, for most humans all over the world, intimate and supportive relationships with others are an essential aspect of happiness.

✓ 2. All Human Beings Are Lovable by Someone

You will need to counteract the belief of many participants that they are unlovable. The idea, however, is not to engage in cognitive modification to get clients to see their own lovable characteristics. Although this may work sometimes, it often fails if the persons do not believe that they are currently loved (or have ever been loved) or are connected to someone somewhere by love. Thus it is easier to point out that, in essence, all people are indeed lovable by someone. That is, by virtue of inclusion in the human race, participants are lovable. Participants will often try to disprove this by bringing up individuals who have committed horrible crimes (e.g., torture, or murder followed by cannibalism). Point out how after these people are put in prison for life without parole, some woman or man on the outside will very often correspond with them and fall in love with them.

✓ B. Proximity Favors Friendship[7]

Say to participants: "A first step in forming new relationships is to find opportunities to make casual but regular contact with people in your everyday environment. There are many ways to do this. If you share an office with a lot of people, turn your desk to face the middle of the room instead of the wall. Use elevators or the coffee machine when lots of other people are also there. Go to parties when invited; stay after activities for a while to chat with others; gravitate to where other people are. Given a choice of a class, job, or housing, you can opt for more or fewer opportunities to make contact with others. Mundane as it sounds, a lot of people find many of their friends among class-mates, members of groups or churches they join, and work colleagues. Online dating sites may be good for finding romantic partners, but they may not be as useful for finding nonromantic friends. That said, there are many other online opportunities to find potential friends. For example, a hiker can go online to find hiking partners; a music buff can go online to find other people who like the same music."

We make friends with people we see most often. Researchers at the University of Leipzig found that students were more likely to become friends with people sitting next to them than to others in a class, even when they were randomly assigned to their seats in the classroom.[8] There is now a large body of research that adds weight to these findings. It does not seem to matter why people are brought together; in one study, it was because their names began with the same letter of the alphabet.[9]

✓ **C. Similarity Tends to Increase Liking**

Tell participants: "A second step in making friends is to mix with people whose attitudes are similar to yours. When you discover them, be sure to let them know that's the case. It may be true occasion-ally that 'opposites attract,' but for most of us most of the time, it isn't. Instead, birds of a feather have a great tendency to flock together. Almost always we like those who share our attitudes to issues like politics, lifestyle, morals, and so on. These attitudes are the ones that matter. Groups based on characteristics (such as age or single parenthood) that are unrelated to these attitudes are often only partly successful."

> **Note to Leaders:** The belief that "opposites attract" may be hard to shake. If so, describe some of the research described below to make your point.

✓ > **Research Point:** There is a lot of research showing that similarity increases attraction. Similarities not only in attitudes, but also in personality traits, activities, age, education, ethnic background, religion, socioeconomic status, and occupations, have each been shown to increase attraction between people. In sum, we seem to like people who remind us of ourselves.[10–15] The tendency to like those who are similar to us shows up very early in development. For example, one study showed that children as young as 3 years old chose puppets whose food preferences matched their own and also preferred to play with an-other child who shared their toy preferences.[16]

✓ > **Research Point:** Similarity and liking do not always go together, however, and similarity can sometimes actually be threatening.[17] For example, it has been found that if people who are similar to us also have something unattractive about them (such as having been in prison or in a mental hospital), we tend to like them less than we do people who are dissimilar, but have nothing unattractive about them. In this case, the similarity is threatening; it does not really validate our view of the world, and suggests that we too are vulnerable to the aspect that is unattractive. This is one reason why it can be effective for people not to reveal personal problems very early in forming new relationships.

✓ **D. Conversation Skills Are Important**

Three behaviors are typical of people who are rated as "good conversationalists": They ask plenty of questions; they give "positive feedback" (indicating that they have heard, understood, and appreciated what the other person says); and they carry their end of the conversation. Carrying one's end of a conversation means speaking roughly half of the time—not all the time, but also not so little that the other person is under pressure to keep the conversation going.

1. Ask and Respond to Questions

There is a thin line between asking questions skillfully and turning a conversation into an interrogation session. If both speakers are skilled, the questions tend to be reciprocated.

✓ 💬 **Discussion Point:** Read the following two conversations, and then have participants discuss which one sounds like the better conversation.

Conversation 1

Person A: Do you know many people here?

Person B: No, but I am a friend of Bill's. Do you know him?

Person A: No, but I work with his sister, Susan. How do you know Bill?

Person B: We went to high school together. Are you a musician like Susan?

Conversation 2

Person A: Do you know many people here?

Person B: No, I don't.

Person A: Are you a friend of Susan's?

Person B: Yes.

Person A: How do you know her?

Person B: We work together.

Note that one reason why the first exchange seems altogether smoother and easier (and results in greater liking) is that A and B are not only asking each other questions, but also volunteering more information than is actually asked for, which quite naturally leads to more questions. Discuss.

2. Make Small Talk

Conversations do not have to be deeply meaningful to be enjoyable. The value of "small talk" or "chit-chat" should not be underestimated. Good conversationalists can participate actively in small talk. Students in one experiment who were asked to get to know each other without using small talk found the task impossible. They simply didn't know where to begin.

3. Self-Disclose Skillfully[18]

Appropriate and skillful self-disclosure—not too much and not too little—requires social sensitivity and social judgment. As relationships progress, there is a tendency to disclose more and more about ourselves, but too little or too much at the wrong time can decrease liking. People seem to like each other best when they disclose roughly the same amount and kind of information.

4. Don't Interrupt

Skillful conversationalists also do not interrupt. Explain to participants: "Interrupting does not always mean breaking into someone's sentences. Starting to talk just fractionally before or instantly after someone has finished risks giving the impression that you are not really listening to them, only waiting for them to be quiet so that you can have your say!"

5. Learn What to Talk About

Good conversationalists learn what to talk about by observing which topics are being discussed and how people react to them. Sometimes the problem is not knowing what to talk about. For some people, this means not being sure which topics are appropriate for which situations. Although there are no rules for this, observing others is a good idea. For other people, the "what to talk about" problem has more to do with lack of activity: If these persons have few hobbies, do not keep abreast of current affairs, rarely venture out to the theatre or the cinema, or rarely travel, they might have little to contribute to a conversation.

💬 **Discussion Point:** Many individuals feel very socially inadequate; understandably, they also find it very difficult to talk about this publicly. Ask in a matter-of-fact way who has low self-confidence about their conversation skills. Then ask who has trouble knowing what topics are appropriate to talk about, and who has trouble thinking of anything to say. Remind participants that their difficulties are most likely situation-specific. Elicit the situations that are most difficult. Then have participants brainstorm ideas for topics of conversation, or activities to help them know what to talk about (e.g., reading newspapers, watching new movies).

> **Note to Leaders:** This skill can be difficult to teach if you yourself have social difficulties or social anxiety in some situations. If you do, now is the time to confess it publicly! You can be a very useful role model if you also practice homework assignments and then discuss them with participants.

✓ E. Express Liking Selectively

It is a lot easier to like someone who likes us than someone who does not. We can communicate liking and caring for others in many ways. We can tell them. We can praise or compliment them. We can seek their company. We can listen to them. We can be supportive of their needs. We can support their causes or people they care about. However, there are a number of important caveats about expressing liking to others, and these should be discussed with participants.

✓ 1. Don't Remark on Obvious or Nonexistent Characteristics

Instruct participants: "Don't remark on totally obvious positive characteristics, particularly if they are obvious to everyone or are common among the people you are with. For example, don't comment on how pretty a person is when she has just won a beauty pageant, or on how well an immigrant reads English when he has been in an English-speaking country for 20 years. Also, don't tell people they have skills they don't possess. For instance, don't compliment the driving skills of someone who has just failed the road test for the third time. We tend to react most positively to people who praise us for attributes we would like to have but are not quite sure we possess—not for attributes we and everyone else know we have, or for ones that we wished we had but know very well we haven't."

✓ 2. Don't Praise Everyone for Similar Characteristics

To be liked by someone who likes everyone is no great honor. Similarly, to be praised by someone for characteristics nearly everyone has is not likely to increase attraction. Going overboard with praise for everyone, in fact, can have unintended negative consequences. The absence of praise can then be construed as disapproval, and that may reduce liking. Excessive praise can also make others question a person's sincerity and wonder whether he or she has an ulterior motive. The person may be seen as ingratiating (i.e., praising someone to get something). Ingratiating people are generally disliked. Expressing liking, therefore, is not always a straightforward process.

✓ F. Join Conversation Groups

If we wait for people to approach us, we may never have friends. Sometimes we must make the first move in finding friends. To do this, we need to find new groups of people to be around. When we are invited to a party at someone's home where we know none of the guests, it is reasonable to expect that the host or hostess will introduce us to at least one person or one group of people. But this does not always happen, and even when it does, we usually cannot stay with the same person or group for the entire party, meeting, or event.

There are two important skills for joining ongoing conversational groups. First, we need to know how to tell whether a group of people having a conversation is open or closed to new people. Second, if the group is open, we need to learn how to join the conversation.

✓ 1. Figuring Out Whether a Group Is Open or Closed

It is important to determine whether a group is open or closed. Open groups will be receptive to our entering the conversation; closed groups may not welcome new members.

In open groups:

- Everyone is standing somewhat apart.
- Members occasionally glance around the room.
- There are gaps in the conversation.
- Members are talking about a topic of general interest.

In closed groups:

- Everyone is standing close together.
- Members attend exclusively to each other.
- There is a very animated conversation with few gaps.
- Members seem to be pairing off.

2. Figuring Out How to Join an Open Group Conversation

Usually the best way to join conversations in open groups is to wait for a lull in the conversation, move close to or stand beside a friendly-looking member of the group, and say something like "Mind if I join you?"

✓ G. Join Organized Groups

One of the most important reasons for joining groups is to meet others. Thus joining ongoing groups that meet regularly can be an effective way of making friends.

1. Find a Group That Meets Frequently

Explain to participants: "The more frequently the group meets, the more likely you are to become friends with someone in the group."

2. Find a Group Where Members Are Similar to You

Tell participants: "It may be more difficult to make friends in groups based on characteristics such as age, sex, or occupation that are not associated with attitudes; in this case, the larger the group, the greater the chance of finding people who share your values. Imagine, for instance, a small local club for divorced people or for single parents. The people in it may have so little in common other than their singleness that meetings become a strain rather than a pleasure."

3. Find a Group That Has Cooperative Aims

In a group organized around a shared interest, it is better to find a group emphasizing mutual help or one aimed simply at having a good time, rather than a competitive group where members are always pitting their skills against one another. Cooperation is conducive to liking. People ordinarily appear more attractive to one another if they are cooperating rather than competing.

Practice Exercise: Give Interpersonal Effectiveness Handout 11a: Identifying Skills to Find People and Get Them to Like You to participants. Explain the task, and give participants time to check the more effective response in each pair. Discuss answers. If time permits, ask participants whether they have been in other situations where it was not clear to them what would be the better course of action between two options.

Correct responses for Handout 11a are as follows: 1A, 2B, 3A, 4A, 5A, 6B, 7B, 8B, 9B, 10B, 11B, 12A.

XII. MINDFULNESS OF OTHERS (INTERPERSONAL EFFECTIVENESS HANDOUTS 12–12A)

Main Point: Friendships are easier to form and last longer when we remember to be mindful of the other persons in these friendships.

Interpersonal Effectiveness Handout 12: Mindfulness of Others. Notice that the three mindfulness skills described here (B, C, and D) are the three core mindfulness "what" skills taught in the Mindfulness module. Under each of the "what" skills are the three core "how" skills also taught in the Mindfulness module. This handout can be taught didactically or very interactively, depending on time.

Interpersonal Effectiveness Handout 12a: Identifying Mindfulness of Others (Optional). Use this handout if you have extra time in the session, or give it out as homework and then discuss it at the next session. The correct responses can be found at the end of this section of the teaching notes, as well as at the end of the introduction to this chapter.

Interpersonal Effectiveness Worksheet 9: Mindfulness of Others. Review this worksheet with participants. Tell participants to check off any of these skills they attempted, whether they completed them successfully or not. Remind them that the idea is to practice, not to be perfect. As in previous worksheets, remind participants to use the mindfulness "what" skill of describing (see Mindfulness Handout 4) when describing events and what they or others have said or done.

✓ A. Why Be Mindful of Others?

Relationships last longer when we remember to be mindful of the other persons in these relationships.

Mindfulness of others is an extension of the relationship effectiveness (GIVE) skills taught earlier in this module (see Section VI of this chapter, plus Interpersonal Effectiveness Handout 6).

✓ **Mindfulness of others is also a reiteration of the core mindfulness "what" and "how" skills** (see Chapter 7, plus Mindfulness Handouts 4 and 5). The skills here include observing and paying attention to others, describing what is observed rather than judging it, and participating in the flow of interactions.

Note to Leaders: A good way to teach these skills is to have participants first read Interpersonal Effectiveness Handout 12 and check the boxes on this handout next to all of those they find difficult and need to work on. Ask each participant to share which boxes they have checked. Afterward, teach each of the points, then go back and discuss. If you are worried about time, you can save this exercise for last.

B. Observing and Attending to Other People

Observing and attending to other people involves several subskills.

✓

1. Pay Attention with Interest and Curiosity

The first subskill is to pay attention with interest and curiosity to others around us. Im tant words here are "interest" and "curiosity." When we have such an attitude, we are open getting to know someone new. We are also open to learning new information about others. This is, of course, critical, since all people and events are in a state of constant change.

2. Be Open to New Information about Others

Approaching people with interest and curiosity is the opposite of being rigid, or unwilling to change our minds about a person when we discover that we have been wrong. It is also the opposite of holding a person to what they said, believed, felt, or wanted yesterday or even 5 minutes ago. People often change their beliefs or what they want. When we are mindless, pouting, or willful, we often cannot or will not acknowledge that a person has changed—even when we want the changes.

✓ 💬 **Discussion Point:** Elicit from participants times when others have been closed to new or corrective information about themselves. How did they feel? What did they want from the other persons?

✓

3. Let Go of Overfocusing on Self

Say to participants: "You can miss much of what the other person is saying or doing when you are overly focused on yourself. Although you want to be aware of yourself during interactions, a problem arises when you are overly focused on yourself. It is hard to be empathic to others or validate what they are saying or doing when you are not focused on them."

Two things can happen when we overfocus on ourselves. First, it can lead to our talking mostly about ourselves. Although some of this is good, too much makes others feel that they are not very important. This does not ordinarily lead to positive interactions. Second, focusing on ourselves during interactions can lead to anxiety[19] about how we are doing and what people are thinking. Anxiety can lead us either to avoid being with people or to stay very quiet when we are with them. Avoiding people and keeping our mouths shut when around others are not effective ways to make or keep friends.

✓ **Research Point:** Data on social phobia[20, 21] show that individuals who are highly anxious about joining groups or talking in groups are often overfocused on themselves and on how they appear to others. Part of an effective treatment is to get these individuals to practice throwing their complete attention toward the other people they are interacting with. This may need to be practiced many times, but ordinarily it is very helpful in reducing anxiety when with others.

👥 **Practice Exercise:** Conduct two role plays where you ask clients to manipulate the focus of their attention. In the first role play, ask the clients to demand a high standard of themselves—that is, to imagine that they need to appear witty and intelligent at all times and to constantly monitor how they're fulfilling that standard. In the second role play, ask the clients to reduce expectations and only focus on what the other persons say. After the role plays, ask the clients about their subjective experience of anxiety and how they would rate it (on a scale of 0–100), and also give feedback on performance. You can ask the other group members to give feedback as well.

4. Stay in the Present

Another important subskill is to stay in the present. That is, we need to listen to other persons in real time, instead of planning what we will say next or thinking about the future consequences of what the persons are saying.

✓ ### 5. Stop Multitasking

Say to participants: "It's essential not to start multitasking when you are interacting with someone else. Don't text others, or answer and start phone conversations with others, during a face-to-face conversation with someone else. It can even mean turning off your cell phone if a conversation is important. In groups, don't look over a person's shoulder when you are talking with him or her, to see if there is someone else you would rather talk to. It is difficult for other people to feel that they are important to you or that you care about them when you frequently turn their attention away from them."

💬 **Discussion Point:** Elicit from participants times when other people have paid attention to something or someone else during interactions. How did this feel?

✓ ### 6. Give Up Judgments and Always Being Right

Judgmental thinking, voice tone, and statements are off-putting to others and spring from an attitude that we are right and others are wrong. This is an ineffective attitude in interpersonal relationships. Always attempting to be right can be lethal in making and keeping friends. Others don't want to always be wrong. It makes them feel that we don't respect their point of view, and they then want to avoid us.

💬 **Discussion Point:** Elicit from participants which of the relationship-observing skills they have most difficulty with. Discuss ways to practice being more observing of others.

✓ ## C. Describing

In regard to mindfulness of others, observing involves several things.

✓ ### 1. Describe What You Observe in a Matter-of-Fact Way

The key words in the heading above are "describe" and "matter-of-fact." When we describe, we state what we observed: the "who," "what," and "where." We might be describing thoughts, feelings, or sensations of our own—how something smells or tastes to us, or what we have seen, heard, or done. The key to describing, as noted in the discussions of the mindfulness skills in Chapter 7, is to distinguish what we are observing within ourselves (e.g., thoughts, feelings, sensations, images) from what we are observing outside of ourselves.

2. Put Aside Judgmental Thoughts and Statements

Judgmental thoughts and statements very often get in the way of describing. Rather than just noticing what someone is doing or saying, we add an evaluation of "good" or "bad" onto what we observe. In addition, we usually then assume not only that we are correct, but also that the entire universe should operate on our rules of what is correct and right. The best way to keep friends and increase emotional closeness with others is to replace judgmental thoughts and words with descriptive words.

3. Don't Make Assumptions about Others

We need to avoid assuming what others are thinking, how they are feeling, what they must be doing, or what they really want or don't want. Such assumptions and interpretations of others can cause no end of trouble in relationships. This is especially true when we don't bother to check the facts. If we want to make and keep relationships, it is essential to treat assumptions and interpretations as hypotheses to be tested, instead of as known facts.

Remind participants: "Remember, you can only describe what you observe through your senses (touch, taste, smell, hearing, seeing). No one has ever observed another person's thoughts, motives, intentions, feelings, emotions, desires, or personal experiences. What we can observe, and thus describe, are all of these things in ourselves."

Interpersonally sensitive people can often correctly infer what is going on with a person even when the other person says nothing about what is going on. As we will see later in the section on validation, being able to "read" other people correctly from knowledge of who they are, things that have happened, and nonverbal communication is very important. However, even when we know people very well or know all that has happened with respect to a certain situation, we still must be open to being wrong. We can check the facts by asking questions and sometimes by watching how people react to what we say and do.

4. Don't Question Others' Motives and Intent

Another thing that can be very damaging to relationships is questioning other people's motives or intentions. People feel pushed away when we question their motives. The most common example is assuming that if words or actions have a certain effect, then that effect must have been intended. For example, it is all too easy to assume that "if I feel manipulated by what you said or did, then you must have intended to manipulate me," or that "if I feel angry about what you did, then you intended to make me feel angry."

Questioning other people's motives is also common in people who have trouble trusting others. Mistrust of specific people without good reasons, however, delays forming friendships and gets in the way of intimacy and closeness.

✓   ### 5. Give Others the Benefit of the Doubt

Giving other people the benefit of the doubt is a very effective skill for maintaining relationships. Even when there is some justification for inferring that another person has some negative intention, usually there is at least some small chance of another possibility. Remembering to give the benefit of the doubt can make it easier to follow up with checking the facts. As with opposite action, it is important to give the benefit of the doubt all the way—that is to really open up to the possibility that your thoughts about the other person's intentions could really be wrong and that there could be other benevolent motivations.[22]

💬 **Discussion Point:** Elicit from participants situations where they inferred that someone else had a negative intention, only to find out later that they were mistaken. Have participants consider whether others have afforded them the benefit of the doubt.

6. Allow Others to Earn Your Trust

Many individuals who struggle with trust have mistaken notions about the process of building trust. For example, some will insist that building trust takes time, as if time itself leads to increased trust. In reality, trust is built when one takes risks with others by choosing to give them opportunities to prove themselves trustworthy; when such individuals act in trustworthy ways, then trust is earned. Without mindfulness, it may take months or even years before opportunities to earn trust are given, reinforcing the notion that trust "takes time." On the other hand, participants can actively practice choosing to allow others to earn their trust. Of course, when others respond in untrustworthy ways (e.g., deliberately taking advantage), then decisions to stop trusting them are reasonable.

💬 **Discussion Point:** Have participants reflect on examples in which either they gave others opportunities to earn trust and examples in which they did not. Elicit also examples of others' giving them a chance to earn their trust.[22]

Too little and too much trust can both be problems. Paranoia is the persistent belief that others are out to harm us or manipulate us, when there is little or no objective evidence that this is so. Clearly, paranoia does not bode well for building close personal relationships. The opposite of paranoia, however, can be thought of as "trust disorder." This involves believing everything that people tell us and never doubting them or their motives, despite evidence that they might not be trustworthy.

Entering relationships naively with untrustworthy or dishonest people can also interfere with finding friends and building closeness and intimacy. Once we are hurt by someone like this, it can be difficult to start over again in a new relationship. Mindfulness does not require being naive to the facts of human nature, discounting negative information about someone, or ignoring warning signals that a relationship may not turn out as well as we hope.

✓ D. Participating with Others

In regard to mindfulness of others, participating means "jumping into the relationship." In other words, it means completely "buying into" or throwing ourselves completely into a conversation, group activity, or relationship. It means letting go of standing outside a group or relationship.

✓ 1. Throw Yourself into Interactions

We can throw ourselves into a conversation or completely "buy into" it without simultaneously throwing ourselves into an ongoing relationship. Staying in the present means participating in the present.

2. Go with the Flow

We need to "go with the flow" of the other person in an interaction or of a group activity, rather than trying to control every activity, decision, and interaction as if our lives or well-being depended on it.

Going with the flow does not mean giving up control of everything. When relationships are abusive, or when groups want us to do things that violate our morals or that make us feel extremely uncomfortable, staying in control of at least what we do is important.

Having at least some control of what others do can be very important when those others are our children, children in our care, or people who report to us whose work we are responsible for. Having some control can also be important with people who could potentially hurt us (such as those who spend our money, take or dispose of our property, write untrue things about us online, etc.).

3. Become One with Group Activities and Conversations

Once we have become involved in a conversation or group activity, we need to "become one" with the interaction by letting go of self-focus and resisting efforts to pull back after we throw ourselves in.

Practice Exercise: Give Interpersonal Effectiveness Handout 12a: Identifying Mindfulness of Others to participants, and explain the task. Give participants time to check the more mindful response for each pair. Discuss answers. If time permits, ask participants if they have other situations where it is not clear to them what would be the more mindful course of action between two options.

Correct responses for Handout 12a are as follows: 1B, 2B, 3A, 4A, 5A, 6A, 7B, 8B, 9B, 10A, 11B, 12B.

XIII. HOW TO END RELATIONSHIPS (INTERPERSONAL EFFECTIVENESS HANDOUTS 13–13A)

Main Point: Ending destructive relationships and those that interfere with pursuing important goals can sometimes be more difficult than forming relationships in the first place.

Interpersonal Effectiveness Handout 13: Ending Relationships. The skills for ending relationships described on this handout are drawn from mindfulness (wise mind), emotion regulation (problem solving, cope ahead, opposite action), and interpersonal effectiveness (DEAR MAN, GIVE FAST) skills. The only new skill is that of practicing safety first when ending abusive or life-threatening relationships. The key to teaching these skills is to make them relevant to participants by discussing relationships they have ended, ones they are considering ending, or ones they wish they had already ended.

Interpersonal Effectiveness Handout 13a: Identifying How to End Relationships (Optional). You can use this handout if you have extra time in the session, or give it out as homework and then discuss it in the next session. It can also be skipped. Correct responses are listed at the end of this section's teaching points, as well as at the end of this chapter's introduction.

Interpersonal Effectiveness Worksheet 10: Ending Relationships (Optional). Assign this worksheet only to those thinking about ending a relationship. If they are trying to leave an abusive or dangerous relationship, review it with them and highlight the necessity of calling a domestic violence hotline (either a local one or, in the United States, the National Domestic Violence Hotline; see the end of this section). As with previous worksheets, remind participants to use the mindfulness "what" skill of describing (see Mindfulness Handout 4) when describing events and what they or others have said or done. Spend some time helping participants figure out how to concisely state the core problems leading to their wish to leave a relationship.

Interpersonal Effectiveness Worksheet 1: Pros and Cons of Using Interpersonal Skills (Optional). This worksheet can also be used in teaching this skill set.

✓ A. Ending Important Relationships Requires Clear Thinking and Interpersonal Finesse

Important relationships come in all varieties: friendships, marriages or other committed life partnerships, parent–child relationships, sibling relationships, work relationships, and psychotherapy or counseling relationships, to name a few of those ordinarily most important. Each of these relationships can vary in the degree to which they enhance or reduce the quality of our lives.

✓ B. Decide to End Relationships in Wise Mind, Never in Emotion Mind

Even in a good relationship, it is not uncommon to have momentary wishes to end it when we are frustrated, angry, or otherwise unhappy. Ordinarily these feelings pass and we forget them. Unfortunately, many people end relationships in emotion mind. If they had waited until the emotion passed, the value of the relationships might have looked very different.

1. Strong Negative Emotion Can Lead to Rash Actions in Interpersonal Situations

When we are highly aroused, our behavior is likely to be mood-dependent, and our ability to take a balanced long-term view of our relationships deteriorates. In addition, our ability to think clearly, communicate effectively, or problem-solve issues in our relationships becomes limited. High negative arousal can also fuel judgmental thinking, which can then further escalate conflict. With conflict escalating, we may find ourselves walking out of a relationship in a fit of extreme anger or frustration. In retrospect, we may regret leaving. It may also be impossible to resurrect the relationship.

2. Think Through the Reasons for Ending a Relationship before Ending It

It may be useful to write out the pros and cons of staying versus ending the relationship before making a decision.

3. It Makes Sense to End Destructive Relationships

Tell participants: "A relationship is destructive when it destroys either the quality of the relationship or aspects of yourself, such as your physical body and safety, your self-esteem or sense of integrity, or your ability to find happiness or peace of mind."

4. It Makes Sense to End a Relationship That Seriously Interferes with Your Quality of Life

Continue: "A relationship interferes with your quality of life when it blocks or hinders your pursuit of goals that are important to you, your ability to enjoy life and do things you like, your relationships with other persons (which a very jealous partner or friend may resent), or the welfare of other people you love."

5. It Makes Sense to Stay in a Relationship When the Cost of Leaving Is Greater Than the Cost of Staying

An example of a relationship in which the cost of leaving might be greater than that of staying might be this: One person is caring for a partner who has a degenerative brain disorder, which results in a complete change of personality. The partner who was once loving is now angry, frequently out of control, incapable of self-care, and unable to recognize the caregiving partner. The caregiver may regard staying within such a relationship as a moral duty, and ending the relationship may result in intense remorse and guilt. In such a situation, however, it will be important for the caregiver to find ways to create sufficient separation to maintain some quality of life both within and outside of the relationship.

6. It Is Important to Differentiate between Justified and Unjustified Guilt in Deciding Whether to End a Relationship

"Justified guilt" is feeling guilty when a completed or intended action violates our important moral values. "Unjustified guilt" is feeling guilty for something that does not in reality violate our moral values. Unjustified guilt is often a result of paying attention to what we believe others will think, rather than to what we ourselves think. (See Emotion Regulation Handouts 8a and 11.)

✓ C. Try Problem Solving to Repair a Difficult Relationship

Problem solving may be effective in repairing a relationship when the relationship is important and there is reason for hope.

1. Problem Solving May Involve Doing Some Serious Work on the Relationship

Tell participants: "In a relationship with a friend, partner, or other person you are very close to, the two of you may need to do some serious work on the relationship. To get started with problem solving, review the problem-solving steps in Emotion Regulation Handout 12. Using a relationship workbook or other set of guidelines may be helpful here also. For example, *The High-Conflict Couple,* a book written for couples by Alan Fruzzetti,[23] gives many guidelines that can be useful in any high-conflict relationship."

2. Problem Solving May Require Getting Other People Involved to Help

In a marriage or a committed partnership, problem solving may require couple counseling. In a relationship with a relative, it may require asking other relatives to help out. In a work setting, it may require working with a mediator. When the decision is to maintain the relationship, but also to increase personal time and separation, joining a support group may be of help.

✓ **D. Use Cope Ahead Skills to Plan How to End a Relationship**

See Chapter 9, Section XVI, and Emotion Regulation Handout 19 for further details on cope ahead.

1. Decide Whether to End the Relationship in Writing, on the Phone, or in Person

Tell participants: "The decision about how to end the relationship will depend greatly on the type of relationship you have, how long you have had the relationship, and the degree of intimacy with the other person."

2. Write a Script in Advance

Say to participants: "Write out ahead of time exactly what you want to say and how you want to explain your decision. If you are ending the relationship in writing, such as through a resignation letter at work or by e-mail with a long-distance e-mail friend, ask someone you trust to read what you have to say before sending it. It is very easy for judgmental, condescending, or insensitive comments to creep into writing, despite your best efforts to send a different message. A second reader can often pick this up for you."

3. Practice What to Say

Continue: "If you are going to end the relationship on the phone or in person, practice in your imagination what you will say, how you will say it, and when you will tell the other person you want to end the relationship. Practice in front of a mirror saying what you want to say. Practice with close friends and get their feedback on how you sound."

4. Troubleshoot Ahead of Time

Tell participants: "Troubleshoot ahead of time what you will say or do in response to what the other person might say or do. It is important here to try to predict what the other person will actually say or do, and then be prepared with a variety of responses."

✓ **E. Be Direct: Use DEAR MAN, GIVE FAST Skills**

Important relationships ordinarily cannot be ended with a simple DEAR MAN, GIVE FAST statement as outlined in Interpersonal Effectiveness Skills Handouts 5–7. However, these steps can guide how a conversation about ending a relationship is approached.

1. DEAR

Say to participants: "Most important at first is to be direct and clear. Describe the relationship problems that have led you to want to end the relationship. Express clearly how you feel about it, and assert that you now want to end the relationship. Have the other person confirm his or her understanding that the relationship is over, and if possible, reinforce by letting the other person know how ending the relationship will be good for both of you. If this is not the case, focus on how a good ending will be in both your interests."

2. MAN

Encourage participants: "Stay mindful, and appear confident. If you are sure that ending the relationship is in your interests, it is important not to give in to entreaties to stay in the relationship. This may be particularly important if you are more important to the other person than he or she is to you. Be careful not to go to extremes, however, unless you really do want to end all contact with the person. For example, if you want to get a divorce, end a sexual relationship, or move out of a place you share with a roommate, you may still want to be friends. Thus it is important to not burn any more bridges than you have to. Although you may not be willing to negotiate whether to end the relationship or not, be ready to negotiate *how* to end it, if that is at all possible."

✓ **3. GIVE**

The person ending a relationship is generally the person in the high-power position. Thus the GIVE skills are particularly important in these situations. Tell participants: "Be gentle. Inhibiting attacks, threats, judgments, and condescending words and expressions can be extremely helpful in smoothing an ending to the relationship. This can be very difficult to do when guilt about ending can easily lead to blaming and judging the other person. Although you may know that you will end the relationship no matter what the other person says, listen to and validate the person's point of view. This can make it easier for both of you to work out an ending that causes the least hurt for the other person."

4. FAST

Say to participants: "Finally, be fair, and make no apologies. Leaving a relationship with your self-respect intact requires you to be truthful about the problems (even if you are tactful about how you frame them) and not to sacrifice your values or integrity. This can be particularly difficult when the reason for ending is that you have changed, rather than that the other person is doing things that make the relationship impossible for you."

✓ **F. Practice Opposite Action for Love If Needed**

Tell participants: "Even though you may know that a relationship must end, at times that does not coincide with an end of love. This is often the case when you love a person but finally realize that the relationship is either destructive or incompatible with your life goals. Incompatible values, career demands, the well-being of children, unwillingness to move to distant locations, and many other considerations may make an alliance impossible between two people, even though there is great love."

Continue: "The central question here is whether or not loving the other person enhances or damages your life. Many times, continuation of love is life-enhancing. At other times, it is not. For example, a woman addicted to drugs who loves a drug addict may need the relationship to get her own drugs. Even though her partner may pimp her out to other men to make drug money, she may still love him and find it very difficult to end the relationship. This also happens often in relationships with abusers. Being mistreated does not always end love. In these situations, to keep from returning to destructive relationships, opposite action for love (as described in Emotion Regulation Handout 11: Figuring Out Opposite Actions) may be called for."

✓ **G. Practice Safety First!**

Emphasize to participants: "It is very important to realize that in a physically abusive relationship or one where you fear for your life, it is very important to get appropriate advice about how to leave the relationship safely. In many abusive relationships, the time of ending and leaving the relationship is a time fraught with danger. Thus the threat of danger should not be taken lightly if your partner in a relationship has been physically abusive or has threatened your life. In these cases, safe housing and a plan for safely leaving the relationship may be necessary. Call the local domestic violence hotline in your city or county for help. It is also important to get advice from a professional who is trained and experienced in working with individuals in abusive relationships."

Note to Leaders: In the United States, you can also refer participants to the National Domestic Violence Hotline website (*www.thehotline.org/tag/safety-planning*). You can find non-U.S. hotlines via your search engine. In addition, if you are not trained and experienced in working with abused and battered individuals in relationships, it is important to refer participants to an expert who has such training and experience (or to get consultation from such a person).

👥 **Practice Exercise:** Give Interpersonal Effectiveness Handout 13a: Identifying How to End Relationships to participants, and explain the task. Give participants time to check the more effective response for each pair. Discuss answers. If time permits, ask participants if they have other situations where it is not clear to them what would be the more effective course of action between two options.

Correct responses for Handout 13a are as follows: 1B, 2B, 3B, 4A, 5B, 6B, 7B, 8B.

XIV. OVERVIEW: WALKING THE MIDDLE PATH SKILLS (INTERPERSONAL EFFECTIVENESS HANDOUT 14)[1]

> **Main Point:** This set of skills helps participants effectively manage themselves and their relationships through (1) dialectics, or balancing acceptance and change; (2) validation, or working on acceptance; and (3) behavior change strategies, or working on change by managing cues and consequences.
>
> **Interpersonal Effectiveness Handout 14: Overview: Walking the Middle Path.** Briefly review this overview handout. Stay on it longer if you are using it to review skills already taught. If you are only teaching some of the skills on this handout, consider skipping it entirely. Do not teach the material while covering this handout unless you are skipping the related handouts.
>
> **Worksheet:** None.

✓ A. Walking the Middle Path

The middle path is one of harmony with reality as it is. The middle path requires the fine-tuning of opposites that in turn produce life's movement, speed, and flow—for example, accepting reality, and also working to change reality; validating ourselves and others, and also pointing out errors; working and resting; or tightening and loosening strings on a violin.

Walking the middle path does not mean 50% of one point of view and 50% of another. Nor does it mean a centerpoint between two extremes. To walk the middle path is to move away from extreme emotional responses, actions, and thinking, and toward balanced and integrative responses to life situations. Walking the middle path allows moving to an extreme and then returning to a state of balance.

B. Dialectics

Dialectics teaches us that all things are interconnected and in a constant state of change. It paves the way to the middle path—that is, the path of balancing extremes.

C. Validation

Validation skills are necessary in all relationships. They communicate that a person's feelings, thoughts, and actions are understandable, given the person's past or current situation. On the other hand, validation does not validate the invalid. The skills taught here review and add more detail to the validation skills taught earlier in this module as part of the relationship effectiveness skills. In other words, they involve increasing the V in GIVE.

A corollary of the point above about validation is that experiencing high levels of *invalidation* can be traumatic. When that happens, self-validation is needed for recovery.

✓ D. Behavior Change Skills

Behavior change skills use behavioral principles of contingency management (i.e., use of consequences) and stimulus control to increase desired behaviors or to decrease undesired behaviors.

XV. DIALECTICS (INTERPERSONAL EFFECTIVENESS HANDOUTS 15–16C)[1]

Main Point: A dialectical stance is essential for walking the middle path, because it decreases a sense of isolation, conflict, and polarities.

Interpersonal Effectiveness Handout 15: Dialectics. This handout briefly outlines the basics of a dialectical perspective.

Interpersonal Effectiveness Handout 16: How to Think and Act Dialectically. This is an extension of Handout 15 and gives examples of specific ways to act dialectically.

Interpersonal Effectiveness Handout 16a: Examples of Opposite Sides That Can Both Be True *(Optional).* This handout can be very useful for in-session discussion to demonstrate how opposites can indeed both be true.

Interpersonal Effectiveness Handout 16b: Important Opposites to Balance *(Optional).* This handout can be very useful during a discussion of how to balance life patterns and in doing homework to identify what life patterns need better balance.

Interpersonal Effectiveness Handout 16c: Identifying Dialectics *(Optional).* Use this handout if you have extra time, or give it out as homework and then discuss it at the next session. The correct responses are listed at the end of this section's teaching points, as well as at the end of this chapter's introduction.

Interpersonal Effectiveness Worksheet 11: Practicing Dialectics; Interpersonal Effectiveness Worksheet 11a: Dialectics Checklist; Interpersonal Effectiveness Worksheet 11b: Noticing When You're Not Dialectical. These worksheets offer three different formats for recording dialectics practice. Worksheet 11 asks participants to practice their dialectical skills only twice between sessions. Worksheet 11a instructs participants to practice and gives multiple opportunities for each skill, as well as multiple check boxes for each skill. Worksheet 11b is aimed at increasing participants' awareness of *not* being dialectical in their interactions, and of the negative outcomes that often follow nondialectical behavior. This worksheet takes the place of a pros-and-cons worksheet, in that the objective is to motivate dialectical behavior.

✓ A. Why Be Dialectical?

✓   **Dialectics helps us stay away from extremes and walk the middle path** in our thinking and actions. It is a world view, and also a way of resolving disagreements and searching for the truth.

✓ B. Dialectics: What Is It?

There are four main ideas in the dialectical perspective.

✓   **1.** *The Universe Is Filled with Opposing Sides and Opposing Forces*

For everything that exists, there is an opposite. If there is a box, there is a "not box"; if there is light, there is dark; if there is up, there is down; there is fat and there is thin; there is male and there is female; there is a positive electrical charge and a negative charge; there is something and there is nothing; physicists trying to identify the most fundamental element of existence found matter, and then they found antimatter. Every part has a whole, and every whole has a part. It is impossible to understand something without knowledge of its opposite.

Everything that exists is made of opposing forces that both hold things together and create constant change. Without gravity, we would fly away from the earth. Electrons are bound together to the nucleus of an atom by electromagnetism.

✓   **Dialectics tells us that opposing points of view can both be true.** When we consider what is left out of our own point of view (i.e., when we consider opposing points of view), we can find a synthesis of both perspectives. This is how we can get unstuck from where we are and change occurs.

Discussion Point: Discuss with participants the idea that everything in the universe includes an opposite.

✓ **2. Everything and Every Person Is Connected in Some Way**

Dialectics reminds us of our connection to the universe. Understanding the interconnectedness of all things increases our understanding of our influence on others and theirs on us. It becomes easier to understand and validate both others and ourselves.

This statement can be taught from three different perspectives, described below.

a. We Are All Connected to Each Other Physically

To make this point, ask participants to notice that the air they are breathing in and out is in turn being breathed in and out by others. Ask them to notice that their feet are touching the floor that is touching every other person in the room. This floor is also touching the hallway; the hallway is touching the steps down to the street; the street is touching blocks far away, which in turn are touching roads going to mountains; the mountains in turn are touching the sky; and so on. The idea is that we can make a direct link between ourselves and the farthest star.

b. Each of Us Has Parts, and Each Is Part of a Greater Whole

Each of us has parts (e.g., arms, legs, blood vessels, cells), and each of us is part of a greater whole (e.g., a family, a workplace, a city). The parts participate in creating the whole (e.g., the leg contributes to the whole body), and simultaneously the whole body (e.g., blood vessels, hip bone) contributes to the parts.

Example: It is not possible for the participants of the skills training program to avoid altering the program within which they interact. The program would not exist without them. It is certainly also the case that they will simultaneously be affected by the program.

✓ ### c. Separation Is an Illusion

Modern physics tells us that separation is an illusion produced by the tendency of our brains to perceive objects as separate. Quantum physics, for example, finds that when we get down to the very smallest molecule and keep going to even smaller bits of matter, we ultimately find that matter dissolves into emptiness.

Documented spiritual experiences suggest that from the beginning of recorded human history, individuals have had profound experiences of reality as a unity—of the universe as one.

Discussion Point: Many individuals have had experiences of unity (i.e., of being one with their surroundings or with the entire universe). Sometimes these experiences take place in a spiritual context, but at other times they occur in definitely secular circumstances. Elicit from participants whether they have ever had such an experience. Discuss the impact, if any, of each experience on the life of the participant who had it.

Note to Leaders: It is important to validate experiences of unity or oneness. These can take many forms. The usual problem is that such an experience is invalidated or deemed unimportant by a participant. Frequently the person may not have told anyone about the experience. Remind participants with such experiences to remember these. Thinking about the experiences can remind them that, indeed, they are not alone and are not unconnected to others and to the universe. For characteristics of spiritual experiences, look at the criteria outlined in Mindfulness Handout 7: Goals of Mindfulness Practice: A Spiritual Perspective.

✓   **3. Change Is the Only Constant**

Dialectics helps us radically accept the changes that are continually occurring. This in turn helps us become more flexible. Such flexibility makes it easier for us to go with the flow, which in turn makes peak experiences more likely.

Everything in the universe is always changing. Indeed, reality itself is a process of continuous transformation. Some changes are fast (such as light waves moving through the air, or our abdomens going in and out as we breathe); others are very slow (such as the wearing down of a river rock as water washes over it, or mountains being pushed up out of the earth). Each day is either shorter or longer than the day before. Flowers come up, bud, bloom, die, and decay. Stars move slowly across the sky. The earth moves around the sun.

✓   *Example:* We are all older than we were a second ago. Our bodies are in a constant process of change: Cells are falling off; new air with new particles is entering our bodies; food we have eaten is being digested; the position of our teeth in our mouths is changing, even if very slightly. If we had a powerful magnifying device, we would see the components of the molecules in our bodies flying around. Our brains are changed with each new experience we have; neurons are constantly firing and sending messages along the neural network, thus permanently changing the overall network.

💬 **Discussion Point:** Discuss the sayings "You can't step in the same river twice" and "Even one vote changes the outcome."

Meaning and truth also evolve over time. What was true for a person in the past may no longer be true, simply because both the person and the environment are changing over time. What existed yesterday, last year, or 5 years ago does not exist now in exactly the same way. From what exists now, something new will emerge. Reality itself evolves transactionally over time. Truth is neither absolute (and never changing) nor relative (and dependent only on who is looking at it). Instead, it evolves over time.

✓   *Example:** Mary, Helen, and Judy each have a daughter. Each has held a set of values that have guided how they have raised their daughters. As their daughters become adults, however, they are rejecting many of their mothers' values.

■ Mary decides that either (1) her own values are right, and thus she has failed in raising her daughter; or (2) her daughter's values are right, and thus the core values guiding her own life are wrong and she is unlikely to get her daughter's respect. **This is a view of truth as absolute.**

■ Helen decides that her daughter's having different values is not important. She believes that all people have their own values, and that there are no right or wrong values. It is important to respect others' values rather than judge them, and she respects her daughter's values. **This is a view of truth as relative.**

■ Judy reasons that values change over time as they interact with changing environmental circumstances. As we all act on our values, the environment changes and as the environment changes, our values develop further. Judy respects her daughter's values as arising out of both the values she taught her daughter and the experiences her daughter has had that Judy never had. Judy does not see either herself or her daughter as wrong, and decides to try to see whether she can learn from her daughter's values just as her daughter learned from hers. **This is a dialectical view of truth as evolving over time.**

Example: Mark, Howard, and George are college juniors who are fed up with constant tests, paper assignments, and grading. They are losing their love of learning.

---

*This example (Mary, Helen, and Judy) and the next one (Mark, Howard, and George) are adapted from Basseches, M. (1984). *Dialectical thinking and adult development*. Norwood, NJ: Ablex. Copyright 1984 by Ablex Publishing Corporation. Adapted by permission of ABC/CLIO.

■ Mark's experience is that he learns more when he has freedom to pursue his own intellectual interests. He also believes, however, that university professors must know what they are doing, and that required courses and standardized tests and assignments must be the soundest educational method. **This is a view of truth as absolute.**

■ Howard believes that students should be able to pursue courses they want to take. He does not accept that it is educationally legitimate for teachers to dictate what students should learn. In his view, giving standardized tests and assignments is a subjective decision made by professors—and he believes that by requiring them, his teachers are using their power to impose on students how to learn. He decides to cultivate the fine art of pleasing professors by giving them what they want. **This is a view of truth as relative.**

■ George recognizes that colleges perform both a certification function for society and an educational function. The conflict between these two functions is at the core of the frustration with exams and standardized assignments. The certification function requires tests and grades; the education function requires opportunities free of arbitrary tests and writing assignments. George recognizes that change will require an evolution in the relationship between the university and society over time. He decides to learn what he can so as to contribute to this evolution. He also recognizes that in the meantime, he will have to make compromises between what is needed for certification that he has learned and what is needed for his own education. **This is a dialectical view of truth as evolving over time.**

Example: Adults often look back on the hard work and sacrifices they made when young to get ahead, and then they impose the same hard work and sacrifice on the young people around them now. For these adults, the meaning of hard work and sacrifice was learned over time in specific circumstances. Its meaning for those who are younger will also evolve over time in specific circumstances, and it is likely to be different, particularly if sacrifices are forced upon them.

✓ **4. *Change Is Transactional***

Dialectics helps us analyze how we are being influenced by our environment and how we are influencing our environment. This in turn leads to a better understanding of our own behavior and or our relationships. Dialectics leads to understanding, not to blame.

The world is one large system with many interacting parts. The sun, the trees, the water, the fruit, the farmer, the grocer, the teacher, the friend, the parent, the sibling—these things are all interconnected and influence one another. So at any given moment, things are never the same as the moment before or the moment after.

Each individual influences his or her environment, just as each environment influences the individual. Reciprocity is the key word here. A affects B, which alters B, which in turn alters A, and so forth. Each person has a completely different "family" that has a unique impact on his or her life. The "family" can consist of partners, children, parents, grandparents, siblings, teachers, peers, therapists, coaches, and others. The impact that these people in the environment have on the individual is just as varied as the impact the individual has on those in the environment.

Example: A relatively new and successful school teacher gets a new student who has a learning disability. Not having had much experience with this, she does a lot of extra work to figure out how best to teach him, and he progresses well through her class. The student comes out of the class not only learning the material, but also feeling more secure in his abilities. At the same time, the teacher has evolved from the experience and is now much better prepared for teaching the next student she encounters with a similar learning disability, and feels more secure in her ability to learn about different learning styles. Student and teacher have both grown and evolved as a result of the experience.[24]

Emotion dysregulation is a good example of the transactional nature of change and of learning. Two functions of emotions are to activate behavior and to communicate to others so that they will respond. When the functions are discouraged or blocked by the environment, the emotions may escalate. This in turn can lead to stronger efforts by the environment to block the emotions. After a time, a vicious cycle can occur.

💭 **Discussion Point:** Describe the following situation: Mom takes Catalina (age 6) to a Yo-Yo Ma concert with seats in the center of the orchestra section. As Yo-Yo Ma plays the cello, Catalina looks up at the stage and thinks she sees a small fire behind the stage. She whispers to Mom that there is a fire. Mom looks and does not see it. [Ask participants what they think Mom will say back to Catalina.] Mom whispers back that there is no fire. Catalina looks again and sees the fire again. [Ask participants what they think Catalina will do now.] Catalina whispers louder, "There's a fire!" Mom still does not see the fire. [Ask participants what they think Mom will do now.] Mom whispers even louder, "No, there is not!" Seeing it again [ask, "What will Catalina say?"], Catalina says loudly, "Mom! Fire!" Mom says [ask, "What and how?"] loudly, "BE QUIET!" After a few more rounds, Mom scoops Catalina up and carries her out of the concert hall. She feels safer and calms down. [Ask, "Did Mom reinforce Catalina for escalating?"] Alas, Mom has just reinforced Catalina for escalating. [Ask, "Did Catalina calming down reinforce Mom for escalating when she took her out of the concert hall?"] Catalina has reinforced Mom for the escalated action of taking her out of the concert.

C. How to Think and Act Dialectically

Review Interpersonal Effectiveness Handout 16 with participants.

> **Note to Leaders:** At either the beginning or end of discussing this handout, it can be helpful to ask participants to check off which dialectical strategies they most need to work on. Or you can ask them to circle those skills they are most interested in practicing. The list of strategies is quite long, and it is not necessary to go over every one. Select and focus on those giving the most trouble to participants.

✓ ### 1. There Is Always More Than One Side to Anything That Exists; Look for Both Sides

a. Ask Wise Mind: What Am I Missing?

Example: Demanding adherence to rules that were correct when a person was a child misses that the person is no longer a child.

Example: Following guidelines for appropriate behavior set by one's previous employer misses that appropriate behavior may be different in another company or at a higher rank in the same company.

Example: Screaming at a boyfriend, "You never think about me! You only care about yourself!" when he turns on a TV football game instead of talking to her.

💭 **Discussion Point:** Ask group members to consider what's being left out in the third example above. Generate more balanced alternative explanations for the boyfriend's turning on the football game. If the group fails to generate any examples, you may choose to give the following: The woman realizes that football is her boyfriend's passion, and that watching one game does not mean he does not care for her. She also remembers that her boyfriend does think about her quite often. This "both–and" perspective synthesizes the "either–or" stance so commonly held by emotionally dysregulated individuals. (See "Move Away from Extremes," below.)

b. Ask "Where Is the Kernel of Truth in the Other Side?": Find the Truth in Both Sides

Say to participants: "Practice looking at all sides of a situation and all points of view. Remember that no one, including you, has the absolute truth. There is wisdom to be gained from examining the truth in opposite perspectives." You can use the examples on Interpersonal Effectiveness Handout 16a (e.g., "You are tough, AND you are gentle") as illustrations.

Each person has unique qualities, and different people have different points of view. This point normalizes and accepts differences among people, rather than seeing differences as cause for conflict. Some people believe that anything that deviates from their own point of view is wrong.

Example: On a driving vacation to Europe, Mary wants to get up early in the morning to go out exploring and see everything. Bill wants to sleep in and enjoy the free breakfast the hotel provides. The truth from Mary's perspective is that this is a once-in-a-lifetime opportunity to see Europe, and they can always sleep and eat breakfast at home. Sleeping is wasting time on the trip. The truth from Bill's perspective is that he is mentally fatigued from his full-time job and responsibilities at home, and that sleeping in and relaxing over breakfast are what vacations are all about.

💬 **Discussion Point:** If you have time, ask each participant to check off the dialectical oppositions on Interpersonal Effectiveness Handout 16a that they have the most trouble with. Also ask participants to write in any other oppositions they have trouble with. Discuss how to find the syntheses of each of the opposites.

✓ **c. Move Away from Extremes**

Encourage clients to let go of seeing the world in "black-or-white," "all-or-nothing" ways. Many individuals think in extremes and rigidly hold to a single point of view. Life is black or white, viewed in dichotomous units. Such people often have difficulty receiving new information; they search instead for absolute truths and concrete facts that never change. The goal of dialectics is not to get participants to view reality as a series of grays, but rather to help them see both black and white, and to achieve a synthesis of the two that does not negate the reality of either.

Example: A man was extremely concerned about his wife's habit of running up debt on their joint credit cards. He was afraid that she would run up so much debt that they would go bankrupt. The first thing he thought to do was to try to take away her credit cards. But doing that would alienate his wife, and this would only increase his distress. So he started to ignore the topic of money completely, in order to avoid his emotional distress—the opposite extreme of trying to keep her from having any access to credit cards. Rather than opting for either one of these two extreme positions, he decided to consider both. This led him to find a third option, a "middle path" synthesis: to speak calmly to his wife about how to create a budget for both of them that they could monitor together.

💬 **Discussion Point:** Discuss the role of emotions in making extreme statements, such as when a teenage boy comes home after curfew, and his father tells him, "You're grounded for the rest of the school year!" Ask participants for other examples of extreme behavioral responses.

d. Balance Opposites

Say to participants: "Work to balance the opposites in your life. For instance, validate yourself as well as others. Accept reality, but also work to change it. Hold someone close, while also letting the person go."

💬 **Discussion Point:** If you have time, review Interpersonal Effectiveness Handout 16b, and ask participants to check off the dialectical oppositions that they have the most trouble balancing. Also ask participants to write in any other dichotomies they have trouble balancing. Discuss.

✓ **e. Make Lemonade Out of Lemons**

Making lemonade out of lemons is the art of taking something that seems apparently problematic and turning it into an asset. From another perspective, it is finding the silver lining in the darkest cloud. For example, suffering can enhance empathy and allow one to understand others who are suffering. Problems in everyday life are an opportunity to practice skills. Indeed, from the point of view of learning new skills, not having problems would be a disaster, since there would be nothing to practice on! The key idea here, of course, is not to act as if the lemon was actually lemonade all along. Such a position is invalidating and oversimplifies the difficulties of turning something very painful and difficult into something valuable or useful.

💬 **Discussion Point:** Elicit from participants times when they have been able to make lemonade out of a lemon. What personal difficulties have they had that they learned from or that somehow influenced them in a positive way? Discuss.

✓ **f. Embrace Confusion**

Embracing confusion, or entering the paradox, is entering into the world of "yes and no" or "true and not true" and allowing it to be what it is. It is becoming comfortable with paradox and confusion. Say to participants: "It is possible for a person to want you to be happy, but also refuse to do what you want. I can be right that it is too cold, and you can be right that it is too hot. I can do my best and still do better."

💬 **Discussion Point:** Read over and discuss the opposites that can both be true on Handout 16a at this point, or come back to this point when you teach the handout. If you are not using the handout, elicit from participants paradoxes in their own lives.

g. Play Devil's Advocate

Playing devil's advocate is arguing against a cause or position simply for the sake of argument or to determine the validity of the point of view. Using this strategy can make it easier to find the truth in both sides of an argument. Tell participants: "When you are working with your own sets of beliefs, it can be helpful to use the two-chair technique. Put two chairs near each other. Sit in one chair to make one side of the argument; sit in the other to take the opposing view; and switch back and forth until clarity is obtained about both points of view." (See Chapter 7 of the main DBT text for a fuller discussion of this strategy.)

👥 **Practice Exercise:** Elicit from participants various dilemmas or conflicts they have had in their lives. Select one to use as a practice case, and ask the person to play the devil's advocate for both sides of the dilemma, using the two-chair technique. Discuss.

h. Use Metaphors and Storytelling

Metaphors and stories have been used throughout history to convey complex events that can have multiple meanings. Stories are also an avenue of clarifying what a person is leaving out in his or her understanding of something. For example, a person may be focused on not wanting to come to the skills training group and decide that skills are not needed to get to his or her goals. You can point out that this is like getting in a boat to go across a river when the boat has no bottom on it. Trying to be what others want a person to be is like a tulip's trying to be a rose just because it happens to have been planted in a rose garden. Finding a tulip garden is an alternative. Learning acceptance is like a gardener's learning to love the dandelions that come into the garden year after year, no matter what the gardener does to keep them out. Moving slowly across a mountain ledge without looking down can be both life-threatening and the only way to survive when edging across the ledge is the only route to safety.

💬 **Discussion Point:** Elicit from participants any stories they have been told or have heard that have helped them hold complexity and opposites in their mind at once. Discuss.

✓ *2. Be Aware That You Are Connected*

✓   **a. Treat Others As You Wish Them to Treat You**

     Tell participants: "Remember that if you are harsh, critical, or invalidating, you are likely to be treated the same way."

💬 **Discussion Point:** Discuss the sayings "What goes around comes around," and "The waves and the ocean are one." Discuss how awareness of connection fits with the values of the "golden rule." Discuss how using GIVE skills over time is like investing in a bank that will pay dividends—even if there is no immediate return on every act of kindness.

     b. Look for Similarities among People Instead of Differences

     It is easy to feel separate from people when we think they are different from us. It is also much easier to be judgmental and critical of those we see as very different from ourselves. We tend to feel closer to people who seem to be like us.

💬 **Discussion Point:** Elicit from participants people they feel close to and people they feel distant from. Ask, "Are you more similar to people you feel close to or people you feel distant from?" Discuss.

     c. Notice the Physical Connections among All Things

     Say to participants: "Once you actually pay attention to the physical world, you find that everything is indeed connected to everything. Each part of your body is connected to another part, your body is connected to the floor, which is connected to the outside (even if by being connected to many things in between), and so on and so on."

👥 **Practice Exercise:** This can be a good time to do the "Acceptance by the Chair" mindfulness exercise. For a description, see Section VI, Part E (the final exercise there) in Chapter 7 of this manual.

✓ *3. Embrace Change*

     a. Throw Yourself into Change

     As long as change is a fact of life, we might as well not only allow it, but also embrace it by throwing ourselves into it.

💬 **Discussion Point:** Elicit from participants times when they have allowed change, even when it was difficult. When has it been easy to embrace change? Discuss.

     b. Practice Radical Acceptance of Change

     Tell participants: "When people and relationships begin to change in ways you don't like, practice radical acceptance of those changes. Allow those you care about to grow, develop, and change over time. Be patient with gradual changes; prepare for sudden changes."

💬 **Discussion Point:** Many individuals have trouble with change. Elicit from participants what types of change they have difficulties with. Discuss how to radically accept change. (See Distress Tolerance Handout 11.)

     c. Practice Getting Used to Change

     Encourage participants to get used to change by purposely making changes in small ways. Note that for people who don't like change, this will be practicing opposite action. (See Emotion Regulation Handouts 9–11.) The idea is to get comfortable with change by practicing it.

💬 **Discussion Point:** Ask who likes change and who does not. For those who do not like change, discuss how they could get more comfortable with it.

✓ **4. Remember That Change Is Transactional**

a. Observe How Everything Affects Everything Else

Say to participants: "Pay attention to the effects of what you do and say on others, and to how what they do and say affects you. Notice how your mood affects others around you, and how others' moods affect you. Seeing your own and others' behaviors as arising from transactions occurring over time can help you let go of blame."

✓ ### b. Practice Letting Go of Blame

Encourage participants to remind themselves that all things are caused by many interactions over time. Dialectics is incompatible with blame, primarily because it focuses on how all things are caused and how those causes are transactional over time. Note also how this is similar to what is taught in nonjudgmentalness.

👥 **Practice Exercise:** If you have time, give Interpersonal Effectiveness Handout 16c: Identifying Dialectics to participants, and explain the task. Give participants time to check the most dialectical response in each group. Discuss answers. If time permits, ask participants if they have other situations where it is not clear to them what would be the most dialectical course of action between two or more options.
Correct responses for Handout 16c are as follows: 1A, 2B, 3B, 4B, 5A, 6C, 7B, 8B.

XVI. VALIDATION SKILLS (INTERPERSONAL EFFECTIVENESS HANDOUTS 17–19A)[1]

Main Point: Validation of others' feelings, beliefs, experiences, and actions is essential in building any relationship of trust and intimacy. To recover from invalidation, we can use the same skills to validate ourselves, along with checking the facts and acknowledging that invalidation hurts.

Interpersonal Effectiveness Handout 17: Validation. The handout reviews the reasons for validation, what validation is, what is most important to validate, and cautions about validation. It is important to address these issues, but unless there is misunderstanding of validation, this handout can usually be reviewed rather quickly.

Interpersonal Effectiveness Handout 18: A "How To" Guide to Validation. Spend most of your time on this handout. It is very important to have participants practice the different types of validation and discuss problems in validating others. This handout is based on the six levels of validation that are taught to therapists and skills training leaders. The skills can also be taught to participants as a review of the GIVE skills.

Interpersonal Effectiveness Handout 18a: Identifying Validation (*Optional*). Use this handout if you have extra time, or give it out as homework and then discuss it at the next session. The correct responses are listed at the end of Section E below in the teaching points, as well as at the end of this chapter's introduction.

Interpersonal Effectiveness Handout 19: Recovering from Invalidation. Review the main points on this handout. If you do not have time to review this handout, give as one of the homework assignments Interpersonal Worksheet 3, and instruct participants to use the same validation strategies they learned to validate others with themselves.

Interpersonal Effectiveness Handout 19a: Identifying Self-Validation (*Optional*). Use this handout if you have extra time, *or* give it out as homework and then discuss it at the next session. The correct responses are listed at the end of Section F below, as well as at the end of this chapter's introduction.

Interpersonal Effectiveness Worksheet 12: Validating Others. Participants are to fill out this worksheet whenever they have an opportunity to practice their validation skills, even if they did not validate. The first section of the worksheet asks participants to check off what validation skills they practiced "on purpose" with others. The phrase "on purpose" is emphasized, so that participants will put some effort into actually trying out the skills with others. The next part of the worksheet asks participants to write down validating statements they made to others, as well as any invalidating statements they made. The ability to notice invalidating statements that participants make themselves is every bit as important as the ability to craft and make a validating statement. The worksheet also asks participants to describe a situation where they practiced validation, including writing down exactly what was said, the interpersonal outcome of what was said, and how they felt after the interaction. The worksheet then asks participants to rehearse validating statements by writing down what they would do differently next time (if anything). Remind participants that they are unlikely to remember exactly what they did and said in a situation if they don't write it down near the time of the interaction.

Interpersonal Effectiveness Worksheet 13: Self-Validation and Self-Respect. As with Worksheet 12, remind participants to fill this sheet out whenever they have an opportunity to practice their self-validation skills, whether or not they actually practiced. Adapt the instructions for Worksheet 12 for self-validation.

✓ A. What Is Validation?

✓ 1. Validation Is Finding the Kernel of Truth in Another Person's Perspective or Situation

When we validate others' experiences, emotions, thoughts, words, or actions, we are verifying the facts of the situation.

Example: If a friend says his arm hurts, we can sympathize with him or offer help—validating that indeed his arm does hurt.

Example: If a person feels intensely sad following the death of her dog, we can both acknowledge her feelings, and also verify that it makes sense and is reasonable to feel so sad following the death of a beloved dog.

Example: When we are going out for dinner, if one person says he doesn't have much money to spend, we can validate that we hear and understand this by suggesting an inexpensive restaurant for a meal.

Example: If a knowledgeable person is taking us on a tour, we can follow her, validating that she knows what she is doing and where she is going. Her behavior makes sense.

2. When We Validate, We Communicate That We Understand the Person's Perspective

✓ We acknowledge that all emotions, thoughts, and behaviors have a cause, even if we don't know what the cause is.

Example: If George forgets an appointment with Mike, Mike can acknowledge that it is understandable, given how much is going on in George's life right now.

Example: If Sara drops and breaks something very valuable that Ruth owns, Ruth can acknowledge that it was an accident.

Example: If Dave has an alcohol problem and keeps relapsing, his friend Keisha can communicate that she understands that urges to drink can feel irresistible, and that it can be really hard to get off of alcohol.

✓ ### 3. Validation Does Not Equal Agreement

Validation does not necessarily mean liking or agreeing with what the other person is doing, saying, or feeling. It does not mean agreeing with what you do not agree with. lt means understanding where the other person is coming from.

Example: A friend had two beers at a concert; then, when driving home an hour after the second one, he was stopped and given a DUI citation. We might say, "I understand how it made complete sense to you to think you would be safe driving after waiting an hour."

💬 **Discussion Point:** How can we validate without agreeing? Many people get this point confused. Elicit ideas from participants for how to validate the other person in the following situations, or in situations the individuals bring up. (1) In a political discussion, a person says something we strongly disagree with (e.g., "I can see you and I come from very different political sides"). (2) A person wants to go to a movie we don't want to go to (e.g., "I see why you would want to go to that movie. I am really hoping we can go to this other movie").

✓ ### 4. Validation Does Not Mean "Making" Something Valid

Validation does not mean endorsing or verifying that which is invalid.

Example: "If someone is angry at you for eating the last piece of cake, and you did not eat it, you might validate that the person is angry, but you would not validate that you actually ate the cake."

B. Why Validate?

1. Validation Improves Our Interactions with Others

It shows that:

- We are listening and understand.
- We are being nonjudgmental.
- We can see the facts or truth of a situation.

2. It Improves Interpersonal Effectiveness

It reduces several obstacles to effectiveness:

- Pressure to prove who is right.
- Negative reactivity.
- Anger.

3. It Makes Problem Solving, Closeness, and Support Possible

It also makes others more receptive to what we have to say.

💬 **Discussion Point:** Elicit times when participants have felt invalidated, and contrast those with other times when they felt validated. How were the two times different? How did they feel each time? How did it affect their behavior each time?

4. Invalidation Hurts

✓ *Example:* Bill is sitting in an important meeting, listening to a presentation by a visitor to his company, when he accidentally knocks his notebook computer off the edge of the table, making a loud noise on the floor. His team leader stops, turns, and says, "Geez, stop multitasking! We've got an important guest." Bill feels extremely embarrassed and angry, since he'd been paying close attention to the talk and was using his computer to take notes for the team. He later recounts the story to his partner when he gets home, who replies, "Why do you keep doing this to yourself? You're never going to get a promotion at this rate."

💬 **Discussion Point:** Ask participants what they think Bill must be feeling after his team leader's and partner's responses. Why are these responses so hurtful? What is missing from their responses? Highlight that what is missing is any understanding of Bill, his behavior, and his feelings.

💬 **Discussion Point:** Ask participants what would be a validating thing the team leader could do. A reasonable response here would be for the team leader simply to ignore the dropping of the computer, since ignoring it would imply that it is insignificant and nondeliberate. Next, ask, "What would be a validating response Bill's partner could give?" If group members have trouble generating a validating response, then offer an example of one, such as "Oh, Bill, that must have been so upsetting and frustrating for you, especially since you were doing everyone a favor by taking notes." If participants say that this sounds too "sappy," encourage them to put into words a validating response they would welcome from someone.

✓ **C. Important Things to Validate**

✓ **1. Validate Only the Valid**

Validating only what is valid is very important, because when we validate something we are not only verifying it; we are also reinforcing the experiences, emotions, thoughts, words, or actions that we validate.

2. Validate the Facts of a Situation

3. Validate a Person's Experiences, Feelings/Emotions, Beliefs, Opinions, or Thoughts

✓ *Example:* If Antwan says his arm hurts and therefore he should not go to school on an important testing day, Mom might validate the pain in the arm, but invalidate the idea that staying home is necessary.

Example: If Maria feels intensely afraid of going to bed without her shoes on, Emma may validate that it makes sense (given that Maria was attacked by an intruder in her bed), but not validate that going to bed without shoes on is dangerous.

Example: If Jorge is upset, saying he failed an important exam, Juan may look at his passing score and validate that he didn't do as well as he wanted to, but invalidate that he failed the exam.

4. Validate Suffering and Difficulties

In the three examples above, Mom, Emma, and Juan all validate the other person's suffering or difficulties.

✓ **D. How Can You Tell What Is Valid?**

Something is valid when it is any or all of the following.

1. Relevant and Meaningful to the Case or Circumstance

Example: When asked whether you think Bill Jones has been a good leader, it is relevant and meaningful to discuss Bill Jones' leadership skills and beliefs; ignoring Bill Jones and talking instead about how terrible you think Susan Smith is as a leader is irrelevant.

✓ **2. Well Grounded or Justifiable (in Terms of Empirical Facts, Logically Correct Inference, or Generally Accepted Authority)**

Example: It is valid to say it is raining when it in fact is raining, but not when the sky is clear.

✓ **3. Appropriate to the End in View (i.e., Effective for Reaching the Individual's Ultimate Goals)**

Example: If Joanne (who has a drinking problem) says that drinking makes her feel better immediately, we can validate the fact that alcohol has this effect, but also invalidate that drinking to solve problems will be effective when Joanne wants to go up the corporate ladder.

✓ **E. How to Validate**

The levels of validation below and on Interpersonal Effectiveness Handout 18 are the same as those that therapists use in individual DBT treatment, and that all team members use on DBT teams. For the most part, they build on each other. At each subsequent level from 1 to 6, the validation is stronger.

> **Note to Leaders:** Review Handout 18 and read the examples. If time permits, ask participants for other examples.

✓ **1. Pay Attention**

Tell participants: "When you pay attention, you treat the individual and what he or she is saying or doing as relevant and meaningful—as requiring serious attention. It communicates that the person, in the moment, is visible, seen, and important to you. Be mindful of your own nonverbal reactions in order to avoid invalidation—for example, rolling your eyes, sucking your teeth, walking away, or saying, 'I don't care what you say.'"

As noted in the discussion of the mindfulness-of-others skills (see Section XII, above), one of the most important characteristics of a good relationship is that people pay attention to each other. People will stop bringing us flowers if we ignore them when they do. People will stop wanting to be around us if we ignore them when they are around.

Even when we disagree or don't understand, we need to pay attention to people's behavior, beliefs, and feelings. How would we ever learn anything new or get to know others if we ignored them whenever we disagree?

Emphasize to participants that paying attention is *not* agreeing or approving of a person's activities, emotions, beliefs, or other experiences. It simply says that the person is alive and counts.

When we *ignore* a person, we communicate that the person's activities, feelings, beliefs, or experiences are not relevant, meaningful, or important to us. Although in the grand scheme of things all beings are important, much of what people do and say is either unimportant, irrelevant, or ineffective. When this is the case, it makes sense to ignore them temporarily, particularly if we want them to stop what they are doing or saying.

Examples: We might ignore people when they throw a tantrum and only pay attention to them when they ask for what they want. We might ignore a person who is insulting us rather than attack back. If a person keeps changing topics or changing his or her mind about something, we might ignore that also and just keep doing whatever we are doing. If a TV commentator is known for exaggerating facts, we might ignore that show and watch something else.

Practice Exercise: If this has not already been done, use the exercise for paying attention described in the GIVE skills (see Section VI, B, 2, "[Act] Interested").

✓ **2. Reflect Back without Judgment**

Say to participants, "The goal at the next level of validation is to communicate that you have accurately heard what the other person has said. Be open to correction. It is important not to add your own assumptions and interpretations."

Example: A person might say in a desperate voice, "She hates me." To validate, we might say,

"So you are feeling desperate and really certain that she hates you . . . " (leaving off the statement "That's silly, because you should know by now that she does not hate you").

Emphasize to participants that reflecting back does *not* imply approval or encouragement. Nor does it imply evaluation of effectiveness or value. To validate does not mean that we necessarily agree or think that this is the only perspective possible. Validation at this level does not require us to add, in word, deed, or nonverbal response, that the other person's responses correspond to the empirical facts when they may not.

Example: We can validate that a person thinks someone is threatening them without agreeing that they are actually being threatened. We can validate that a person feels angry without agreeing on what the person is angry about.

Discussion Point: Elicit from participants times when others have not heard what they had to say accurately. How did it feel? Discuss.

Practice Exercise: Pair participants up. Ask one person in each pair to describe a situation in the last week from his or her life or skills practice. Instruct the other person to listen and then reflect back to the talker. At first, the person's reflecting should try to offer an accurate understanding of what was said. Then halfway through, they are to reflect back a misunderstanding of what the person said. Instruct the talker to keep going, trying to explain the situation to the listener. After some time, ask participants to switch roles and have the listener talk and the talker listen. Discuss how it felt to be understood and to be misunderstood.

✓ **3. "Read Minds"**

Explain to participants: "Level 3 validation is figuring out what is going on with a person without his or her telling you in words.

In everyday language, this is known as 'interpersonal sensitivity.' There are a number of ways to read what is going on with another person. Voice tone and body language, including facial expression, can communicate aspects of experience that a person has not put into words. Observe the person's posture, face, and behavior. Put that information together with what is happening and what you already know about the person. At times just knowing the situation, such as when a loved one has died suddenly or a person has just gotten engaged, may be enough to enable you to read what is going on with the person. Then express how you think the person may be feeling, wishing, or thinking. When someone knows how you feel or think without your having to tell them directly, it is almost always experienced as validating. At a minimum, such validation communicates that you know the other person—that you are validating the individual as him- or herself."

To practice this level of validation, ask participants to find a word to describe the feeling they are seeing in the other person, and then tell the other person what they see, as in these examples.

Example: "I can see you are really excited about this idea."

Example: "I'm so sorry you didn't get the loan for the mortgage on that wonderful house. That must be really disappointing." (This is more validating than paying attention without saying anything or saying only, "I'm sorry about that.")

Example: "You must be wondering what is going on with us changing the schedule so radically."

a. Use Caution and Be Open to Correction

Level 3 validation can be fraught with danger and can have the potential for great harm. The chief danger is that an incorrect or only partially correct description of the other person's private experiences will be shoved down the person's throat. Say to participants: "Do not use consequences or observed functions of behavior as proof of another's private intent. If you feel manipulated by what someone says or does, do not assume that the intention was to manipulate you. If a friend is late picking you up, do not assume the person doesn't care about you. Effective Level 3 validation requires you to accept that you might have misread the other person."

b. Offer a Reading of the Other Person a Little Tentatively

It is a good idea to offer a reading of another person as a hypothesis or guess—for example, "I'm guessing that you were really disappointed about that," instead of "You're really feeling disappointed about that." Remind participants: "Remain open to being corrected by the other person. Remember, no one can actually observe another's internal thoughts and feelings."

Discussion Point: Elicit from participants times when others asked them for something or said no to a request, with no apparent understanding of how it would affect the participants. How did it feel? What do they wish others had said or done differently? Discuss.

✓   **4. *Communicate an Understanding of the Causes***

Say to participants: "Look for how the feelings, thoughts, and actions of a person make sense, given the other person's history and current situation, even if you don't approve of the behaviors, emotions, or actions themselves. The goal is to communicate to the person that his or her behavior is understandable in light of previous events or circumstances. In essence, you are saying, 'Given your history of X, how could your experience/behavior be other than Y?'"

The important point to make here is that all behavior is ultimately understandable and sensible if we consider the causes.

a. Learning History

We can communicate that a person's behavior makes sense because of the person's learning history, even if it does not make sense in terms of current events.

Example: We can say that it makes sense to be afraid of walking down an alley if a person was assaulted in a dark alley last week, even if this particular alley is well lighted, it is daytime, and the neighborhood is a safe place to walk.

Example: We can say to a recent immigrant to the United States that it makes sense that the person makes a lot of mistakes in English if he or she never spoke English before.

Example: We can tell someone we understand the person's anger at us, given that someone told the person we stole his or her money, even when we are not the ones who stole it.

Example: We can communicate that it makes sense to be somewhat hopeless about a new weight loss program if every program the other person has tried before failed.

b. A Previous Event

We can communicate that a person's behavior makes sense because of a previous event, even if it does not make sense in terms of present facts.

Example: We can say that it makes sense to carry an umbrella walking to work if the weather report said it will be raining today, even if it is sunny and bright all day.

✓   *Example:* A friend hears that others got invitations and went to another friend's birthday party and he did not. We can say it makes sense for him to wonder whether he was left out on purpose. This makes sense even if the facts are that (unknown to both of you) his invitation was eaten by the dog.

c. A Mental or Physical Disorder

We can communicate that a person's behavior makes sense because of a mental or physical disorder, even if it does not make sense in terms of facts.

Example: We can say it makes sense that another person would get tired easily (and much more tired than others) after even light exertion if the person is just getting over cancer treatments.

Example: We can say it makes sense that a person would feel hopeless if the person has depression, even if the situation is not hopeless.

Example: We can tell someone that his or her interpretation that we are angry makes sense, given our gruff voice tone, even if we are anxious instead of angry.

✓ **5. Acknowledge the Valid**

Level 5 validation is communicating that a person's experiences make sense because they fit the present facts, are well grounded, are logically correct, or are effective for their ultimate goals. This level of validation is at the heart of DBT. It is the answer of yes to the question "Can this be true?" It involves looking for how the person's behavior makes sense because it is a reasonable or normative response to a current situation.

Example: Sharon is sometimes shy in groups. Now she is attending a DBT skills training group. When she occasionally speaks up in the group, John on the other side of the table gives her an angry, threatening look. After one group session, Sharon says to a friend in the group with her, "John was giving me really mean looks. I don't want to sit anywhere near him next time." A response that would validate Sharon in terms of what actually happened would be "Boy, I really understand, and I wouldn't want to sit near him either if I were you. He gave you quite a look when you spoke up."

✓ Tell participants: "At Level 5, also *act* on what you view as valid. Often *not acting* on what a person says or does is invalidating. For example, a person is screaming for help in a house on fire; the responding firefighter just looks up and says, 'I see you need saving,' but doesn't try to save the person. This would be enormously invalidating."

Examples: "If you are criticized for not taking out the garbage on your day, admit that it is your day and take it out. If someone presents a problem, help the person solve it (unless they just want to be heard). If people are hungry, give them food. Acknowledge the effort a person is making."

Again, however, caution is needed. We can insult and invalidate a person if we try to validate something because of past causes or personal characteristics, when the present circumstances make a response valid.

✓ *Example:* "You are criticized for not taking out the garbage on your day, and you respond by saying, 'You are just upset with me because you had a bad day,' or you say that the other person's upset is due to events in childhood. These are both Level 4 validation. But using such personal or past events avoids acknowledging that it is reasonable for the other person to want you to take out the garbage when it is your turn." Not only is it not validating, it is often insulting as well.

✓ **6. Show Equality**

Say to participants: "Respond to the other person as having equal status with yourself and as being entitled to equal respect. Level 6 validation is the opposite of treating the person in a condescending manner or as overly fragile. It is responding to the individual as capable of effective and reasonable behavior, rather than assuming that he or she is either inadequate or superior. It implies being your genuine self within the relationship."

Practice Exercise: One at a time, have each participant briefly describe a difficult or frustrating part of his or her day or week; have the person to their left say something validating (and brief) to the speaker. Then that person shares with the person to his or her left, who in turn says something validating, and so on. Continue until all participants (including the leaders) have shared and been validated. Then list on the board all the validating behaviors people noticed, and match them with the methods of validating listed on Interpersonal Effectiveness Handout 18.

Continue: "It can be very hard to validate when you do not understand the other person's point of view, or when the other's feelings or behaviors make no sense to you. In these situations, you can do one of two things: Either validate the person's feelings or point of view but not what the person does; or admit that you don't understand but want to understand. This is an example of being authentic and treating the person as an equal."

Example: Some people might say that they cannot understand why a person engages in dysfunctional behavior. The key here is to recognize that most dysfunctional behavior is a response to emotional pain when a person cannot find another way to reduce the pain. In these situations, a validating response could be "I can see that you are obviously in a lot of pain." In this case, we are validating the emotion, though not the behavior.

Example: An alternative strategy that can be very effective is to say, "I know you want me to understand this, and, believe me, I want to understand this, but I just can't get it. Let's keep talking. Tell me again." This alternative strategy, presented in a nonjudgmental way, communicates that our lack of understanding is the problem in the conversation, not the invalidity of the other person's emotions or behavior. It also communicates deep interest in the other's difficulties.

Practice Exercise: If you have time, distribute Interpersonal Effectiveness Handout 18a: Identifying Validation, and explain the task. Give participants time to check the more effective validating response for each pair. Discuss answers. If time permits, ask participants if they have other situations where it is not clear to them what would be the more effective validating course of action between two options.

Correct responses for Handout 18a are as follows: 1B, 2A, 3A, 4B, 5A, 6B, 7B, 8B.

F. Recovering from Invalidation

Review Interpersonal Effectiveness Handout 19: Recovering from Invalidation with participants.

Begin by saying: "Recovering from invalidation can be just as important as validating others. There are several types of invalidation. Some are helpful and some are harmful."

1. Helpful Invalidation

Say to participants: "When your opinions, beliefs, or behaviors are invalidated, and they are in fact based on false or inaccurate information, then invalidation can be helpful. When done with respect, these interactions are usually not distressing and may even be sought. For example, giving and receiving corrective feedback and engaging in debates about opinions can be critical to intellectual stimulation and personal growth."

a. Corrective Feedback

Continue: "Corrective feedback is information that clearly shows that your facts are wrong, or your beliefs don't make logical sense in terms of the facts, or your behavior is not effective for reaching your goals. When the feedback is correct and given in a nonjudgmental manner that is open to discussion and to your point of view, you may agree, change your mind, feel fine, and go forward."

💬 **Discussion Point:** Elicit from participants times when they have been told that their facts are incorrect (and they actually were incorrect). Elicit times when they have been shown that their opinion on something does not make logical sense.

b. Opinion Debates

Go on: "Opinion debates can occur when a person disagrees with your opinions or beliefs, such as a political point of view, religious beliefs, philosophical positions, or other beliefs that another person could reasonably disagree with. The person may argue strongly against your point of view. Whether you feel invalidated usually depends on whether the other person treats your views with respect and listens to you even when disagreeing. It is easy to feel fine after a hearty but respectful discussion or debate and continue on your way."

💬 **Discussion Point:** Elicit from participants times when they have heated political debates with friends, family members, or colleagues. Discuss who disagreed with them and how they felt about it.

2. Corrosive Invalidation

Say to participants: "But invalidation can be exceptionally distressing when your point of view is disregarded while the other person's validity is unquestioned. How distressing this is depends on the importance of the person invalidating you and the importance of your own position to your self-respect and ability to trust yourself. There are as many levels of harmful invalidation as there are levels of validation. Here are several examples of harmful invalidation."

a. Being Ignored

"Others do not pay attention to what you do or have to say, even when what you are doing or want to say is valid and relevant. You are treated as an unimportant and irrelevant person. This is particularly harmful if this pattern is persistent and long-lasting. The problem is that you can easily start feeling unimportant and irrelevant."

b. Not Being Understood

"Others don't understand what you have to say, what you think, or how you feel, even when you keep trying to tell them. What you say about yourself or your experience simply does not get through to the other person. It may be that the person is insensitive, unable to 'get' where you are coming from, or has his or her own opinions about you, no matter what you say or do.

The problem is that you may start to question your ability to communicate to others. You can even begin to worry that they are right about you and you are wrong."

c. Being Misread

"Others not only misread you, but are insensitive to what is going on with you unless you spell it out for them in clear A-B-C language. The problem is that in these cases, it is easy to feel as if you and your responses must be very different from others. You may also start to believe that the other persons are sensitive to you but just don't care about you. This can lead to believing that you are inadequate or that there is something wrong with you."

d. Being Misinterpreted

"Other persons give understandable but incorrect causes for your behavior and your experiences. You say how you feel, and the other persons say, 'No, you don't feel that way.' Or they may misinterpret with great certainty your intent for doing or saying things. Their inferences about your intent are often pejorative and hurtful, and may be based on how your behavior affects them: 'I feel manipulated; therefore, you must have intended to manipulate me.' Your reasons for doing or not doing things are misconstrued often in ways that make you look motivated to be incorrect, ineffective, or otherwise problematic. Valid reasons for your behavior, such as previous learning or biological characteristics, are ignored. It is assumed that if you wanted to be different, you would be different. The problem is that it is hard to feel accepted and cared about when people often misinterpret you."

e. Having Current Facts Ignored or Denied

"Facts that explain your reasonable behavior are discounted, rendered unimportant, or distorted. For example, you are late because of traffic, and your friend responds, 'Oh, you are always late; don't give me that.' Responses that make perfect sense under present circumstances are explained in terms of the past. For example, a current boss who repeatedly fails to come through with promised support says, 'You mistrust me because your previous boss made promises she didn't keep.' The problem is that when current facts are ignored or denied, it can sometimes lead to serious consequences—for example, when you are abused but the abuser denies it, or you are innocent but are found guilty of a crime."

f. Receiving Unequal Treatment

"Others treat you as very different from them in essential ways, even when you are not so different. You are treated as inferior, a child, fragile, or unable to really understand the other person. The problem is that when you are treated as different from others, it is hard to feel that you are part of the group."

3. Traumatic Invalidation

> **Note to Leaders:** The following discussion is particularly appropriate for groups of clients who have suffered from physical or sexual abuse or other traumatizing events, and/or who have a formal diagnosis of PTSD. Personalize the discussion as appropriate for a particular group.

Traumatic invalidation is extreme or repetitive invalidation of individuals' significant private experiences, characteristics identified as important aspects of themselves, or reactions to themselves or to the world. Traumatic invalidation can be focused on individuals' perceptions of themselves and of their environment, sensory experiences, thoughts and beliefs, emotions and desires, and/or actions. There is frequently a violation of the persons' familiar ideas about themselves and the world, and of the integrity of their own perceptions about themselves and their environments.

Typically, traumatic invalidation comes from a very important person, group, or authority whom an individual is or was dependent on for his or her sense of personal integrity and well-being. It can occur only once, as when a mother refuses to believe that her daughter is telling the truth when she reports sexual abuse by her father, or when a witness falsely testifies that a person committed a crime. Or it can be an accumulation of oversights and misreadings of emotions, motives, and actions by an important person or institution, or by part or all of a family or other important group, that leads to psychological exclusion or perception of the individual as an outsider.

The problem with such extreme or pervasive invalidation is that it results in a threat to the person's psychological integrity and a confused sense of internal veracity and credibility, putting the person in a state of pervasive insecurity. Common sequelae of such invalidation include intrusive thoughts and memories; reexperiencing of the invalidation; intense shame, confusion, anger, and defensiveness; markedly increased interpersonal sensitivity to subsequent invalidation; intense efforts to get validation from the invalidator, as well as persistent efforts to obtain validation from others; and avoidance of contact with invalidators and difficulties in trusting other people.

4. Recovery from Harmful Invalidation

Give Interpersonal Effectiveness Handout 19 to participants. Say to them: "There are many things you can do to recover from harmful invalidation. Here are some of them."

✓ **a. Check the Facts**

"Check *all* the facts in a nondefensive way. Check them out also with another person you can trust to validate the valid. This is a critical step after invalidation, so that you do not reexperience invalidation."

b. Acknowledge and Work to Change Your Invalid Responses

"If your responses were incorrect or ineffective, admit it and try to change what you are thinking, saying, or doing. Also, stop blaming; it rarely helps a situation."

c. Drop Judgmental Self-Statements

"Even if you did make a mistake or believed something that is not correct, it does not mean you are 'stupid' or even to blame for not knowing the facts. Remember that there are often many valid reasons for invalid behavior."

d. Remind Yourself That All Behavior Is Caused

"It is also important to remind yourself that all behavior is caused, and that this is true of your responses also. Remember that you are and have always been doing the best you can, given the circumstances and your personal history."

"Admit that it hurts to be invalidated by others even if they are right."

e. Be Compassionate toward Yourself. Practice Self-Soothing. Admit That It Hurts to Be Invalidated by Others Even If They Are Right.

"Keeping a stiff upper lip may be needed while around the person invalidating you, but on your own, there is every reason to be compassionate and self-soothing. It does hurt to be invalidated."

f. Remind Yourself That Invalidation, Even When You Are Right, Is Rarely a Catastrophe

"Keep in mind that invalid responses—either someone else's or your own—are generally not the end of the world."

g. Acknowledge Your Valid Responses

"If your responses were valid under the circumstances, acknowledge that you are correct, or that your responses are reasonable and normal for the situation. Self-validation can take a lot of work and a lot of verbal processing with others. But it is well worth the effort."

h. Describe Your Experiences and Actions in a Supportive Environment

"Describing your experiences and behaviors can be vital in letting go of invalidation. The describing process is similar to exposure therapy for trauma and anxiety disorders. Through the experience of nonreinforced shame and personal invalidity evoked in describing, you can gradually learn that your responses are understandable and valid in important ways."

✓ 👥 **Practice Exercise:** Ask participants to check off on Interpersonal Effectiveness Handout 19 each set of behaviors they have difficulty with. Then read each one and ask who checked it off. Consider using this information to give homework assignments for the week.

✓ **i. Use All the Steps for Validating on Yourself**

"Validating yourself may seem like a very simple point, but people often forget this. Each level of validation we have talked about can be used on yourself."

- "*Pay attention* to your own behavior (thoughts, feelings, and actions)."
- "*Reflect* by describing to yourself your own private (thoughts and feelings) and public (actions) behaviors."
- "*Be mindful of your own emotions and situation.* Be sensitive to what your emotions and the situation may be telling you about what you need."
- "*Try to understand* your deepest thoughts and feelings. Again, recognize that all of your behavior is caused, and therefore inherently understandable. Remember that you are doing the best you can."
- "*Acknowledge the valid* by standing up for yourself when your behavior is valid, even if others don't see it."
- "*Treat yourself with respect.* See yourself as equal to others."

✓ **j. Practice Radical Acceptance of Yourself**

"Practicing radical self-acceptance requires acknowledgment that being invalidated by others hurts. It requires compassion toward yourself and self-soothing. It will ultimately be much easier if you can also practice radical acceptance of the person who has invalidated you." Encourage participants to use some of the reality acceptance exercises in Distress Tolerance Handout 11b: Practicing Radical Acceptance Step by Step and Distress Tolerance Handout 14: Half-Smiling and Willing Hands. For example, imagining the invalidating person with a half-smile and willing hands can be very useful.

Practice Exercise: If you have time, distribute Interpersonal Effectiveness Handout 19a: Identifying Self-Validation, and explain the task. Give participants time to check the more effective validating response for each pair. Discuss answers. If time permits, ask participants if they have other situations where it is not clear to them what would be the more effective validating course of action between two options.

Correct responses to Handout 19a are as follows: 1A, 2B, 3A, 4B, 5A, 6B.

XVII. STRATEGIES FOR CHANGING BEHAVIOR (INTERPERSONAL EFFECTIVENESS HANDOUT 20–22A)[1]

> **Main Point:** There are very effective strategies for increasing behaviors that we want in ourselves or others (reinforcement, shaping) and for decreasing behaviors that we do not want (extinction, satiating, punishment). The secret to being effective at behavior change is to learn these strategies and put them into action.
>
> **Interpersonal Effectiveness Handout 20: Strategies for Increasing the Probability of Desired Behaviors.** Review the main points on this handout. It is important that participants understand the concepts of reinforcement (a consequence that increases behavior), shaping (reinforcement of small steps leading to a larger change), and intermittent reinforcement (occasional reinforcement that makes a behavior persist).
>
> **Interpersonal Effectiveness Handout 21: Strategies for Decreasing or Stopping Undesired Behaviors.** This handout teaches extinction, satiation, and punishment. It is very important to teach clearly the distinction between extinction and punishment.
>
> **Interpersonal Effectiveness Handout 22: Tips for Using Behavior Change Strategies Effectively.** This handout outlines important issues in selecting and implementing consequences.

Interpersonal Effectiveness Handout 22a: Identifying Effective Behavior Change Strategies *(Optional)*. Use this handout if you have extra time, or give it out as homework and then discuss it at the next session. The correct responses are listed at the end of this section's teaching points, as well as at the end of this chapter's introduction.

Interpersonal Effectiveness Worksheet 14: Changing Behavior with Reinforcement; Interpersonal Effectiveness Worksheet 15: Changing Behavior by Extinguishing or Punishing It. It is important that participants actually try the behavior change strategies they are learning in this module. Be sure to assign one or both of these worksheets as homework. Review the instructions on the worksheet with participants and carefully review their homework in the next session. These skills are often difficult for therapists and skills trainers to learn. It may also take some time for participants to learn and use them.

Note to Leaders: One of the best and easiest books to read on behavior change is a book titled *Don't Shoot the Dog,*[25] which lists both effective and ineffective ways to promote change. The examples are very good, and assigning this book can be very helpful. It is routinely assigned for parents in our adolescent DBT programs. Many of the adolescents also read it.

A. Strategies for Increasing the Probability of Desired Behaviors

✓ ### 1. What Is Reinforcement?

Reinforcement is *any* consequence that increases the frequency of a behavior. **All human beings, as well as other animals, are influenced by the consequences of their behaviors.**

Note to Leaders: It is essential that participants get the main point here: Reinforcement is a consequence that increases a behavior. Have them repeat it to you. Tell participants to memorize this definition. Throughout teaching these skills, periodically ask them to tell you what reinforcement or a reinforcer is.

💬 **Discussion Point:** Ask participants what behavior of their own they would like to increase. Suggest writing it down on the line at the top of Interpersonal Effectiveness Handout 20.

✓ ### a. It Is Not Necessary for People to Be Aware That Their Behavior Is Being Influenced by Consequences

What is required for a reinforcer to work is that an individual is aware of the reinforcing event's having occurred (e.g., sounds would not reinforce a deaf person; visual pictures would not reinforce a blind person). What is *not* required is that the person be aware of the connection between the reinforcer and his or her own behavior.[26, 27]

✓ ### b. People Commonly Reinforce Others' Behavior without Realizing That They Are Doing It

Example: "If every time a person gets angry and attacks you, you give the person what he or she wants, you will see that over time the tendency of the other person to get angry goes up."

Example: "If whenever you bring up a painful topic, a friend of yours with an alcohol problem starts feeling an intense urge to have an alcoholic drink and tells you of the urge, and then you immediately sidestep talking about the painful topic, you can predict that the friend's urges to drink will become more frequent when you start discussing painful topics the friend wants to avoid."

c. Reinforcement Is the Most Effective Way to Increase the Frequency of a Behavior

Reinforcement tells a person what will be rewarded in specific situations (and what will not be rewarded).

If a maladaptive behavior is being reinforced, it is very common for others to believe that the person behaves this way on purpose to get the reinforcer. This is based on the premises that individuals know what is reinforcing their own behavior, and that reinforcement of behavior is associated with behavioral intent. Neither of these is necessarily true; however, these beliefs are the genesis of much pain and suffering. Crying, suicide attempts, tantrums, and pouting are written off as attempts to get attention. Anger, tiredness, anxiety, and fear are written off as attempts to avoid doing what is needed. A cry for help is viewed as manipulative, and so on. Alas, such inferences are pejorative, often wrong, and very hurtful.

We need to remember the point made above: **People are often not aware of what reinforcers are actually controlling their behavior.** Although an individual has to experience a reinforcer, the individual does not have to be aware of the connection between the consequence and his or her own behavior for reinforcement to work. Statements about what is controlling one's own behavior are opinions. Alas, opinions can be based on many things other than the facts.

✓ 2. Why Reinforce?

Some people think that behavior should occur on its own—that we should not have to reinforce to get individuals to do the "right" thing. This is a basic misunderstanding of human (and animal) behavior. One of the most important tasks of rearing children, for example, is systematically reinforcing effective behaviors. In essence, knowing what is "right" is learned. Doing the right thing is also learned. Reinforcement is an important way that we learn. The idea that people "should" do the right thing just because it is right ignores the fact that all behavior is caused.

> **Note to Leaders:** This point can be very controversial. Discuss with participants. Use as many examples as needed to get the points across. If necessary, bring up a lot more examples. If you find it useful, go to very extreme examples of how effective reinforcement can be, such as in "brainwashing."

✓ 3. Two Types of Reinforcement

a. Reinforcement as Reward

Reinforcement as reward (sometimes called "positive reinforcement") increases the frequency of behavior by adding a positive consequence.

Examples: Praise, frequent flyer miles on an airline, an earned privilege, money, a smile, or a satisfying outcome to an interpersonal situation can each increase behavior when it occurs as a consequence of a specific behavior.

✓ 💬 **Discussion Point:** Ask participants what things would be rewards or positive consequences for the behavior they have chosen to increase. That is, what would make them more likely to engage in the behavior? Suggest writing down individual reinforcers on the handout.

> **Note to Leaders:** Guide participants to keep reinforcers realistic, safe, and appropriate for the goal behavior. For instance, a new car is not a realistic reinforcer for exercising 5 days a week for a month; drinking alcohol, using drugs, and letting go of responsibilities are not effective; going to Africa on a safari may be unrealistic. Also encourage participants to search for meaningful reinforcers beyond just money, such as time spent with a parent, a child, or a friend.

b. Reinforcement as Relief

Reinforcement as relief (sometimes called "negative reinforcement") increases the frequency of behavior by removing an unpleasant condition.

Examples: "A headache goes away if you take an aspirin; your boss stops nagging you when you get your reports in on time; people stop bothering you for information if you throw a tantrum; an annoying noise stops when you buckle your seatbelt in your car; feelings of sadness and fear lessen when you drink a lot of alcohol; a back pain gets relieved when you get a massage."

✓ 💬 **Discussion Point:** Elicit from participants consequences of specific behaviors that provide relief in their lives. Suggest writing these down on the handout. Ask what kinds of behaviors—their own or others'—are maintained by ending unpleasant and/or painful conditions.

> **Note to Leaders:** Negative reinforcement can be a touchy topic to discuss in a group setting. Often dysfunctional behaviors, such as self-cutting, drinking, using drugs, or lying, are reinforced by subsequent relief of emotional suffering. Telling someone, "I am suicidal," can be reinforced by the listener's responding with greater sympathy or switching from a painful topic of conversation to focusing on the suicide ideation.

💬 **Discussion Point:** Ask participants to identify negative situations or sources of discomfort that they would like relieved or removed.

Example: A teenage girl might mention a parent's nagging her to clean her room. What new behavior might help reduce this discomfort? For instance, if the teen's cleaning her room led to a reduction in the parent's nagging, the adolescent might be more likely to pick up after herself in the future. Elicit one or two other examples from the group.

💬 **Discussion Point:** Elicit from participants times when they have given people they love much more time when the loved one is in trouble than when the person is not.

✓ ### 4. *What Is Shaping?*

Shaping is reinforcing small steps that lead toward a bigger goal. Each successive step toward a larger goal needs to be reinforced until the new behavior is stable. This increases the chances of continuing to work toward the goal.

✓ *Example:* "You can take small, reinforced steps toward finding a job. Apply online for one job on Monday and reinforce that. Apply for two jobs on Tuesday and reinforce that. Continue until a good part of every day is spent looking for a job."

Example: "If your goal is to get up early five mornings a week to exercise for half an hour, you can first reinforce yourself for getting out of bed early, then reinforce yourself for exercising for 10 minutes, then 20 minutes, and so on."

5. *Why Use Shaping?*

Shaping is useful because some behaviors are very difficult to learn in one step, particularly behaviors that are complex and require a lot of steps.

💬 **Discussion Point:** Ask participants whether they or family members have ever been frustrated with themselves for not starting a large project until the night before. How would shaping apply? Elicit examples. Examples for writing a report might include deciding on these steps: Step 1 would be to sit down and outline the report the week before the due date and then, once that's done, to allow some TV time. Step 2 would be to write the introduction and provide a small reinforcement for that, and so on.

💬 **Discussion Point:** Ask participants to identify one or two steps on the way to changing a behavior of their own that they want to change.

✓ **6. *Timing Counts in Reinforcement***

Tell participants: "Reinforce immediately following the desired behavior. If you wait too long, the reinforcer won't be connected with the behavior."

✓ *Example:* "You are trying to improve your backhand in tennis, and your coach is observing 30 swings. Would you prefer your coach to tell you, 'That's the swing! Nice job!' immediately after you use the right form, or would you prefer the coach to wait until you are done and then say, 'Your 14th swing—I liked that one'?

👥 **Practice Exercise:** Play the "clicker game." To play this game, you need to bring a loud clicker (or whistle) to the skills training group. You then ask one person to volunteer to play the role of the learner (which we call the "dog") and one person to play the role of the "dog trainer." The task of the dog will be to learn new behaviors taught by the trainer. Once a person is selected to play the dog, that person goes out of the room. The trainer's task is to teach the dog new behaviors by reinforcing successive steps toward the behavioral sequence that is being taught. Before bringing the person playing the dog back into the room, the group decides on what sequence of behaviors to teach the dog. Examples might be for the dog to walk to a whiteboard, turn around two times, and then go sit down, or for the dog to walk in and then go to a window and close the blinds. An easier task might be to train the dog simply to turn around or just walk to the window. Do not make the task too easy or too hard. Instruct the person who is playing the dog that when he or she comes into the room, the trainer is going to try to teach him or her new behaviors by clicking the clicker every time he or she is engaging in the behaviors wanted. The task of the trainer is to click the clicker (or blow the whistle) immediately after every time the dog takes a step toward the desired behavior. The trainer should *not* use the clicker or whistle when the dog is not engaging in the correct sequence of behaviors. If the person playing the dog gets off track, the trainer can ask the dog to go back to the door and start over. Starting over can be done multiple times in one game. Once the game is over, discuss how it went and what participants learned.

Note to Leaders: It is essential that you practice playing the clicker game before you teach it.

7. *Reinforcement Schedules*

Say to participants: "When and how often a behavior is reinforced are very important if you want the behavior to persist without your having to reinforce it every time it occurs. There are several different types of reinforcement schedules."

✓ **a. Continuous Reinforcement**

Say: "In continuous reinforcement, every instance of a designated behavior is reinforced. This can be important at the beginning when you are trying to shape and establish a new behavior. Continuous reinforcement will get a behavior to occur at very high frequency. However, if that is all you do, the behavior will disappear quickly as soon as you stop reinforcing it."

✓ *Example:* "If your car starts every time you turn the ignition key but one day it does not, you may try to get it going a few times, but you will quickly stop. If you have a car that often does not start but usually does after many tries, you may keep trying for a really long time."

Example: "If your sick mother always answers the phone but does not today, you may drop everything and run over to her home. If she only intermittently picks up the phone, you may keep calling her for several days."

✓   *Example:* "Putting money into a vending machine ordinarily produces the soda you want. Once the vending machine does not work once or twice, you are unlikely to keep trying that machine."

b. Intermittent Reinforcement

Continue: "In intermittent reinforcement, the designated behavior is reinforced only some of the time. You can make a behavior almost indestructible (that is, impervious to change) by putting it on an intermittent reinforcement schedule and then gradually lengthening the number of responses required for reinforcement or increasing the length of the interval before responses are reinforced. This is particularly likely to work if you make the length of time between reinforcements variable (and therefore unpredictable). Behaviors that are otherwise incomprehensible can often be explained by principles of intermittent reinforcement."

✓   *Example:* Addiction to gambling occurs because of intermittent reinforcement.

Example: Staying with and feeling love for an abusive partner are often on a very thin intermittent reinforcement schedule; the abusive partner perhaps reciprocated love frequently in the beginning of the relationship, and then gradually lengthened the time between expressions of love.

Example: A parent can inadvertently put a child on an intermittent reinforcement schedule by responding to tantrums only episodically.

B. Strategies for Decreasing or Stopping Undesired Behaviors

Review Interpersonal Handout 21 with participants.

✓ ### 1. What Is Extinction?

Extinction is the reduction of a behavior by removing ongoing reinforcement.

Example: "When attention is reinforcing an unwanted behavior, you instead ignore it."

Example: "When your child's demands are reinforced by your giving in to the demands, you instead do not give in."

Tell participants: "Extinction works best when an alternative behavior replaces the unwanted behavior. In particular, you can extinguish a behavior and at the same time soothe."

Example: "Your child throws a tantrum to get you to take him with you on a walk. You can say, 'I know this is hard for you, and I am sorry you are so distressed, but you will have to stay home and I will be home before long.' Then leave the child at home and go out for a walk."

a. Be Aware of the "Behavioral Burst"

When a behavior has been reinforced and then reinforcement is stopped, the behavior will initially increase; that is, there will be a "behavioral burst." (If there is not a behavioral burst, the wrong reinforcer may have been withheld.) If the reinforcement remains stopped and is not restored, the behavior will decrease over time.

✓   *Example:* If a little girl begins to throw a tantrum in the supermarket because she wants Cocoa Puffs cereal, a parent is likely to give in to stop the escalation of the tantrum. Giving in, however, reinforces the tantrum and makes it more likely to occur during the next supermarket visit. By contrast, if after reinforcing tantrums repeatedly the parent withholds reinforcement—that is, does not buy the Cocoa Puffs—the tantrum is likely to escalate in the moment (making everyone unhappy!). However, if the parent holds the line by not giving in during this and subsequent shopping trips—that is, tolerates the behavioral burst of the escalating tantrum—the tantrum behavior is likely to extinguish over time. Extinction is helped along by positively reinforcing any efforts by the little girl to walk calmly through the store.

b. Beware of Intermittent Reinforcement

If the parent in the example above says no the first three times, but the fourth time gives in and buys the Cocoa Puffs, then the parent has created a much bigger problem. The tantrum is now on an intermittent reinforcement schedule. As noted previously, an intermittently reinforced behavior is the most difficult to extinguish. So it is important not to give up in the face of a behavioral burst, but instead to ride it out.

Emphasize to participants: "If you are trying to change someone else's behavior rather than your own, **be sure to orient the person whose behavior you are changing.** Explain that you are beginning to work to extinguish the behavior, so that it does not seem arbitrary or punitive. And don't forget to reinforce alternative, adaptive behaviors."

💬 **Discussion Point:** Elicit examples from group members of behaviors that might be reduced or eliminated through extinction. Ask each participant to state what reinforcer will be eliminated or given to the individual at times not connected to the behavior (i.e., noncontingently).

✓ ### 2. What Is Satiation?

Satiation is providing a reinforcer before it is needed.

Example: "A baby who cries when hungry will not cry if you give the baby food before he or she cries."

✓ *Example:* "Giving more attention to the baby when he or she throws tantrums might be reinforcing the tantrum behavior. Giving just as much attention when the baby is not throwing a tantrum will lessen that impact."

Example: "If you talk to your sister longer when she is lonely, you might be reinforcing her feelings of loneliness. You can stop having that impact by talking to her for just as long when she is not lonely."

Example: "A spouse who gets angry if you forget to buy the toothpaste will not get angry if you keep the toothpaste on hand."

a. How Satiation Works

When the reinforcer is given before the unwanted behavior occurs, it reduces motivation for the behavior and thus the behavior decreases in frequency.

b. An Advantage of Satiation over Extinction

Tell participants: "An advantage of satiation over extinction is that you do not get the behavioral burst you get with extinction. A disadvantage is that you must provide more potential reinforcers than you may want to provide."

c. The Use of Satiation in DBT

The concept of satiation is why DBT therapists take phone calls even when their clients are not in a crisis. DBT therapists want clients to recognize that they do not have to be suicidal to get attention from their therapists. This is important because if clients have to be suicidal to talk to their therapists, it would make sense that the clients who very much want to talk with their therapist would, despite their best efforts, get more suicidal.

💬 **Discussion Point:** Elicit examples from group members of behaviors that might be reduced or eliminated through satiation with the reinforcer *before* the problematic behavior occurs. Discuss the pros and cons of this strategy versus extinction.

✓ ### 3. What Is Punishment, and How Is It Different from Extinction?

Punishment is adding a consequence that decreases a behavior. The consequence can be adding something negative (e.g., time out for a child, traffic tickets, verbal criticism) or taking away something positive (but not previously a reinforcer of the behavior). The difference between this and extinction is that extinction involves taking away a reinforcer for a behavior, while punishment involves taking away something unrelated to reinforcement.

Example: "Let's say that your sister harasses you to spend more time taking care of your mother, who is sick. Your sister does this by nagging, criticizing, or 'guilt-tripping' you. So far, you have given in and spent more time with your mother. Extinction of this harassment would involve defining this behavior for your sister as unwanted and unhelpful, and then never, ever agreeing to spend more time helping out with your mother when your sister harasses you. Punishment might involve withdrawing warmth, refusing to meet with your sister, calling your sister names, bringing up past transgressions, and making her feel criticized and guilty."

Example: "Your son throws tantrums when you tell him he has to go to bed. Usually, in the face of tantrums, you give in and let him stay up for a little more time. Extinction would be to not give in and not let him stay up when he throws a tantrum—that is, removing the reinforcer. Punishment would be taking away an hour of TV every time he throws a tantrum—a consequence not related to your previous reinforcing behavior."

Note to Leaders: Emphasize that punishment may make a person stay away from the punisher, hide a behavior, or suppress the behavior when the punisher is around. Punishment may at times be necessary, but it is essential to keep it specific, time-limited, and appropriate to the "crime," as well as to reinforce an alternative behavior. Otherwise, punishment will not work. Punishment by itself does not teach new behavior, and it may even lead to self-punishment.

💬 **Discussion Point:** Elicit from participants some examples of behaviors that appear necessary to punish rather than extinguish. For each example, debate the possible advantages versus disadvantages of punishment.

a. The Relative Ineffectiveness of Punishment

Punishment is one of the least effective ways to change behavior over the long term. Punishment suppresses the punished behavior when the person punishing is nearby, but the behavior tends to recur when the punisher is not present. It also doesn't teach any new behaviors to replace the punished ones.

b. The Need for Alternative Behaviors

When punishment is used, alternative behaviors must be reinforced to replace the behavior being extinguished. Neither extinction nor punishment teach new behaviors. People cannot unlearn old behaviors. It is not in any person's (or animal's) evolutionary interest to be able to wipe out old behaviors easily. One never knows whether behavior that is problematic now will be very useful in some new, as yet unimagined context. Thus, although punishment can get a person to stop behaving a particular way, the capability for the behavior is always present. In sum, people can learn new behaviors, but they can't unlearn old behaviors.

c. Overcorrection

Research Point: A form of punishment called "overcorrection" has been found in several studies to stop various types of dysfunctional behaviors.[28] Overcorrection is both a form of punishment and a form of repair that fits the "crime." Studies have found that overcorrection is more effective than correction alone.[29] Instructions need to be explicit; the rationale of overcorrection needs to be clearly stated; and there should be positive consequences for engaging in the overcorrection, which are also clearly laid out. The required corrective behavior is thus dialectically related to the problem behavior.

There are three steps in overcorrection when it is used as a punishment following the occurrence of a problem behavior.

- *First, the person punishing withholds something the punished person wants, or adds an unpleasant consequence.* The most effective consequence is one that expands a natural but undesirable (from the punished person's point of view) effect of the behavior.
- *Second, the punisher requires the person to engage in a new behavior that both corrects and overcorrects the harmful effects of the problem behavior.* (This requires, of course, that the person figure out clearly what harm was actually done.)
- *Third, once the new "overcorrecting" behavior occurs, the punisher immediately stops the punishment by undoing the negative conditions or stopping the withholding.* Thus the punished person has a ready way to terminate the behavior. The challenge, of course, is to devise outcomes and overcorrection behaviors that are undesirable enough, without being trivial or unrelated to the behaviors the punisher wants to teach.

Example: "Your son has friends over when you are gone, and they leave the living room a mess. You then withhold permission for his friends to come over, and also for his going out with friends. The required correction is to clean up the living room completely, and overcorrection is to clean up the entire downstairs. As soon as this is done, his friends can come over again, and he can visit his friends."

Example: Several clients left a group session early and trashed the entrance to our clinic. This damaged not only the clinic entrance, but also my ability to be relaxed about leading a group if someone left early. The consequence I put on them was that they could not come back to the group until they organized and paid for repairs; the overcorrection was to make it more beautiful than before. Correction and overcorrection to my loss of faith were to hire and pay for a person to sit in the clinic's reception area during group sessions until the clients were out of the group.

Example: "A person spills something on your floor. Correction would be to clean it off the floor, and overcorrection would be to clean the entire floor."

Example: "If a couple is persistently late for dinner engagements, they could correct by finding a way to meet you on time, and overcorrect by offering to pick you up or pay for your parking."

Example: "You drop and break a vase at your friend's house. Correct by replacing the vase. Overcorrect by filling it with beautiful flowers."

C. Tips for Using Behavior Change Strategies Effectively

Review Interpersonal Effectiveness Handout 22 with participants.

1. Summarize Behavior Change Strategies Learned So Far

Go over the strategies participants have learned thus far, particularly reinforcement, extinction, and punishment.

✓ ### 2. Not All Consequences Are Created Equal

The power of something to be a reinforcer or a punishment depends on a number of things—for example, the intrinsic value of the consequence to the person, the setting, and how sated or deprived the person is of something desired.

a. The Value to the Person Counts

"One person's poison can be another person's passion." A reinforcer is something a person will change his or her behavior to get (positive reinforcement) or get relief from (negative reinforcer). If the person does not care one way or the other about a consequence, it will not work as a reinforcement.

Example: A fresh plate of broccoli normally won't do it for most people. Some examples of motivating reinforcers might include a nice dinner in a special restaurant, time with a really special friend, or downloading some new music after the completion of a major project.

Observing what happens when various consequences are applied is the best strategy for figuring out what will work as a consequence. Observing as a strategy, however, can be difficult, since changing consequences can take a lot of time and effort, and it is not always possible to start and stop. An alternative is to ask the person what consequences he or she would work to get (reinforcement) or work to avoid (punishment).

b. The Context Counts

It is also important to assess the potency of consequences in different situations. A reinforcer in one situation (hugging a teenager at home) may be punishment in another (hugging a teenager in front of a group of friends). Bringing chocolates to a person on a diet can be punishing, but can be reinforcing when a person is not dieting. Money is a reinforcer for working, but not for love given.

c. The Quantity of a Reinforcer Counts

Satiation, or having a desire for something satisfied completely, can make people feel as though they have had too much. This can make something unpleasant that would otherwise be reinforcing.

Examples: "Food is not a reinforcer after a really big meal; affection is not a reinforcer if you receive plenty of that. Something is only a reinforcer if it is given in appropriate doses. This is also true with praise." (Elicit other examples from participants.)

If people are deprived of something they like, it is more likely to be an effective reinforcer than something they can have whenever they want it.

Examples: "Water may not be a reinforcer if you have enough, but it is definitely a reinforcer if you have been in the heat without liquids for a long time. Food is a reinforcer when you have not had any for a long time. If access to a cell phone or a computer has been taken away, getting it back can be a reinforcer. An opportunity to spend time with a close friend you have not seen in a long time is more reinforcing than time with a friend you see every day."

Discussion Point: Finding powerful reinforcers can be a problem. Many people already have most of what they want or need—or if they do not, they cannot afford to get it even as a reinforcer. In these cases, an effective strategy is to take something away (e.g., access to a cell phone) for a period of time and then restore its use following the desired behavior. Something else can then be taken away (e.g., coffee in the morning, shoes other than the pair hated the most) and then restored following the desired behavior. Participants can keep changing what they are depriving themselves (or another person) of, or can rotate through two or three different things over time. This approach works best if the participants know (or the other person knows) the expected deprivation and reinforcement schedule. The key idea is first to use deprivation to make an item highly desirable, and then to use it as a reinforcer. Discuss with participants how they might use this strategy on themselves or others.

d. Natural Consequences Are More Effective in the Long Run Than Arbitrary Consequences

Natural consequences can be reinforcing or punishing. One type of effective punishment is to let natural negative consequences happen. For example, a nasty hangover is a natural consequence of drinking too much. Staying up very late at night may cause a person to be too tired to focus at work, and then to get in trouble for slacking off. If a behavior doesn't have natural consequences or the natural consequences are too dangerous, then arbitrary consequences may be necessary. A teen who violates curfew one weekend may be grounded for the following weekend. Although it is common for parents to ground children for various infractions, staying at home on a weekend is not a natural outcome of staying out late on a previous day or weekend. In these cases, punishment should be specific, should be time-limited, and should fit the "crime."

> *Example:* "If you're an employee who misses a deadline, you might be punished by losing the chance to present a report to your supervisor because you don't have it ready in time—a natural consequence of missing the deadline. In contrast, an ineffective punishment is one that isn't specific, lasts too long, and/or doesn't fit the behavior. For instance, if you miss a deadline, your boss may give you a bad evaluation, move you to a new work group, and remind you of the missed deadline constantly."

In a similar manner, natural positive consequences can be powerful. Preparing well for job interviews at a law firm can result in a job offer; smiling at people on the street can result in an immediate smile back; approaching people at parties can lead to interesting conversations, cleaning up the kitchen can result in a hug or thank-you; dieting can result in losing weight.

✓ ### 3. Behavior Learned in One Situation May Not Happen in Other Situations

New behaviors have to be learned in all relevant contexts. Learning is highly associated with situations. We learn, for example, that we might be punished for talking while in church, but are likely to be rewarded for talking in social situations. We learn that when a certain person is present, we might be punished for a specific behavior; when that person is absent and other people are present, we might be rewarded, or the behavior might be ignored. Behaviors reinforced at work may not be rewarded at home. Behaviors rewarded at home may be punished at work.

💬 **Discussion Point:** Elicit from participants behaviors of theirs that are rewarded in one situation and ignored or punished in other situations.

To change our own or another person's behavior, we need to pay attention to the situation. It is very important when learning or teaching a new behavior not to assume that if behavior is learned in one situation, it will transfer to another situation. It is easy to be judgmental of people who can do something in one context, but then can't do it in another. For example, we might find it easy to strike up conversations with people we know, but be completely stumped about doing it with strangers. Playing the piano might be easy when we are alone, and very difficult when others are listening. A person might be able to abstain from drinking too much at home, but not when out with friends.

👥 **Practice Exercise:** If you have extra time, distribute Interpersonal Effectiveness Handout 22a: Identifying Effective Behavior Change Strategies. Explain the task, and give participants time to check the more effective response for each pair. Discuss answers. If time permits, ask participants if they have other situations where it's not clear to them what would be the more effective change strategy.

Correct responses to Handout 22a are as follows: 1B, 2B, 3A, 4A, 5B, 6B, 7B, 8A.

References

1. Miller, A. L., Rathus, J. H., & Linehan, M. M. (2007). *Dialectical behavior therapy with suicidal adolescents.* New York: Guilford Press.

2. Merriam-Webster. (2014). Definition of "skill." *www. merriam-webster.com/dictionary/skill?show=0&t= 1393001274*

3. Linehan, M. M. (1997). Validation and psychotherapy. In A. Bohart & L. Greenberg (Eds.), *Empathy reconsidered: New directions in psychotherapy* (pp. 353–392). Washington, DC: American Psychological Association.

4. Bower, S. A., & Bower, G. H. (2004). *Asserting yourself: A practical guide for positive change.* New York: Da Capo Press. (Original work published 1980) The idea for the four DEAR skills (Describe, Express, Assert, Reinforce) was suggested by Bower and Bower's "DESC scripts" (Describe, Express, Specify, Consequence). Their excellent self-help book is very compatible with DBT and can be used by both skills trainers and participants.

5. Hauser-Cram, P. (1998). I think I can, I think I can: Understanding and encouraging mastery motivation in children. *Young Children, 53*(4), 67–71.

6. Linehan, M. M., & Egan, K. J. (1985). *Asserting yourself.* New York: Facts on File.

7. Festinger, L., Schachter, S., & Back, K. (1950). *Social pressures in informal groups: A study of human factors in housing.* Stanford, CA: Stanford University Press.

8. Back, M. D., Schmukle, S. C., & Egloff, B. (2008). Becoming friends by chance. *Psychological Science, 19*(5), 439–440.

9. Segal, M. (1974). Alphabet and attraction: An unobtrusive measure of the effect of propinquity in a field setting. *Journal of Personality and Social Psychology, 30*(5), 654–657.

10. Newcomb, T. M. (1961). *The acquaintance process.* New York: Holt, Rinehart & Winston.

11. Byrne, D. (1961). Interpersonal attraction and attitude similarity. *Journal of Abnormal and Social Psychology, 62,* 713–715.

12. Byrne, D. (1971). *The attraction paradigm.* New York: Academic Press.

13. Byrne, D., & Griffith, D. (1966). A developmental investigation of the law of attraction. *Journal of Personality and Social Psychology, 4,* 699–702.

14. Condon, J. W., & Crano, W. D. (1988). Inferred evaluation and the relation between attitude similarity and interpersonal attraction. *Journal of Personality and Social Psychology, 54,* 789–797.

15. Heine, S. J., Foster, J.-A. B., & Spina, R. (2009). Do birds of a feather universally flock together?: Cultural variation in the similarity–attraction effect. *Asian Journal of Social Psychology, 12*(4), 247–258.

16. Fawcett, C., & Markson, L. (2010). Similarity predicts liking in 3-year-old children. *Journal of Experimental Child Psychology, 105,* 345–358.

17. Novak, D., & Lerner, M. J. (1968). Rejection as a consequence of perceived similarity. *Journal of Personality and Social Psychology, 9*(2, Pt. 1), 147–152.

18. Cozby, P. C. (1972). Self-disclosure, reciprocity, and liking. *Sociometry, 35,* 151–160.

19. Spurr, J. M., & Stopa, L. (2002). Self-focused attention in social phobia and social anxiety. *Clinical Psychology Review, 22,* 947–975.

20. Clark, D. M., & Wells, A. (1995). A cognitive model of social phobia. In R. Heimberg, M. Liebowitz, D. A. Hope, & F. R. Schneier (Eds.), *Social phobia: Diagnosis, assessment, and treatment* (pp. 69–93). New York: Guilford Press.

21. Rapee, R. M., & Heimberg, R. G. (1997). A cognitive-behavioral model of anxiety in social phobia. *Behaviour Research and Therapy, 35,* 741–756.

22. Axelrod, S. (2012). Personal communication.

23. Fruzzetti, A. (2006). *The high-conflict couple: A dialectical behavior therapy guide to finding peace, intimacy and validation.* Oakland, CA: New Harbinger.

24. Axelrod, S. (2012). Personal communication.

25. Pryor, K. (1985). *Don't shoot the dog: How to improve yourself and others through behavioral training.* New York: Bantam Books.

26. Lieberman, D. A., Sunnucks, W. L., & Kirk, J. D. J. (1998). Reinforcement without awareness: I. Voice level. *Quarterly Journal of Experimental Psychology, 51B*(4), 301–316.

27. Bizo, L. A., & Sweeney, N. (2005). Use of an ESP cover story facilitates reinforcement without awareness. *Psychological Record, 55,* 115–123.

28. Marholin, D., Luiselli, J. K., & Townsend, N. M. (1980). Overcorrection: An examination of its rationale and treatment effectiveness. *Progress in Behavior Modification, 9,* 186–192.

29. Azrin, N. H., & Wesolowski, M. D. (1974). Theft reversal: An overcorrection procedure for eliminating stealing by retarded persons. *Journal of Applied Behavior Analysis, 73*(4), 577–581.

Chapter 9

Emotion Regulation Skills

Difficulties in regulating painful emotions are central to the behavioral difficulties of many individuals. From these individuals' perspective, painful feelings are most often the "problems to be solved." Dysfunctional behaviors, including suicidal behaviors, substance use disorders, overeating, emotion suppression, overcontrol, and interpersonal mayhem, are often behavioral solutions to intolerably painful emotions.

Individuals with high emotional sensitivity and/ or intensity, or frequent emotional distress, can benefit from help in learning to regulate their emotions. Emotion regulation skills, however, can be extremely difficult to teach, because many individuals have been overdosed with remarks to the effect that "If you would just change your attitude, you could change your feelings." Some individuals come from environments where everyone else exhibits almost perfect cognitive control of their emotions. Moreover, these very same others have often exhibited both intolerance and strong disapproval of the individuals' inability to exhibit similar control. Some people will at times resist any attempt to control their emotions, because such control would imply that other people are right and they are wrong for feeling the way they do. Thus emotion regulation skills can be taught only in a context of emotional self-validation.

Like interpersonal effectiveness and distress tolerance, emotion regulation requires application of mindfulness skills—in this case, the nonjudgmental observation and description of one's current emotional responses. The theoretical idea is that much emotional distress is a result of secondary responses (e.g., intense shame, anxiety, or rage) to primary emotions. Often the primary emotions are adaptive and appropriate to the context. The reduction of this secondary distress requires exposure to the primary emotion in a nonjudgmental atmosphere. In this context, mindfulness to one's own emotional responses can be thought of as an exposure technique. (See Chapter 11 of the main DBT text for a fuller description of exposure-based procedures.)

As noted in Chapter 1, the DBT model of emotion regulation is transdiagnostic, with data suggesting efficacy of DBT across a range of emotional disorders. As such, it is highly compatible with the similar transdiagnostic model underlying the Unified Protocol,[1, 2] developed by David Barlow and his colleagues. Similar to DBT, the Unified Protocol addresses deficits in emotion regulation that underlie emotional disorders by (1) increasing present-focused emotion awareness, (2) increasing cognitive flexibility, (3) identifying and preventing patterns of emotion avoidance and maladaptive emotion-driven behaviors, (4) increasing awareness and tolerance of emotion-related physical sensations, and (5) utilizing emotion-focused exposure procedures.[1]

The specific DBT emotion regulation skills taught in this module are grouped into the following four segments: understanding and naming emotions; changing unwanted emotions; reducing vulnerability to emotion mind; and managing extreme emotions.

Understanding and Naming Emotions

The first segment of the module (Sections I–VI) focuses on understanding and naming emotions: identifying the functions of emotions and their relationship to difficulties in changing emotions; understanding the nature of emotions by presenting a model of emotions; and learning how to identify and label emotions in everyday life.

Understanding the Functions of Emotions

Emotional behavior is functional to the individual. Changing ineffective emotional behaviors can be extremely difficult when they are followed by reinforcing consequences; thus identifying the functions and reinforcers for particular emotional behaviors can be useful. Generally, emotions function to communicate to others and to motivate one's own behavior. Emotional behaviors can also have two other important functions. The first, related to the communication function, is to influence and control other people's behaviors. The second communication function is alerting oneself. In this latter case, emotions function like an alarm, alerting the person to pay attention to events that may be important. Identifying these functions of emotions, especially of unwanted emotions, is an important first step toward change.

Identifying Obstacles to Changing Emotions

Many factors can make it hard to change emotions, even when a person desperately wants to. Biological factors can increase emotion sensitivity, intensity, and time needed to return to emotional baseline. All of us—even those with sunny dispositions—at times have intense emotional reactions, however, and when this happens we need adequate skills to modulate our emotions. Inadequate skills can make this regulation very difficult. Emotion regulation is even more difficult when others in the environment are reinforcing dysfunctional emotions. This is particularly true when concurrent emotion overload, low motivation, or myths about emotions get in the way.

Identifying and Labeling Emotions

An important step in regulating emotions is learning to identify and label current emotions. Emotions, however, are complex behavioral responses. Their identification often requires the ability not only to observe one's own responses, but also to describe accurately the context in which the emotion occurs. Thus learning to identify an emotional response is aided enormously if one can observe and describe

(1) the event prompting the emotion; (2) the interpretations of the event that prompted the emotion; (3) the history prior to the prompting event that increases sensitivity to the event and vulnerability to responding emotionally; (4) the phenomenological experience, including the physical sensation, of the emotion; (5) the expressive behaviors associated with the emotion; and (6) the aftereffects of the emotion on other types of functioning.

Changing Unwanted Emotions

The second segment of the module (Sections VII–XII) has to do with changing emotional responses by learning how to check the facts, take opposite action when the emotion does not fit the facts, and engage in problem solving when the facts of the situation are the problem.

Check the Facts

Emotions are often reactions to thoughts and interpretations of an event, rather than to the actual facts of an event. Checking the facts, and then changing appraisals and assumptions to fit the facts, are basic strategies in cognitive therapy as well as in many other forms of therapy.

Problem Solving

DBT assumes that most people feel painful emotions for good reasons. Although all people's perceptions tend to become distorted when they are highly emotional, this does not mean that the emotions themselves are the results of distorted perceptions. Thus an important way to control emotions is to control the events that set off emotions. Problem solving for emotional situations, particularly when the problematic events are painful, unexpected, or unwanted, can be extremely useful. Often an unwanted emotion is entirely justified by the situation, but the situation can be changed if the person takes active steps to solve the problem at hand. Solving problems also requires a very thorough assessment of the facts, and checking the facts is often the first step in problem solving.

Opposite Action

Actions and expressive responses are important parts of all emotions. Thus one strategy to change or regulate an emotion is to change its action and expressive components by acting in a way that opposes or is inconsistent with the emotion. This should include both overt actions (e.g., doing something nice for a person one is angry at, approaching what one is afraid of) and postural and facial expressiveness. With respect to the latter, however, clients must learn that the idea is not to block expression of an emotion; rather, it is to express a different emotion. There is a very big difference between a constricted facial expression that blocks the expression of anger and a relaxed facial expression that expresses liking.

Most effective treatments for emotional disorders ask clients to reverse the expression and action components of problem emotions. Some psychotherapy researchers believe this is why these treatments work. The following are some examples.

Behavioral activation, an opposite-action technique, can be an important treatment for depression. It is natural for a person who feels sad and is no longer finding pleasure in activities that were previously enjoyed to attempt to cope by withdrawing socially, ceasing to engage in activities, and "shutting down." The problem is that such coping strategies do not help alleviate depression; they make it worse.

Behavioral activation targets avoidance. Originally developed as a comparison treatment to CBT, it has gained empirical support from a multisite trial showing it to be as effective as CBT and medication at a 6-month follow-up.[3] What is interesting about behavioral activation is that avoidance behaviors (such as inactivity and rumination) are viewed as the key factors underlying and maintaining depression, and treatment aims to combat clients' use of such maladaptive behaviors.

Similarly, exposure-based treatments where clients do the opposite of avoiding and escaping feared events are the most effective treatments for anxiety disorders. Avoidance of or escape from feared stimuli maintain anxiety disorders and prohibit new learning from taking place. Exposure involves confronting situations, objects, and thoughts that evoke anxiety or distress because they are unrealistically associated with danger. Response prevention is conceptualized as blocking avoidance or escape from feared situations. By encouraging the individual to approach and remain in the feared situation, response prevention allows the realization that the fear is unrealistic. Exposure and response prevention are commonly used in the treatment of obsessive–compulsive disorder (OCD). Foa and colleagues demonstrated the importance of using both exposure and response prevention in treating patients with OCD; exposure leads to reduction in the anxiety response, and response prevention leads to a reduction in escape behaviors.[4]

Effective treatments for anger stress a number of opposite actions, such as learning to identify the cues to frustration and/or anger and then leaving the situation to cool down, as well as changing thoughts to understand the other person and reduce the demand that reality be different.

Reducing Vulnerability to Emotion Mind

The third segment of the module (Sections XIII–XVII) focuses on reducing vulnerability to negative emotions (emotion mind) and preventing efforts to overcontrol emotions by accumulating positive emotions, building mastery, learning how to cope ahead of difficult situations, and taking care of the body. All people are more prone to emotional reactivity when they are under physical or environmental stress,[5] are in situations where they are out of control,[6] or are living in a state of deprivation,[7] particularly when the deprivation extends to many areas of life. Accordingly, the behaviors targeted here include three major sets of skills: accumulate positive emotions, build a sense of mastery/"cope ahead," and build a resilient biology.

Accumulating Positive Emotions

Increasing positive emotions can be accomplished in a number of ways. Increasing the number of pleasurable events in one's life is one approach. In the short term, this involves increasing daily positive experiences. In the long term, it means building a "life worth living" and making necessary changes so that pleasant or valued events will occur more often. To do this, it is often necessary to spend some time figuring out what one really wants out of life, what one's values are. This is particularly important with clients for whom an uncertain identity is part of their problem. It is very difficult to have a life that is experienced as worth living if one's life is out of sync with one's most important values. Building a life worth living is important because it improves one's sense of resilience. It can be much easier to cope with a loss or a negative event when it is balanced with positive experiences in one's life.[8] Losing a dollar may be traumatic for a poor and starving person, but for a well-fed rich person it may be inconsequential. Having a friend move away can be devastating if it is a person's only relationship. In addition to increasing positive events, it is also useful to work on being mindful of pleasurable experiences when they occur, as well as being unmindful of worries that the positive experience will end.[9]

Building Mastery and Learning to Cope Ahead

In building a sense of mastery, there are two focal points: (1) engaging in activities that build a sense of self-efficacy, self-control, and competence; and (2) learning to cope ahead of time with difficult situations via imaginal rehearsal. The goal of building mastery in DBT is very similar to activity scheduling in both cognitive therapy and behavioral activation for depression.[10, 11]

Taking Care of the Body (PLEASE Skills)

To build a resilient biology, the focus is on balancing nutrition and eating, getting sufficient but not too much sleep (including treating insomnia and nightmares, if needed), getting adequate exercise, treating physical illness, and staying off nonprescribed mood-altering drugs or misusing prescribed medications.

Poverty can interfere with balanced nutrition and medical care, and can put many goals out of reach that individuals might wish to work toward. Although these targets seem straightforward, making headway on them can be exhausting for both clients and their therapists and skills trainers. With respect to insomnia, many of our clients fight a never-ending battle. Nightmares, anxious rumination, and poor sleep hygiene are often the culprits. Work on any of these targets requires an active stance by clients, as well as persistence until positive effects begin to accumulate. The typical problem-solving passivity of many clients can create substantial interference here.

Managing Extreme Emotions

The fourth segment of the module (Sections XVIII–XX) deals with how to manage very difficult emotions. Decreasing emotional suffering through mindfulness to the current emotion is an important skill here, as well as learning how to identify one's

skills breakdown point and then turning to the distress tolerance skills when that happens.

Mindfulness of Current Emotions

Mindfulness of current emotions means experiencing emotions without judging them or trying to inhibit them, block them, distract from them, or hold on to them. The basic idea here is that exposure to painful or distressing emotions, without association to negative consequences, will extinguish their ability to stimulate secondary negative emotions. The natural consequences of judging negative emotions as "bad" are feelings of guilt, shame, anger, and/or anxiety whenever distressing feelings arise. The addition of these secondary feelings to an already negative situation simply makes the distress more intense and tolerance more difficult. Frequently, a distressing situation or painful affect could be tolerated if only a person could refrain from feeling guilty or anxious about feeling painful emotions in the first place.

Identifying the Skills Breakdown Point

When emotional arousal is so extreme that complicated skills cannot be used, the person has reached the skills breakdown point. It's important for participants to learn to recognize when they have reached this point, and then to turn to the crisis survival skills covered in Chapter 10 of this manual. I do not discuss them here.

The final segment of the module (Sections XXI–XXII) covers troubleshooting when emotion regulation skills aren't working, and revisits the model of emotions described earlier with the addition of DBT skills where relevant.

Selecting Material to Teach

As with the other modules, there is a great deal of material for each skill in the emotion regulation teaching notes that follow. You will not cover all the content the first several times you teach specific skills. The notes are provided to give you a deeper understanding of each skill, so that you can answer questions and add new teaching as you go. For each skill, I have put a checkmark (✓) next to material I almost always cover. If I am in a huge rush, I may skip everything not checked. Similarly, on this manual's special website (*www.guilford.com/skills-training-manual*), I use stars (★) for core handouts I almost always use. Also as in chapters on earlier modules, I have summarized research in special "Research Point" sections. The great value of research is that it can often be used to sell the skills you are teaching.

It is important that you have a basic understanding of the specific skills you are teaching. The first several times you teach, carefully study the notes, handouts, and worksheets for each skill you plan to teach. Highlight the points you want to make, and bring a copy of the relevant teaching note pages with you to teach from. Be sure to practice each skill yourself, to be sure you understand how to use it. Before long, you will solidify your knowledge of each skill. At that point you will find your own favorite teaching points, examples, and stories and can ignore most of mine.

··· | **Teaching Notes** | ···

I. GOALS OF THIS MODULE (EMOTION REGULATION HANDOUT 1)

> **Main Point:** The overall goal of emotion regulation is to reduce emotional suffering. The goal is *not* to get rid of emotions. Some individuals will always be more emotional than others.
>
> **Emotion Regulation Handout 1: Goals of Emotion Regulation.** Briefly review the goals on this handout. Provide enough information and discussion to orient participants to the module, link the module to participants' goals, and generate some enthusiasm for learning the emotion regulation skills.
>
> **Emotion Regulation Worksheet 1: Pros and Cons of Changing Emotions** *(Optional)*. This worksheet is designed to help participants (1) decide whether they want to regulate a current emotion, and (2) decide whether it is in their interest to learn to regulate their own emotions or stay in emotion mind much of the time. Its major use is to communicate that the goal of this module is to regulate emotions they want to change, not to change their emotions just because others want them to. This worksheet can also be used as an exercise to improve the likelihood of being effective when a person is overcome with emotions (e.g., when the person just wants to yell and scream or completely avoid a situation or person). It can also be used as a teaching tool for how to figure out goals. For instructions in teaching pros and cons, see the teaching notes for the Distress Tolerance module (Chapter 10, Section V) on reviewing pros and cons as a way to make behavioral decisions. Assign this worksheet as optional if you teach other handouts in the session that have associated worksheets.

Orient participants to what is meant by "emotion regulation," to the skills to be learned in this module, and to the rationale for their importance.

✓ A. What Is Emotion Regulation?

Say to participants: "Emotion regulation is the ability to control or influence which emotions you have, when you have them, and how you experience and express them."[12]

Go on to explain that **regulating emotions can be automatic as well as consciously controlled.** Tell participants: "In this module, we will focus first on increasing conscious awareness and control of emotions. Second, we will provide so much practice regulating emotions that you will overlearn the skills. Ultimately, the regulation should become automatic."

Continue: "Emotions are out of control or 'dysregulated' when you are unable, despite your best efforts, to change which emotions you have, when you have them, or how you experience or express them."

✓ 💬 **Discussion Point:** Either before or after reviewing Emotion Regulation Handout 1, ask participants to check off each goal that is important to them in the boxes on the handout and then share their choices.

✓ 💬 **Discussion Point:** At some point, ask each person to name the emotions that he or she most wants to change. Write the list on a whiteboard (if possible). Discuss similarities and differences.

Explain that the goals of emotion regulation are as follows.

✓ B. Understand Your Own Emotions

Say to participants: "Before you can regulate your own emotions, you need to understand them. You can do this by learning to do two things."

✓   ***1. Identify Your Own Emotions***

"The simple act of naming your emotions can help you regulate your own emotions."

✓   💬 **Discussion Point:** Some people always know what emotion they are feeling. Others have no idea most of the time. For some, trying to figure out how they feel is like looking down into a fog. Elicit from each participant which type of person he or she is.

✓   ***2. Understand What Emotions Do for You***

"It can be very hard to change emotions when you do not understand where they come from or why they are there."

✓   ## C. Decrease the Frequency of Unwanted Emotions

Continue: "Once you understand your own emotions, you can learn how to cut down on the frequency of the ones you don't want. You can do this in several ways."

✓   ***1. Stop Unwanted Emotions from Starting***

"You can't stop all painful emotions—but you can make changes in your environment and in your life to reduce how often negative emotions occur."

💬 **Discussion Point:** Ask participants what kinds of emotional situations they have the most trouble solving or changing.

✓   ***2. Change Painful Emotions Once They Start***

People often believe myths about emotions—that changing emotions is inauthentic, on the one hand, or that all emotions should be suppressed, on the other hand.

💬 **Discussion Point:** Ask participants whether they are afraid of losing all their emotions, hoping to get rid of all their emotions, or both. Discuss.

Note to Leaders: It is essential to highlight that the point is to change the emotions participants themselves want to change, not the emotions other people want them to change. Remind participants that emotion regulation skills will not be crammed down their throats. At each point and for each skill, it is up to the participants to consider the pros and cons of maintaining an emotion or a particular emotional intensity. When the emotion or the intensity of the emotion is ineffective or too painful to bear, change may be desirable, and emotion regulation skills will be useful. If the emotion is not one a participant wants to change, or if the intensity, even though painful, is effective, then changing the emotion or the intensity of the emotion may not be useful.

---

3. Emotions Themselves Are Neither Good nor Bad

In and of themselves, emotions are not good or bad. They just are. Evaluating our emotions as either good or bad is rarely helpful. Thinking that an emotion is "bad" does not get rid of it. It may lead us to try to suppress the emotion.

4. Suppression of Emotions Makes Things Worse

Suppressing emotions is a temporary solution that causes greater problems in the long run.[13] Emotions may be comfortable or uncomfortable, wanted or unwanted, excruciatingly painful or ecstatically pleasurable. Judging emotions as "bad" can make painful emotions even more painful.

5. *Emotion Regulation Is for Ineffective Emotions Only*

Say to participants: "Emotion regulation strategies are for emotions that are *not* effective in helping you achieve your own goals in life. Emotions are effective when certain things are true:

- "Acting on the emotion is in your own self-interest."
- "Expressing the emotion will get you closer to your own goals."
- "Expressing your emotion will influence others in ways that will help you."
- "Your emotion is sending you a message you need to listen to."

💬 **Discussion Point:** Elicit from participants when emotions have been useful and when they have been destructive. Have participants discuss the emotions that give them the most trouble.

✓ D. Decrease Vulnerability to Emotion Mind

Explain to participants: "Emotion regulation will help you decrease your vulnerability to emotion mind. It won't take away your emotions, but it will help you balance emotion mind with reasonable mind to get to wise mind. And it will also increase emotional resilience—in other words, your ability to bounce back and cope with difficult events and emotions."

✓ E. Decrease Emotional Suffering

Say: "Finally, emotion regulation will enable you to decrease your emotional suffering. Specifically, you'll learn to do these things:

- "Reduce suffering when painful emotions overcome you."
- "Manage extreme emotions so you don't make things worse."

> **Note to Leaders:** Be sure to highlight that although it may take a *lot* of work at the start for participants to regulate and control their emotions, over time they will get better and better at it. If they practice a lot, at some point regulating their emotions effectively will become automatic and often easy.

II. OVERVIEW: UNDERSTANDING AND NAMING EMOTIONS (EMOTION REGULATION HANDOUT 2)

> **Main Point:** It is difficult for people to manage their emotions when they do not understand how emotions work. The point of this section is that knowledge is power.
>
> **Emotion Regulation Handout 2: Overview: Understanding and Naming Emotions.** When you are teaching this module for the first time or when time is of the essence, you can use this handout to teach the key points for What Emotions Do For You (Emotion Regulation Handout 3) and What Makes it Hard to Regulate Your Emotions (Emotion Regulation Handout 4). Handouts 3 and 4 can be skipped if it is easier to teach the material without handouts. The information itself is critical, but the handouts are not. Orient participants to the content of the model for describing emotions (Emotion Regulation Handout 5), but do not teach Handout 5 yet.
>
> **Worksheet:** There is no assigned worksheet for this handout. Emotion Regulation Worksheets 2–4a cover the topics in this section.

Orient participants to the skills taught in this part of the module and the rationale for their importance.

✓ A. What Emotions Do for You

There are reasons why humans (and other mammals) have emotions. The purpose of regulating emotions is *not* to get rid of them. We need them for survival!

There are three major functions of emotions:

- To motivate action.
- To communicate to others.
- To communicate to ourselves.

> **Note to Leaders:** If you skip Emotion Regulation Handout 3, pick up key points in the teaching notes for this handout and provide them here.

Knowing what emotions do for us can help us figure out how to regulate them, and also how to appreciate them even when they are painful or difficult.

✓ B. Factors That Make Regulating Emotions Hard

Regulating emotions is like regulating temperature. We want to be able to raise the intensity of emotions when needed (like making a room warmer), and to decrease the intensity of emotions when needed (like making a room cooler).

Factors that can make it very difficult to get our emotions under control include these:

- Biology.
- Lack of emotion regulation skills.
- Reinforcing consequences of emotional behaviors.
- Moodiness that makes the effort to manage emotions difficult.
- Emotional overload.
- Emotion myths.

Understanding each of these factors can be critical for troubleshooting emotions.

> **Note to Leaders:** If you skip Emotion Regulation Handout 4, pick up key points in the teaching notes for this handout and provide them here.

✓ C. A Model for Describing Emotions

Emotions are complex, full-system responses. Changing any part of the system can change the entire response. Assure participants: "Once you know all the parts of the emotion system, you can decide where to try to change it first."

✓ D. Ways to Describe Emotions

Conclude: "Learning to observe, describe, and name your emotions can help you regulate your emotions."

III. WHAT EMOTIONS DO FOR YOU (EMOTION REGULATION HANDOUT 3)

> **Main Point:** There are reasons why humans (and many other animals) have emotions. They have three important functions, and we need all of them!
>
> **Emotion Regulation Handout 3: What Emotions Do for You.** If you teach the content from this handout, it can be useful as you talk to write the three major functions of emotions on the board: (1) to motivate action, (2) to communicate to others, and (3) to communicate to ourselves. If time is short, skip this handout and summarize the information when introducing the module or this skills section with Handout 2.
>
> **Emotion Regulation Worksheet 2: Figuring Out What My Emotions Are Doing for Me; Emotion Regulation Worksheet 2b: Emotion Diary.** Skip both of these worksheets (as well as Worksheets 2a

and 2c, which are examples of how to fill these out) for participants starting the Emotion Regulation module for the first time. Adding them will almost always require extra time (which you may not have), and the worksheets can be overwhelming to beginners. Use these worksheets with individuals who have gone through the module at least once or have been in skills training for a while. The worksheets can also be very useful in individual therapy, together with individual coaching. Use Worksheet 2 first. If necessary, instruct participants in how to rate intensity of emotions (0 = no emotion, no intensity to 100 = maximum intensity). When participants become practiced at filling Worksheet 2 out, then move to Worksheet 2b.

Worksheet 2b is for participants who want to identify how their emotions are functioning over time. Knowing the function of an emotion can be extremely helpful in changing it. For example, this worksheet can be very useful for assessing whether a participant's own emotions are being reinforced by people in the environment. If they are being reinforced, and the emotion is one the participant is trying to reduce, then it may be very important to ask those others to change how they react to the emotion's expression—or how they are *not* responding when the emotion is not expressed. (The DEAR MAN, GIVE FAST skills described in Chapter 8 and in Interpersonal Effectiveness Skills Handouts 5, 6, and 7 should be used for such requests.)

Orient participants to the functions of emotions, and give a rationale for their importance.

✓ A. Emotions Have Functions That Help Our Species to Survive

Emotional behaviors evolved as immediate, automatic, and efficient ways to solve common problems that humans and other emotional animals must solve to survive. **There are three primary functions of emotions.**

✓ B. Emotions Motivate (and Organize) Us for Action

1. Emotions Prepare Us Physically for Action

Emotions prepare our bodies to act. The action urges connected to specific emotions are largely hard-wired in our biology.

2. Emotions Save Time

Emotions save time in getting us to act in important situations. We don't have to think everything through. We can react to situations extremely fast.

✓ *Example:* "Imagine that there is a tsunami, and a huge wave of water 20 feet high is coming at you and your family on the beach. You, however, are the only one who sees it coming. Ask yourself: How likely is it that you and your family will survive if you walk up to them and calmly say, 'A tsunami is coming; let's all run up the hill to save our lives'? How fast do you think each member of your family will run if there is no emotion? To save yourself and your family, you will run and scream, 'TSUNAMI!! RUN! RUN! COME ON!' That is your only hope."

Example: When people are physically attacked, anger can energize them quickly to attack back and protect themselves. Similarly, anger on a football field can energize players to play harder.

Example: Students often do not want to reduce test anxiety, because they are afraid that if they do, they will quit working so hard and then fail their tests.

Example: People are sometimes afraid to reduce guilt, because they are afraid that without guilt, they may start doing dishonest and harmful things.

Example: If there were no emotions, one would not feel the need to comfort a crying baby.

✓ ### 3. Emotions Can Be Hard to Change

Emotions can be very hard to change when the associated behavior is very important. This is because emotions are to an extent biologically "hard-wired" responses to important events.

✓ *Example:* "If your house is on fire and you need to run for your life, it would be very hard to stop being afraid before you get away from the fire."

Example: "If your child has been molested by a neighbor, and you want him locked up in jail and away from your child, it will be very hard to reduce contempt for the molester before you have reported it to police and he is arrested and put in jail."

Example: "If someone is threatening to 'steal away' the person you want to take to the prom, and he or she is interested in the other person, it will be hard to get jealousy to go down before you have done what is needed to get your intended date to say yes to going to the prom with you."

💬 **Discussion Point:** Elicit from participants what they think would happen if people could really shut down emotions. For example, who would survive if we could actually eliminate fear or love?

4. Functions of Specific Emotions in Our Lives

> **Note to Leaders:** If there is not enough time to review all of the emotions listed below, review several, selecting those most relevant to your participants.

a. Fear

Fear organizes our responses to threats to our life, health, or well-being. It focuses us on escape from danger.

b. Anger

Anger organizes our responses to the blocking of important goals or activities or to an imminent attack on the self or to important others.[14] It focuses us on self-defense, mastery, and control.

c. Disgust

Disgust organizes our responses to situations and things that are offensive and contaminating.[15] It focuses us on rejecting and distancing ourselves from some object, event, or situation.

d. Sadness

Sadness organizes our responses to losses of someone or something important, and to goals lost or not attained.[16] It focuses us on what is valued and the pursuit of goals, as well as on communicating to others that we need help.

e. Shame

Shame organizes responses related to personal characteristics or our own behaviors that are dishonoring or sanctioned by our own community.[17] It focuses us on hiding transgressions and, if these are already public, engaging in appeasement-related behaviors.

f. Guilt

Guilt organizes responses related to specific actions that have led to violation of values.[17] It focuses us on actions and behaviors that are likely to repair the violation.

g. Jealousy

Jealousy organizes responses to others who threaten to take away relationships or things very important to us.[18, 19] It focuses us on protecting what we have.

h. Envy

Envy organizes our responses to others' getting or having things we do not have but want or need.[19] It focuses us on working hard to obtain what other people have.

i. Love

Love organizes our responses related to reproduction and survival.[20] It focuses us on union with and attachment to others.

j. Happiness

Happiness organizes our responses to optimal functioning of ourselves, others we care about, or the social group we are part of.[21] It focuses us on continuing activities that enhance pleasure and personal and social value.

> **Note to Leaders:** You can create more examples by reviewing Emotion Regulation Handout 6: Ways to Describe Emotions, or Emotion Regulation Handout 11: Figuring Out Opposite Actions.

💬 **Discussion Point:** Elicit and discuss other examples, especially examples having to do with anger. Suggest an emotion, and then go around the group and ask participants what they have an urge to do when experiencing the emotion. Do this with different emotions, and then highlight the different action urges associated with different emotions.

💬 **Discussion Point:** Suggest various actions, and then ask participants to imagine engaging in the action with emotion and without emotion. Discuss the differences. Here are some sample actions:

- Soothing a baby or child with and without affection.
- Running away from or avoiding a dangerous situation with and without fear.
- Apologizing for one's own behavior with and without a sense of guilt.
- Lying about one's own behavior with and without guilt (or with and without fear).

✓ C. Emotions Communicate to (and Influence) Others

✓ 1. Facial Expressions Are Biologically Hard-Wired Aspects of Emotions

Among both humans and animals, facial expressions can communicate faster than words.[22, 23]

2. Some Emotional Expressions Have an Automatic Effect on Others

Several facial expressions of emotion have automatic effects on other people. That is, these effects are not learned. For example, an infant reacts spontaneously to an adult's smile or look of fright.[24] This automatic reaction serves infants well until they learn to use words.

Even after children can use words, facial expressions are still very helpful. Having both verbal and nonverbal forms of emotional expression means having two ways of communication for important situations.

✓ 3. Emotional Expressions Influence Others (Whether We Intend It or Not)

Examples: Expressions of warmth and friendliness toward an acquaintance may result in a later favor; disappointment expressed by a supervisor may result in improved work by an employee; anger may result in one person's giving another his or her rightful due instead of withholding it.

Example: Communicating agonizing sadness and despair may influence a therapist or another person to reassure, give help, or otherwise make efforts to take away the pain.

Example: Expressed anger may stop others' behavior.

💬 **Discussion Point:** Ask participants for examples of their emotions' influencing others and of their being influenced by others' emotions. Discuss these examples. Also, elicit examples of times when this strategy boomeranged—that is, when participants' expressions of emotion got them something they didn't want.

💬 **Discussion Point:** The point that emotions can influence others even when we don't consciously intend them to do so is extremely important to make. This can happen even when we are not aware that our emotions are having such effects on others. Discuss this point with participants. Elicit examples of when their automatic emotional expressions have had an impact on other people, even though they did not consciously intend to have such an effect.

✓ **4. Emotions Can Be Very Hard to Change When a Communication Is Important**

As noted earlier, emotions can be extremely hard to change when a communication is important. This is because emotions are to an extent "hard-wired" responses to important events.

Example: John asks Kathy to stop behaviors that are really annoying to him, but she does not change unless he gets really angry. If this is almost always the case, and Kathy only responds to expression of anger, then it will be very hard for John to stop feeling and acting angry when Kathy does annoying things. Kathy is reinforcing John's expressions of anger.

Example: Julie wants her son, Billy, to realize how dangerous a situation is. When Julie is trying to communicate this to Billy, it will be hard for her to stop being afraid. Otherwise, Billy may think the situation is not as dangerous as it is.

Example: If Maria wants Terry to know what she likes, she may want to communicate happiness or joy when he does things that make her happy. In fact, it would be hard for her to stop being happy around someone who often does loving things that she likes. It also would not be in her best interest. This is one reason why communication of happiness or joy is often automatic (i.e., not under our immediate control).

Note to Leaders: Be sure that you understand the examples above before you teach them. The point being made is that if we want to communicate our anger, fear, or joy to someone, it is difficult to do this if we have to consciously organize not only what we say, but our facial expressions, our voice tone, our posture, and so on. And because communication of emotional responses is so important, it is also not in our best interest (from an evolutionary point of view) to be able to shut off emotional communications easily.

💬 **Discussion Point:** Elicit ideas about what different emotions communicate.

✓ **5. What Happens When Verbal and Nonverbal Expressions of Emotion Don't Match?**

Research Point: When nonverbal expressions of emotion (e.g., actions, facial and body expressions, voice tone) don't go with what a person says, other people almost always will trust the nonverbal expressions over the verbal ones.[25]

> **Note to Leaders:** This point about verbal and nonverbal expressions is very important. A major premise of DBT is that the nonverbal emotional expressions of many individuals with emotion regulation difficulties do not accurately indicate what they are experiencing; thus the individuals are often misread. See the discussion of apparent competence in Chapter 3 of the main DBT text.

💬 **Discussion Point:** Ask participants for examples of being misread or of misreading others because of mismatched nonverbal communication.

✓ **D. Emotions Communicate to Ourselves**

✓ **1. Emotions Can Be Signals to Check Things Out**

✓ Emotions can be signals or alarms that something is going on in a situation. This is what is meant by the saying "Listen to your gut." Likewise, when we say that a person has a "good feel for a situation," we are referring to emotions as signals.

2. Information about Situations, Based on Emotions, May or May Not Be Accurate

Sometimes signals picked up from a situation are processed out of our awareness.[26] This processing sets off an emotional reaction, but we cannot identify what it is about the situation that set off the emotion.[27] Through trial and error—that is, experience—people learn when to trust these emotional responses and when to believe they do not provide accurate information.

💬 **Discussion Point:** Ask participants for examples of when their "feel" for a situation proved to be correct. Discuss how people often ignore their own "sense" or "feel" for a situation simply because they can't put into words their reasons for this "sense" or "feel," or because once they say what they are sensing, other people disagree.

✓ **3. Treating Emotions as Facts Leads to Difficulties**

When carried to extremes, emotions are treated as facts: "If I feel incompetent, I am," "If I get depressed when left alone, I shouldn't be left alone," "If I feel right about something, it is right." People use their emotions as evidence that what they believe is correct.

Example: "If you had a needle phobia and treated the fear as fact, then you might try to get rid of all of the needles in the world."

💬 **Discussion Point:** Ask participants for examples of times when the intensity of their emotions seemed to validate their own view of events. Draw from them instances when emotions have been self-validating and when changing negative emotions has been invalidating. Have them give personal examples if possible. Discuss.

> **Note to Leaders:** The points above—that emotions function to communicate to ourselves, and that these communications may not always be accurate—are crucial and very sensitive for many individuals. This is particularly true for individuals who have experienced pervasive invalidating environments. In the absence of validation from others, a primary function of negative emotions can sometimes be self-validation.
>
> The way this works is as follows: When feelings are minimized or invalidated, then it is difficult for individuals to get their concerns and needs taken seriously. One way they counteract this is to increase the intensity of their emotions. Sooner or later, highly emotional people will probably be attended to. If at a later point, these persons do not get very emotional under the same circumstances, this proves other people right: The original emotions weren't valid in the first place. If a situation is not as bad as a person said it was, then he or she feels shame for having caused so much trouble to others. After enough of these

instances, the person begins to believe that his or her integrity is on the line with emotions. Ergo, the function of negative emotions gradually evolves to that of self-validation.

Getting these points across to highly emotional individuals is fraught with difficulty, because the very idea is invalidating. Care, patience, and skill are needed here.

IV. WHAT MAKES IT HARD TO REGULATE EMOTIONS? (EMOTION REGULATION HANDOUTS 4–4A)

Main Point: Regulating emotions is very hard. Biology, lack of skills, reinforcing consequences, moodiness, mental overload, and emotion myths can each make regulating emotions very difficult.

Emotion Regulation Handout 4: What Makes It Hard to Regulate Your Emotions. Review this handout reasonably fast, validating that emotion regulation is very difficult. You can revisit it later to troubleshoot difficulties in using skills successfully.

Emotion Regulation Worksheet 16: Troubleshooting Problems in Emotion Regulation (Optional). This worksheet is designed to work with Emotion Regulation Handout 24: Troubleshooting Emotion Regulation Skills. However, it can be given to participants earlier if you do not think it will overwhelm them or interfere with practicing other skills. The worksheet can also be used individually in skills coaching.

Emotion Regulation Handout 4a: Myths about Emotions (Optional). If this handout is used, the best way to work with it is simply to ask participants to read the myths and circle the ones they believe are true. It can be helpful and interesting to ask them to circle the statements they agree with in *emotion mind only*, and to put a checkmark by the ones they agree with when in *wise mind*. Once this is done, and before you move on to any teaching points, use the devil's advocate strategy described below under F, "Emotion Myths." (For a fuller description of this technique, see Chapter 9 of the main DBT text.) If you skip reviewing this handout, you can describe several myths about emotions when introducing the Emotion Regulation module.

Emotion Regulation Worksheet 3: Myths about Emotions (Optional). You can assign this worksheet whether or not you review Handout 4a. The worksheet is very similar to the list of myths in Handout 4a, but each myth on the worksheet already has one challenge written in. The homework is to develop new challenges or rewrite the challenges already there in more personal language. It is not uncommon for participants to like the challenges as written. If these have personal value for them, this is fine. The important point is for the participants to "own" a challenge, not to necessarily think up a new one. There are also spaces for participants to write in and challenge their own myths.

Orient participants to the following factors that interfere with emotion regulation.

✓ A. Biology

Biological factors can make emotion regulation harder. Some babies are born more emotionally sensitive than others, and they may remain that way as children and adults.[28] Emotional intensity also differs across people.[29] High emotional sensitivity and intensity can get in the way of learning emotion regulation strategies and of using already learned strategies.

💬 **Discussion Point:** One way to think about biological differences in emotionality is to consider the children we know or have known. Most parents with multiple children talk about the amazing differences among their children in emotional temperament—differences that become evident shortly after birth. Elicit such experiences in participants' own lives. Are they more or less emotional than siblings? Have they always had difficulties in emotion regulation, or have the difficulties only shown up recently?

✓ B. Lack of Skill

Say to participants: "When you have skill deficits, you actually don't know how to change or regulate your emotions and emotion-related actions. You also may not know how to get yourself regulated enough to even want to lower the intensity of your emotions."

✓ **Not having a skill is very different from not having motivation.** People learn emotion regulation starting in infancy.[30] The back-and-forth exchange of emotions between mother and baby is the start of emotion regulation training.[31, 32] Child rearing is, in many ways, a task of teaching children how to regulate their emotions. Some parents are very good at this. Some try hard but do not have the necessary skills. Some don't have the time or the desire to do it. Some parents can't regulate their own emotions, and thus find it extremely difficult to teach their children how to do it.[33] Because of biological sensitivity, some children have much more difficulty learning to regulate their emotions than others.

Example: Learning to regulate emotions is like learning to play golf. Although everyone can learn the skill somewhat, it is much easier for some people than for others to get really good at it.

✓ **Skills and their use are frequently context-dependent.** That is, a person can have skills in one set of situations, but not in others; or in one mood, but not in another; or in one frame of mind, but not in another.

💬 **Discussion Point:** Elicit descriptions of participants' experiences in learning emotion regulation.

✓ C. Reinforcement of Emotional Behaviors

As discussed above, emotions have functions. When the functions of certain emotions are reinforced in a particular situation, it can be extremely difficult to change these emotions.

Example: "If every time you are angry, people give you what you want, it will be very, very difficult for you to learn how to regulate your anger. Getting what you want when you are angry can reinforce angry outbursts."

Example: "If people only listen and help you when you get very sad and depressed and cry a lot, it will be very hard for you to stop being sad."

Example: "If you are afraid but walk down a dark alley anyway, and then you are attacked, you will have a tough time getting yourself not to be afraid the next time you are tempted to walk down an alley."

Explain: "Sometimes your emotions do you much good, even when they are very painful or get you in trouble. When this is the case, it can be very hard to change your emotions. You may not even realize that you can't change your emotions, because they are doing too many good things for you. When this happens, your emotions are being reinforced even if you don't want them to be. Emotions are reinforced when they do various things for you:

- ▪ "They may communicate important messages or cause people to do things for you."
- ▪ "They may motivate your own behavior, so that you do things that are important to you."
- ▪ "They may validate your beliefs about what is going on in a situation."
- ▪ "Or they may make you feel better than you would feel without them."

✓ D. Moodiness

Regulating emotions takes a lot of effort and energy.[34, 35] It also takes willingness (a distress tolerance skill; see Distress Tolerance Handout 13). Say to participants: "Moodiness and lack of energy can interfere with your willingness to do the work emotion regulation takes. You may have the capability, but it may be interfered with by your current mood."

✓ **E. Emotional Overload**

Continue: "At times, your emotions can be so extreme that you simply cannot get into wise mind in order to figure out what to do. When you are highly aroused, worry thoughts and ruminations[36, 37] can keep the emotion firing like a computer program that is automatically started when you get highly emotional. Worries like 'Why did I do that?' and 'What will I do?' get started and trick your brain into thinking that there is actually an answer to the worries.[38] Usually, however, there is no answer, so the worries go round and round and round.[39] Often worries function as a way to escape your emotions.[40] Escaping your emotions, however, keeps you from attending to them effectively.[41, 42] You may have the skills, but ruminating interferes with using your skills."

Example: Although crying or sobbing can often be reparative, at other times it can become an out-of-control vortex: The more we cry, the more distressed we become, and the more we cry. In these situations, concurrent rumination and rehearsal of all that is wrong repeatedly elicit tears and sobs, so that the reparative function of the emotion is blocked.

✓ *Example:* Extreme anger or other intense emotions can be like falling into a sea of dyscontrol. Reasonable mind does not have a chance to surface and moderate the influence of emotion mind.

✓ **F. Myths about Emotion**

Faulty beliefs about emotions, the value of expressing emotions, and the ease of recognizing and controlling emotions can cause much trouble when we are trying to learn emotion regulation. Some myths invalidate emotional experiences, such as believing that negative emotions are selfish, or that we can control all our emotions if we just use willpower. What is invalidating is that these myths in no way resonate with our experience of our own emotions. Other myths overvalue emotions. These beliefs ignore the effectiveness of emotions and their expressions, and assert that if we have them, we should not change them. Both sets of beliefs can interfere with emotion regulation.

Example: The myth "Emotions won't go away" can be replaced with the following: "An emotion can be like being on a surfboard. You will ride up and down on the wave until it finally goes away."

👥 **Practice Exercise:** If you are using Handout 4a, distribute it and ask each person to *circle* myths they believe when in emotion mind, and to put a *check* by those they believe when in wise mind. Ask which myths they circled and which they checked. Use the devil's advocate technique to dispute myths about emotions. In this technique, you play the role of the devil's advocate, who believes in the myth even more than the participants do. (This can take a fair amount of acting skill on your part.) The task of participants is to develop challenges or counterarguments to the myths. These challenges can be used as cheerleading statements later to help the clients feel better. Have everyone write challenges down as participants think them up. Even when people have been through the myths before and know that you do not really believe your devil's advocate position, the strategy can still be used, because it provides an opportunity to practice challenging dysfunctional beliefs.

Note to Leaders: For a more expanded set of instructions for this exercise, see Interpersonal Effectiveness Handout 2a: Myths in the Way of Interpersonal Effectiveness. If you only get through a few of the myths on Emotion Regulation Handout 4a, then assign it instead of Worksheet 3 as homework, asking participants to come up with challenges for the rest of the myths.

V. A MODEL OF EMOTIONS (EMOTION REGULATION HANDOUTS 5–6)

Main Point: Emotions are complex, full-system responses. Changing any part of the system can change the entire response. Knowing the parts of an emotion can guide efforts to change the emotion.

Emotion Regulation Handout 5: A Model for Describing Emotions. This handout shows the components of an emotional response in the form of a flow chart. With some exceptions, the component categories match those on Emotion Regulation Handout 6 and Worksheets 4 and 5. Make every effort to review Handout 6 and at least the basics of the accompanying teaching notes (Section VI, on p. 345) in the same session as Handout 5. Otherwise, it will be very difficult for participants to fill out the worksheets.

Emotion Regulation Handout 6: Ways to Describe Emotions. This long handout lists typical components for 10 specific emotions. It gives participants ideas when they have trouble describing characteristics of their own emotions. It does not have to be gone over in detail. You might go over one or two pages in detail (choose your favorites); you can then go through the rest briefly, explaining what they are, and have clients read them between sessions. Some will find this very helpful, others not so helpful. It is essential to convey that the features listed on the handout are not necessary to each emotion. These are typical features, but because of culture and individual learning, features may differ from person to person.

If you must split Handouts 5 and 6 into two sessions, you can assign the reading of Handout 6 as homework, and then instruct participants how to use it to figure out their own emotions and fill out Worksheet 4 or 4a. Alternatively, it might be preferable to put off assigning worksheets until after reviewing Handout 6.

Emotion Regulation Worksheets 4 and 4a: Observing and Describing Emotions. These two worksheets have different formats for filling in the same information—the components of a participant's emotion. Worksheet 4 uses the same graphic format as the model of emotions in Handout 5. Worksheet 4a asks for the components of a specific emotion in a list format. Participants should refer to Handout 6 for ideas when they have trouble describing their own emotions. If necessary, instruct them in how to rate intensity of emotions (0 = no emotion to 100 = most extreme emotion). Common problems in filling out these worksheets are described in the next section.

A. Characteristics of Emotions

Note to Leaders: If you did not review Emotion Regulation Handout 3, review the seven points below either here or later after describing the model of emotions.

✓ ### 1. Emotions Are Complex

Emotions are complex; they generally consist of several parts or different reactions happening at the same time.[43]

✓ ### 2. Emotions Are Automatic

Emotions are involuntary, automatic responses[44] to internal and external events.

✓ ### 3. Emotions Cannot Be Changed Directly

We can change the events that cause emotional experiences, but we cannot change emotional experiences directly. We cannot instruct ourselves to *feel* a particular emotion and then feel it. We cannot use willpower to stop an emotional experience even when we desperately want to.

✓ **4. Emotions Are Sudden, and They Rise and Fall**

Emotions ordinarily occur suddenly,[45] although the intensity of a particular emotion may build up slowly over time. They are also like waves in the sea, because they rise and fall. Most emotions only last from seconds to minutes.

✓ **5. Emotions Are Self-Perpetuating**

Once an emotion starts, it keeps restarting itself. We might even say that "emotions love themselves." This is because emotions sensitize us to events associated with the emotions.

Examples: When we are in a house at night alone and are afraid, every little sound seems like it may be someone breaking in. When we are in love, we see only the positive points of the person we love. Once we are jealous, every time our loved one looks at someone else, it is proof of betrayal.

6. Emotions Have Components

Emotions have components.[42] These components are interrelated, and each component influences all others. Thus, although an emotion can be thought of as a complete and transactional systemic response to external and internal events, it can also be very helpful to examine each component separately. A very important take-home message here is that changing just one component can often change the entire emotional response.

7. Some Emotions Are Universal

There are probably about 10–12 universal emotions (e.g., anger, disgust, fear, guilt, joy, jealousy, envy, sadness, shame, surprise, interest, love[46]). People are born with the potential, the biological readiness, for these. Others are learned and are usually some combination of the basic emotions.

✓ **B. Components of Emotions**

> **Note to Leaders:** As you review the components of emotions, it is useful to start drawing the model for describing emotions on the board, using Emotion Regulation Handout 5 as your guide. (Take a copy of the handout with you to the board. I always do.) This way, the model unfolds as you talk about it, and participants don't get confused about where you are.
>
> The flow of teaching goes much better if you go in the order listed below (points 1–10). You can mention Prompting Event 2 when first presenting prompting events (saying that an emotion just experienced can also be a prompting event), and also as a final comment when completing the explanation of the model.
>
> For each component, give a definition, an example, and one way you can change your emotion by changing that component. (For names of skills that fit each emotion component, see Emotion Regulation Handout 25: Review of Skills for Emotion Regulation.)

✓ **1. Prompting Events**

Prompting events are events or situations that occur right before an emotion starts. They are the cues that set off the emotion at that particular moment instead of at some other moment. (Prompting events are not the events that led up to the prompting event.) Prompting events can be external (outside the person, in the environment) or they can be internal (inside the person).

> **Note to Leaders:** You can help participants remember the meaning of the word "cue" by referring to cue cards in a play which are held up to prompt actors to say their lines.
>
> "Prompting event" is the term used here instead of the word "trigger." The word "trigger" implies an invariably automatic effect, as when a bullet comes speeding out of a gun when the trigger is pulled.

> "Prompting event" is a softer term, implying an easier route to change and the possibility that the event does not always result in an emotional response.

✓ **a. Prompts Can Be Internal**

A person's own thoughts, behaviors, and physical reactions can prompt emotions. One emotion can prompt another secondary emotion.

✓ *Example:* "When you feel sad, you can then feel angry that you feel sad."

✓ **b. Prompts Can Be External**

Events in the environment, including things that people do, can prompt an emotion.

Examples: "Rain on your wedding day, or a friend's saying something mean, can make you feel sad."

✓ **c. Events Can Prompt Emotions Automatically**

An external event can prompt an emotion automatically. That is, a person can have an automatic reaction without any thoughts about the event.

Examples: "You may feel fear when looking down from a high place, or joy when seeing a beautiful sunset."

💬 **Discussion Point:** Elicit other examples. Get examples of both primary emotions and secondary emotions. (Remember, a secondary emotion is an emotional response to a preceding emotion.)

✓ **d. When Prompting Events Change, Emotions Can Change**

Say: "You can change emotions by changing prompting events. You can avoid these events, or you can take action to change them through problem solving."

2. *Attention/Awareness*

Tell participants: "A prompting event will not prompt an emotion if you are not aware that it actually happened. The event has to grab at least part of your attention to have an effect."

Example: "Your mother says something mean, but your cell phone has died and you do not hear it, and she does not say it again."

a. There Is No Emotion without Awareness

Say: "Even when an event is internal—for example, an emotion, an infection, or tense muscles—it will not prompt an emotion if you are not aware of it at some level. The attention grab can be very rapid, but it has to be there at least a little."

✓ **b. When Attention Is Distracted, Emotions Can Change**

"You can change emotions by *distracting your attention away* from prompting events." (See Distress Tolerance Handout 7: Distracting.)

✓ **3. *Interpretation of Events Can Be the Prompting Event***

Continue: "Often what really sets off your emotion is your interpretation of the prompting event, not the event itself. Interpretations are thoughts, beliefs, or assumptions about an event, or appraisals of the event."

> **Note to Leaders:** It is very important to get this point on interpretation across to participants. The more examples you give, the better. It can be particularly effective to tell a story in which at first a person would

> misinterpret the situation because of inadequate information, and then change the interpretation when more information is given.

Example: "Your best friend, Jacob, is walking down the mall across from you with another friend of his. You wave and shout his name. He keeps on walking without saying anything. You interpret this as meaning that he likes his other friend more than you, and you feel hurt. If, however, you interpreted it as meaning that the mall was crowded and Jacob did not see or hear you, you would probably not feel hurt."

Example: Mary doesn't like Susan or Jenny. Susan gets very angry at Mary for not liking her; Jenny gets very afraid. Why? Susan is thinking how much she has done for Mary; Mary should appreciate it and like her. Jenny thinks that if Mary doesn't like her, then maybe no one will ever like her.

a. Interpretations Can Contribute to Complex Emotions

Interpretations, as well as the beliefs and assumptions on which they are based, may become part of very complex emotions. For example, despair is sadness combined with a belief that things are terrible and will not get better.

b. Many Interpretations Are Based on Learned Beliefs

Example: People would not be afraid of guns if they did not believe guns can kill.

Practice Exercise: Have participants think up events and interpretations that set off different emotions. One way to do this is to get one person to give a situation or event, have another give an interpretation, and have a third give the emotion. Then, for the same event, have a fourth person give another interpretation and a fifth figure out the emotion that would go with that interpretation. This can be repeated many times with the same event. Go through a number of events. The important point to make is that often people are responding to their own interpretations of an event, not to the event itself.

✓
c. When Interpretations Change, Emotions Can Change

Say: "You can change emotions by checking the facts and changing your interpretations, beliefs, and assumptions accordingly. (Or you can put on 'rose-colored glasses.')"

4. Vulnerability Factors

Vulnerability factors are conditions or events that make an individual very sensitive to a prompting event, more likely to make emotional interpretations, and more biologically reactive to specific events. These can occur shortly before the prompting event, or they can occur in the distant past.

✓
a. Events from the Near Past Can Make Us Vulnerable

If we have not had enough sleep, have not eaten, are sick or recently disabled, have drunk alcohol or used mood-altering drugs, or have just been through very stressful events, we are likely to be more vulnerable to emotions than at other times.
In addition, sometimes a prompting event is the "straw that breaks the camel's back."

Example: We are more likely to get angry at someone who is asking us for the tenth time for a loan when we have no more money than we are the first time the person asks.

Example: If we are rejected by one person and then rejected by another, we may have a much stronger reaction to the second rejection than we had to the first.

Example: If we go through a very stressful situation that we don't handle very well and feel ashamed about it, we are more likely to say yes if we are offered a drink, drugs, or another way of escaping from ourselves.

Example: If we are in a lot of physical pain or have had many unfair demands placed on us lately, we are much more likely to get very angry if anyone puts one more demand on us.

✓ **b. Events from the Distant Past Can Make Us Vulnerable**

Events from the distant past can make us more vulnerable to events in the present. This is particularly true if we have not processed or resolved the prior events.

Example: A person who has had a traumatic experience may respond to similar situations as if the traumatic event is happening again, even when it is not. When a person is so traumatized that he or she develops PTSD, for example, the person often responds to even very small events that are associated with the traumatic event as if the trauma is happening again. Thoughts of being shot at, raped, or in a car wreck, or any reminder of such an event in the environment, can evoke the very same reaction as the original experience of being shot at, raped, or in a car wreck.

Example: Many adults find that they sometimes react emotionally to another person in the same way that they reacted to one of their parents, even though the person is in most ways not at all like their parent. Usually the other person has done or said something similar to what a parent said or did. Something in the present can evoke a response from the past, even when we are not consciously aware that the current event is a reminder of the past event.

✓ **c. When Vulnerability Factors Change, Emotions Can Change**

Say: "You can reduce negative emotions by reducing your current vulnerability factors. For instance, you can do this by getting more sleep; by building a life with less stress; and by increasing resiliency factors in other ways, such as using strategies to desensitize yourself to cues linked to past events."

✓ **5. *Biological Changes***

When emotions fire, several complex biological changes occur so quickly as to be simultaneous.[43]

a. Emotions Involve Brain Changes

Emotions involve neurochemical changes in the brain.[47, 48] Some parts of the brain (e.g., the limbic system) appear to be very important in regulating emotions. The brain changes can then have effects on the rest of the body.

Note to Leaders: It is important to note that brain differences between people with a disorder and people without the disorder are not necessarily permanent. It is also not true that the only ways to change the brain are medications or direct stimulation of some sort, such as electroconvulsive treatment (ECT). We now know that the brain can also change when behavior changes![49] For example, one study found that individuals with major depression treated with an antidepressant or with interpersonal therapy showed the same regional brain changes after 12 weeks of treatment.[50] It is thought that psychotherapy is a learning experience and produces change in synaptic plasticity through a retraining of implicit memory systems.[51–53]

Research Points:

- *Emotional brain circuits.* There appear to be many emotional brain circuits. Different circuits (or systems) appear to be associated with different broad groups of emotions. Examples include the rage/anger system, the fear/anxiety system,[54] the lust/sexuality system,[55] the care/nurturance system, the panic/separation system, and the play/joy system. Different parts of the brain (e.g., the amygdala, hypothalamus, and anterior cingulate) and different neurochemicals (e.g., serotonin, norepinephrine, oxytocin, and prolactin) are associated with the firing of emotions and the regulation of emotions. Some people have difficulties regulating all of their emotional circuits. Others have difficulties in only one or a few circuits.[56]

- *Brain asymmetry.* Differences in activation of left and right regions of the brain are related to a predisposition for positive emotional states (right activation low compared to left activation) and negative emotional states (left activation low compared to right activation). For example, some studies have shown that people with clinical depression, compared to people without depression, had decreased left brain activation. Differences in right-brain versus left-brain activation can influence vulnerability to various emotional states. High or low activation in various parts of the brain can make it easier or harder for some individuals to regulate their emotions.[57–61]

- *Problems in brain chemistry.* Some researchers believe that one reason some people have trouble regulating emotions is that they have a problem in their brain chemistry.[62]

✓   **b. Emotions Involve Nervous System Changes**

The nerves that are peripheral to the brain and spinal cord send signals to the muscles to contract or relax, and also control autonomic activity—for example, the action of the heart and glands, breathing, digestive processes, and reflex actions. All these responses are also part of emotional responding.

There are two nerve systems controlling autonomic processes that act in opposite directions from each other: an *activating* system and a *deactivating* or quieting system.

When we are under stress, the activating system kicks in. Called the "sympathetic nervous system," it *increases* heart rate and blood pressure, cools the skin, causes sweating, increases the rate of breathing, and activates the production of sugar to give us energy. It prepares us for actions *now*.

The other system, called the "parasympathetic nervous system," counteracts these actions by slowing down the body. When we are relaxed, this quieting aspect of the system takes over.

✓   **c. When Biological Processes Change, Emotions Can Change**

We can change our emotions by targeting biological processes with medications, neurofeedback, ECT, behavioral skills aimed at evoking the parasympathetic nervous system, yoga, and many other approaches or techniques.

Psychoactive drugs work to control emotions by changing brain chemistry. Putting drugs into the brain system can have powerful effects on our emotions. However, once the brain knows the drugs are there, it often changes the chemistry again to compensate, and then the drugs quit working.

d. Dysfunctional Behaviors Can Also Regulate Emotions through Biology

Many dysfunctional behaviors (such as using illicit drugs, overusing alcohol, or self-cutting) also regulate emotions by regulating biology. In these cases, however, the behaviors take a great toll on us in other ways.

6. Experiences

Emotions are almost always associated with the experience of feeling sensations and with urges to do something. Both our feelings and our urges prompt us to act in some way.

✓ **a. Sensations (Feelings)**

When we have emotions, we are actually sensing our body and brain changes. This is usually what is meant by an "emotional experience." Sensations are an important part of emotions and are the reason we often call emotions "feelings."

Example: Sadness involves sensations of low energy, heaviness, and emptiness.

Example: Anger involves sensations of high energy and agitation.

✓ **The experience of sensations cannot be changed directly.** If sensations we don't like could be changed directly, we would all get rid of physical pain and of emotions we find painful. But what would happen then? We would not avoid dangerous situations. If a child was lost, we would not go out and try to find the child. We would not feel jealousy and thus might not protect what we have. We might decide to give up on anger and not defend ourselves or fight for the rights of others. This would be a disaster. Without feeling emotions, how would we survive? From an evolutionary point of view, the feelings and experiences of emotions are critical for survival.

✓ **The experience of sensations can only be changed indirectly. For example, we can focus our attention on something else through distraction, or we can change our biology to block the sensations.**

💬 **Discussion Point:** Say: "When people tell you to quit feeling an emotion, it is like telling you to quit feeling the rain come down on your head or the pain when someone hits you over the head with a skillet. The only way to 'quit feeling' it is to divert your attention or change some other aspect of your emotion. Although that is sometimes easy to do, it is sometimes next to impossible. Telling a person to divert attention when his or her foot is in a fire, for example, would not be effective." Discuss this idea.

> **Note to Leaders:** If participants have been through the Distress Tolerance module already, they may believe that this point contradicts the distraction skills they learned as part of crisis survival. The point to be made is that no skill works for every situation. Problem solving ("getting your hand out of the fire") and radical acceptance ("when you can't get your hand out of the fire") may sometimes be more effective than distraction.

✓ 👥 **Practice Exercise:** If you have not done this previously, lead participants in a series of exercises where they try to quit feeling/sensing something *without* diverting their attention (e.g., their hands on the table, their arms on their chair arms). Then instruct them to try to stop feeling something by diverting their attention.

💬 **Discussion Point:** Say: "Sometimes the problem with emotion is that you cannot sense your body and its changes. To regulate emotions, you have to be skilled in sensing your body. If you have been practicing shutting off all sensations for years, this can be difficult." Get feedback from clients: Which participants have difficulty sensing their bodies? Which have difficulty pinpointing exactly what part of their bodies they are sensing? Discuss the notion that for some people, emotions are like a fog; they can't see (sense) what exactly an emotion is.

✓   **b. Action Urges**

An important function of emotions is to prompt behavior (e.g., fight in anger, flight in fear). Many of the nervous system changes described above are designed to activate the body to be ready for action. As the body gets ready for action, very strong urges to act can arise.

💬 **Discussion Point:** Discuss the action urges of several emotions. Elicit feedback from participants. For ideas on actions that go with various emotions, see Emotion Regulation Handout 6: Ways to Describe Emotions.

7. *Expressions*

One of the most important functions of emotions is to communicate.[63] If it is to do that, an emotion has to be expressed.

✓   **a. Facial Expressions Communicate Emotions**

The facial expression of primary or basic emotions is "hard-wired" into human beings.[64, 65]

> **Research Point:** Research shows that in all cultures, there are some facial expressions that are linked to the same basic emotions. (Many actions that express emotions are also hard-wired.) A change in facial muscles when emotions are activated is universal. People are extremely sensitive to facial expressions from early childhood onward.[66, 67] During infancy, emotional expressions are especially important social signals at a time when verbal communication is not possible.[68–71] Researchers now think that changes in the facial muscles play a very important role in actually *causing* emotions. We humans have more nerves in the face than anywhere else in the body. Facial expressions for many of our basic emotions are the same across cultures. The importance of facial expressions in communicating with others is likely very important to our survival.

✓   **b. Body Language Communicates Emotions**

Even when our faces cannot be seen, our bodies can communicate emotions. Our posture can be relaxed, tense, drooping, or shoulders back. Our hands can be clenched and tight, or open and relaxed. Each different posture sends a message to others about how and what we are feeling.

People can learn to inhibit emotional expressions or to express them differently. For complex emotions that are learned, the expressions are also learned.

Some facial expressions and behaviors may express different emotions, depending on one's overall culture;[72] one's regional culture (e.g., the South vs. the Northwest in the United States); and one's family culture, school culture, and individual differences.[73]

💬 **Discussion Point:** Discuss the fact that each family, town, state, and so on is a "miniculture." Expressiveness that is OK in one miniculture may not be OK in another. Get examples from participants' own experience.

💬 **Discussion Point:** Discuss the point that what an expression means can vary from time to time and person to person. Thus reading emotions is easy in some ways, but very difficult in others. People often misread other people's emotions. The same behavior can express many different emotions, and the same emotion can be expressed by many different behaviors. Discuss how one behavior can mean many things and how different behaviors can mean the same thing. Get examples from participants' own lives.

💬 **Discussion Point:** Many individuals have learned to hide their emotions by controlling the facial muscles and body language that express emotions. This is a natural result of social learning in an emotionally invalidating environment. The hiding is usually automatic; that is, the individuals do not intend it, or are not aware of it. This is a major reason why others often do not know that these persons are as upset as they are—they don't look it! Discuss how participants have learned to conceal their emotions in this way.

💬 **Discussion Point:** It is also possible that some individuals are born with emotional systems that are less obviously expressive than the systems of others. It may be that this initial tendency to under-express emotions (e.g., through facial expressions) sets up a situation where others do not get the feedback they need to interact with these persons appropriately. Thus the environment becomes less responsive to the *emotional* expressions of these individuals, setting up an invalidating pattern. Discuss this hypothesis with participants.

👥 **Practice Exercise:** Go around the room and have participants try to express a particular emotion nonverbally with their facial expressions or just with their bodies. Ask other participants to try and guess what emotion they are expressing.

✓   **c. Words Communicate Emotions**

Telling other people how we feel about them, ourselves, or a particular event, or how we feel in general, can be very powerful (e.g., "I love you," "I hate you," "I am sad," "I'm sorry"). It can improve others' understanding of us and also elicit reactions in others.

💬 **Discussion Point:** Some people have learned never, or hardly ever, to tell other people how they really feel. This can be an advantage in situations where others will punish them for their feelings, or where their true feelings will unnecessarily hurt others. However, this can create a lot of problems with trustworthy people. Discuss when telling the truth about participants' emotions has been hurtful and when it has been helpful. When has concealing emotions been helpful or hurtful?

✓   **d. When Facial and Body Expressions Change, Emotions Can Change**

We can change emotions by changing our facial and body expressions. In particular, the connection among our bodies, faces, and emotions is so tight that we can change our emotions simply by changing our facial expressions. This is called the "facial feedback hypothesis."[74] We can also change our emotions by changing our posture, how we hold our hands, and the tightness of our muscles.

Example: If we are very afraid or anxious, we can feel calmer by relaxing our muscles.

> **Research Point:** In a study examining the facial feedback hypothesis,[75] each participant was asked to hold a pencil in the mouth to either facilitate or inhibit smiles. Those participants in the "facilitate smile" condition reported more positive experiences when pleasant scenes and humorous cartoons were presented to them. These results support the theory that our emotions change to match our facial expressions.

Emphasize that **changing emotional expressions is different from suppressing emotion.** Explain to participants: "When you suppress an emotion, you are working hard to restrain, stifle, or hold back a natural expression. It is like trying to smother the expressive part of your emotion. Suppressing emotions can actually lead to more extreme emotions. In contrast, when you change an emotional expression, you are replacing one expression with another. You are actively altering your muscles to modify your expression. Generally, this is very hard to do if your face and body are very tense, as they usually are when you are trying to suppress an emotion."

💬 **Discussion Point:** The relationship among facial expression, body language, and each individual's actual emotional experience is not an exact correspondence. This is particularly so when what we say does not match our voice tone, our facial expression, and/or our body posture. When this happens, almost everyone will pay attention to the nonverbal communication and ignore the words. This, of course, is a real problem for those of us whose words are more accurate than our nonverbal expressions. Go around the group and have participants discuss ways in which their emotions have been misread, as well as ways in which they have misread others' emotions.

8. Actions

✓ **a. Emotions Prepare the Body for Action**

One of the primary functions of emotions is to prepare the body for action (e.g., kissing, hitting, running toward someone, withdrawing passively, avoiding, doing cartwheels). Thus an action itself can be thought of as a part of an entire emotional response. Emotions in general can be thought of as a rapid response system. Tell participants: "Remember, emotions evolved in order to prompt actions necessary for survival. Later in this module, we will review how particular types of action typically go with specific emotions."

💬 **Discussion Point:** One of the most important tasks in development is to learn when to inhibit emotional actions and when not to. People who are very impulsive often have great difficulty here: When they act in accord with their emotions, and this is viewed by others as inappropriate, it is often called "acting out." Other individuals may be so inhibited that they rarely engage in emotional actions. Discuss who is overly impulsive and who is overly inhibited. Often the same person is impulsive in some situations and inhibited in others. Again, discuss.

✓ **b. When Actions Change, Emotions Can Change**

Say to participants: "You can change emotions by acting opposite to the emotion's action urge. Again, this is something we will work on later in this module."

9. Emotion Names

a. Naming Emotions Is Universal and Helpful

Every culture gives names to emotions. To name an emotion also requires **awareness** of the emotion. When we are communicating to others how we feel, it is important to be able to identify what emotion we are actually feeling, so that our communication will be accurate. There is also some evidence that people who can give an emotion a name experience less negative emotion.[76] How to name emotions is learned.[77] Obviously, it is easier to name simple emotions than complex ones.

✓ **b. Through Awareness and Naming, Emotions Can Change**

Tell participants: "You can change emotions by learning to be aware of and to name your emotions. Again, we will work on this later in this module."

10. Aftereffects

Intense emotions have powerful aftereffects on memory, thoughts, the ability to think, physical functioning, and behavior.

✓ **a. "Emotions Love Themselves"**

One of the most important aftereffects of emotions is that we become hypervigilant to cues and events that could set off the same emotions and attention is narrowed to information that is incompatible with our emotion. In this way, emotions organize us in such a way as to continue (or keep "refiring"). An emotion that feels as if it has gone on for a very long time is one that is refiring over and over again.

Example: When we are afraid, we often become hypersensitive to any threat to our safety.

Example: When we are angry, we often become hypersensitive to any insulting behavior of others or to behaviors that threaten to interfere with our goals.

Example: When we are in love we ordinarily see all the positives in the person we love and do not see the negative.

b. Monitoring Aftereffects of Intense Emotions Can Help Us Change Subsequent Emotions

Tell participants: "Once you know that intense emotions narrow attention and increase sensitivity to cues for the same emotion, you can remind yourself to check the facts. Knowing you may be seeing things through the lenses of the emotion you are trying to change rather than the lenses of present reality can be helpful at this point.

C. Primary and Secondary Emotions (*Optional*)

> **Note to Leaders:** This section on the differences between primary and secondary emotions is likely to overload people taking this module for the first time. It can be useful new information for people going through the module a second time.

1. Primary Emotions Are Our Immediate, First Reactions

Our spontaneous emotional reactions to events outside of ourselves are examples of primary emotions.

2. Secondary Emotions Are Usually Reactions to Our Primary Emotions

Sometimes secondary emotions follow primary emotions so quickly that we do not even notice the primary emotions. Sometimes we have spent so many years suppressing our primary emotions that we automatically "jump over" the primary emotions and never even experience them. That is, we develop a habitual secondary emotional response.

Example: Anger is often a secondary emotion to fear. In fact, for some people, anger is a secondary emotion to many primary emotions. Fear can also be a secondary emotion—for example, when a person is very fearful of anger.

✓ ### 3. Secondary Emotions Can Make Identification of Primary Emotions Difficult

If we cannot identify and describe a primary emotion, we will have trouble changing it. Thus problem solving in regard to the primary emotions is difficult. This topic will come up again and again in working with emotions.

💬 **Discussion Point:** Elicit examples from participants of occasions when they have a secondary emotional reaction to a primary emotion (e.g., getting depressed about being depressed, getting angry or feeling ashamed for getting angry). Ask which usually causes them more trouble and pain—the primary or the secondary emotion?

VI. OBSERVING, DESCRIBING, AND NAMING EMOTIONS (EMOTION REGULATION HANDOUT 6)

> **Main Point:** Learning to observe, describe, and name emotions can help with regulating emotions.
>
> **Emotion Regulation Handout 6: Ways to Describe Emotions.** This handout gives participants ideas when they have trouble describing characteristics of their own emotions. It does not have to be gone over in detail. It is essential to convey that the features listed on the handout are not necessary to each emotion. These are typical features, but because of culture and individual learning, features may differ from person to person.

Emotion Regulation Worksheets 4 and 4a: Observing and Describing Emotions. These two worksheets differ in format, but ask for exactly the same information and have the same instructions. Let participants choose which one they want to use, and then review them with participants.

Common problems and errors on these worksheets include the following:

- *Prompting Event:* Participants often want to write an entire story for "Prompting Event." However, this section should just describe the few moments immediately before the emotion fired. The "story" goes in the "Vulnerability Factors" section.

- *Vulnerability Factors:* The history preceding the prompting event can be communicated under "Vulnerability Factors." This section is here so participants can tell the story that explains their reaction to the prompting event. Here participants can list events from the distant past (to explain their learning history), as well as events in the immediate past that may have increased their vulnerability to emotion mind. Participants often forget to put in physical illness or pain, alcohol or drug use, lack of sleep, over- or undereating, and stressful events in the 24 hours before the prompting events; it is often important to remind them to do this.

- *Biological Changes and Expressions:* It is easy to confuse "Face and Body Changes and Experiences" as part of "Biological Changes" with "Face and Body Language" as part of "Expressions." Biological body changes refer to physical changes (blushing, muscles tensing, sweating, hair follicles standing up, etc.). These are the automatic physiological changes that take place with emotions. Describing the experience of body sensations (feelings) sounds similar to describing biological changes (e.g., feeling muscles tensing, feeling hairs standing up). The point to make to participants here is this: "These very same things can also happen without your feeling them, so it is important to note whether you do feel these changes. Face and body language is expression visible to others. It is sometimes the result of face and body changes, as when blushing makes your face visibly red. It can also include such things as frowning, grimacing, smiling, slumping, clenching hands, slinking back, looking down, staring, and crossing arms."

A. Why Observe and Describe Emotions?

 ### 1. To Improve the Ability to Regulate Emotions

Research Point: Research shows that in processing an emotional experience, it is more effective to be very specific about the emotion and emotional events than to try to regulate the emotion in overly general or nonspecific ways.[78, 79] For example, anxiety is reduced by observing and describing the specific fear-producing cues, in contrast to general impressions regarding cues prompting fear and anxiety.[80]

2. To Learn to Be Separate from Emotions

Explain to participants: "By learning to observe your emotions, you learn to be separate from them and not to be identified with them. In order to control your emotional responses, you must be separate from your emotions so that you can think and use coping strategies."

3. To Learn to Be at One with Emotions

Continue: "Nevertheless, you also need to be one with your emotions, in the sense that you identify them as part of yourself and not something outside of yourself."

Example: To the extent that a rider is "one" with a horse, he or she can control the horse. If the rider is separate, fighting the horse, the horse will fight back, and the rider cannot control it smoothly. On the other hand, if the rider is mindless, so to speak, and has no identity separate from the horse, he or she will just cling to the horse for dear life, and the horse will assume all control.

✓ **B. Steps in Observing and Describing Emotions**

Review the organization of Emotion Regulation Handout 6: Ways to Describe Emotions with participants. The emotions on this handout are grouped in families, and each emotion family has one page describing its characteristics. The sequence of emotions is alphabetical except for guilt, which is put after shame because they are often confused. (Shame is a response to evaluating one's entire self as bad or unworthy; guilt is a response to evaluating one's specific behaviors as bad or immoral.) Although the word "jealousy" is commonly used to mean both jealousy and envy, they are separated here, because instructions for changing these emotions are different from each other. Explain to participants: "Jealousy is when you have something of value and someone else is threatening to take it away; envy is when someone else has something you want but don't have."

The key idea to convey to participants is this: "**You can figure out what your emotion is by matching events and your responses to sets of events and responses on Handout 6**. If you can't identify your own emotion—either a current emotion or a past emotion—you can figure it out by systematically reviewing each emotion component and writing it down if necessary. When the components are put all together and you can see your responses in their totality, it can be much easier to figure out your emotion. If necessary, you can review Handout 6 to see which group of emotion components matches your emotion the best."

> **Note to Leaders:** Depending on the group you are teaching, it may be important to provide some discussion of each of the emotions on Emotion Regulation Handout 6 *as you review how to describe and name emotions*. Some are very easy to understand; others may be more difficult. Many of the descriptions in this handout were made up by ordinary people in response to questions about their emotional experiences. Identify each of the following components when reviewing a specific emotion from Handout 6. In my groups, I usually review two or three emotions and assign reading the entire handout as homework.

In reviewing one or several of the emotions on Handout 6, use the outline below to highlight each of the characteristics of these emotions. Note that each of these characteristics map onto the model of emotions previously described.

✓ *1. Prompting Events*

Tell participants: "For each specific emotion, these are typical prompting events that set off the emotion—events that occurred right before the emotion started." Here is a place to remind participants that the story of what led up to the event goes under vulnerability factors, which are unique to each person and are not on Handout 6.

✓ *2. Interpretations of Events That Prompt Emotion*

Say: "For each specific emotion these are typical interpretations, thoughts, and assumptions about the event that prompt the emotion."

3. Biological Changes and Experiences

Continue: "For each specific emotion these are typical biological changes and experiences, feelings, body sensations, and action urges. Focus here on body changes that you sense (or that you can sense if you pay attention). Note that changes and experiences are similar across some emotions and very different for others."

4. Expressions and Actions

Continue: "Expressions and actions are typical facial expressions, body language, verbal communications, and actions associated with specific emotions. Remember that a primary function of emotions is to elicit actions to solve specific problems. Attend to the actions associated with each emotion."

5. Aftereffects of Emotion

Say: "Aftereffects are what happened to your mind, your body, and your emotions just after your first emotion started."

6. Name of the Emotion

As you review various emotions described on Handout 6, check in with participants at the end of each review to be sure that they are correctly identifying and naming this emotion in themselves.

Note to Leaders: Remind participants to use the "Other:" blanks to write in idiosyncratic prompting events, interpretations, biological changes, experiences, expressions and actions that are typical for them for the various emotions. But check the items to be sure that they really do go with the emotion listed. Some participants may not understand their primary emotion, or may not realize that what they are experiencing is a secondary emotion occurring so quickly they do not even realize they have skipped over (or simply avoided experiencing) the primary emotion associated with the prompting event.

💬 **Discussion Point:** As you go through Emotion Regulation Handout 6, ask participants to give their own ideas about characteristics of emotions. Suggest that all write down new ideas on their handouts.

👥 **Practice Exercise:** First, ask each person to think of an emotional situation to role-play, or use one of the following situations.

- ▪ "Interacting with a friend who gets very angry at you during the interaction."
- ▪ "Being afraid of a very shady-looking person who moves in very close to you at a bus stop."
- ▪ "Meeting a loved one at the airport."
- ▪ "Sitting next to a person you find disgusting."
- ▪ "Talking with a friend about something very sad."

Second, give instructions on how to do a role play. Have two clients role-play the situation, or you can role-play it with one client. The client who chose the emotional situation needs to communicate as much as possible his or her emotions during the role play.

Third, have everyone observe the role play and describe the nonverbal expressive behavior of the role players. Guide clients to pay special attention to faces.

Fourth, have the role players describe how they actually felt and what they were expressing in the role play.

Note to Leaders: For further suggestions regarding role-play techniques, see Chapter 8, Section V (the Practice Exercises for the DEAR MAN skills).

C. Factors That Interfere with Observing and Describing Emotions

Note to Leaders: The points in the section below are usually best made during homework sharing. Participants should fill out as many homework sheets (Emotion Regulation Worksheets 4 or 4a) as there are prompting events. Thus, if a person has a secondary emotional reaction prompted by the original emotion or set of emotions, he or she should fill out a second worksheet. You need to be particularly vigilant about this during homework sharing; it can be very difficult to sort out.

1. Secondary Emotions (Emotional Reactions to Emotions)

As noted earlier, when a secondary emotion comes on the scene, it can cover up or confuse the primary emotional reaction. Sometimes the only way to sort this out is to pay significant attention to the prompting event and the interpretations of the event. You might ask participants: "What emotion would most people have following that emotion?" or "If you were not afraid [guilty, ashamed] of your own emotions, what emotion would you have experienced after that prompting event?" or "Is there any emotional response you were probably avoiding?"

2. Ambivalence (More Than One Emotional Reaction to the Same Event)

Explain to participants: "People often experience two or more emotions at almost exactly the same moment. This can confuse the situation. For example, you might love your parents, and at the same time be furious with them and want to get as far away from them as possible. When moving to a new town, you might be excited and afraid at the same time. To sort this out, complete a worksheet for each emotion experienced, and don't worry about which is primary and secondary before completing the worksheet. It will probably be less confusing to figure this out after completing the worksheet, even if it is difficult to separate the primary and secondary emotions."

VII. OVERVIEW: CHANGING EMOTIONAL RESPONSES (EMOTION REGULATION HANDOUT 7)

> **Main Points:** To change unwanted emotions, we must first check the facts. Sometimes this is all that is needed. When the emotion does not fit the facts, we need to practice acting opposite to our emotion. When the emotion fits the facts and the situation is the problem, we need to do problem solving.
>
> **Emotion Regulation Handout 7: Changing Emotional Responses.** Review this handout even if only briefly, so that participants know that besides checking the facts (covered next in Section VIII), there are two other skills for changing emotional responses: opposite action (covered in Section X) and problem solving (covered in Section XI). Section IX covers how to decide which of the two latter skills to use after checking the facts. This overview, then, orients participants to the three emotion change strategies and prepares them for Section IX and the flow chart in Emotion Regulation Handout 9. Teach the individual skills in Sections VIII–XII, using the handouts described there.

✓ A. Check the Facts

Say to participants: "Changing beliefs and assumptions about a situation to fit the facts can help you change your emotional reactions to it. This requires that you first check out the facts. Checking the facts is a basic strategy in cognitive therapy as well as in many other forms of therapy."

✓ B. Opposite Action

Continue: "When emotions do not fit the facts, and knowing the facts does not change your emotion, then acting opposite to your emotions—all the way, repeatedly—will change your emotional reactions. This is similar to the old adage 'If you fall off a horse, get right back on.'"

✓ C. Problem Solving

Go on: "When your emotions fit the facts of the situation and you want to change your emotions, then the situation is the problem. Solving problems will reduce the frequency of negative emotions."

✓ D. The "Yes, But" Barrier to Changing Emotions

Doing what is needed to change emotional responses can be very difficult. It requires effort, willingness, and an ability to determine what is in one's own best interest. "Yes, but" is a typical response to efforts to help a person change emotions, particularly when emotional intensity is high and changing emotions is experienced as admitting that the person's own feelings are invalid. The problem is that "yes, but" does not lead to feeling better or to solving emotional problems. When "yes, but" rears its head, it can be useful to remind participants that there are only four possible responses to any problem:

1. "*Solve the problem* by changing the situation or by leaving the situation."

2. "*Change your emotional reaction to the situation,* so that painful emotions are reduced even though the problem remains."

3. "*Radically accept the situation.* That is, acknowledge that the situation can't be helped and you can't change how you feel either, but that completely and willingly accepting this state of affairs can give you a sense of freedom and reduce your suffering."

4. "*Stay miserable.* (Or you can make things worse.*)"

Note to Leaders: The four options above are presented in the orientation to DBT skills (see Chapter 6). If you have reviewed these steps, remind participants. If this is the first time you are covering these points, see Chapter 6 for a fuller description. If time permits, you might also want to give out General Handout 1a: Options for Solving Any Problem.

VIII. CHECK THE FACTS (EMOTION REGULATION HANDOUTS 8–8A)

Main Point: We often react to our thoughts and interpretations of an event rather than to the facts of the event.[81] Changing our beliefs, assumptions, and interpretations of events to fit the facts can change our emotional reactions.[82]

Emotion Regulation Handout 8: Check the Facts. If you have a lot of time, this handout may be easier to teach if you have participants pull out Emotion Regulation Handout 6: Ways to Describe Emotions and look at the sections on prompting events and interpretations of events that prompt feelings of specific emotions. If time allows, it can also be helpful to have participants take out copies of Worksheet 5; then, using situations from participants' own experiences as examples, you can have people fill in a worksheet as you go. The principal strategies used and taught here are those of cognitive modification (see Chapter 11 of the main DBT text).

Emotion Regulation Handout 8a: Examples of Emotions That Fit the Facts *(Optional).* This handout can be skipped if you are not going to teach opposite action after checking the facts. The same information is also included in Emotion Regulation Handout 13: Reviewing Opposite Action and Problem Solving. However, for many participants, understanding opposite action is much easier if you have first reviewed how emotions fit with facts.

Emotion Regulation Worksheet 5: Checking the Facts. It is important to review this worksheet with participants. It can be particularly useful to fill out one of these worksheets while teaching Check the Facts to both demonstrate what is meant by each instruction and to demonstrate how to do it. If necessary, instruct in how to rate intensity of emotions (0 = no emotion, no intensity; 100 = maximum emotion intensity). The "Before" and "After" spaces are for rating emotions before and after checking the facts. If participants have trouble figuring out what emotion they are feeling, instruct them to review Handout 6 and/or fill out Worksheet 4 or 4a. Notice that each step in checking the facts has two sections: one for writing down the descriptions of the situation and of thoughts and interpretations that are probably setting off the emotional response; and one section for considering alternative thoughts, interpretations, and descriptions of the facts.

---

*Again, the fabulous idea of adding on "you can make things worse" was sent to me in an e-mail from a person who had gone through DBT skills training. Unfortunately, I cannot find the e-mail to give proper credit to this person. I hope to hear from her for a correction in the future.

✓ **A. Why Check the Facts?**

> **Note to Leaders:** Review only a few of the points in Section 1 below, using examples where needed. This section gives the theory behind checking the facts, and you will have many opportunities to teach this material when reviewing homework and when teaching subsequent skills where checking the facts is an integral component.

1. *Thoughts and Interpretations of Situations and Events (Instead of the Facts) Can Set Off Painful Emotions*[83]

   a. **Beliefs about Reality Can Cause Powerful Emotions**

   Example: A person who believes that a loved one has died in a car accident will feel deep sadness and grief, even if the information the person was given was incorrect and the loved one did not in fact die.

   Example: A person who believes that someone is trying to hurt him or her may feel very afraid, even if the facts are completely different and the other person is trying to help, not hurt.

   b. **Faulty Beliefs about What We Think We Need Can Lead to Emotional Misery**

   Example: "I need illicit drugs to control my pain," instead of "I need to find an effective, nondestructive way to deal with my pain."

   Example: "I must be in control!" instead of "I like being in control better than being out of control."

   Example: "You should be different [e.g., nicer, on time, more understanding, willing to give me more pay]," instead of "You are who you are. Something caused you to be this way. But I want you to be different."

   c. **Faulty Beliefs about Events Can Cause New Problems**

   Example: "I can pass a test without studying for it beforehand," when the person has a low grade point average.

   Example: "I have enough gas in the car to get where I am going," when the fuel gauge is on empty.

   Example: "Your spending time with your friends means that you do not love me and I should move out of the house."

   Example: "Your not inviting me to the party means that you do not like me."

   d. **Thinking in Absolutes Can Set Off Extreme Emotions**

   "Thinking in absolutes" means extreme thinking, black-and-white thinking, all-or-none thinking, and either–or thinking.

   Example: "He hates me," instead of "He is pretty annoyed with me."

   Example: "This job is terrible! I can't stand it!" instead of "Some parts of this job are difficult, but other parts are not so bad. I can tolerate this."

   Example: "If I don't make straight A's in this course, I am a failure," instead of "I may want an A, but less than an A is not a failure."

   Example: "You are either vulnerable or invulnerable," instead of "A person can be tough at times and vulnerable at times."

✓ 👥 **Practice Exercise:** Ask participants to imagine the following scene: "Your car has had a flat tire on the expressway. You are parked on the side of the road right after a ramp. You are standing by your car and hoping someone will stop. You see your best friend [mother, father, sister, teacher] coming up the ramp onto the expressway, in the car alone. You wave and jump up and down. Your friend [or whoever it is] looks right at you, but then speeds up and goes by. How would you feel? Would you feel angry? Hurt? Disappointed?" Ordinarily participants will say one of these emotions. Elicit their thoughts about the situation, suggesting interpretations (such as "What a mean thing to do!"), unrealistic demands on reality ("Friends always stop for a friend in need"), absolute thinking ("He hates me"), and so on. Then continue the story: "You discover later that a small child was in the car that you didn't see, and the child was seriously hurt and your friend was desperately trying to get to the hospital to save the life of the child. Knowing this new fact, how would you feel?" Ordinarily, feelings will change. Point out to participants that the only thing that really changed was their interpretation of the event.

💬 **Discussion Point:** Elicit examples of times when participants' interpretation of an event or thoughts running through their minds have influenced how and what emotion they feel. Check for examples of thinking and interpretations that did not fit the facts, unrealistic demands on reality, and thinking in absolutes.

✓ **2. *Our Emotions Can Affect* What *We Think about Events and* How *We React to Thoughts***

Temporary moods, for example, can influence ideas, memories, perceptions,[84] and interpretations of important events, particularly when the events are complex and ambiguous.[85] The very same information can take on very different coloring, depending on our current emotional state.[86]

Example: When we are angry or annoyed, the cheery friend who calls us up seems more like a pest than a loyal friend.

Example: When we are anxious or afraid, the sound of the wind rattling our bedroom window sounds like someone breaking in.

Example: When we are in a happy mood, even a sour friend can seem like a great person to get together with.

Example: When we are ashamed of making a mistake at work, we may interpret two co-workers laughing in the hall as making fun of our job performance.

Example: When we are sad, we may think a bad grade means we'll never graduate from college.

💬 **Discussion Point:** Elicit examples of times when participants' mood or current emotions have colored how they interpreted events.

Note to Leaders: Relate the fact that emotions can influence thoughts to the concept that "emotions love themselves" and thus perpetuate themselves, discussed both earlier and below.

✓ **3. *Believing That Our Thoughts Are Absolute Truths Can Be a Recipe for Disaster***

It is important to keep these things in mind:

- No one has the absolute truth.
- Believing that "I have a hold on the absolute truth" ordinarily leads to conflict and can even precipitate wars.
- Different opinions on the facts can be valid even if we don't agree with them.
- There is always more than one way to see a situation, and more than one way to solve a problem.

■ Two things that seem like (or are) opposites can both be true.
■ Meaning and truth evolve over time.

> **Note to Leaders:** The points listed above are also covered in Chapter 8, Section XV, in the discussion of dialectics as part of the skills for walking the middle path.

✓ **4. Knowing the Facts Is Essential for Solving Problems**

Incomplete knowledge of the facts, or faulty beliefs about them, can interfere with problem solving.

Example: Believing that my roof is not leaking when it is leaking means that I will not get the roof fixed.

Example: Believing that I failed my exam because the grading was unfair, when in reality it was because I did not study, means that I may not study for the next exam.

✓ **5. Examining Our Thoughts and Checking the Facts Can Change Our Emotions**

When we respond to incorrect facts, learning the correct facts can change our emotions. In addition, knowing the actual facts of a situation can help us problem-solve emotional situations. That is, knowing the facts can help us change the facts.

> **Note to Leaders:** It may be useful to point out that several effective mental health treatments are based on helping people change cognitions (i.e., thoughts, beliefs, interpretations). One of the major treatments for depression is cognitive therapy. Various forms of CBT (which focuses on changing both cognitions and behaviors) have been developed for treating anxiety disorders, eating disorders, substance use disorders, and many others.[87] Two of the major treatments for personality disorders—Schema Therapy[88] and Mentalization-Based Therapy[89]—also target changing cognitions.

✓ **B. How to Check the Facts**

✓ **1. Ask: What Is the Emotion I Want to Change?**

Tell participants: "It is much more difficult to change an emotion when you don't know what emotion or set of emotions you are actually feeling. Facts about a situation might fit one emotion but not another. Reviewing Emotion Regulation Handout 6 can be very helpful to you here. Pay careful attention to current thoughts, physical sensations, posture, action urges, actions, and verbal statements when you are reviewing ways to describe emotions."

✓ **2. Ask: What Is the Event Prompting My Emotion?**

Say to participants: "Describe the facts observed through the senses. Just the facts! Challenge judgments, extremes, and absolute black-and-white descriptions. A more balanced view of the facts may change your emotions."

Explain that a prompting event can be an event outside of ourselves or an internal event such as a previous emotion, series of thoughts, or an ability or inability to do a task. A prompting event can be a secondary reaction to a previous emotion (e.g., anger at ourselves for feeling afraid), thought (e.g., feeling guilty at judgmental thoughts about someone), or lack of ability (e.g., feeling ashamed at our inability to remember someone's name). Our emotions can also be elicited by our own actions (e.g., joy at playing well in a piano recital).

One problem in figuring out emotions is that we often describe situations and our own emotions, thoughts, and actions in judgmental language, with absolute black-and-white statements. Usually this is not an effective way to describe an event, because it can evoke strong negative emotional reactions. Indeed, our mental description of the event, rather than the event itself, may be the actual prompting event.

✓ ### 3. Ask: What Are My Interpretations, Thoughts, and Assumptions about the Event?

Often we add to what we observe and then react to what we have added, rather than to what we observed. We jump to a conclusion and then act on that.

Say to participants: "Think about some erroneous interpretations you might make (and then act on) when feeling particular emotions." Or use these illustrations:

- *Anger:* "Listening to a person express disappointment in something you do (fact) and thinking the person is trying to control you (interpretation)."
- *Disgust:* "Seeing a man looking in your window from the street (fact) and thinking he is a sexual predator (interpretation)."
- *Envy:* "Observing someone receiving a hug (fact) and thinking that this person gets a lot more love than you do (interpretation)."
- *Fear:* "Hearing a creaking sound in the night (fact) and thinking someone is breaking into your house (interpretation)."
- *Happiness:* "Seeing no clouds in the morning sky (fact) and believing it won't rain on your way home (interpretation)."
- *Jealousy:* "Watching the person you love sitting close to someone else (fact) and believing he or she is now in love with that person (interpretation)."
- *Love:* "Realizing a person wants to have sex with you (fact) and assuming the person is in love with you (interpretation)."
- *Sadness:* "Finding out that a person made plans without you (fact) and deciding the person does not love you (interpretation)."
- *Shame:* "Dropping the ball in a game (fact) and then thinking of yourself as being a loser (interpretation)."
- *Guilt:* "Not wanting to share your food with someone (fact) and deciding that you are being selfish (interpretation)."

✓ "**Consider all the other possible interpretations.** Other reasonable interpretations, particularly if they are more benign, can be an effective way to regulate your emotions. Practice looking at all sides of a situation and all the various points of view."

✓ ### 4. Ask: Am I Assuming a Threat?

Say to participants: "Ask yourself whether you are imagining a threatening event or outcome. Painful emotions are almost always related to some type of threat. What negative outcomes might you be anticipating from the event?" Explain that often we are not even aware that we are assuming some sort of threat. The threat is implicit in our minds. It can be important to really search for the threat we are associating with the prompting event. This is particularly important when we have checked all the facts and still are having very intense emotions. This is a clue that our current emotion may be a secondary emotion, and that it may be very important to figure out what implicit (i.e., nonverbal) threat we are actually reacting to.

✓ #### a. Label the Threat

The first thing to do is to label the threat, which involves labeling the emotion. Here are the types of threat we may sense when we are feeling particular emotions:

- *Anger:* Being attacked or important goals being blocked.
- *Disgust:* Being contaminated.
- *Fear:* Encountering danger to life, health, well-being.
- *Sadness:* Losing something permanently or not attaining goals.
- *Shame:* Being kicked out of the community.

■ *Guilt:* Violating one's own values.

■ *Jealousy:* Someone else's taking away a valued person and/or thing.

■ *Envy:* Not attaining what is wanted or needed because others have substantially more power, influence, and belongings.

✓ **b. Evaluate the Chances That the Threatening Event Will Really Occur**

It is important to be in wise mind when considering the likelihood that a threatening event will occur. Often what seems threatening at first glance is not so threatening once we think about it.

Example: "You think, 'I'm going to be robbed,' when seeing two men walking towards you on a street at night. Evaluate the chances that the threatening event will really occur by observing if there are other people around, if the men are carrying weapons, and so on."

Now present the following points to participants, and give the examples that follow:

■ "Consider: What was the outcome previous times you had a similar thought?"

Example: "When having a headache, you think, 'I probably have some terrible disease.' Remind yourself that you have had many headaches in the past that were not serious and went away before long."

■ "Ask questions; seek more information; check and review the known facts of the situation."

Example: "When a co-worker walks by you at the mall without saying hi, you think, 'She doesn't like me.' Seek information: Ask the co-worker whether she saw you at the mall."

■ "Observe the problem situation, after first calming yourself down so as to see clearly."

Example: When your son tells you he had an accident while driving your car, you think, 'My car is destroyed.' Observe by checking out the car yourself."

■ "Perform experiments in the real world to see if your predictions come true. How factual are your worries and predictions about events?"

Example: "You think, 'I can't get a job.' Conduct this experiment: Apply for lots of jobs that you qualify for, and see what happens."

✓ **c. Think of Other Possible Outcomes**

Tell participants: "Now imagine as many other possible outcomes as you can. The simple act of generating alternative outcomes can itself increase your belief that other outcomes are possible."

Example: "When told by your boss that he would like to meet with you, you think, 'I'm going to be fired.' Generate alternative outcomes: 'He's going to ask me for the status of the project I'm working on,' 'He's going to ask me if I can stay late to help him with the project that's due tomorrow,' 'He's going to give me a bonus for all the overtime I put in this year.'"

✓ **5. *Ask: What Is the Catastrophe?***

What if the threatening event actually does occur?

a. If the Worst Outcome Does Occur, What Are the Realistic Consequences?

Sometimes the facts are every bit as bad as we think they are. However, we often make a bad situation even worse when we catastrophize the facts. "Catastrophizing" is exaggerating the negative characteristics of the facts, and focusing on the worst possible outcome (e.g., "It's terrible and it's never going to get any better," "I'm going to die"). Panic induced by the thought "Oh my God, I'm dying" can constrict the blood vessels and actually increase the probability of having a heart attack.[34] Catastrophizing can increase both physical pain and emotional pain.[90–92]

> **Note to Leaders:** Help participants see that catastrophizing thoughts are just that: thoughts and images arising and falling within the mind. This can be a difficult concept for them to grasp at first. Refer to the skill of mindfulness of current thoughts (Distress Tolerance Handout 15).

💬 **Discussion Point:** Ask: "Can anything really be a catastrophe?" Dr. Albert Ellis, a famous therapist who was well known for telling people to stop catastrophizing, was once in a debate with someone who tried to get him to admit that some things really are catastrophes. The person said to Ellis: "What if you are in a plane, and all of a sudden it goes into a nose dive, and it is falling to the earth with you in it? What about that? What would you say then?" Ellis replied very calmly: "Hmm, if you die, you die." Discuss this with participants. Is there really any fact that one could not accept with equanimity? Even if real catastrophes occur, does catastrophizing (i.e., focusing on the most distressing or hopeless parts of the catastrophe) help anything?

✓ **b. Imagine Coping Well with Catastrophes**

Encourage clients to imagine that they are coping well with catastrophes in various ways:

- *Problem solving* (see Emotion Regulation Handout 12)
- *Cope ahead* (see Emotion Regulation Handout 19)
- *Radical acceptance* (see Distress Tolerance Handouts 11–11b)

> **Note to Leaders:** At times, participants may find it difficult if not impossible to stop catastrophizing. They may begin fighting you, resisting any attempts on your part to help them move to alternative responses to very painful facts. At these times, it can be very helpful to move to the next point below.

✓ **6. Ask: Does My Emotion and/or Its Intensity Fit the Facts?**

Encourage clients to check out whether the emotion they are trying to change fits the actual facts of the situation. As noted earlier, emotions evolved as a way for individuals to respond effectively to common problems. There are common situations likely to elicit each of the basic emotions. When such a situation occurs, the corresponding emotion is likely to be useful in the situation—it is likely to fit the facts.

Examples of situations that fit the facts of particular basic emotions are listed in Emotion Regulation Handout 8a. Be sure to note that these are not the only valid prompting events for the emotions in question. Often the problem is not with the specific emotion; it is with the intensity of the emotion. You can also give these examples:

Example: "You get laid off from work and react as if you have been sent into a lifetime of poverty."

Example: "A person cuts ahead of you into a grocery line, and you react as if the person had physically attacked you and your child in line with you."

> **Note to Leaders:** It can be very difficult for intensely emotional persons to see through irrational, non-factual descriptions, faulty interpretations, unrealistic worries, and catastrophic versions of the facts. Once again, it is important to remember that "emotions love themselves." The aftereffects of emotions include narrowing of attention and sensitivity to threat, which can also make it very difficult to change thoughts and images. At these points, participants might be better advised to first use crisis survival skills (e.g., actively working to change body chemistry, using TIP skills, distracting, self-soothing, and doing pros and cons of remaining so emotional [see Distress Tolerance Skills Handouts 5–8]).

💬 **Discussion Point:** It can be helpful to discuss with participants the concept of "middle-of-the-night thinking." This is the type of thinking that occurs when we wake up at night with worries and catastrophizing thoughts about our lives. When we wake up in the morning, we often wonder how we could worry so much and believe such catastrophic thoughts. In the middle of the night, it can be helpful simply to say to ourselves: "These are middle-of-the-night thoughts. I am going to ignore them until morning." Elicit from participants times when they have had "middle-of-the-night thinking" that in the morning did not seem nearly as distressing. Elicit and provide ideas on skills that might be helpful in the middle of the night: "For example, it can be helpful to splash very cold water on your face, and then use paced breathing to distract from your thoughts for a time." (See Distress Tolerance Handout 6a for a description of how cold water works.)

✓ **C. Examples of Emotions That Fit the Facts** (*Optional*)

Review Emotion Regulation Handout 8a with participants.

> **Note to Leaders:** Handout 8a can be a helpful review of prompting events for various emotions. It also is good for clarifying what emotions fit what facts. Review one or two of the items on this handout, and suggest that participants review the rest of the handout between sessions.

✓   Handout 8a gives examples of basic emotions that fit the facts. In general, the situations listed fit the emotions they are linked to. They are not the only valid prompting events, however. Most important in deciding whether or not to try to change an emotion is to ask wise mind whether specific emotional responses are effective in the specific situation for advancing important personal goals.

Explain to participants that **emotions function to solve problems of common situations we encounter.**

1. Fear

Fear functions to keep us safe by urging us to escape danger through avoiding, running away, or hiding from anything that threatens us.

2. Anger

Anger functions to protect us from assault or loss of important people, things, or goals by urging us to threaten and attack those who might hurt us.

3. Disgust

Disgust functions to keep contamination away from us. It urges us to get rid of or away from whatever we find disgusting. Emphasize that disgust is related to people (including the self), as well as to things such as foods, bodily fluids, or excrement. Consider the words we use sometimes to describe such people or things ("slimy," "greasy," "smarmy," "scumbag," etc.).

Example: Disgust keeps us from eating foods that will poison us, getting into water that is so polluted it will kill us, and picking up or touching things that might cause a disease.

4. Envy

Envy functions to motivate us to work hard to obtain what others have, in order to improve our lives and those of people important to us. It can also mobilize us to try to reduce what others have (when they have a lot more than we do), in order to equalize the distribution of resources. In this way, envy can be thought of as the emotion that redistributes wealth and power.

Envy often fits the facts when others may have a lot more than we do in areas that are very important to us, and it is ultimately unfair that we have less. The problem is that envy is so often corrosive of the mind and spirit that it does us little good. Bitterness is a common outcome of envy. Thus, because it does us little good, it can be ineffective.

> **Research Point:** Research suggests that happiness is not determined by the absolute value of an event or a person's situation, but by its value in relation to other events or situations both interpersonally (among those in the person's environment) and intrapersonally (compared to the person's experience in the past).[93] When others have more than we do, not only does this generate envy, but it also adds to our unhappiness. This is why envy is often ineffective, and why we might want to bring it down even when it is justified.

5. Jealousy

Jealousy is justified when someone is threatening to take away relationships or things very important to us. Jealousy is the emotion that ensures we do everything possible to protect these relationships or things. We often do this by trying to control the actions of people we want close to us, or by refusing to share what we have with others.

> **Note to Leaders:** It can be very difficult to know when a relationship is threatened and when it is not. Many people can give examples of situations where they felt very safe within a relationship, only to have the person they loved suddenly leave for another person, without apparent warning signs. Checking the facts (Emotion Regulation Handout 8) can itself be a form of jealous behavior. The important question to ask here is this: "Is it effective to act jealous?"

6. Love

Love functions to motivate us to find, be with, and attach ourselves to other people and things. It is justified when those we love enhance our survival and well-being. Although one can argue that everyone and everything are lovable (and therefore love is always justified by the facts), one can also easily argue that sometimes we love the "wrong" people or things. This can be the case when we are in love with a person who does not love or care for us—or when the person we love actively harms us (such as in violent or otherwise abusive relationships, in friendships with individuals who require co-dependence on addictive behaviors to sustain the relationship, or in friendship groups that threaten to abandon us if we improve our lives more than they do or want to).

7. Sadness

Sadness functions to pull us into ourselves so that we can figure out what is really important to us and what to do when we have lost important things. It also signals to others that help is needed.

8. Shame

Shame has two important functions. First, it prompts us to hide behaviors that would elicit rejection from others and lead to our being rejected from the community. Second, if our behavior somehow becomes public, shame prompts us to grovel and appease those we have offended so that we are not rejected.

Shame is a community-based emotion. It is easy to conclude that if behaviors or personal characteristics are not immoral or wrong, then shame is never justified. This is not the case, however. Shame's evolutionary advantage is that if behaviors sanctioned by one's community elicit shame, then shame-based expressions and actions can keep one in the community. Although staying in a community that elicits shame may not be beneficial in many instances, it is not completely useless. It could have made the difference between life and death in earlier times, and may even do so now in some cultures or groups.

Note to Leaders: If participants in skills training have a mental disorder, the discussion of shame can be critical. It is important for these participants to see that identifying themselves as having a mental disorder, especially when this is done before others get to know them, can not only result in rejection but can also increase a sense of shame. In most cultures, shame is a justified emotion with respect to having a mental disorder. Validate that this is not fair.

9. *Guilt*

Guilt functions by urging us to repair behaviors that violate our moral values, and to prevent future violations.

IX. PREPARING FOR OPPOSITE ACTION AND PROBLEM SOLVING (EMOTION REGULATION HANDOUT 9)

Main Point: If checking the facts does not reduce unwanted emotions, we then have to decide which skill to try next: opposite action or problem solving. A flow chart can help us decide what skills to use for changing emotional reactions to situations.

Emotion Regulation Handout 9: Opposite Action and Problem Solving: Deciding Which to Use. This handout is a flow chart to help participants figure out what skill to use to change frequent but unwanted emotions. It can be reviewed here to highlight that sometimes a participant has the facts straight and what has to change is the situation. Alternatively, you can make that point while reviewing opposite action, and then teach this handout as a review after teaching problem solving. The key to teaching and understanding this handout is in the examples, so be sure to give at least one example for each situation. Also, it can be useful to elicit examples at each point from participants.

Emotion Regulation Worksheet 6: Figuring Out How to Change Unwanted Emotions *(Optional).* This worksheet mimics Handout 9, but has instructions for using the flow chart to decide what skills to use for changing emotions. Although this worksheet is optional, it can be extremely useful. You can use it for teaching instead of using Handout 9. If you do so, however, give out an extra copy. If it is given to participants, go over the instructions, and be sure participants understand how to use the flow chart.

✓ A. Three Ways to Change Unwanted Emotions

Remind participants: "In this module, we are focusing on three ways to change unwanted emotions."

✓   ▪ "*Checking the facts* has already been covered. Sometimes just knowing the true facts can change how you feel."

✓   ▪ "*Problem solving* is changing your emotions by avoiding, modifying, or solving the event prompting the emotion." (This skill is covered in Section XI, after opposite action.)

     ▪ "*Opposite action* is changing your emotions by acting opposite to your emotional urge to do something." (This skill is covered next, in Section X.)

✓ B. When to Use Opposite Action versus Problem Solving

Say to participants: "The flow chart in Emotion Regulation Handout 9 is designed to help you figure out when to practice opposite action and when to practice problem solving. For both, you have to check the facts first."

Note to Leaders: It is important to reassure participants that you are not telling them that the way to change all emotions is opposite action. This can seem invalidating when the problem is a serious, ongo-

> ing negative event in their lives. Point out that problem solving is also important and that you will teach it after opposite action.

✓ Now present the following instructions for following the Handout 9 flow chart to participants. As you go through them, ask each of the questions on the flow chart and then give a good example for that particular situation (your own or from below).

Start by asking: "**Does this emotion (and its intensity) fit the facts?**"

1. **If yes (the emotion fits the facts), ask: "Is acting on this emotion effective?"**

    a. **If yes (the emotion fits the facts) and yes (acting on the emotion is effective):**

        ▪ "**Be mindful of the current emotion.** Suppressing or avoiding emotions you do not want is rarely useful, and positive emotions are to be enjoyed."

        Example: "When you are afraid your 3-year-old daughter may be hit by a car as she runs into a street with traffic, experience the fear. Don't try to suppress it, or you may not run out and bring your child back to the curb."

        Example: "When you are in love with a truly wonderful person, enjoy and revel in it."

✓   ▪ "**Act on the emotion. Follow your urges.**"

        Example: "When you are afraid of walking down a very dangerous alley, avoid it."

        Example: "When you are in love with a truly wonderful person, be with the person."

        Example: "When you are ashamed about events in your past that would likely result in social rejection if others knew about them, keep them private."

✓   ▪ "**Engage in problem solving.**"

        Example: "When anxiety about money fits the facts because you are having trouble paying your bills, create a budget and work on ways to cut spending or bring in more money."

        Example: "When you are frequently apart from the partner you love, find a way to get together more often."

        Example: "When you are angry at being denied your apartment deposit unjustly, use interpersonal effectiveness skills to fight to get it back."

✓
✓   **b.** **If yes (the emotion fits the facts) but no (acting on the emotion is not effective):**

        ▪ "**Do not act on the emotion. Consider opposite action.**"

        Example: "You are on a mountain near the top. There was an avalanche behind you, which blocks your ability to go back. There is a crevasse in front of you, which is not impossible to jump over. You are terrified of jumping but have no way to get help. You have waited a long while for help but are now beginning to freeze. Acting on your fear and not jumping will lead to your freezing to death. Opposite action is to summon all your courage and jump."

        Example: "When a car cuts in front of you, you're angry and have an urge to speed up and cut it off. Anger fits the facts, but cutting off the other car is unlikely to be effective; opposite action is to slow down and accept that some drivers cut people off."

        Example: "Your mother is dying, and you are very sad, but your mother cannot tolerate people being sad around her. Give her cheerful news and focus on positive events."

        Example: "You have applied for a lot of jobs, but haven't gotten any offers. You find a job opening you could apply for that is just the job you are hoping for, but you are afraid to apply for it because you think you might not get it. Acting on your fear and not applying will not be effective. Opposite action is to get your courage up and apply for the job."

✓   **2.** **If no (the emotion does not fit the facts) and no (acting on the emotion is not effective):**
✓

        a. **"Do not act on the emotion."**

        b. **"Change your thoughts to fit the facts.** This is the easiest way to change emotions. When it works, nothing else is needed."

✓   c. **"Do opposite action.** At times, even knowing the facts does not change emotions. In these instances, changing your behavior to change your emotions will be more effective."

        Example: "If you fall off a horse that is not dangerous and are afraid to get back on, get back on."

        Example: "You are afraid to apply for jobs, because you think you will never get a job. Extremes, like 'I will never get a job,' are unlikely to fit the facts, and acting on your fear and not applying will not be effective. Opposite action is to get your courage up and start applying for jobs."

✓   **3.** **If no (the emotion does not fit the facts) but yes (acting on the emotion is effective):**

        a. "Be mindful of current emotions. Effectiveness depends on your goals. At times an emotion is viewed as effective simply because it makes you feel good to experience the emotions."

✓   b. **"Gracefully accept the consequences of acting on the emotion.** Once you decide that an emotion that does not fit the facts is effective for your own goals, then it is important to remember that you may not like the consequences of acting on the emotion."

        Example: "If acting on anger is effective because it makes you feel good, then you may need to accept the consequence that it may put a strain on a relationship you value."

X. ACTING OPPOSITE TO THE CURRENT EMOTION (EMOTION REGULATION HANDOUTS 10–11)

> **Main Point:** When emotions do not fit the facts of a situation, or do not lead to effective behavior, acting opposite to these emotions will change the emotions if this is done repeatedly and all the way.
>
> **Emotion Regulation Handout 10: Opposite Action; Emotion Regulation Handout 11: Figuring Out Opposite Action.** Make every effort to review Handouts 10 and 11 in the same session. Without examples, it can be hard for participants to understand what an opposite action would look like. Handout 11 is a multipage guide for identifying opposite actions for nine specific emotions. Although the handout gives suggestions for effective opposite actions, it is important to teach participants how to identify their own action urges and how to figure out effective actions opposite to those urges. Brief versions of the critical points are summarized on Emotion Regulation Handout 13: Reviewing Opposite Action and Problem Solving.
>
> It is not necessary to go over every line of every emotion on Handout 10. You should, however, review several emotions so that participants see how to use the handout. In our experience, helping participants differentiate between jealousy and envy and between shame and guilt can be very important. Because the situation that justifies shame is not intuitively obvious (i.e., the threat of being kicked out of the group if shameful behavior or personal characteristics are made public), it is essential that you review this emotion at least briefly. You can also go over each emotion, make one or two highlighting comments, and then ask for questions. Or you can ask participants which emotions they have questions about. I often assign reading through this handout as homework.
>
> **Emotion Regulation Worksheet 7: Opposite Action to Change Emotions.** The homework is to practice opposite action. Filling out the worksheet is used to record the homework so that it can be discussed. Review the worksheet with participants. If necessary, instruct participants in how to rate intensity of emotions (0 = no emotion, no discomfort; 100 = maximum emotion intensity, maximum discomfort).

> The "Before" and "After" spaces are for rating the intensity of an emotion before and after practicing opposite action. If participants have trouble figuring out what emotion they are feeling, instruct them to review Emotion Regulation Handout 6, and/or to fill out Worksheet 4 or 4a. When analyzing whether the emotion is justified, participants should focus on the prompting event. Thus it is important to remind participants to be very specific in describing the facts surrounding the prompting event. If necessary, review the mindfulness "what" skill of describing.

✓ **A. What Is Opposite Action?**

Opposite action is acting opposite to the emotional urge to do or say something.

✓ **B. Why Act Opposite?**

Opposite action is an effective way to change or reduce unwanted emotions when your emotion does not fit the facts. The old adage "If you fall off a horse, get back on it," is an example of acting opposite to fear's urge to avoid the horse.

Most effective treatments for emotional disorders ask clients to reverse the expression and action components of problem emotions. Some psychotherapists believe this is why these treatments work. Here are some of these treatments:

■ *Behavioral activation*—that is, doing the opposite of avoidance behaviors, such as isolating, inactivity, and rumination—is an effective treatment for depression.[94]

■ *Exposure-based treatments*, which involve doing the opposite of avoiding and escaping feared events, are effective treatments for anxiety disorders.[95]

■ *Effective treatments for anger* stress learning to identify the cues to frustration and/or anger, and then leaving the situation to cool down rather than going on the attack.[96]

> **Note to Leaders:** It is essential to get across to participants the rationale for this technique and to elicit their cooperation. See the section on exposure-based procedures in Chapter 11 of the main DBT text for a more extensive discussion.

C. When Opposite Action Works Best

✓ **1. When Knowing the Facts about a Situation Does Not Work**

Say to participants: "When knowing the facts about a situation does not work to change your emotional responses, then opposite action can be effective."

Example: "Knowing something is not dangerous, but still being very afraid of it. This is very common."

Examples: "Finding out a person did not intend to hurt you, but still feeling angry; knowing your husband loves you and will never leave you, but reacting with jealousy when he looks at beautiful women."

Example: "Being loved and completely accepted by your friends, but still hiding your body out of shame when you are in the locker room with them."

Example: "Knowing that asking your boss for a raise is not a threat to your well-being or safety, but still not getting yourself to ask."

Example: "Knowing intellectually that your behavior in a specific situation was not immoral, but still feeling guilty."

✓ **2. When the Emotion (or *Its Intensity* or *Duration*) Is Not Justified by the Situation**

Tell participants: "When your emotion—or its strength, or the length of time it lasts—is not justified by the situation, opposite action can be effective. Problem solving is needed when an emotion is justified by the situation."

Emphasize that **emotions are *not* justified when they do not fit the facts of the actual situation.**

Note to Leaders: Evaluating whether an emotion is justified by the facts is similar to determining whether a person has an anxiety disorder or not. For example, a diagnosis of specific phobia requires that the fear or its intensity is irrational, given the facts; in social phobia, fear or anxiety must be out of proportion in frequency and/or duration to the actual situation.[97] The term "unjustified by the facts" is used here to avoid using the term "irrational."

Example: "You are told a person said mean and untrue things about you (prompting anger) when in fact he did not."

Example: "When your boss is introducing a new manager to your work group, she praises two of your co-workers, but not you (prompting fear and hurt). Then you find out she didn't say anything about you because she had praised you excessively to the manager just an hour previously."

Example: "The person you love actively harms you, such as in a violent or otherwise abusive relationship, or friends that you love require you to share their dependence on addictive behaviors to sustain the relationship."

Discussion Point: Elicit examples of situations where participants have experienced emotions that they then discovered did not fit the facts.

Note to Leaders: You can say that if an emotion does not fit the facts, the emotion is not justified, and that this means it is not justified by the facts. Asking whether an emotion is justified is a shorthand way of asking if the emotion fits the facts. Some therapists or skills trainers (more clinicians than participants, in my experience) find it difficult to say to a person that the person's emotion is not justified. Generally this is because the clinicians believe that this invalidates the emotion and the person. It is important to remember that a behavior or emotional response can be understandable, while at the same time not being valid. If you or your participants have a lot of trouble with the term "justified," you can substitute "fits the facts" or another term. When you are changing a term, however, it is important not to "fragilize" the participants. "Fragilize" is a word I invented for DBT; it means treating participants as if they are fragile and unable to tolerate, learn, or do what is needed. The idea is that treating a person as fragile can have the unintended effect of increasing fragility.

✓ **Practice Exercise:** Tell the following story: "You are going into your office, and when you open your office door you see a poisonous snake hissing and moving near you. You slam the door and are afraid to open it again." Then ask: "Is fear in that situation justified?" (The answer is yes. Fear fits the facts and is justified.)

Now continue the story. "Overnight, your office manager gets someone to come in and get rid of the poisonous snake. It is no longer in your office, and there are no snakes in your building. You get to the office, but no one tells you that the snake has been removed from your office. You are afraid to open the door to your office." Then ask: "Is fear justified now?" (The answer is no.) Most likely, however, almost all participants will say yes. The reason is that they think if fear is understandable (there is no way of knowing that the snake is no longer in the office), it is also justified. Discuss how an emotion can be understandable but still not justified by the facts.

Note to Leaders: The point that emotions can be understandable and at the same time not justified by the facts can be very difficult for participants (and often for skills trainers also) to grasp. The main problem is that people often think that if a response is reasonable (such as grieving for a son one has been told is dead when he is in fact alive), then it must be justified. Your task here is to disentangle these two ideas. An emotional response can be both reasonable *and* unjustified. Give extreme examples to make your point. Use examples both where someone is told the wrong facts and where a misinterpretation of the facts is reasonable.

💬 **Discussion Point:** Solicit from participants and discuss other times when information appears to fit the facts but does not.

✓ **3. When the Emotion (or _Its Intensity_ or _Duration_) Is Not Effective for Meeting Goals in the Situation**

Continue: "When your emotion—or its strength, or the length of time it lasts—is not effective for meeting your goals in the situation, opposite action works. Sometimes your emotions may fit the facts very well, but experiencing and expressing the emotion may do you little good and may even cause you harm. In considering opposite action, it is important to think through whether your emotional responses are effective."

Example: "Your boss criticizes you in front of people you are trying to impress, and then asks for your opinion on an important point. If you want to impress your boss and others at the meeting with your competence, responding with anger may not be in your best interest, even though anger would be justified."

Example: "You are in the middle of driving on the cliff side of a high, two-lane, winding mountain road. You look down; there is no guard rail, and the road is very narrow. You are suddenly overcome with intense fear; however, panic may actually cause you to go over the cliff rather than keep you safe. Freezing by stopping your car and refusing to go forward is also not an effective option."

Example: "Just before you go for your driver's test, you get news that you did not get into the school you applied to. Intense disappointment and perhaps anxiety fit the facts, but these emotions might also interfere with doing well on the driver's test."

Example: "A car wreck creates a long backup when you are in a hurry to get somewhere, and you get angry. Being angry does not help you safely get to your destination faster."

Note to Leaders: When evaluating whether emotions are effective, participants can use Emotion Regulation Worksheet 1 or 2. If they are unsure of goals, you might introduce Emotion Regulation Worksheet 11 or 11a: Getting from Values to Specific Action Steps.

💬 **Discussion Point:** Elicit examples where an emotional reaction has been well justified by the situation, but experiencing and/or expressing the emotion has been ineffective.

4. When You Are Avoiding What Needs to Be Done

Go on: "Sometimes the issue is not really whether an emotion fits the facts, but rather whether acting on your urges has the outcome of avoiding doing things that you need to do. If you find that you are avoiding doing something for this reason, opposite action can be effective."

Example: "You are depressed and want to stay in bed all day; you want to isolate yourself and avoid everyone and everything. Getting up and active, and engaging with people rather than avoiding them, however, are necessary to reduce the depression."

Example: "You are so anxious that you don't want to engage in a treatment that will reduce your anxiety. Acting on your urge to avoid, however, will lead to more anxiety."

Example: "You borrowed a friend's book with an inscription from a famous person, and you promised to return it. You have lost it on a camping trip, however, and are avoiding going anywhere near where your friend might be, because you don't want to let your friend find out that you lost the book. Unless you want to stop being friends, you will have to tell your friend what happened sooner or later. This calls for opposite action."

Example: "After looking for a job for 2 years, you get a fabulous job offer at a nursing home for elderly people. A small part of your job will be to manage the bodies of people when they die. You are terrified of dead bodies. This calls for opposite action if you want the job."

✓ **D. How to Do Opposite Action, Step by Step**

> **Note to Leaders:** Do not skip any of the steps 1–7, as it is important that participants have a good grasp of how and when to use opposite action.

✓ **1. Identify and Name the Emotion You Want to Change**

Instruct participants: "Use Emotion Regulation Handout 6 or Emotion Regulation Worksheets 4 or 4a, if necessary. Then fill in the emotion's name and rate its intensity (0–100) on Worksheet 7: Opposite Action to Change Emotions."

✓ **2. Check the Facts**

Tell participants: "The second step can be difficult to figure out. Is there any chance you have misinterpreted a situation or missed important facts about the situation? Check the facts to be sure."

a. Ask: Does the Emotion Fit the Facts of the Situation?

Continue: "Ask yourself: 'Is the emotion a reasonable response, given the situation? Is it justified by the facts?' If your answer is no, move to Steps 3 and 4. If you need to, use Emotion Regulation Handouts 8, 8a, or 11. The last two list the major events (or sets of facts) that ordinarily justify specific emotions. You can also use Emotion Regulation Worksheet 5 to check the facts if necessary."

✓ **3. Identify and Describe Your Action Urges**

Say: "Pay attention to your impulses, desires, and cravings. Focus on what you feel like doing or saying. Ask yourself: 'What do I feel like doing? What do I want to say?' Review Emotion Regulation Handout 6 for some ideas if you can't figure it out."

✓ **4. Ask Wise Mind: Is Expressing or Acting on This Emotion Effective in This Situation?**

Go on: "Ask wise mind: 'If I act on my urge, will it make things better or worse? Will acting on my emotion solve the problem I am faced with? Is expressing my emotion a wise thing to do?' If the answer is no, move to Step 5."

✓ **5. Act Opposite to the Emotion's Urges**

Say to participants: "If you have gotten this far in the process, you have decided that your emotion is not justified by the facts or not effective for your goals. So you should do the *opposite* of your action urges. Look over Emotion Regulation Handouts 11 and 13 for ideas on possible opposite actions for various emotions."

a. Do the Opposite of Your *Actual* Action Urges

Instruct participants: "Do the opposite of what your own, *actual* action urges are. Do not blindly follow the actions in Handouts 11 and 13." The reason for this instruction is this: The opposite actions[17] in these handouts assume that emotions are relatively straightforward and have universal and identifiable common action urges. Emotions, however, are often much more complex and may be a blend of several emotions occurring all at the same time. The expression and action urges may be unique to that blended emotion. Even when an emotion is simple and easy to identify, its action urges may be unique to an individual or to the individual's cultural or ethnic group.

Practice Exercise: Ask participants to close their eyes and imagine a situation during the past week when they felt angry. Instruct them to imagine the situation and the interaction as if it were happening in the present moment. Then ask them to notice how they feel. Now, as they continue to imagine, instruct them to relax their fingers and their arms and turn the palms of their hands upward on their thighs (if they are sitting) or at their sides (if they are standing). Suggest that they relax their faces from forehead to chin, smoothing them out as much as possible, and then turn the corners of their mouths slightly up. Ask them to notice their emotions again. It is common for people to report a lowering in anger. Explain: "This is opposite action with the hands and face."

> **Note to Leaders:** In this exercise, you are teaching "willing hands" and "half-smiling" as opposite actions. Both are actions opposite of anger. See Distress Tolerance Handout 14 for a fuller set of instructions and rationale for half-smiling and willing hands.

b. Let Opposite Actions Do the Work; Do Not Suppress Emotions

Go on: "Let your opposite action do the work for you. Don't try to suppress your emotional experiences or feelings. If you try to suppress an emotion while doing opposite action, then you are not letting the strategy work—and it may not work. If you experience your emotion, all the while keeping your eyes, ears, and senses open, then you will learn in a fundamental way that, indeed, the emotion is *not* justified. Once your brain gets that information encoded, you will find your emotional reaction going down, down, down over time. Opposite action is a strategy that works over time to reduce your unwanted emotional reactions. If it does not seem to be working, give it time."

Practice Exercise: Have participants close their eyes and pay attention to sensations in their faces. Guide them in noting any areas of tension. Now instruct participants to imagine a situation during the past week when they felt sad or worried. While thinking about it, they should again notice sensations in their faces. Instruct participants to raise a hand slightly to signal to you when they have the situation in mind. Now, as they continue to imagine, instruct them to try to mask the feelings so that no one else in the room (if anyone was looking) would know what they were feeling. Have them notice the sensations in their faces; have them notice what happens to their emotions. Next, instruct each person to relax the muscles in the face, smoothing them out as much as possible. Have participants notice how their emotions change (or don't change); have them notice how different their faces feel. It is common for people to report that when they relax their faces, they feel much more vulnerable. Explain: "This means you are allowing feelings to come and go. You are not holding them in or pushing them out."

✓ ### 6. *Do Opposite Action* All the Way

Emphasize to participants: "When you do opposite action, do it *all the way*. This means opposite posture, facial expression, thinking, what you say, and how you say it. 'Halfway' opposite action does not work. It is important to work on every part of your response to make sure your opposite action is done *all the way*. See Emotion Regulation Handouts 11 and 13 for ideas."

a. Examples of Halfway Opposite Words and Opposite Thinking

Example: "Going to a party to try to reduce your social phobia, but spending all your time looking down and standing in corners, is halfway opposite action."

Example: "Getting on a plane to reduce your fear of flying, but thinking, 'It's going to crash,' is halfway opposite action."

Example: "Acting kind and sweet to reduce anger or disgust, but thinking, 'You jerk! How disgusting!', is halfway opposite action."

Example: "Answering a question in a group to reduce feeling humiliated when you are talking in these settings, and then saying, 'Oh, that was so stupid!', is halfway opposite action."

b. Examples of Halfway Opposite Facial Expression, Opposite Voice Tone, and Opposite Posture

Example: "Saying, 'I understand your point,' to reduce irritation, but saying it with a sarcastic voice tone, is halfway opposite action."

Example: "Going to the park with your children to reduce sadness, but doing this with a very sad facial expression and slumped posture, is halfway opposite action."

Example: "Slumping and looking like you are trying to hide when you reveal actions you are ashamed of is halfway opposite action."

c. Halfway Opposite Actions Don't Work

Say: "As you can see from these examples, changing your thinking and your emotional expressions without changing your emotional actions very rarely works. The central aspects of this skill are figuring out what your emotional action urge is, figuring out what the opposite action would be, and then *doing it*."

Discussion Point: Elicit from participants examples of times when they or others have done halfway opposite actions. What effect did it have? Check how people felt during and after doing halfway opposite actions.

Practice Exercise: Elicit from participants times they have tried to change their own emotions by acting opposite to the emotion urge—for example, by going to a party they are afraid to go to, or letting a boyfriend or girlfriend out of their sight to get over jealousy. Then have participants role-play or demonstrate acting opposite all the way and then acting opposite halfway. If participants do not want to act scenes out, get them to describe situations where they did opposite actions only halfway.

> **Note to Leaders:** It is important to note again that you are not suggesting suppressing emotions, which many participants may have learned to do quite effectively already. Opposite action, in some ways, is even the opposite action of suppressing emotions.[97, 98]

✓   **7. *Continue Acting Opposite until the Emotion Goes Down***

Tell participants: "Act opposite in a situation long enough for it to work. That is, keep doing it until you notice your emotion coming down in intensity even just a little bit."

Also, emphasize the need for practice: "**Repeat opposite action over and over every chance you have.** Sometimes opposite action works immediately. Most of the time, however, you have to practice a lot to get over habitual unjustified emotions. You also sometimes have to practice a lot to get over an emotion that was justified by a situation for years, but now is not."

Example: "If you are anxious when talking in groups, it may take a lot of times talking in friendly groups to reduce anxiety about it. This is also true of people who do public speaking. It is usual to feel very anxious at first, and then, over time and many practices, to feel much more comfortable."

Example: "If you are ashamed of something you have done, even though you will not be rejected by your friends if they find out, you may have to talk about it multiple times in your group before you stop feeling ashamed."

💬 **Discussion Point:** Elicit from participants examples of times when they have done the opposite of their emotional urges and found that over time their emotional reactions changed. Fear is generally the easiest emotion to work with, so you may want to start with that first. Then ask for other emotions where opposite action has worked.

✓ E. Figuring Out Opposite Actions

Review Emotion Regulation Handout 11 with participants.

> **Note to Leaders:** The justification for each emotion listed in Emotion Regulation Handout 11 and below is related to the evolutionary function of the emotion. Examples of situations that ordinarily elicit the primary emotions are very similar to those listed in Emotion Regulation Handout 8a. (Review this handout with participants, if necessary.) Fear is placed first below, because opposite action when there is no actual danger makes sense to just about everyone. You need to give many examples, starting with the proverbial example of getting back on a horse after falling off. Anger is placed after fear, because people so frequently confuse anger with fear.
>
> Note that for each emotion in Handout 11, there is a line for participants to put in a personal example that may justify the emotion. Although there is much commonality across cultures in eliciting events for basic emotions, there may be variations on the relationship of situations to emotions across cultures, and it is important to be open to these. This can be a good place to ask participants to put down such information, if appropriate.
>
> Do not let participants drift too far off course. Be sure that the situation itself elicits an emotion, *not* an individual's interpretation of the situation. New facts that justify an emotion should be common or normative in the person's culture, not idiosyncratic to a person or family.
>
> Finally, the suggestions for opposite action are just that—suggestions.

1. Fear

Tell participants: "When fear is *not justified*, approach what you fear rather than avoid it. Do what you are afraid to do rather than avoid it."

👥 **Practice Exercise:** The very best practice exercises for opposite action to fear, or to any emotion, are those in which you can get participants to act differently from how they feel right in the group. Over and over across modules, look for opportunities to instruct members to do their best not to act in accord with their emotions of the moment. For example, when people want to leave a session out of anxiety, anger, hurt feelings, or panic, instruct them to stay, orienting them to how staying is practicing acting opposite to their emotions. Periodically ask, "What do you do when you are afraid?" Coach participants until they can always chime out, "Do what you are afraid of!" "What do you do when you're depressed?" "Get active!" "What do you do when you feel guilty?" "Figure out if it is justified, and either repair it (if it is) or do it over and over and over (if not)!" And so on. Drill members until they have this cold.

2. Anger

Say to participants: "When anger is *not justified*, gently avoid the person you are angry with, rather than attacking. Also avoid thinking about him or her, rather than ruminating about all the terrible things the person has done. Distract yourself. Do something kind rather than mean. Try to see the other person's point of view rather than blaming them. Practice half-smiling and/ or willing hands."

Note to Leaders: As mentioned in an earlier note, see Distress Tolerance Handouts 14 and 14a for instructions on how to teach half-smiling and willing (open) hands. Half-smiling here replaces anger's scowling or hostile grinning, so it is particularly important that the face is completely relaxed before a person engages in a half smile.

Practice Exercise: Briefly teach participants how to half-smile if you have not covered it already. Have participants close their eyes and imagine the person they are angry with. Instruct them: "Bring to mind what the person has done that has caused so much anger. Notice your emotions." After a few minutes, instruct participants: "While you continue to think about the person and what he or she has done, relax your whole face. Relax your forehead, relax your eyes, relax your cheeks, and let your jaw relax (teeth slightly apart). Then half-smile ever so slightly. Continue half-smiling, and notice your emotions." Discuss any changes that occurred.

Practice Exercise: Repeat the exercise above. But instead of half-smiling, instruct participants in willing hands if you have not covered it already. Substitute willing hands for half-smiling in the exercise above. Discuss any changes that occur.

Practice Exercise: Repeat the exercise with either half-smiling or willing hands. But now add: "Attempt in your mind to consider the feelings, thoughts, and wishes of the person you are angry with. Try to validate aspects of the other person's behavior, if only in terms of the behavior being caused. Notice your emotions. Discuss any changes that occur. Discuss experiences."

Note to Leaders: No matter which of these three practice exercises you use, it is important to tell participants to choose a person they have been angry with recently, but *not* to choose a person who has abused or traumatized them unless they are very sure they are ready to handle their emotions. This is particularly important if participants have PTSD that has not yet been treated.

3. *Disgust*

Instruct participants: "When disgust is *not justified*—that is, there is no danger of contamination or harm—bring the food or item that you find disgusting very close to you, and keep it close while distracting yourself from irrelevant disgusting thoughts. Or embrace a person you find disgusting, once you find out that your perception was inaccurate."

Note that increased exposure to a person results in increased liking for that person.[100, 102] But add: "The exception here is that this is true primarily for people who are similar to you. If it becomes clear after spending more time with a person that this person is dissimilar to you, liking may decrease."[101]

Discussion Point: Elicit examples of things people have found disgusting in the past that they no longer find disgusting. Discuss what made their disgust go down over time. Examples may include foods participants found disgusting in childhood, changing diapers the first few times, or taking care of a sick relative or another patient.

Practice Exercise: Bring in something very safe (such as durian fruit or fish sauce) that has a terrible odor. Have each person keep smelling the odor until participants acclimate to the smell.

4. *Envy*

Say: "When envy is *not justified*, the opposite action is to count your blessings and inhibit urges to diminish what others have."

5. Jealousy

Say: "When jealousy is *not justified*—in other words, there is no threat at all to what you have or possess—opposite action is to let go of controlling others or the situation and to share what you have with others."

6. Love

Say: "When love is *not justified*—that is, you love an inappropriate or wrong person or thing—opposite action is to avoid and distract from the person or thing that is loved and all reminders, including loving thoughts, and to remind yourself constantly of why love is unjustified."

Example: "The person you love does not love you."

Example: "Friends require you to share their dependence on addictive behaviors to sustain the relationship."

Example: "Friendship groups threaten to abandon you if you improve your life more than the other members do or want to."

Example: "You have difficulties moving away from home, changing schools, jobs, or residences, ending relationships (such as therapy, teacher–student, or boss–employee relationships), or tolerating friends moving away."

Example: "You are overly attached to possessions, rituals, or habits."

💬 **Discussion Point:** Elicit examples of situations where participants have "loved too much" or been too attached to persons, places, or things. How did they "recover"?

7. Sadness

Say: "When sadness is *not justified,* and particularly when you are also depressed, get active. Do things that make you feel competent and self-confident, rather than being passive. Increase rewarding activities and pleasant events. Approach, don't avoid."

Example: "When you lose a credit card, you have to call and get it canceled to move forward, not sit around being sad that you lost it."

> **Note to Leaders:** Sadness and disappointment are normal emotions and are often justified by the facts. They become problematic when they outlive their usefulness. The behaviors of sadness (e.g., slowing down, isolation, ruminating about what is lost) can by themselves create a situation in which it is very difficult to stop feeling sad. This can lead to a vicious cycle of depression, which also slows us down, often includes isolation, and so can keep regenerating over and over the very depression we are trying to get out of.

8. Shame

Say: "When shame is *not justified*, there is no threat of being rejected by others. The opposite action for shame is to stop hiding your behavior with people who you know won't reject you. If your behavior violates your own moral values, but you will not be rejected by others if they know about your behavior, act on the emotion of guilt [see next page]—but do not act on the emotion of shame. For example, instead of avoiding a person when you lost something you borrowed from him or her, meet with the person, apologize, and offer to replace the borrowed item. If, in contrast, your behavior does not violate your own moral values, reduce shame by repeating the behavior over and over in a group that will not reject you."

✓ 💬 **Discussion Point:** Elicit from participants examples of behaviors and personal characteristics that can get people devalued and ejected from groups. Behaviors might include criminal behaviors; personal characteristics might include race, sexual orientation, weight/other physical characteristics, mental disorder, criminal convictions, family origins, and personal history. Discuss how cultural values change, and how with these changes what is "shameful" also changes. Ask about cultural values when participants were children as opposed to now.

> **Note to Leaders:** Remember, behavior and personal characteristics can be moral and valued by the individual, and yet shame can still be justified if others the person cares about will ostracize him or her for that behavior or those personal characteristics. In these situations, it can be important to fight the social norms of the group and advocate to change its values.

9. Guilt

Say: "When guilt is *not justified*—that is, your behavior does not violate your own values or moral code—several opposite actions might be called for. The main opposite action is to continue with the behavior and stop apologizing for it. If your behavior violates other people's values but not your own (so shame is justified but guilt is not), you can either hide the behavior (this might be important if the community is one you want to stay in *and* the community might kick you out if they know about your behavior); leave and join a different community; or try to change your community's values. In the third case, social action to change community values would also be a form of opposite action to shame."

> **Note to Leaders:** If participants don't know what their own values or moral codes are, it can be hard for them to know whether they have actually violated them. See Emotion Regulation Handout 18 for a list of possible values that may be helpful in figuring this out. You can also suggest readings from the commandments and precepts of the world's major religions as a starting point. Remember to be respectful of participants from various religious traditions, as well as of those without a religion. If you are treating a person or group from a single religion, you might want to present only the commandments/precepts of that religion.

a. Differentiating "Values" and "Moral Codes"

Although values and moral codes are very similar, they can be differentiated. As the term is used here, a "moral code" is a set of beliefs about what behaviors are wrong or immoral (or, in some vocabularies, sinful). "Values," in contrast, are what is viewed as important and valuable in one's life. Although there may be an overlap between behaviors that are important to avoid and behaviors that violate one's moral code, they are not identical ideas. Values usually refer to what one wants to do in life. Morals usually refer to what one wants to avoid doing. This, again, is not an absolute truth, but it is useful for teaching these concepts.

People and cultures may have different views about what behaviors are moral and immoral. Morality can be learned by observation, by consequences while being raised, or by indirect teaching. Our personal moral codes may have been learned in school or in attending religious activities. Some people can articulate their own moral codes very clearly. Others who may be just as moral would have difficulties describing their moral codes.

> **Note to Leaders:** Summarize opposite action before going on. Make sure that participants understand the concept clearly and know how to use the skill effectively.

F. Troubleshooting

> **Note to Leaders:** If participants say that opposite action is not working, it is important that you do troubleshooting to figure out the problem. Review all the steps of opposite action above and in Emotion Regulation Handout 10, to be sure the procedures are being carried out according to the directions.

1. Is the Emotion Actually Unjustified by the Facts of the Situation?

If the emotion is really justified by the facts, problem solving could be a better way to reduce the emotion.

2. Are Participants' Actions Really Opposite to Their Action Urges?

Perhaps participants are following Emotion Regulation Handout 11 too closely, rather than paying attention to their own individual action urges.

3. Was Opposite Action Done All the Way?

Check out participants' automatic thoughts during opposite action. You might want to ask them to demonstrate how they did it. Often you will find that voice tone, eye gaze, and posture were really not carried out all the way, even though the participants thought they were.

4. Review "Before" and "After" Emotion Intensity Ratings

Was a person's opposite action so brief that the individual did not learn anything new? Check the person's emotion intensity ratings before and after the opposite action, and discuss whether the person was actually processing the information in the situation.

5. Remind Participants That Opposite Action Can Take Time

Children do not get over their fears of ghosts under the bed by looking under the bed one time. Similarly, opposite action does not work if it is only carried out once or a few times.

XI. PROBLEM SOLVING (EMOTION REGULATION HANDOUT 12)

> **Main Point:** When an emotion is justified by the situation, avoiding or changing the situation may be the best way to change one's emotion. Problem solving is the first step in changing difficult situations.
>
> **Emotion Regulation Handout 12: Problem Solving.** The steps in problem solving are clearly laid out in this handout. Consider starting with one or two sample problems from participants. Put them up on a whiteboard, and then review each step for each problem. If you start by eliciting more than one problem to work on, be sure you have sufficient time to complete all the steps for all problems.
>
> **Emotion Regulation Worksheet 8: Problem Solving to Change Emotions.** The homework for this skill is to practice solving problems that elicit unwanted emotions. Filling out the worksheet can be helpful in figuring out the problem and how to solve it. But actually solving the problem (i.e., taking Steps 5 and 6) is most important for changing emotions. It is useful to review both pages of this worksheet with participants, to be sure they understand what to write where. As with reviewing previous worksheets, tell participants to begin by writing down the emotion name and the starting ("Before") intensity of the emotion. If necessary, remind participants of how to rate the intensity of emotions (0 = no emotion; 100 = maximum intensity). The "After" space is for the intensity rating after implementing a solution. For problems you have worked on in the group, you might want to demonstrate how the worksheet would be filled out.

✓ **A. Why Learn Problem Solving?**

Say to participants: "When an unwanted emotion fits the facts, the facts are the problem, and you need problem solving. In addition, the ability to solve problems is a basic skill that everyone needs in order to build a life worth living. It is one of the core skills necessary for improving emotion regulation or solving emotional problems."

1. Solving Problem Situations Can Change Difficult Emotions

The specific type of problem solving covered here focuses on solving problem situations that elicit unwanted emotions. When the situation is the problem, the problem-solving skills described here are called for. Most importantly, when the emotion that one wants to change is justified by the situation, changing the situation may be the best way to change one's emotions. Problem solving is the first step in changing difficult situations.

✓ ### 2. Problem Solving Is Needed When Acting on an Emotion Is Not Likely to Be Effective

Problem solving as a coping strategy increases the probability of effective coping with a wide range of problematic situations. In contrast to skills that are automatic and effortless (at least after a lot of practice), problem solving ordinarily requires a conscious and focused effort aimed at developing and applying new solutions to the problems one encounters in everyday life.

B. Acknowledge When There Is a Problem to Be Solved

Tell participants: "Before starting problem solving, you have to recognize that there is indeed a problem to be solved."

1. Types of Problem Situations

a. Situations or People That Elicit Painful or Destructive Emotions

Situations or persons that bring out painful or destructive emotions call for problem solving, even if we do not immediately see what could be done to change a situation or to deal differently with a person.

b. Situations or People That Are Habitually Avoided Because They Cause Painful Emotions

Situations or persons that we tend to avoid because they bring out painful emotions definitely call for problem solving—particularly if our avoidance interferes with getting what we want in life.

c. One-Time Problem Situations

One-time problem situations—for example, not having a ride to an important appointment, or having an acute illness—call for problem solving.

d. Repeated Problem Situations

When problem situations tend to occur over and over—such as repeatedly being misinterpreted by a friend, or repeatedly failing important exams—problem solving can break the cycle.

e. Repeated Failures to Inhibit Destructive or Ineffective Behavior

A special type of repeated problem situation involves repeatedly failing to keep from engaging in behaviors that are destructive or ineffective. Such behaviors include self-harm, substance abuse, angry outbursts, missing work or therapy, or not doing therapy or school assignments.

f. Chronic Problem Situations

Ongoing situations that create continual misery in life—such as living with a partner who is abusive, or working in a job one hates—may call for problem solving most strongly of all.

✓ ### 2. Defining Problems: Let Go of Judgmentalness

a. Problems Are Specific to Persons and Situations

Situations that are a problem for one person may not be a problem for another. Also, the very same painful emotion may be caused by very different situations depending on the person.

b. Problems Are Specific to Time and Circumstances

The same situation may be a problem at one time, but not at another time, depending on changing circumstances within the same person.

> **Note to Leaders:** Problem solving is easiest to teach if you try to solve a problem you have (or think up), or a problem offered by one of the participants, assuming that the problem is not too complex. When solving the problem be sure to review and model steps 1–7 below.

✓ C. Seven Basic Steps in Problem Solving[102]

✓ 1. Observe and Describe the Problem Situation

a. Describe the Situation

Tell participants: "First, use the mindfulness 'what' skill of describing to give just the facts of the situation." (Refer them to Mindfulness Handout 4, if necessary.)

b. Describe What Is Problematic about the Situation

Say: "Next, describe just what about the situation is problematic. Include the consequences of the situation that make it a problem for you."

Example 1: "Not having a ride to an important appointment means I can't get to my appointment; I am afraid I will miss it."

Example 2: "Being ill is not only distressing, but makes it hard for me to do a good job at work; I am worried about the quality of my work."

Example 3: "Repeatedly being misinterpreted by my friend creates conflict; it makes me irritated; it makes me want to stop talking with my friend."

Example 4: "Failing important exams might lead to my failing the course; I need the course to graduate; I am afraid I may not graduate."

Example 5: "Destructive and ineffective behavior ensures that I will not be able to build a life I want to live."

Example 6: "Living with a partner who is abusive is very painful and feels threatening; I feel ashamed that I have not done anything about this."

Example 7: "Working in a job I hate is a big factor in my not having a life I want to live; I hate my job more each day."

c. Describe the Obstacles to Solving the Problem

Continue: "Now describe the conflicts or other obstacles making it hard for you to solve this problem."

Example 1: "By the time I find another way to get to my appointment, it will be too late, and I will miss it."

Example 2: "I don't have enough money to get the medicine I need to feel better."

Example 3: "This is just about my only friend, and I am afraid of alienating her and losing her friendship."

Example 4: "I don't know what to do to get better grades. I study, but I can't seem to understand the material."

Example 5: "I don't know what sets off my problem behaviors."

Example 6: "If I leave my abusive partner, I will have no one who loves me."

Example 7: "I don't have another job to go to. I can't afford not to have a job."

👥 **Practice Exercise:** Elicit examples of current problems from participants. Write them on a board. Include a description, the participants' emotions, the problematic consequences of the situation, and any conflicts or other obstacles evident in the situation. When you are doing this in large groups, you can "fill in the blanks" as needed to move the process along.

✓ ## 2. Check the Facts

If necessary, refer participants to Emotion Regulation Handouts 8 and 8a.

a. Ask: Are My Facts Correct?

Often we respond to our interpretations of situations, rather than to the situations themselves. Our interpretations may be correct; they may also be incorrect. It is important to check the facts.

b. Ask: How Distressing Is the Situation?

It is easy to catastrophize a situation and make it into a much bigger problem than it really is. Radical acceptance and other distress tolerance skills are ways to help us reduce emotion, stop catastrophizing, and see the problem situation more clearly.

c. Ask: Do the Conflicts or Other Obstacles I've Described Reflect the Facts of the Situation?

It is also important to check the facts about conflicts or other obstacles. In periods of emotional distress, it is easy to see many more obstacles than are really there. Interpersonal situations that feel like conflicts in one emotional state may feel like minor disagreements in another emotional state.

> **Note to Leaders:** At times it can be extremely difficult for participants to pinpoint what has set off problem behaviors or what is getting in the way of change. When this is the case, it can be useful for participants to do a chain analysis on themselves to trace the events that led up to a problem behavior or painful emotion. If you have not reviewed the section on analyzing behavior in Chapter 6 and have time, review it here. It may be useful to teach here General Handout 7: Chain Analysis and General Handout 8: Missing-Links Analysis. If so, be sure to include a procedure for giving feedback on participants' use of General Worksheets 2 and 3.

👥 **Practice Exercise:** Check the facts for the problem descriptions written on the board in Step 1. If the descriptions are clearly factual, move to the next step. It may also be useful to elicit from participants times when they responded to a situation as if it were a major problem when it really wasn't. Modeling examples of this can be useful as well.

✓ ## 3. Identify Your Goal in Solving the Problem

Go on: "The third step is to identify your goal in solving the problem. Keep it simple and something you can really achieve. Naturally, the ultimate goal is to reduce painful emotions. The major task for this step is to identify what has to happen for you to feel better."

Example 1: "Finding a way to get to the important appointment."

Example 2: "Finding a way to get the treatment needed to feel better—or, if that can't be done, finding a way to improve the quality of my work."

Example 3: "Getting my friend to understand me better, or at least stop misinterpreting me."

Example 4: "Finding a way not to fail my exams."

Example 5: "Getting help for understanding my behavior and a strategy for changing it."

Example 6: "Living without a partner who abuses me."

Example 7: "Finding a way to work and like my job, or at least not hate it."

✓   **4. *Brainstorm Lots of Solutions***

Continue: "The next step is to come up with as many novel ideas as possible for solving the problem."

a. Solutions Can Be Thought of as One or More Actions That Lead to the Goal

Example: To avoid getting harmed by a boss who is mean, solutions may include leaving the job, writing a letter of resignation, or making an appointment with the human resources manager at work.

Example: "Your parents have moved in with you and are driving you crazy. Solutions might include putting a lock on your bedroom door, accepting them for who they are, or getting cable television to distract them."

Example: "You are afraid of failing a hair-coloring exam in your cosmetology course because the instructor said you cannot take home the mannequin to practice. Solutions might include practicing on a friend, doing visualizations of the procedure, buying a large doll to practice on, or arranging to use the mannequin at the school on the weekend."

Example: A first step to managing a drinking problem might be to join Alcoholics Anonymous and get a sponsor as quickly as possible.

b. All Ideas Are Welcome; Don't Evaluate While Brainstorming

It is imperative that ideas not be judged during the brainstorming process. The aim is to generate as many ideas as possible, without censuring any ideas that come to mind—to let thoughts run free and wild. Brainstorming requires an atmosphere of psychological safety. It can take time, but it is important to get every idea anyone can think of down in writing.

> **Note to Leaders:** When demonstrating problem solving it is also important for you as the leader to generate some ideas, particularly if the group's ideas are rigid or noncreative. In these cases, it would be a good idea for you to generate clearly outrageous ideas. You can suggest clearly antisocial ideas (burn the house down) or clearly ineffective ideas (go to bed and ignore the problem). However, if the group is generating primarily impulsive, ineffective solutions, then you can generate a number of possibly effective ideas. The idea is to get the participants to open up their minds to new possibilities. Continue generating ideas until there are no new ideas or until it is clear that all potentially effective ideas have been generated. Remember that it is never too late to add new ideas to the pool.

Some people almost immediately start to evaluate suggestions, analyze the practicality of each solution, or point out problems rather than continuing to generate new ideas. It can be difficult to leave an idea alone and wait until a later time to evaluate it. But this is a necessary condition of brainstorming. Distress tolerance and impulse control are often necessary to achieve this.

Practice Exercise: In a group setting, there are two ways to do brainstorming. One is to have individuals first generate ideas on their own, either by writing them down or by simply thinking about different options. You can then go around the group and have each person share one idea. Keep going around until the ideas run out. Alternatively, you can elicit ideas from the group as a whole. That way, those who cannot think of any ideas are not put on the spot. Interesting research suggests that you will get more and more creative ideas if you let folks think them up on their own and then share them with the group.[102, 103]

✓ **5. Choose a Solution That Fits the Goal and Is Likely to Work**

Although brainstorming can be fun, it is not an end in itself. The point is to generate an effective solution to a problem where no solution was immediately evident. Thus, once many ideas have been generated, it is time to identify which one or two are the best to implement.

a. Prioritize the Suggested Solutions

The potential solutions can be prioritized by organizing them in order of likelihood to work and feasibility of implementation. A solution that might work is useless if it is impossible to put it into action.

b. Do Pros and Cons, and Consult Wise Mind

One or two of the best solutions from the priority list should be chosen. These should be evaluated with wise mind, and a formal pros-and-cons exercise should also be conducted on each.

Practice Exercise: Select solutions generated for one or more of participants' problems. Use the Figure 9.1 schematic to practice pros and cons.

✓ **6. Put the Solution into Action**

The entire enterprise of problem solving is aimed at putting into action an effective solution to the problem at hand. As the tire commercials say, this is where "the rubber meets the road."
The chief problems here are as follows:

- Inertia ("This is too hard!" "I am too tired," "I don't have time," etc.).
- Fear-generating thoughts ("If this doesn't work I will look like a fool," "This won't work and I will be a failure," "People will get mad at me," etc.).
- Willfulness ("I shouldn't have to solve this; they caused it," "If I do something to solve this, I'll look weak," etc.); and
- Impulsiveness (i.e., running head first into the problem with an impulsive, ineffective solution, rather than the one initially thought through).

Discussion Point: Elicit from participants examples of times when they have known a solution that might work, but then did not follow through with implementing it. Remind them that this is just

	Solution 1	Solution 2
Pros		
Cons		

FIGURE 9.1. Chart for figuring out pros and cons of potential solutions to problems.

a new problem to solve. Ask whether the main problem was inertia, fear, willfulness, impulsiveness, or something else. Troubleshoot how to overcome such problems in implementing solutions.

✓ **7. *Evaluate the Results of Implementing the Solution***

Instruct participants to ask themselves: "Am I satisfied with the results of my problem solving? Do I feel better about my situation than before? Were there any negative outcomes for myself or for others?"

The bottom line is that the best-laid plans can go awry. Even when a solution is carried out exactly as planned, it can fail. Unanticipated obstacles can arise, or others can respond in unexpected ways. Thus a critical step in problem solving is to examine how well one's actions work in solving a problem.

Explain to participants: "Once you realize that you have to evaluate your problem solving, you may be more open to the idea that effective problem solving can take multiple efforts with different solutions before you find the one solution or set of solutions that actually solves the problem. Often if a first effort does not solve a problem completely, it will at least improve the situation somewhat. Then applying other solutions to the problem may reduce all or most of the factors that made the situation distressing."

> **Note to Leaders:** It is critical to present problem solving as a process that takes time and patience. The idea that there are simple, one-shot solutions can present a tremendous barrier to the focused, difficult, and time-consuming process that solving some problems can require. The more examples you provide of successful problem solving following extended effort, the better—whether these are from your own life or from the lives of others you know.

> 💬 **Discussion Point:** Elicit from participants examples from their own lives of problems that have been solved with the first solution they tried, and problems that required multiple attempts before getting solved.

XII. REVIEWING OPPOSITE ACTION AND PROBLEM SOLVING (EMOTION REGULATION HANDOUT 13)

> **Main Point:** It is important not only to know when to use opposite action and when to use problem solving, but also to have a clear idea of how these two skills differ in actual practice.
>
> **Emotion Regulation Handout 13: Reviewing Opposite Action and Problem Solving.** This handout summarizes justifying events for each basic emotion, and then lists sets of opposite actions (for unjustified emotions that don't fit the facts, or for justified emotions that are ineffective) and problem solutions (for justified emotions). It is reviewed after problem solving is taught, to clarify the relationship of opposite action to problem solving. If time is short, review only the problem-solving column, as this is information that has not been presented before.
>
> When you are reviewing the problem solutions, it is helpful if you link the solutions to the justifying events. (You can also point out that in these cases, justifying events are the same as prompting events in Emotion Regulation Handout 6, and that both justifying events and opposite actions in this handout are shorthand versions of what is presented in Emotion Regulation Handout 11.)
>
> **Worksheet:** None.

Highlight to participants that the information in the first two columns of Emotion Regulation Handout 13 (justifying events and opposite actions) constitutes a review of what has already been presented in previous handouts (or in previous classes if this is being used in an advanced skills class). Then review different types of problem solutions.

✓ A. Review Problem Solutions

Point out that for each emotion, the first solution is acting on the emotion if that is reasonable. This is followed by solutions aimed at changing the situations, followed by avoiding the situation, and then (when reasonable) changing thoughts about the situation. Be careful not to suggest that this is an exhaustive list of problem solutions. Instead, present it as a starting list of ideas.

Describe the four types of solutions for justified emotion to participants as follows.

✓ 1. Acting on the Emotion

A major function of emotion is to motivate action. Often the action urges associated with the emotion are the same as actions that represent solutions. The actions associated with basic emotions generally function to solve common types of problems.

✓ *Examples:* "If a tsunami is coming in from the ocean, run for high ground; if you love someone, spend time with this person; and so on."

2. Changing the Situation

Say: "At other times, simply acting on an emotion urge may give you only temporary relief when permanent relief is needed. In these situations, you will need to use your problem-solving skills to come up with a strategy for actually changing or solving the situation."

✓ *Example:* "Running away from a rat in your kitchen and jumping up on a chair will temporarily reduce fear and panic, but sooner or later you have to get down from the chair. If you don't get the rat out of the kitchen, you are likely to have a lot more fear. Problem solving in this case might involve getting a rat trap, baiting it, and putting it in your kitchen, or getting a friend or exterminator to come and get the rat out."

3. Avoiding or Leaving the Situation

Go on: "Sometimes you can't change the situation, because other people or situations are more powerful than you are. In these cases, you might choose to avoid the situation altogether."

Example: "If you are a student in a school where you are being bullied, and no amount of complaining to the school or others seems to stop it, you can change schools—or, if possible, avoid walking anywhere near the bullies or block their messages on Facebook."

✓ *Example:* "If you discover that you are really not good in a particular area of school or work and want to stop doing poor work in that area, you can change classes or find a new job in an area you are good at."

4. Changing Thoughts and Interpretations of the Situation

Continue: "Sometimes you can't really change the problem situation, and you can't avoid it either. In these cases, you might try changing how you are thinking about the situation."

Example: "Cheerlead yourself ('I can do this; I am going to be OK') in scary situations where you have to act opposite to your fear, even when there is real danger."

Example: "If you are envious of someone who has a lot more money than you, you can try putting on a pair of rose-colored glasses about your own status, or placing less value on what others have. An example of this might be to join a group advocating simple living, in hopes it will change your attitude."

Example: "If someone breaks up with you, you can remind yourself that it is better to have loved and lost than to never have loved at all."

> **Note to Leaders:** Although many of the problem solutions provided are very clear and easy to understand, some are not so easy and will need clarification and discussion. It is important to note that the

solutions provided are for use when the person actually wants to change an emotion by using one of the problem-solving strategies: acting on emotions, changing the situation, avoiding or leaving the situation, or changing how one views the situation. Some of the points that have been difficult for participants are outlined below. Review as many as you can. Knowing these possible solutions for each of these emotions can also be very helpful when you are coaching clients.

B. Review Typical Solutions for Each Emotion

Review the list of steps covered in Section XI and in Emotion Regulation Handout 12 for solving problem situations. In addition, briefly highlight the following:

1. Fear

Many people do not think of solving fear by doing things that give them a sense of control and mastery. However, this can be very useful over the long run in learning how to respond effectively to events that initially are frightening. (See Emotion Regulation Handout 19: Build Mastery and Cope Ahead.)

2. Anger

It is very important to note here that one should only fight back when that is likely to be an effective response. Say: "An example when fighting back might be needed could be being grabbed from behind when getting into your car at night. If someone only grabs for your handbag or wallet, on the other hand, it might be more effective to give it to the person."

3. Disgust

Imagining understanding a disgusting person, or imagining really good reasons for something disgusting that has happened (problem solving by changing thoughts about it), might not at first glance appear to be a very good idea. As some participants might say, it seems disgusting in itself. You can point out: "However, if you have no choice except to be around people who do disgusting things on occasion—say, on a bus ride or in a school or work group—this might be an alternative to never-ending feelings of disgust. It is also useful if you yourself have done something truly disgusting in your lifetime. It beats hating yourself for life."

4. Envy

Say: "Although many people do avoid others who have more than them, many also believe that you should be able to stop wanting what others have. From their perspective, the problem is that you want things you don't have, not that others have a lot more than you. What is important here is to focus on what is effective problem solving and give up a judgmental attitude."

5. Jealousy

People who are locked into intimate relationships with others whom they depend on for sustenance and therefore cannot leave have become outraged at the thought that they should work at being more desirable to the persons they depend on. As one participant yelled at me, "You mean I should make myself more desirable to my pimp?" The only response one can give to this critique is this: "Becoming more desirable should only be used if the person you depend on is threatening to leave, and you absolutely want to keep the person from leaving you. Note also that I did not put in the option of changing your thought or interpretation of the person leaving you, because if you actually delude yourself that the person will not leave you, you might lose him or her."

6. Love

What is important to make clear here is this: "You only fight to find or get back your beloved when loving the person actually fits the facts—that is, the person has all the qualities that justify love."

7. Sadness

Grieving does not sound at first like a strategy to reduce sadness, but it is. Tell participants: "Grief is necessary to process and comes to terms with loss. If you avoid it, you may end up with long-lasting grief that makes things worse, not better." There is a large overlap between acting opposite to sadness and problem-solving sadness. This is because acting opposite, once grief has subsided, actually reduces sadness through building back a life that is experienced as worth living. See the ABC skills for reducing vulnerability and building a life worth living (Emotion Regulation Handouts 15–19) for more on these topics.

8. Shame

Many participants will be distressed at the suggestions that they hide or change what will get them rejected, avoid a group, or find a new group to be part of, even when they do not agree that they should be rejected in the first place. It is important to remind participants that the only reason to hide behaviors or characteristics or avoid or find new groups in these situations is if they don't want to be rejected. Remind them that they can skip these solutions, and instead become activists and work to change the group's and society's values and beliefs.

9. Guilt

The important point to be made about guilt when it is justified is this: "To repair what you have done or said, you first have to figure out what you have harmed. If out of anger you kick in a wall, figuring out the repair is easy: Fix or replace the wall. If you have told a mean lie about someone, repair by telling everyone the truth in a manner that gets people to believe you now, not the lie you told. It can be much more difficult to repair, however, when you have done something that loses another's trust or destroys or takes something away that you cannot replace or give back. In these cases repair may take a long time. It can also be difficult to repair something when it is important that you keep anyone from knowing that you are the person who has done the damage. In these cases, you may need to repair by helping others, rather than the person you have harmed."

✓ 💬 **Discussion Point:** Be sure to take questions about problem solving for each of these emotions as they arise. For emotions that create a discussion, elicit examples of problem-solving strategies for those emotions from participants, and share any of your own that will clarify the material.

XIII. OVERVIEW: REDUCING VULNERABILITY TO EMOTION MIND (EMOTION REGULATION HANDOUT 14)

> **Main Point:** Emotional distress and anguish can be reduced by decreasing factors that make us vulnerable to negative emotions and moods.
>
> **Emotion Regulation Handout 14: Overview: Reducing Vulnerability to Emotion Mind—Building a Live Worth Living.** This handout is an overview to orient participants to what is coming next. It can be reviewed very quickly, or skipped (with the information written on the board).
>
> **Emotion Regulation Worksheet 9: Steps for Reducing Vulnerability to Emotion Mind.** This is a summary worksheet for all the ABC PLEASE skills. If time is short, or you have a group whose members do not like to write, this is a good worksheet to use. Review each section, and point out that participants

can use it to record their pleasant events, as well as their work on developing long-term goals and values, building mastery activities, coping ahead, and using PLEASE skills.

A. Becoming Less Vulnerable to Painful Emotions

Say to participants: "The skills here are about how to build your life so that you become less sensitive and vulnerable to painful emotions. All of us have times when we are more vulnerable to painful emotions than at other times. When we are vulnerable, we can be much more sensitive to events that prompt painful emotions. Some people lead lives that make them vulnerable to painful emotions almost all the time. Accumulating positive events in your life, and practicing the other skills you will learn here, will help increase your resilience."

✓ B. The ABC PLEASE Skills

Tell participants: "You can remember this set of skills with the term **ABC PLEASE.**"

- "**A is for <u>A</u>ccumulate positive emotions.** When you accumulate positive experiences, events, and valued behavior patterns, you build a wall between you and the sea of emotional dyscontrol."
- "**B is for <u>B</u>uild mastery,** which means doing things that make you feel competent and effective. This is a line of defense against helplessness and hopelessness."
- "**C is for <u>C</u>ope ahead** of time with emotional situations. Before you get into an emotional situation, rehearse a plan so that you are prepared to cope with the situation skillfully."
- "**PLEASE stands for a set of skills that will help you take care of your mind by taking care of your body.**"

> **Note to Leaders:** As noted earlier, DBT assumes that it is often (but not always) the events in life that cause unhappiness, not faulty appraisals of events. This is the opposite of what many therapists assume. However, a reconciliation between the two points of view is possible. A person who gets emotional often begins distorting;[104] thus vigilance for distorting is useful, and reappraisal can be helpful. However, over-focusing on cognitive distortions as the source of difficulty simply further invalidates the behavior, emotions, and thinking processes of the suffering individual. Instead, the goal is to *validate* the individual's responses.

XIV. ACCUMULATING POSITIVE EMOTIONS: SHORT TERM (EMOTION REGULATION HANDOUTS 15–16)

> **Main Point:** Most people who feel painful emotions do so for good reasons. It is usually (but not always) the events in life that cause unhappiness. Increasing positive events now can accumulate into a happier life.
>
> **Emotion Regulation Handout 15: Accumulating Positive Emotions: Short Term; Emotion Regulation Handout 16: Pleasant Events List.** Handout 15 is an overview of building positive experiences now by increasing pleasant events. Move from Handout 15 to Handout 16 in the same session. If there is not a lot of time, ask participants to skim Handout 16 quickly for events that they would find pleasant, and to review the complete schedule during the week. Encourage participants to do as many events as possible that would make them feel happy or joyful, even if only a little bit at first.
>
> **Emotion Regulation Worksheet 10: Pleasant Events Diary.** This worksheet is designed to be filled out daily. It can be useful to have participants write out their plans for pleasant events during the session. During the week, participants should write out what they actually did, and then rate how mindful they were to each event (i.e., how focused and in the moment they were, and how much they participated), how unmindful they were to worries (with no worries = 0), and how pleasant the experience was. Emo-

tion Regulation Worksheets 9 and 13 also have brief sections for tracking pleasant events, along with the other ABC PLEASE skills.

A. Why Add Positive Events to Your Life?

✓ **1. Positive Events Increase Positive Emotions/Decrease Negative Emotions**

First, positive events not only increase positive emotions, but decrease sadness and other negative emotions. In fact, they are so important that they are important components of two of the most effective behavioral interventions for major depression, cognitive therapy[105] and behavioral activation.[10]

✓ **2. All People Need Positive Events in Their Lives to Be Happy**

We all need positive events in our lives. However, each person needs different things to be happy, and the same person can have different needs at different times.

✓ **3. The Absence of Positive Experiences Has Negative Effects**

The absence of positive experiences in life reduces happiness, increases sadness, and creates vulnerability to events prompting painful emotions.[106]

Example: "Positive events are like food: Food does you no good if you don't eat it, and positive events do you no good if you don't experience any."

4. Negative/Aversive Events Have Negative Effects

Too many negative or painful events in life make it very difficult to feel happy and content,[107] particularly when a person is living a life deprived of positive events.

Example: When people diet, they are often in a state of deprivation, which then results in negative emotional states. Too much work and no play can have the same effect.

💬 **Discussion Point:** Elicit examples from participants when a sense of deprivation has had a negative impact on their emotions and moods. Discuss.

5. Both Short-Term and Long-Term Positive Events Are Needed

Building a life worth living requires attention to both short-term and long-term positive events.

- Short-term positive events are those that make us feel better *now*—right this minute.
- Long-term positive events are those parts of our lives that give a lasting sense of happiness or contentment.

6. Pleasant Events Are Possible Even in Deprivation

Even in a very deprived life, a person can find or develop pleasant events that will lift the spirits, at least momentarily, and increase positive emotions, even if only slightly.

7. Avoiding Negative Events Can Result in Avoiding Positive Events

People sometimes accidentally avoid pleasant events because they spend so much energy avoiding painful events. This is a recipe for unhappiness.

8. Developing Pleasant Events Is Worth the Effort

People sometimes don't bother to develop pleasant events, or they are too depressed, tired, overworked, or overwhelmed to make the effort. Often people don't realize how important it is to add "little positives" into their daily routines. The saying "All work and no play makes Jack a dull boy" could be changed to "All blah and no pleasure makes Jack an unhappy boy."

✓ **B. How to Build Positive Experiences Now**

✓ ### 1. Do at Least One Pleasant Thing a Day

Tell participants: "To start with, do at least one thing each day that prompts positive emotions, such as enjoyment, pleasure, serenity, calmness, love, joy, pride, or self-confidence."

Note to Leaders: It can be very important to stress to participants that getting themselves to engage in positive events and to avoid avoiding (see below) often requires a concerted effort to use the skill of opposite action. Problem solving may also be required. I have found it very useful to have everyone check off possible pleasant events on Emotion Regulation Handout 16 and then plan a week of pleasant events on Emotion Regulation Worksheet 10 before the session is over.

---

2. Use Problem-Solving Skills

Say: "Use problem-solving skills to figure out how to increase the positive events in your life. This is particularly important when you have very little money, an inflexible schedule, or many demands. It can be difficult, but it is possible."

3. Plan Pleasant Events Ahead of Time

Go on: "Plan pleasant events ahead of time when they are hard to do. Also, try to agree on the plan with someone else. This can help mobilize you, even when your mood says no to doing anything."

✓ ### 4. Practice Opposite Action When Necessary

Continue: "Practice opposite action when you need to activate yourself. (For ideas, see Emotion Regulation Handout 10.) Once you are unhappy, it can be extremely difficult to activate yourself to increase the pleasant events in your life."

5. Don't Think in Terms of "Deserving" and "Not Deserving"

Say: "Don't think in terms of 'deserving' and 'not deserving.' It is *not* effective. It is also judgmental thinking. If you are a person who thinks this way, you may have to do opposite action by engaging in pleasant events when feeling you don't deserve them. You may also have to practice nonjudgmentalness, one of the mindfulness 'how' skills in Mindfulness Handout 5."

6. Positive Events Are Reinforcers

Go on: "Keep in mind that positive events are reinforcers. That is, they make you want to activate yourself and keep having positive experiences."[108]

✓ ### 7. Avoid Avoiding

Continue: "A special case of taking opposite action is to avoid avoiding events that are pleasant or that will lead to pleasant events. People often avoid pleasant events or taking the sometimes difficult steps that will lead to pleasant events when they are in a bad mood. They say, 'Why bother?' and sometimes just give up. This, of course, does not work in the long run, even though at times it does work for the short term. When this is happening to you, the best strategy is to look at the pros and cons of avoiding, and also consult wise mind."

💬 **Discussion Point:** Ask participants to find three to seven pleasant events listed in Emotion Regulation Handout 16 that they can do in the next week. Ask them to circle these items and write them down on Emotion Regulation Worksheet 10. Ask participants to share what they circle and/or write down.

💬 **Discussion Point:** Elicit little things that participants find pleasant. Be creative. Get new ideas from Distress Tolerance Handout 2: Overview: Crisis Survival Skills (see also Chapter 10 of this manual).

✓ C. Be Mindful of Positive Experiences

A pleasant event that is not attended to will have little effect on our emotions. Often when we think that a pleasant event isn't pleasant, the reality is that we did not pay attention to it.

1. Focus Your Attention on Positive Events As They Happen

Paying attention to positive events can sometimes take a lot of effort. We may be too absorbed with something else to notice the event, or we may have trouble focusing on one thing because there are many distractions. We can also be in the habit of avoiding our own experiences so that we try to suppress even pleasant emotions.

Example: "When you are absorbed in reading a book, it is hard to appreciate that your children are playing right beside you."

2. Refocus on the Positive When Your Mind Wanders to the Negative

When the number of positive events in our lives is much smaller than the number of painful events, it can be hard to tear our minds away from what is painful. This can be particularly difficult when we are angry or bitter and think that feeling better will mean we have "given in." In these situations, refocusing on positive parts of events is an example of opposite action. Completing a pros-and-cons worksheet can motivate doing opposite action and building positive experience (see Emotion Regulation Worksheet 1).

Example: "When you are angry at someone and ruminating about how terribly the person has treated you, it is hard to pay attention to the wonderful meal you are eating with a very good friend."

3. Participate and Engage Fully in the Experience

Boredom is a common problem in trying to increase pleasant events. Boredom, however, is often the result of watching events rather than participating in events. Watching the world go by is nowhere as interesting as participating fully in the flow of life's events. Mindfulness is the practice of being present to our lives. It is difficult to benefit from events we are not present to.

Example: "You go to a party you were once looking forward to, but now sit back and just watch others have fun. This is unlikely to boost your morale as much as it would if you threw yourself into the party and engaged with others."

> **Note to Leaders:** Note that each of the core mindfulness skills is essential to benefit from adding pleasant events to one's life. Observing or noticing the event in the present, describing it as it really is without distortion, participating, and engaging nonjudgmentally, one-mindfully, and effectively are all important to experiencing and integrating the pleasant moment.

💬 **Discussion Point:** Elicit from participants times when they have been completely mindless or "zoned out" when positive events occurred, and times they have been very attentive to positive events. Discuss the differences in experiences.

✓ D. Be Unmindful of Worries

✓ 1. Don't Destroy Positive Experiences by Worrying

It is common for some people to worry about various aspects of a positive experience:

▪ When the experience will end.

    ■ Whether they deserve the experience or not.

    ■ How the experience might cause others to expect more of them.

Worrying about these things, however, only detracts from the positive experience as it is happening.

✓ **2. Refocus on the Positive When Necessary**

Encourage participants: "Refocus your mind on the positive parts of ongoing events when worries come up."

💬 **Discussion Point:** Discuss factors that make it hard to focus attention on positive events when they are happening.

> **Note to Leaders:** Many people have to work hard to get positive emotions to linger. The skills described above are extremely important. Many emotionally dysregulated individuals can experience positive emotions, but these evaporate in a second; they do not last. Often they are afraid that if they feel good, bad things will happen—that is, they have a phobia of positive emotions[109]—or a negative thought intrudes so quickly it erases the positive. These points should be stressed.

✓ E. Be Patient

Tell participants: "Adding one or two small pleasant events is unlikely to make a dramatic difference in the quality of your life. But adding them is helpful in changing emotions a little at a time. For pleasant events to be effective, you have to practice them often and try many different activities. Over time, the small changes they make in mood will add up to a noticeable difference. Be patient, be patient!"

Example: Even a pleasant event as small as noticing enjoyable things while walking from place to place can make a small difference. These small differences add up over time.

XV. ACCUMULATING POSITIVE EMOTIONS: LONG TERM (EMOTION REGULATION HANDOUTS 17–18)

> **Main Point:** It is hard to be happy without a life experienced as "worth living." Building such a life requires attention to one's own values and life priorities over the long term. This can take time, patience, and persistence.
>
> **Emotion Regulation Handout 17: Accumulating Positive Emotions: Long Term; Emotion Regulation Handout 18: Values and Priorities List.** These two handouts should be discussed in the same session. Handout 17 breaks down the process of building a life worth living into seven steps. Handout 18 helps with Step 2 ("Identify values that are important to you"). Remember that the goal of reviewing values is for participants to get to Steps 5 ("Choose one goal to work on now"), 6 ("Identify small action steps toward your goal"), and 7 ("Commit to taking one action step now"). If you wish to accomplish each of these steps in one session, you cannot linger too long on identifying values.
>
>   Some individuals know what values are and have a clear sense of their own values. However, many people don't know what you are talking about when you mention values, and they are unable to articulate their own values. Rather than spending much time trying to define what a value is, just give them Handout 18's listing of values. Ordinarily this is sufficient to get the point across. Values on Handout 18 are grouped into 14 general categories, A through N. Under each general value are more specific values for a total of 58 specific values. Let participants know that they can choose the more general values, the more specific values, a combination of both, or values not on the list (in which case they should write them down on the lines provided under O for "other").

> **Emotion Regulation Worksheets 11 and 11a: Getting from Values to Specific Action Steps.** Both these worksheets are designed for working out what steps are needed to build a life worth living. Worksheet 11 is linear, provides more space, and also emphasizes attending to relationships as a value. Worksheet 11a is much briefer and works well with adolescents. It can also be reviewed at the same time you are teaching Handout 17. Having participants fill out Worksheet 11 or 11a during a group session is a good way to teach this skill if you have time. Alternatively, select one or two group members to guide others through the worksheet on the board. Note that doing the homework on this skill is not designed to have an immediate effect on the quality of participants' lives. Such work may improve a sense of mastery (see Emotion Regulation Handout 19: Build Mastery and Cope Ahead), but major shifts in the quality of life take time.
>
> **Emotion Regulation Worksheet 11b: Diary of Daily Actions on Values and Priorities.** Worksheet 11b is an advanced worksheet for keeping track of actions taken across different life goals and values. This sheet is ordinarily too advanced for most participants at the beginning of skills training, but can be useful for experienced participants who are working on several different goals at once. This worksheet is often very useful in individual therapy. Working on values is also tracked on Emotion Regulation Worksheet 9, which covers all of the other ABC PLEASE skills.

✓ A. Long-Term Happiness Means Experiencing Life as Worth Living

✓   Tell participants: "It is hard to be happy without a life worth living. This is a fundamental tenet of DBT. Of course, all lives are worth living in reality. No life is *not* worth living. But what is important is that you *experience* your life as worth living—one that is satisfying, and one that brings happiness."

1. Accumulating Positive Events May Require Changing Your Life

✓   Say: "If positive events do not occur in your life very often, you may need to make changes in your life so that positive events will occur more often. Accumulating events that build a life worth living is like saving pennies in a piggy bank."

2. A Life Worth Living Is a Life That You Value and That Contains Things You Value

Go on: "Two things are important here. First, you need to go into Wise Mind to find and describe your most important values. Second, you may need to push yourself to overcome fear, regret, shame, guilt, and hopelessness in identifying the values you want to pursue in your life."

✓ 3. Building a Life Worth Living Takes Time and Patience

a. Short-Term Pleasures versus Long-Term Happiness

Short-term pleasures can sometimes interfere with building a life of stable happiness and contentment. Always seeking things that make us feel different or better *right this minute* can at times get in the way of building permanent positive events into our lives. Sometimes we seek a pleasant event to avoid working on long-term goals that will make permanent changes in our lives. If there are not permanent positive events in our lives, pleasant feelings will probably be temporary rather than lasting.

b. Permanent Positive Events

Permanent positive events are related to the following:

- Living our lives according to our own personal values.
- Achieving goals that are important to us.
- Developing lasting and loving interpersonal relationships.

✓ **B. Building a Life Worth Living, Step by Step**

✓ **1. Avoid Avoiding**

The central problem for many people in building a life worth living is that they avoid doing what is needed to build such a life. Factors that can interfere include not knowing what they want in life; moodiness; emotional overload; and inability to accept that life is often unfair. Although these factors and others may be very understandable reasons for avoiding the hard work necessary to build a life worth living, getting to work on the task is what is needed now. Ultimately, each of us has to build our own lives worth living.

✓ **2. Identify Values That Are Important to You**

a. What Are Values?

▪ *Values are things that really matter.* Say: "Values are the things that are important to you, what you cherish about life. They are your highest priorities in life."

▪ *Values are not goals; they are not outcomes, and they are not in the future.* "Values are ways of living; they are about engaging in activities that you value. It is keeping priorities straight when you make life decisions—big ones and little ones. Values are like a 'pathless path.' They give your life direction and meaning, but they do not have an endpoint. Values are like guideposts that remind you of what you care about. Values may tell you that a specific goal is important to work on, but achieving the goal does not mean you can forget that value in your life."

Example: "You can work on relationships, achieving things in life, and having integrity. But there is no date in the future when you can say, 'I have achieved that value and don't need to keep it a priority in my life any longer.' "

▪ *Values change over time and often are not simple to figure out.* "Values can change during your lifetime and as a result of major life events. Values can also be in conflict with each other. Figuring out which values are most important at any given point in your life can be very important."

Example: "Having a good time, seeking fun and things that give pleasure, and having free time may be very important when you are young and fancy-free, with few obligations. But, once you are married and have a baby, having a family, staying close, and spending time with your spouse and child may be far more important."

Good questions to ask participants (and to have them ask themselves) in figuring out values include the following:

▪ "What in life are your highest priorities? What in life really matters to you?"
▪ "What is the direction you want your life to go in?"
▪ "What is in your life now that you do not want to lose?"
▪ "What things of value are *not* in your life right now?"

And add: "Simply affirming your own values in this way has been found to buffer psychological stress responses."[110]

✓ 👥 **Practice Exercise:** Ask participants to review Emotion Regulation Handout 18, and to check off values that are important to them. Be sure to remind them that they can also write down any important values not included in this handout. Then have each person count up the number of values he or she checked. Share the number of values checked and some of the most important ones with the group. Ask, "How many checked 1–10 values?" How many checked 11–20? How many 21–35? 36–45? Over 45?" My experience is that almost always there is a typical curve, with few at the extremes and most in the middle. Give participants a chance to share one or two values, as well as any new values they wrote out.

> **Note to Leaders:** Be prepared for some distress when participants are looking at the list of values. The list will make many people aware of how far their own lives are from their values. To head this off, you might want to ask participants first to identify one or two important values that are already present in their lives. These might include things that they already have (such as having people to do things with or secure and safe surroundings) or things that they are already doing in their lives (such as working toward goals or treating people equally).

> **Note to Leaders:** If you ask participants to check off only values they believe are really important, or if you suggest an arbitrary number of values to check, you may be waiting a very long time for them to finish the task. It takes a lot of thought to figure out which values are *most* important. When you are responding to participants' values, remember, it is not to suggest or recommend values. It is your task to help participants find their own values.

> **Research Point:** This emphasis on values and their role in building a life worth living is similar to the emphasis on values in Acceptance and Commitment Therapy,[42] a form of CBT that is very similar to DBT. Most of the values in Handout 18 were adapted from research done in Europe comparing values across different countries.[111] Thus these values are very general and are widely shared, at least in Western cultures. Similar lists of general values, however, come up in many different research studies on values.

b. Decide Whether Values Are Really Your Own

Often we have made other people's values our own values without really thinking about them. Sometimes we speak and act as if we value things that, in fact, we don't value. We value others' opinions of us, and so we live according to their values to get their approval. Most of us do this some of the time. Some of us do this all of the time. It can be hard to live according to our own values when what we really want is to fit in with others. This is especially difficult if the group we want to fit in with has values different from our own. To have a life worth living, however, we have to live according to our own values. Of course, if we also highly value having others love and approve of us, we may also have to live at least some of our life according to others' values. It's important to know when our highest value is getting love and approval from others and when it's living according to other wise mind values. This can take a lot of thought—and a lot of checking the facts.

Good questions to ask participants (and to have them ask themselves) to see whether a value is really their own value include the following:

- "If you could act according to a particular value but could not tell anyone about it, would you do it? For example, if being an educated person is an important value, but you could not tell anyone that you are taking courses to further your education, would you still take the courses?"
- "If anything were possible, what direction would you want your life to go toward? (This is not about what you think is realistic or what others may think you deserve.)"

💭 **Discussion Point:** Ask each participant to think of one value he or she currently struggles with that has mostly or completely come from others. Then have participants select one they themselves are ambivalent about or have already rejected. Discuss how difficult it can be for participants to live according to their own values when they have been punished for not living up to other people's values, or when they have been promised great rewards for living according to other people's values.

✓ ### 3. *Identify One Value to Work On Now*

Tell participants: "Most people have many important values. Focus on just one that is your highest priority. Otherwise, the task will feel too big and overwhelming. Be sure to pick a value you actually want to work on at this time in your life. Look at what is in your life now that you really value, and at what valuable things are not in your life right now."

Good questions to ask participants (and to have them ask themselves) include the following:

- ■ "Which value is your highest priority right now?"
- ■ "In what areas does your current life not match your values very well?"
- ■ "Is your own behavior in accord with your wise mind values?"
- ■ "Are there things you really value that are not in your life enough?"
- ■ "Are you doing things that you value?"
- ■ "Are you doing things that go against your core values?"
- ■ "Where do you need to make changes in your life so that it will match what is most important to you?"

✓ **4. Identify a Few Goals Related to This Value**

a. Goals Are Something Specific That You Can Achieve

Say to participants: "Identify a few goals that will get you closer to your values. Once you have achieved a goal, you don't have to work on it any more."

Example: "If you value being powerful and influencing others, you can work on increasing that over your entire life. In contrast, a goal that could help you get more power and influence would be to get a college degree. Once you get it, you don't continue to work on it."

Example: "If your highest value is contributing to the larger community, you can continue to do that all your life. Goals that could get you closer to that value would be to get a part-time volunteer job or to donate time to a neighborhood spring cleanup. Once you have done these things, you have achieved those goals."

b. What Goals Will Get You Closer to Living Your Value?

Goals need to be very specific. Good questions to ask participants (and to have them ask themselves) include the following:

- ■ "What is one thing you could accomplish that would be in accord with the value you are working on?"
- ■ "What is one thing about your behavior that you could change to be living in accord with the value you are working on?"
- ■ "Are there major impediments that must be overcome before you can accomplish your goal?"

Examples:

- ■ "If your value is to make a great deal of money, your goals might include first to get an education, and then to look for a high-paying job or one with potential for advancement."
- ■ "If your value is to live in secure and safe surroundings, a goal might be to get an apartment in a safe area of town."
- ■ "If your value is to have a steady income that meets your basic needs, a goal might be to get a job."
- ■ "If your value is to care for nature and the environment, a goal might be to keep your room or apartment clean and well maintained."
- ■ "If your value is to have close and satisfying relationships with others, a goal might be to make one friend."
- ■ "If your value is to be courageous in facing and living life, a goal might be to do something that you are afraid of or that you are avoiding."

■ "If your value is to be a healthy person, a goal might be to lose or gain weight when your doctor recommends it."

c. Remember the "Art of the Possible" in Setting Goals

Continue: "Be sure that your goals are reasonable. There is no point in setting up goals that cannot be achieved. If the value is to compete successfully with others, setting a goal to be a national tennis champion in 2 years when you have never had tennis lessons is unrealistic. It is also important to avoid goals that will reduce your quality of life if they are met. For example, if your value is to make sacrifices for others, giving away your college education savings to a friend who wants a new car is likely to cause long-term harm that is much greater than the benefits of solving the friend's temporary transportation needs."

✓ ## 5. Choose One Goal to Work on Now

a. Put Goals in Order of Importance and Reasonableness

Go on: "You cannot work on every goal related to a value at once. It can be very helpful to organize goals in a list, with the most important and realistically possible goal at the top of the list. This will enable you to set your priorities, so that you know which goal to work on first."

b. Select One Goal

Select the one goal that is reasonable and important to work on now.

✓ ## 6. Identify Small Action Steps toward Your Goal

Say to participants:

■ "Figure out what small steps will move you toward your goals."
■ "Ask yourself what you have to accomplish to get to the goal."
■ "Break the task into small steps you can take now."
■ "Break it down again if the steps are too big."

✓ ## 7. Take One Action Step Now

Example: Value: Be part of a group.

Possible goals:

■ Reconnect with old friends.
■ Get a more social job.
■ Join a club.

Pick one goal to work on right now:

■ Join a club.

Figure out a few action steps for moving toward the goal:

■ Look for clubs on craigslist.
■ Go to the bookstore by my house and ask about book groups.
■ Join an interactive online game or chat room.

Take one step:

■ Turn on the computer.

Practice Exercise: Participants often have trouble telling the difference among values, goals, and action steps. Ask participants to work on Worksheet 11 or 11a during session time, and then share what they filled out on the sheet with each other. This also provides you with an opportunity to provide feedback before participants leave the session.

XVI. BUILD MASTERY AND COPE AHEAD SKILLS FOR EMOTIONAL SITUATIONS (EMOTION REGULATION HANDOUT 19)

> **Main Point:** Feeling competent and adequately prepared for difficult situations reduces vulnerability to emotion mind and increases skillful behavior.
>
> **Emotion Regulation Handout 19: Build Mastery and Cope Ahead.** As its title indicates, this handout covers the steps for building mastery, as well as for coping ahead with emotional situations. Both skill sets are ordinarily taught in the same session.
>
> **Emotion Regulation Worksheet 12: Build Mastery and Cope Ahead.** On this worksheet, participants are to schedule activities to build a sense of accomplishment and then report on what they actually did. Remember that doing activities to build mastery is the target. The point of scheduling is to increase the probability that participants will actually do the homework assignment. However, in reviewing the homework it is important to not penalize participants if they did something other than they planned.
> There is space on this worksheet to report two practices of coping ahead. This assignment is hard to do if no difficult situation comes up. In this case, you can assign practice on past situations that were not handled very well.
>
> **Emotion Regulation Worksheet 13: Putting ABC Skills Together Day by Day.** This worksheet has a brief section for tracking <u>A</u>ccumulate positive emotions, <u>B</u>uild mastery, and <u>C</u>ope ahead. These skills are also tracked on Emotion Regulation Worksheet 9.

✓ **A. Build Mastery**

1. What Is Mastery?

Tell participants: "Mastery is doing things that make you feel competent, self-confident, in control, and capable of mastering things. Human babies have a natural tendency to increase mastery. This tendency can be lost over time, however, if efforts to increase mastery are not reinforced."

✓ ### 2. Why Build Mastery?

Doing things to build mastery is an important component of two of the most effective treatments for depression, cognitive therapy and behavioral activation.[3] Building a sense of confidence and competence makes a person more resistant to depression and other negative emotions.[112, 113]

Building mastery usually requires doing something that is at least a little bit hard or challenging. The idea is to generate a sense of accomplishment. Over time, a series of accomplishments leads to a more positive self-concept, higher self-esteem, and an overall greater level of happiness.[114, 115]

> **Note to Leaders:** In teaching how to build mastery, it can be helpful to draw lines like those in Figure 9.2. The heavy line two-thirds of the way up on a whiteboard represents the point at which a task becomes impossible. Trying to do a task above this line leads to failure (and a consequent sense of failure and a lowered sense of mastery and competence). Doing tasks at the bottom third of the board, below the dotted line, does not increase mastery. The best place to be trying to master something is midway up, in a space that is difficult but possible. Accomplishing that type of task will give a sense of mastery.

3. How to Build Mastery

a. Do at Least One Thing Each Day

Tell participants: "Do at least one thing each day to build a sense of accomplishment."

✓ **b. Plan for Success, Not Failure**

Say: "Do something difficult, but possible. Lives of failure are lives where expectations are too high."

Example: "When you are starting to work out, it is not a good idea to try to run 5 miles the first day just because you heard that a person who is in good shape can do that."

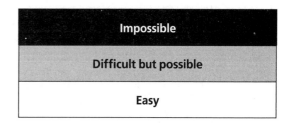

FIGURE 9.2. Different levels of task difficulty for Building Mastery.

✓ **c. Gradually Increase the Difficulty over Time**

Continue: "Once you have mastered the first task, try something a little more difficult each time. However, if any task is too difficult at first, do something a little easier next time."

Example: When I was learning how to go camping, I started by setting up a tent in the front yard; then I started sleeping in a sleeping bag in the bedroom; then I tried doing both at a car camping site.

d. Look for a Challenge

> **Note to Leaders:** It is extremely important to give examples of very small things that can give a sense of mastery, either from your own life or from the lives of others. An academic bookworm, for example, can get a tremendous jolt of mastery from something as simple as learning how to light a campfire. A person who has never exercised seriously before can get a high from going from lifting 5-pound weights to 10-pound weights. A person with a phobia can increase mastery through taking small steps of opposite action.

💬 **Discussion Point:** Describe a time in your own life when you had a surge of mastery from an accomplishment. Ask participants for examples from their own lives. Discuss how it felt to succeed at something.

💬 **Discussion Point:** Elicit activities that give participants a sense of mastery. These will probably differ for each person.

B. Cope Ahead

✓ **1. What Is Cope Ahead?**

Say to participants: "Coping ahead is figuring out which situations are likely to cause you trouble, and then not only planning ahead how to cope with expected difficulties, but also imagining being in the situation and coping effectively."

✓ **2. Why Cope Ahead?**

> **Research Point:** There is a large amount of research showing that we can learn new skills simply by imagining and practicing new skillful behavior in our minds. This is true for all sorts of skills from sports (e.g., tennis players can improve their tennis by practicing their tennis service in their minds[116]) to interpersonal skills (e.g., individuals can improve their assertion skills by practicing assertive behaviors in their minds[117]). As it turns out, imagining an activity fires many of the same regions of the brain as actually engaging in that activity does.[118] Not only does coping ahead help us in planning how to deal with emotionally pro-

vocative situations, but it also increases the likelihood that we will more automatically respond with the skillful sequence of behaviors we have practiced.

✓
✓ **3. When to Use Cope Ahead**

Tell participants: "Cope ahead is useful in many types of emotional situations. Here are some of them."

✓
- "In any situation coming up where there is a threat or you feel afraid."
- "When you know your emotions may get so high that you will forget your skills, or you will be unable to put skillful actions together."
- "In a new situation where you are very unsure of your skills, and your insecurity may elicit an emotional reaction that will make it very difficult for you to manage the situation effectively."
- "When you may have difficult urges—such as to run away, hit someone, or say yes to using alcohol or drugs—which would get in the way of skillful behavior if you followed them."
- "When you could get so emotional or your destructive urges could be so high that you don't even want to behave skillfully."

✓ **4. How to Cope Ahead**

✓ **a. Describe a Problem Situation**

Say: "Start by describing a problem situation for which you are worried about coping well."

- "Once you have described the situation, check the facts to be sure that the problem you perceive would be an actual problem if it occurred. (If you need to, use Emotion Regulation Handout 8.)"
- "Then name the emotions and urges likely to interfere with using your skills."

✓ **b. Decide What Skills to Use**

Continue: "Next, decide what coping or problem-solving skills you want to use in the situation. Be specific. Write it out in detail. You may need to use problem-solving skills to figure out how to cope effectively. Mindfulness, distress tolerance, and interpersonal effectiveness skills may also be useful."

✓ **c. Imagine the Situation**

Go on: "Now imagine the situation in your mind as vividly as possible. Be sure to imagine yourself *in* the situation, not watching the situation. Also, be sure to imagine in the present tense—not the future or the past."

✓ **d. Rehearse in Your Mind Coping Effectively**

- "Rehearse in your mind exactly what you could do to cope effectively, including rehearsing your actions, your thoughts, what you can say, and how to say it."
- "Rehearse coping with new problems that come up."
- "Rehearse coping with your most feared catastrophe."

✓ **e. Practice Relaxation after Rehearsing**

Note to Leaders: Some participants may not have visual imagery. With individuals whose imagery is primarily verbal, suggest that they rehearse verbally, in their minds, going over the strategies they will use. Suggest that they give themselves subvocal instructions in what to do. Other participants may find kinesthetic imagery (a sense of body place) or audio imagery useful.

✓

Example: I suddenly became afraid of driving in tunnels. To reduce this fear, I started driving in every tunnel I could find, reassuring myself that there was no danger of its falling in on me. When this didn't work (because the fact is that a tunnel could fall in on me, since earthquakes are possible in Seattle), I asked myself, "What's the threat?" I realized that telling myself the tunnel wouldn't fall in was avoiding the threat. Next I drove in tunnels and imagined that one *did* fall in on me. I then imagined jumping out of the car, putting on my Wonder Woman outfit and rushing to save others, and then running out of the tunnel to safety. I noticed that my fear came down a lot (from 80 to 30 on a 100 scale), but it did not come down to zero. I asked myself again, "What's the threat?" and realized that the primary fear was that the tunnel would not only cave in, but I would be trapped in the tunnel in extreme pain with a fire raging and no one who could get to me to save me. I then practiced radical acceptance of pain and death, and after several practices my fear went away completely.

> **Note to Leaders:** Note that in this story I've included imagery of saving others and radical acceptance, both of which have allowed me to imagine the event ending with me in a peaceful state. In other words, it may be useful to end imaginal practice with a behavior that solves a problem or provides a positive outcome for self or others. If you are using this strategy, it is important to discuss with each participant what positive event as an outcome of their behavior would bring them a sense of peace. It is also important to notice that I used fantasy (jumping out of my car in my Wonder Woman outfit). See Emotion Regulation Handout 20a: Nightmare Protocol, Step by Step for another example of this strategy.

💬 **Discussion Point:** Give either my example above or one of the following examples in segments, and at each coping point ask participants what they think the protagonist in the example should be practicing in his or her imagination.

Example: Joe is getting ready to sing solo for the first time at a recital given at his university. He has had a cold, and he is afraid his voice might give out for a minute or two in the middle of his performance. To cope ahead, he imagines first singing with no troubles. This is helpful, but he is still anxious. Then he practices in his mind walking out on stage with a glass of water in his hand, bending over, and putting it on the floor before he starts. Then he imagines singing, having his voice go out suddenly, bending over to gather his wits together, picking up his glass of water, taking a sip of water, and then continuing to sing when he is ready. In this real life example, Joe's anxiety went all the way down, and he sang his solo without incident.

> **Note to Leaders:** It is very important to help participants figure out what the emotion cue actually is in a situation. This is particularly true where the emotion is fear; it is typical for individuals to misperceive what they are actually afraid of.

Example: Sharon is addicted to drugs, and her bus stop to work is on a street where there are a lot of drug dealers. Many of them know her, and when they see her, they approach and offer to sell her drugs. She cannot move to a safer neighborhood right now. She practices cope ahead skills every morning before going to work by imagining herself waiting for the bus, having a dealer approach her, and then telling the dealer in a determined voice, "No! Stay away from me!" With her therapist, she imagines standing at the bus stop with cravings, reviewing her pros and cons in her mind, and telling the dealer, "No! Stay away!" At a later point, she practices this at home.

👥 **Practice Exercise:** Elicit several problem situations, and then select one or two to practice with participants. Discuss possible ways to cope with each situation, and have participants write out specific steps. Then encourage the participants to sit back, close their eyes, and rehearse in imagination using the coping skills to manage the situation. At the end, lead participants through a brief relaxation exercise. Get feedback and discuss.

> **Note to Leaders:** It is important throughout skills training to look for situations where participants can practice cope ahead. Add it as an individual homework assignment where appropriate.

XVII. TAKING CARE OF YOUR MIND BY TAKING CARE OF YOUR BODY (EMOTION REGULATION HANDOUT 20)

> **Main Point:** An out-of-balance body increases vulnerability to negative emotions and emotion mind. Taking care of one's body increases emotional resilience. The mnemonic PLEASE covers treating Physica**L** illness, balanced **E**ating, avoiding mood-**A**ltering substances, balanced **S**leep, and **E**xercise.
>
> **Emotion Regulation Handout 20: Taking Care of Your Mind by Taking Care of Your Body.** It is rare that a participant has difficulty understanding this handout. If pressed for time, you can usually go through this handout rather quickly. Emotion Regulation Worksheet 14 (see below) is used for recording practice.
>
> **Emotion Regulation Worksheet 14: Practicing PLEASE Skills.** On this worksheet, participants are to record their use of the PLEASE skills during the week. There is a row for each day, and participants can record how they practiced each of the PLEASE skills that day. At the bottom of each column is a space for checkmarking whether each specific skill was helpful over the week.

✓ **A. The Body's Influence on the Mind**

Tell participants: "An out-of-balance body increases vulnerability to negative emotions and emotion mind. If you use the skills in this part of the module to take care of your body, this will increase your emotional resilience."

✓ **B. The PLEASE Skills**

Explain to participants: "You can remember these skills with the term PLEASE. This stands for the following: Treat Physica**L** illness, balance **E**ating, avoid mood-**A**ltering substances, balance **S**leep, and get **E**xercise."

✓ **1. Treat Physica**L** Illness**

Say to participants: "Being sick lowers your resistance to negative emotions. The healthier you can become, the better able you will be to regulate your emotions."

Many individuals fear going to a physician or do not have the behavioral regulation to get themselves to doctor appointments. Others do not have the self-regulation to take prescribed medications (either psychotropics or general medication).

✓ 💬 **Discussion Point:** Discuss any illnesses participants have had. What interferes with treating illness? Common obstacles may include embarrassment about the problem (as in the case of sexually transmitted diseases), lack of assertion skills, lack of money, problems with self-regulation, fear of medical treatment, and negative previous experiences of seeking medical care.

✓ **2. Balance **E**ating**

Say: "Try to eat the amounts and kinds of foods that help you feel good—not too much or too little. Both eating too much[119] and excessive dieting[107] can increase your vulnerability to emotion mind. When and how often you eat and your daily eating routine can be especially important for some individuals, such as those diagnosed with bipolar disorder. Stay away from food that makes you feel overly emotional."

💬 **Discussion Point:** Encourage people to avoid foods that make them feel bad. Ask participants for foods that make them feel good (e.g., chocolate), calm (e.g., milk), or energized (e.g., sugar, meat); stress the role of such foods, in moderation.

> **Research Point:** Research on restrained eaters on self-imposed diets shows negative effects of eating too little. For example, restricting food intake has been shown to lead both to eating binges and to psychological problems (such as preoccupation with food and eating, increased emotionality and dysphoria, and distractibility).[107]

> **Note to Leaders:** Do not try to convince participants that foods they think are bad for them are not actually harmful. This is likely to become a losing battle.

✓ ### 3. Avoid Mood-<u>A</u>ltering Substances

Explain: "Alcohol and drugs, like certain foods, can lower resistance to negative emotions. Stay off illicit drugs. Use alcohol in moderation, if at all."

💬 **Discussion Point:** Use this as an opportunity to discuss alcohol and drug problems participants may be having. Discuss the effects of mood-altering substances on emotions,[120] as well as difficulties in staying off these substances.

✓ 💬 **Discussion Point:** Mood-altering substances alter moods! This is why it is not a good idea to drink alcohol or use drugs before a job interview, or before or during other events where behavioral and emotional control is very important. Elicit other examples from participants of when it has been important for them not to use alcohol or other drugs.

✓ ### 4. Balance <u>S</u>leep

Continue: "Try to get the amount of sleep that helps you feel good—not too much or too little, usually between 7 and 9 hours. Keep to a consistent sleep schedule, especially if you are having difficulty sleeping."

> **Research Point:** An increasing amount of research suggests that lack of sleep is related to a wide variety of emotional difficulties.[121]

💬 **Discussion Point:** Elicit participants' troubles with sleep. This is usually an important problem for emotionally dysregulated individuals. Too little sleep, especially, can make them particularly vulnerable to negative emotions; it may be part of a depression syndrome. What has helped? What has made things worse?

5. Get <u>E</u>xercise

Explain: "Aerobic exercise, done consistently, is an antidepressant.[122] In addition, a regular exercise schedule can build mastery. Do some sort of exercise 5 to 7 days per week. Try to build up to 20 minutes of exercise each time."

💬 **Discussion Point:** Ask what forms of exercise participants engage in. An important problem here is that consistent exercise requires self-management skills, and most emotionally dysregulated individuals have few such skills. This discussion is an opportunity to discuss principles of self-management, especially reinforcement principles. (For information on reinforcement, see Interpersonal Effectiveness Handout 20: Strategies for Increasing the Probability of Behaviors You Want.)

> **Note to Leaders:** The nightmare and sleep hygiene protocols are ordinarily not reviewed in skills training groups unless the participants are in the group specifically to deal with nightmares or sleep disturbances. I ordinarily assign these handouts as reading material and suggest that if needed they ask their individual therapist to work with them on the protocols. I have not put any checkmarks on these protocols. If you teach them, each numbered step in each protocol should be reviewed.

XVIII. NIGHTMARE PROTOCOL (EMOTION REGULATION HANDOUT 20A)

> **Main Point:** Recurrent nightmares are not only highly distressing but they also interfere with adequate and restful sleep.
>
> **Emotion Regulation Handout 20a: Nightmare Protocol, Step by Step** *(Optional).* This optional handout, together with Worksheet 14a (see below), can be used when participants have recurrent nightmares.
>
> **Emotion Regulation Worksheet 14a: Target Nightmare Experience Forms** *(Optional).* If Handout 20a is used, it is very important to go over this worksheet in detail. Note that this worksheet consists of three forms. On the Target Nightmare Experience Form, the participant describes in detail the distressing dream. For some individuals, this may be very difficult, and you might want to have such a participant fill it out in the presence of a therapist. Some therapists in our group have skipped this first form and started the protocol with the second form, the Changed Dream Experience Form. Here, the participant describes a changed dream in detail. The changed dream scenario should be reviewed with each individual to be sure he or she follows the instructions exactly. When practicing the nightmare protocol, participants track their progress on the third form, the Dream Rehearsal and Relaxation Record.

> **Research Point:** The nightmare protocol described below and outlined in Emotion Regulation Handout 20a is based on the Imagery Rehearsal Therapy (IRT) for chronic nightmares developed by Barry Krakow and colleagues.[123] Several controlled clinical trials of IRT have shown that it is effective in reducing the frequency of nightmares.[124, 125]

✓ Explain to participants that this treatment is based on the following ideas:

- **Nightmares are behaviors that are learned,** often as a result of traumatic events. Once learned, they may be maintained by habit.
✓ - **Habitual nightmares can be changed by practicing new dreams to replace them.**
✓ - **New dreams are learned by rehearsing a changed dream**—one without the negative and traumatic events in the old nightmare—and following the rehearsal with relaxation.
- **In developing new dreams, it is important to put in changes that elicit a sense of mastery and control. In nightmares people ordinarily feel not only terrified but also out of control. Current clinical thinking is that this factor—the increase in personal mastery in the dream—appears to be important in how IRT works.**

Point out as well that the nightmare protocol is very similar to the skill of cope ahead. Both focus on writing out a script and rehearsing it mentally. Thus both seek to change problem behaviors by imaginal rehearsal of coping and mastery behaviors.

✓ **A. Practice Necessary Skills**

Tell participants: "Practice necessary skills first to be sure you are ready to work on changing nightmares."

1. Relaxation

Say: "Practice relaxation. Decide what relaxation method you want to use while working on your nightmares. Practice it to be sure that you can do it, and that when you practice you do become more relaxed."

2. Pleasant Imagery

Go on: "Practice pleasant imagery to be sure that you can evoke imagery."

3. Coping Skills

Continue: "Decide on and rehearse coping skills in case you become distressed when thinking about your nightmares." Explain that TIP skills (see Chapter 10 and Distress Tolerance Handout 6) may be useful if arousal gets very high. Other distress tolerance skills, such as temporary distraction or self-soothing, may also be useful. Problem solving (see Section XI of this chapter) may be necessary to determine whether the target nightmare is too severe to work on at the moment.

B. Choose a Recurring Nightmare

Tell participants: "Choose a recurring nightmare to work with. Select one you are prepared to manage. Do not start with your most severe or traumatic nightmare unless you are very prepared. First practice on easier ones, and work up to harder ones."

C. Write Down the Target Nightmare

Say: "Now write down your target nightmare in moment-to-moment detail. Include events in the environment, as well as thoughts, feelings, and assumptions about yourself during the dream."

> **Note to Leaders:** The step of writing down the nightmare can be skipped for individuals with PTSD, for whom the nightmare is itself traumatic. The key event in this protocol is developing a sense of mastery, not exposure to the nightmare itself.

D. Choose a Changed Outcome for the Nightmare

Continue: "Next, choose a way to change the outcome of the nightmare. This can be any change before anything traumatic or bad happens. It can be anything you want it to be, as long as it prevents the bad outcome of the usual nightmare from occurring. There are some people who believe that the more outrageous the change (for instance, a gun turning into a banana), the better the protocol works."

Explain that the outcome can include insertion of new information. For example, a male veteran who feels ashamed of his own behavior in war and believes he has let down his troops can stand up in the dream and see a huge group of people whose lives have been saved by his behavior. A woman who has been raped and feels weak for not fighting back can imagine her arms and legs bulging with muscles and an auditorium of people giving her a standing ovation for speaking up and admitting the rape.

> **Note to Leaders:** It is important to work with participants to be sure that any new ending has the desired effect of making them feel competent and good about themselves.

E. Write Down the Full Nightmare with the Changes

Go on: "Now write down the full nightmare, with the changed outcome and any other changes you have made."

F. Rehearse and Relax Each Night

Say: "Rehearse the entire changed dream by visualizing it each night *before* practicing relaxation. The relaxation should be something that is effective; each person might use a different strategy."

> **Note to Leaders:** Suggest mindfulness practices, or progressive relaxation as described in Distress Tolerance Handout 6b: Paired Muscle Relaxation, Step by Step.

G. Rehearse and Relax during the Day

Conclude: "Finally, rehearse the new dream as often as possible during the day, followed by relaxation. The key idea here is to remember that changing nightmares takes practice, practice, practice. But, in general, the effects should show up within a few weeks."

> **Note to Leaders:** See *www.huffingtonpost.com/belleruth-naparstek/getting-rid-of-repeating_b_487024.html* for variations on this protocol as used with veterans. The basic idea here is to follow the protocol as described, but also to add to the dream an ending that will allow the person to wake up in a peaceful state. In other words, the aim is to add an ending where the dreamer engages in a behavior that solves a problem or provides a positive outcome for others. If you use this strategy, it is important to discuss with each participant what positive event as an outcome of his or her behavior would bring the participant a sense of peace.

XIX. SLEEP HYGIENE PROTOCOL (EMOTION REGULATION HANDOUT 20B)

> **Main Point:** Adequate sleep on a daily basis is essential for both mental and physical health. Difficulties in sleeping can often be solved by using a series of sleep-inducing strategies.
>
> **Emotion Regulation Handout 20b: Sleep Hygiene Protocol** *(Optional)*. This optional handout, together with Worksheet 14b (see below), can be used when participants have these particular sleep difficulties.
>
> **Emotion Regulation Worksheet 14b: Sleep Hygiene Practice Sheet** *(Optional)*. If Handout 20b is used, review this worksheet with participants.

> **Research Point:** There is an enormous amount of research showing that both quantity and quality of sleep are related to physical and mental health.[126] Length of sleep is also related to longevity: Either too little or too much sleep is associated with a shorter lifespan.[127]
>
> Evidence for the particular importance of sleep in the mood disorders has mushroomed over the past decade. Among adolescents and adults with a mood disorder, sleep disturbance:
>
> - Is a risk factor for mood disorder episodes.
> - Can contribute to relapse.
> - Has an adverse impact on emotion regulation.
> - Has an adverse impact on cognitive functioning.
> - Compromises health.
> - May contribute to substance use comorbidity and suicidality.
>
> Sleep disturbance is now seen as an important but underrecognized mechanism in the cause and main-

tenance of the mood disorders.[128] Because the biology underpinning the sleep and circadian system is an open system, readily influenced by inputs from the environment, there are now several powerful, simple, and inexpensive treatments.

The suggestions for good sleep hygiene in the following protocol are, for the most part, extremely common in most sleep hygiene lists.

Steps 1–6 in this protocol are intended to increase the likelihood of restfulness/sleep.

✓ **1. Develop and Follow a Consistent Sleep Schedule Even on Weekends**

Explain to participants: "When it comes to sleep, ritual is everything. Go to bed and get up at the same times each day. Engage in the same ritual each night when it is time for bed. Avoid anything longer than a 10-minute nap during the day. The idea here is to get time of day to be a prompting event for sleep."

2. Do Not Use the Bed for Daytime Activities

Say: "Do not use your bed for activities such as watching TV, talking on the phone, or reading during the day. This will make you more likely to associate your bed with sleep."

3. Avoid Certain Things before Bed

Continue: "Avoid caffeine, nicotine, alcohol, and heavy meals late in the day, and exercising for 3–4 hours before going to bed. Also, do not watch TV before bed if a show is emotionally arousing (for example, it is election night and your candidate is losing)."

4. Prepare the Room for Sleep

Continue: "Turn off the light, keep the room quiet, and make the temperature comfortable and relatively cool when you are preparing to sleep. Try an electric blanket if you are cold; putting your feet outside the blanket or turning on a fan directed toward your bed if you are hot; or wearing a sleeping mask, using earplugs, or turning on a 'white noise' machine if needed."

5. Give Yourself Half an Hour to an Hour to Fall Asleep

Say: "Give yourself from 30 to 60 minutes to fall asleep. If this doesn't work, evaluate whether you are calm, or whether you are anxious or ruminating, and follow the appropriate steps after Step 6."

✓ **6. Do Not Catastrophize about Not Sleeping**

Explain: "Catastrophizing about not sleeping is sure to keep you awake. Worrying about not sleeping is one of the major factors in continuing insomnia.[129] If sleep is completely elusive, rest in bed, reminding yourself that you will be OK with reverie and resting. Do not decide to give up on sleeping for the night and get up for the 'day.'"

Steps 7–9 are for use if participants are calm but wide awake.

7. Get Out of Bed and Pursue a Quiet Activity

Say: "Go to another room and read a book, or do some other quiet activity that will not wake you up further."

8. Listen to Public Radio

"With eyes closed, listen to public radio (BBC, NPR, or the like) at low volume. Public radio is a good choice for this, because there is little fluctuation in voice tone or volume." (Do not listen to news that will disturb you.)

9. Eat a Light Snack

"Eat a light snack of complex carbohydrates[130] (such as an apple)."

Steps 10–15 are for use if participants are anxious or ruminating.

✓ **10. Use TIP Skills**

Say: "Splash your face with cold water, or put your face in a bowl of ice water or cold water on your eyes and upper face (this will reduce arousal for a brief time). Then get right back in bed. To block ruminating, practice paced breathing as soon as you lie back down. Remember, if you have any medical condition, get medical approval before using cold water." (See Distress Tolerance Handout 6a: Using Cold Water, Step by Step.)

✓ **11. Try the 9–0 Meditation Practice**

"Try the 9–0 meditation practice, to put a slight burden on your memory that will interfere with worries. Breathe in deeply and breathe out slowly, saying in your mind the number 9. On the next breath out, say 8; next, say 7; and so on until you are saying 0. Then start over, but this time, instead of starting with 9, start with 8 as you breathe out, followed by 7 and so on until you reach 0. Next, start with 6 and so on to 0; then start with 5; then with 4 and so on until you have gone all the way down to starting with 1. Continue with the practice, starting over as often as necessary until you fall asleep. There are other similar strategies, such as counting to 10 at least 10 times, first pausing after the count of 1, the next time pausing after the count of 2, then pausing at 3, 4, and so on to 10. Then, if you are not out like a light, start over."

12. Focus on Bodily Sensation

"Focus on the bodily sensation of the rumination if you find yourself ruminating."[38, 131]

13. Read an Emotionally Engrossing Novel

"Read an emotionally engrossing novel for a few minutes until you feel somewhat tired. Then stop reading, close your eyes, and try to continue the novel in your head."

14. Reassure Yourself

"Remind yourself that what appear to be very big problems in the middle of the night often do not seem so worrisome in the morning. In the middle of the night, remember those times and tell yourself, 'These are just middle-of-the-night thoughts, and in the morning I will think and feel differently.' "

15. If Rumination Doesn't Stop . . .

"If rumination doesn't stop, follow these guidelines. If it's solvable, solve it. If it is insolvable, go deep into the worry all the way to the 'catastrophe'—the very worst outcome you can imagine—and then imagine coping ahead with the catastrophe."[132] (See Emotion Regulation Handout 19: Build Mastery and Cope Ahead.)

💬 **Discussion Point:** Discuss with participants how using these strategies for combating rumination can be useful at others times of the day—not just when they are trying to sleep.

✓ 💬 **Discussion Point:** Elicit from participants difficulties they have with sleep and any strategies they have used that were helpful. Discuss use of prescription medications for sleep, and emphasize that really good sleep hygiene practices can be as helpful in the long run. Do not hesitate to share sleep strategies you have found helpful.

XX. OVERVIEW: MANAGING REALLY DIFFICULT EMOTIONS (EMOTION REGULATION HANDOUT 21)

> **Main Point:** At times, the intensity of negative emotions can be so high that special skills are necessary to manage them.
>
> **Emotion Regulation Handout 21: Overview: Managing Really Difficult Emotions.** This handout is an overview to orient participants to what is coming next. Review it quickly. It can also be skipped and the information written on the board.

✓ **A. Mindfulness of Current Emotions**

Say to participants: "Suppressing emotion increases suffering. Mindfulness of current emotions is the path to emotional freedom."

✓ **B. Managing Extreme Emotions**

Say: "Sometimes emotional arousal is so high that you can't use any skills, particularly if the skills are complicated or take any thought on your part. This is a skills breakdown point. Crisis survival skills, like the ones described in Distress Tolerance Handouts 6–9a, are needed."

✓ **C. Troubleshooting Emotion Regulation Skills**

Remind participants: "Troubleshooting emotion regulation skills helps you figure out why a skill isn't working. When you are learning many new skills, it is easy to forget many of them or forget how to practice them."

✓ **D. Reviewing Skills**

Point out that reviewing emotion regulation skills can also be helpful. The flow chart model of emotions (see Section V of this chapter, and Emotion Regulation Handouts 5 and 25) puts the skills in order so that they are better understood and remembered.

XXI. MINDFULNESS OF CURRENT EMOTIONS (EMOTION REGULATION HANDOUT 22)

> **Main Point:** Suppressing emotion increases suffering. Mindfulness of current emotions is the path to emotional freedom.
>
> For advanced groups, or participants who you feel confident can experience their own emotions without trauma, mindfulness of current emotions can be moved up and taught before Emotion Regulation Handout 6: Ways to Describe Emotions.
>
> **Emotion Regulation Handout 22: Mindfulness of Current Emotions: Letting Go of Emotional Suffering.** Do not try to skip over this handout or rush through it. Mindfulness of current emotions is a critical skill underpinning many if not most of the skills in DBT. Avoiding emotions interferes with using almost every other skill in this module.
>
> **Emotion Regulation Worksheet 15: Mindfulness of Current Emotions.** The worksheet allows participants to check off what skills they have used in practicing mindfulness of emotions. This can be very helpful, because participants often forget exactly how to practice the skill. If necessary, remind participants how to rate intensity of emotions (0 = no emotion; 100 = maximum intensity). The "Before" and "After" spaces are for rating the intensity of the emotion before and after practicing mindfulness of current emotions. If participants have trouble identifying what emotion they are feeling, instruct them to review Emotion Regulation Handout 6, and/or to fill out Emotion Regulation Worksheet 4, 4a, or 5. Worksheet 15 ends with a section for comments and a description of experiences while practicing.

✓ **A. What Is Mindfulness of Current Emotions?**

Mindfulness of current emotions means observing, describing, and "allowing" emotions without judging them or trying to inhibit them, block them, or distract from them.

✓ **B. Why Be Mindful of Current Emotions?**

1. To Learn That Emotions Are Not So Catastrophic

Tell participants: "By exposing yourself to emotions, but not necessarily acting on them, you will find that they are not so catastrophic. You will stop being so afraid of them. Once you are less afraid, the fear, panic, and anger that you feel in response to your own emotions will dissipate. Observing emotions works on the same principle as exposure does in treating phobias and panic."

✓ **2. To Find a Path to Freedom**

Say: "Over time and with practice, you will gradually feel more and more free, less controlled by your emotions. Letting go of controlling emotions is a path to freedom. Many people believe that they have to control their emotions at all times. When you believe this, it is easy to become controlled by your own rules about emotions. You lose your freedom to be and feel as you do. Other people believe that they simply cannot bear painful emotions—that they will fall into the abyss or they will die if they do not control their emotions. This is the road to losing freedom. Wisdom and freedom require the ability to allow the natural flow of emotions to come and go, experiencing emotions but not being controlled by emotions. Always having to prevent or suppress emotions is a form of being controlled by emotions."

✓ **3. To Decrease Suffering**

Explain to participants that accepting painful emotions eliminates the suffering, leaving only the pain. At times, acceptance even reduces the pain. Fighting emotions ensures that they stay.[13] This is simply a restatement of the principles of mindfulness (see Chapter 7 of this manual) and of distress tolerance (see Chapter 10), but these points are extremely important to get across.

4. To Accept Painful Emotions as Part of the Human Condition

There are valid reasons for negative emotions. Short of making tremendous life changes, people probably cannot get rid of a lot of them; even then, negative emotions will always be a part of life. Ergo, the trick is to find a new way of relating to negative emotions so that they do not induce so much suffering. The way is through acceptance.

💭 **Discussion Point:** Learning to let go of emotions is extremely difficult. It takes a lot of practice. Discuss the role of acceptance of emotional suffering. Usually, you can expect participants to get this point. Get feedback.

✓ **C. How to Let Go of Emotional Suffering**

✓ **1. Observe Your Emotion**

Tell participants: "Start by just observing your emotion. Acknowledge its presence. Step back. Get unstuck from the emotion."

✓ **a. Experience the Emotion as a Wave**

Say: "Try to experience your emotion as a wave, coming and going. Imagine that you are on a beach and that emotions, like the waves of the ocean, are coming in and out, in and out. Dig your toes into the sand and allow them to come and go."

✓ **b. Imagine Surfing the Wave**

Continue: "Now imagine you are on a surfboard, riding the waves of your emotions. Try to keep your balance and just ride the surfboard."

Explain that surfing emotions is very similar to surfing urges in the treatment of substance use disorders.[133] Surfing urges and surfing emotions are similar if not identical skills. Surfing emotions can be extremely useful when it is important to inhibit the action linked to the emotion.

✓ **c. Try Not to Block or Suppress the Emotion**

Go on: "Open yourself to the flow of the emotion. Do not try to get rid of the emotion. Don't push it away. Don't judge or reject it."

d. Be Willing to Have the Emotion

Trying to build a wall to keep emotions out always has the effect of keeping emotions in. It is like trying to keep the ocean off the beach by building a wall of sand. The ocean inevitably seeps through, but it pools behind the wall because it is unable to go back out to the ocean quickly.

✓ **Research Point:** More and more research shows that trying to block or suppress emotions actually makes them worse.[97, 134] In fact, avoiding emotional sensation appears to be at the root of generalized anxiety disorder. Thus it is important to practice tolerating emotional sensations, without either trying to shut them down or to avoid them by going in circles with worry.

e. Do Not Try to Keep the Emotion Around

Say: "Don't cling to the emotion. Don't rehearse it. Don't hold on to it. Don't amplify it."

2. Practice Mindfulness of Body Sensations

Tell participants: "Pay attention to your physical sensations. It can be very useful here to concentrate on just physical parts of the emotion."

- "Notice where in your body you are feeling emotional sensations."
- "Experience the sensations as fully as possible."
- "Watch to see how long it takes for the emotion to go down, or the quality of experience to change. Adopt a curious mindset."

✓ **3. Remember: You Are Not Your Emotion**

Remind participants: "You are not your emotion. Do not necessarily act on the emotion. Continue to observe it. Also, remember times when you have felt different."

4. Practice Loving Your Emotions

- "Respect your emotion. Don't assume that it is irrational or based on faulty perceptions or distortions."
- "Let go of judging your emotion."
- "Practice willingness to have the emotion."
- "Practice radical acceptance of your emotion."

Note to Leaders: See Distress Tolerance Handout 11: Radical Acceptance and Distress Tolerance Handout 13: Willingness. If necessary, comment on the meaning of willingness and radical acceptance, for those who have trouble understanding the concepts.

Point 4 above is of course a difficult one. "Loving" in this context means "acceptance." The idea of loving and accepting emotions does not mean increasing or augmenting them. Fighting emotions does not make them go away. Accepting emotions allows a person to do something about them.

> **Note to Leaders:** These general instructions for mindfulness of current emotion often do not appear useful to participants at first. Remind participants that the point of mindfulness is to become free so that even intense emotions are not so disturbing. This takes a lot of practice. It is important to practice this skill with participants. Throughout skills training in this and other modules, often refer back to mindfulness of current emotion.

The following story is adapted from one I was told by a Zen teacher, who read it in a book by another spiritual teacher, Anthony de Mello.[135] The story is a very helpful one in teaching the concept of loving one's emotions.

✓   ⚘ **Story Point:** A man bought a new house and decided that he was going to have a very beautiful lawn. He worked on it every week, doing everything the gardening books told him to do. His biggest problem was that the lawn always seemed to have dandelions growing where he didn't want them. The first time he found dandelions, he pulled them out. But, alas, they grew back. He went to his local gardening store and bought weed killer. This worked for some time, but after summer rains, alas, he found dandelions again. He worked and pulled and killed dandelions all summer. The next summer he thought he would have no dandelions at all, since none grew over the winter. But, then, all of a sudden, he had dandelions all over again. This time he decided the problem was with the type of grass. So he spent a fortune and had all-new sod put down. This worked for some time, and he was very happy. Just as he started to relax, a dandelion came up. A friend told him it was due to the dandelions in the lawns of his neighbors. So he went on a campaign to get all his neighbors to kill all their dandelions. By the third year, he was exasperated. He still had dandelions. So, after consulting every local expert and garden book, he decided to write the U.S. Department of Agriculture for advice. Surely the government could help. After waiting several months, he finally got a letter back. He was so excited. Help at last! He tore open the letter and read the following: "Dear Sir: We have considered your problem and have consulted all of our experts. After careful consideration, we think we can give you very good advice. Sir, our advice is that you learn to love those dandelions."

This story can be told as often as necessary. The idea is to get to the point where clients say to you, "I know, this is a dandelion."

💬 **Discussion Point:** Have participants share times when radical acceptance of emotions has reduced suffering. Share your own experiences. Discuss the idea of "loving" one's emotions.

👥 **Practice Exercise:** Play a few minutes of emotion-generating music. This can be dissonant jazz fusion (e.g., Track 1 of John Coltrane's album *Meditations*) or other emotional music (such as Carl Orff's Carmina Burana, Dimitri Shostakovich's Symphony No. 10, or Samuel Barber's Adagio for Strings). Instruct participants to experience their emotions while listening. Elicit reactions.

👥 **Practice Exercise:** It can sometimes be very hard to get participants to have emotional responses just when you want to practice mindfulness of current emotions. A current emotion is needed to practice on! Be creative and try exercises that are very likely to generate some sort of emotion. For example, go around in a circle and have everyone sing one line of a song. Interrupt them periodically to redirect them to pay attention to their bodies and not escape into self-judgment, or into thinking about what they're going to sing. Or ask everyone to yell as loudly as they can at the same time, for about 10–20 seconds. Instruct participants to pay close attention to their emotional responses while engaging in the exercise.

✓   👥 **Practice Exercise:** Review Emotion Regulation Worksheet 15 with participants, and ask them to check off the ways they are willing to practice mindfulness of current emotions. Discuss.

XXII. MANAGING EXTREME EMOTIONS (EMOTION REGULATION HANDOUT 23)

> **Main Point:** Knowing one's own skills breakdown point is important. It signals the need first to use crisis survival skills (see Chapter 10 and Distress Tolerance Handouts 6–9a) and then to return to emotion regulation skills.
>
> **Emotion Regulation Handout 23: Managing Extreme Emotions.** This handout teaches participants how to identify their skills breakdown point. Crisis survival skills are listed on this handout, and you can give brief descriptions from the teaching notes below. You may be tempted to stop teaching emotion regulation skills and go to the crisis survival skills. Don't! Simply mention that set of skills, and spend time helping participants know when they should use emotion regulation skills first and when they should try crisis survival skills first.
>
> **Worksheet:** None. If needed, refer participants to the appropriate Distress Tolerance Worksheets.

✓ A. What Is the Skills Breakdown Point?

Tell participants: "You are at your skills breakdown point when your emotional distress is very high—so extreme that you go into overload."

- "You are completely caught in emotion mind. You can't focus on anything but the emotion itself."
- "You are emotionally overwhelmed."
- "Your mind is shutting down. Your brain stops processing information."
- "You can't solve problems or use complicated skills."

Go on: "Knowing at what point emotional distress interferes with your own coping and problem solving can be very important. In these times of crisis, special skills may be needed."

✓ B. Identify Your Personal Skills Breakdown Point

Continue: "When you are *not* in a crisis situation, think back on previous emotional episodes, and figure out how emotionally distressed you were when you 'hit the wall' and simply could not use your emotion regulation skills. This is your skills breakdown point."

1. How Distressed Were You?

"At what level of distress were you when you couldn't focus your mind on anything but the emotion, couldn't solve problems, or couldn't use any other complicated skills? Think back."

✓ 2. Check the Facts

"Check the facts. Do you really 'fall apart' at this level of arousal? Check to be sure the problem is not that although you could use skills, you just don't want to because they seem too hard. If you really do want to use skills but just can't figure out how to do it at this level, then this is indeed your personal skills breakdown point."

> **Note to Leaders:** It is important to note that reaching the point where their skills have broken down does not mean that participants themselves have broken down.

✓ C. What to Do at the Skills Breakdown Point

> **Note to Leaders:** Ordinarily I do not teach what to do at the skills breakdown point during the emotion regulation module. Instead I tell them they will get these skills in the next module, distress tolerance skills. If you need to teach these skills here, use the distress tolerance skills handouts and worksheets listed below.

✓ 1. *Use Crisis Survival Skills*

Tell participants: "The first thing to do when you know you have reached your skills breakdown point is to use the crisis survival skills covered in Distress Tolerance Handouts 6–9a."

a. TIP Skills for Changing Body Chemistry

- ▪ "Change your body temperature by putting cold water on your face, or by having a warm bath or foot soak."
- ▪ "Do intense aerobic exercise for 20 minutes or more."
- ▪ "Do paced breathing."
- ▪ "Focus on your body to tense and then relax muscles, one group at a time."

b. Distraction from the Event Prompting the Emotion

- ▪ "Shift your attention: Move your mind away from what is distressing you."
- ▪ "Focus your mind on something else—anything else."
- ▪ "Leave the situation completely."

c. Self-Soothing through the Five Senses

- ▪ "Look at something pleasant (vision)."
- ▪ "Listen to soothing music or other pleasant sounds (hearing)."
- ▪ "Touch something soft or soothing."
- ▪ "Smell something pleasant."
- ▪ "Eat or drink something good (taste)."

d. Improving the Moment You Are In

- ▪ "Imagine being somewhere else or in a different situation."
- ▪ "Pray."
- ▪ "Find relaxing things to do."
- ▪ "Encourage yourself."
- ▪ "Find some kind of meaning in the present moment."
- ▪ "Focus your entire mind on one thing in the moment."
- ▪ "Take a short vacation from the moment by briefly avoiding the situation."

2. *Return to Mindfulness of Current Emotions*

Go on: "At times the most useful thing to do, even with very extreme emotions, is to just 'sit' with them. Sooner or later they always go down. It may be difficult, but it can keep you out of trouble for now."

3. *Try Other Emotion Regulation Skills*

Say: "If nothing seems to be working, go to Emotion Regulation Handout 24: Troubleshooting Emotion Regulation Skills."

XXIII. TROUBLESHOOTING EMOTION REGULATION SKILLS (EMOTION REGULATION HANDOUT 24)

> **Main Point:** When one or more emotion regulation skills do not seem to work, it is important not to give up on the skills. Instead, participants should troubleshoot how they are being applied.
>
> **Emotion Regulation Handout 24: Troubleshooting Emotion Regulation Skills.** This handout helps participants figure out what is interfering with their efforts to control or regulate difficult and ineffective emotions. Worksheet 16 provides much of the same information. Teaching works best if participants have Worksheet 16 out, as well as Handout 24, while you go over it. If you are tight for time, teach this section by only going over the worksheet, or have participants use the worksheet during the week and then discuss it during homework review in the next session.
>
> **Emotion Regulation Worksheet 16: Troubleshooting Emotion Regulation Skills.** For many, this worksheet teaches itself.

✓ **A. Questions for When Skills Aren't Working**

✓   **1. Ask: Am I Biologically More Vulnerable?**

   Advise participants to check for temporary changes in biology, such as physical illness, menstrual cycle (for women), too little or too much food, effects of mood-altering drugs or alcohol, too little or too much sleep, too little exercise or movement or over-exercise, or biological imbalance caused by some mental disorders (such as bipolar disorders or schizophrenia). If biological disruptions are suspected, then it is important to get the body back in balance. At times, with some mental disorders, taking psychotropic medications may also be important.

✓   **2. Ask: Did I Use My Skills Correctly?**

   The first step in answering the second question is for participants to carefully read over the instructions for each skill tried. If this does not help, the next step is for them to get some coaching in how to use the skills or in how to select the skill(s) likely to be the most effective.

✓   **3. Ask: Is My Environment Reinforcing Intense Emotionality?**

   Say to participants: "If you have tried everything else to change your emotions and nothing has worked, then it is reasonable to suspect that your emotions are giving you some hidden benefit. Outside of your awareness, something might be reinforcing your emotions. To find out, these activities can be very useful."

   ■ "Review Emotion Regulation Handout 3."
   ■ "Fill out Emotion Regulation Worksheet 2 and/or 2b."

✓   **4. Ask: Am I Putting in the Time and Effort That Regulating My Emotions Will Take?**

   ■ "Do a pros and cons (Emotion Regulation Worksheet 1)."
   ■ "Practice radical acceptance and willingness skills (see Distress Tolerance Handouts 11 and 13)."
   ■ "Practice the mindfulness skills of participating and effectiveness (see Mindfulness Handouts 4c and 5c)."

   5. Ask: Am I Too Upset to Use Complicated Skills?

   Say to participants: "Trying complicated skills when you are at your skills breakdown point can lead to intense frustration and eventually giving up on skills altogether. However, you may be so far into emotion mind that you don't even know you have hit your skills breakdown point.

The secret is to practice your most important skills intensely when you are *not* in emotion mind. However, sometimes even when you have practiced the skill, your skills simply don't help. When this happens, try the following steps."

- "If the problem can be easily solved now, then immediately begin problem solving (see Emotion Regulation Handout 12)."
- "If the problem cannot be solved now and you are worrying about it, practice mindfulness of current emotions (see Emotion Regulation Handout 22). Worries often are just your mind's way of trying to escape from painful emotional sensations.[41] Escape, however, often does not work. It is hard to escape your own self. It may be paradoxical, but it appears to be true that if you simply focus your mind on experiencing your sensations, neither trying to suppress them or enlarge them, they will start to fade away before too long. Watch and see how long it takes for intense sensations to go down. Pay attention to which physical sensations you are actually feeling. Focus on physical sensations rather than on emotional thoughts or images."
- "If the emotional intensity is too high for you to think straight or use any skills, then use TIP skills or other crisis survival skills (see Emotion Regulation Handout 23 and Distress Tolerance Handouts 6–9a)."

✓ **6. Ask: Are Emotion Myths Getting in the Way?**

Conclude: "Finally, are myths about emotions getting in your way? For example, are you being judgmental about your emotions ('My emotions are stupid')? Or do you believe that your emotions are who you are? If so, complete Emotion Regulation Worksheet 3. Or simply check the facts, challenge the myths, and practice thinking nonjudgmentally."

XXIV. REVIEW OF SKILLS FOR EMOTION REGULATION (EMOTION REGULATION HANDOUT 25)

Main Point: Modifying any part of the emotion system will have an effect on the emotion. Specific DBT skills are aimed at specific components of emotions.

Emotion Regulation Handout 25: Review of Skills for Emotion Regulation (*Optional*). This optional handout is an overview of the major groups of DBT skills. The flow chart is very similar to the one in Emotion Regulation Handout 5: A Model for Describing Emotions. The handout can be used in a number of ways to summarize what has been learned in the entire module. It can be pinned up to remind participants of their emotion regulation skills (this works even better if the handout is laminated). It can also be distributed to other providers working with participants as an aid in figuring out what skills to use. When time is short, reviewing this handout with participants should be skipped.

Worksheet: None.

Briefly go over the model of emotions on Emotion Regulation Handout 25, reminding participants of the skills they have learned.

References

1. Farchione, T. J., Ellard, K. K., Boisseau, C. L., Thompson-Hollands, J., Carl, J. R., Gallagher, M. W., et al. (2012). Unified Protocol for transdiagnostic treatment of emotional disorders: A randomized controlled trial. *Behavior Therapy, 43,* 666–678.

2. Barlow, D. H., Farchione, T. J., Fairholme, C. P., Ellard, K. K., Boisseau, C. L., Allen, L. B., et al. (2010). *Unified protocol for transdiagnostic treatment of emotional disorders.* New York: Oxford University Press.

3. Dimidjian, S., Hollon, S. D., Dobson, K. S., Schmal-

ing, K. B., Kohlenberg, R. J., Addis, M. E., et al. (2006). Randomized trial of behavioral activation, cognitive therapy, and antidepressant medication in the acute treatment of adults with major depression. *Journal of Consulting and Clinical Psychology, 74,* 658–670.

4. Foa, E. B.,Wilson, R. (2001) *Stop obsessing!: How to overcome your obsessions and compulsions.* New York: Bantam Books.

5. Bolger, N., DeLongis, A., Kessler, R. C., & Schilling, E. A. (1989). Effects of daily stress on negative mood. *Journal of Personality and Social Psychology, 57,* 808–818.

6. Thompson, S. C., Sobolew-Shubin, A., Galbraith, M. E., Schwankovsky, L., & Cruzen, D. (1993). Maintaining perceptions of control: Finding perceived control in low-control circumstances. *Journal of Personality and Social Psychology, 64,* 293–304.

7. Misanin, J. R., & Campbell, B. A. (1969). Effects of hunger and thirst on sensitivity and reactivity to shock. *Journal of Comparative and Physiological Psychology, 69*(2), 207–213.

8. Bonanno, G. A. (2004). Loss, trauma, and human resilience: Have we underestimated the human capacity to thrive after extremely aversive events? *American Psychologist, 59,* 20–28.

9. Hayes, A. M., & Feldman, G. (2004). Clarifying the construct of mindfulness in the context of emotion regulation and the process of change in therapy. *Clinical Psychology: Science and Practice, 11,* 255–262.

10. Martell, C. R., Dimidjian, S., & Herman-Dunn, R. (2010). *Behavioral activation for depression: A clinician's guide.* New York: Guilford Press.

11. Beck, A. T., Rush, A. J., Shaw, B. F., & Emery, G. (1979). *Cognitive therapy of depression.* New York: Guilford Press.

12. Gross, J. J. (2014). *Handbook of emotion regulation* (2nd ed.). New York: Guilford Press.

13. Campbell-Sills, L., Barlow, D. H., Brown, T. A., & Hofmann, S. G. (2006). Effects of suppression and acceptance on emotional responses of individuals with anxiety and mood disorders. *Behaviour Research and Therapy, 44,* 1251–1263.

14. Lemerise, E. A., & Dodge, K. A. (2008). The development of anger and hostile interaction. In M. Lewis, J. M. Haviland-Jones, & L. Feldman Barrett (Eds.), *Handbook of emotions* (3rd ed., pp. 730–741). New York: Guilford Press.

15. Rozin, P., Haidt, J., & McCauley, C. R. (2008). Disgust. In M. Lewis, J. M. Haviland-Jones, & L. Feldman Barrett (Eds.), *Handbook of Emotions.* (3rd ed., pp. 757–776). New York: Guilford Press.

16. Barr-Zisowitz, C. (2000). Sadness: Is there such a thing? In M. Lewis & J. M. Haviland-Jones (Eds.), *Handbook of emotions* (2nd ed., pp. 607–622). New York: Guilford Press.

17. Rizvi, S., & Linehan, M. M. (2005). The treatment of maladaptive shame in borderline personality disorder: A pilot study of "opposite action." *Cognitive and Behavioral Practice, 12,* 437–447.

18. Buss, D. M., Larsen, R. J., Westen, D., & Semmelroth, J. (1992). Sex differences in jealousy: Evolution, physiology, and psychology. *Psychological Science, 3,* 251–255.

19. Salovey, P., & Rothman, A. (1991). Envy and jealousy: Self and society. In P. Salovey (Ed.), *The psychology of jealousy and envy* (pp. 271–286). New York: Guilford Press.

20. Hatfield, E., & Rapson, R. L. (2000). Love and attachment processes. In M. Lewis & J. M. Haviland-Jones (Eds.), *Handbook of emotions* (2nd ed., pp. 654–662). New York: Guilford Press.

21. Averill, J. R., & More, T. A. (2000). Happiness. In M. Lewis & J. M. Haviland-Jones (Eds.), *Handbook of emotions* (2nd ed., pp. 663–676). New York: Guilford Press.

22. Darwin, C. (1998). *The expression of the emotions in man and animals* (3rd ed., P. Ekman, Ed.). New York: Oxford University Press.

23. Ghazanfar, A. A., & Logothetis, N. K. (2003). Neuroperception: Facial expressions linked to monkey calls. *Nature, 423,* 937–938.

24. Peltola, M. J., Leppanen, J. M., Palokangas, T., & Hietanen, J. K. (2008). Fearful faces modulate looking duration and attention disengagement in 7-month-old infants. *Developmental Science, 11,* 60–68.

25. Mehrabian, A., & Wiener, M. (1967). Decoding of inconsistent communications. *Journal of Personality and Social Psychology, 6*(1), 109–114.

26. Sweeny, T. D., Grabowecky, M., Suzuki, S., & Paller, K. A. (2009). Long-lasting effects of subliminal affective priming from facial expressions. *Consciousness and Cognition, 18,* 929–938.

27. Monahan, J. L., Murphy, S. T., & Zajonc, R. B. (2000). Subliminal mere exposure: Specific, general, and diffuse effects. *Psychological Science, 11,* 462–466.

28. Sheese, B. E., Voelker, P., Posner, M. I., & Rothbart, M. K. (2009). Genetic variation influences on the early development of reactive emotions and their regulation by attention. *Cognitive Neuropsychiatry, 14,* 332–355.

29. Larsen, R. J., Diener, E., & Emmons, R. A. (1986). Affect intensity and reactions to daily life events. *Journal of Personality and Social Psychology, 51,* 803–814.

30. Calkins, S. D. (1994). Origins and outcomes of individual differences in emotion regulation. In N. A. Fox (Ed.), The development of emotion regulation:

Biological and behavioral considerations. *Monographs of the Society for Research in Child Development, 59*(2–3, Serial No. 240), 53–72.

31. Kaitz, M., Maytal, H. R., Devor, N., Bergman, L., & Mankuta, D. (2010). Maternal anxiety, mother–infant interactions, and infants' response to challenge. *Infant Behavior and Development, 33,* 136–148.

32. Moore, G. A., Hill-Soderlund, A. L., Propper, C. B., Calkins, S. D., Mills-Koonce, W. R., & Cox, M. J. (2009). Mother–infant vagal regulation in the face-to-face still-face paradigm is moderated by maternal sensitivity. *Child Development, 80,* 209–223.

33. Moore, G. A. (2010). Parent conflict predicts infants' vagal regulation in social interaction. *Development and Psychopathology, 22,* 23–33.

34. Muraven, M., Tice, D. M., & Baumeister, R. F. (1998). Self-control as limited resource: Regulatory depletion patterns. *Journal of Personality and Social Psychology, 74,* 774–789.

35. Goldberg, L. S., & Grandey, A. A. (2007). Display rules versus display autonomy: Emotion regulation, emotional exhaustion, and task performance in a call center simulation. *Journal of Occupational Health Psychology, 12,* 301–318.

36. Lyubomirsky, S., & Nolen-Hoeksema, S. (1995). Effects of self-focused rumination on negative thinking and interpersonal problem solving. *Journal of Personality and Social Psychology, 69,* 176–190.

37. Nolen-Hoeksema, S. (2000). The role of rumination in depressive disorders and mixed anxiety/depressive symptoms. *Journal of Abnormal Psychology, 109,* 504–511.

38. Borkovec, T. D., & Inz, J. (1990). The nature of worry in generalized anxiety disorder: A predominance of thought activity. *Behaviour Research and Therapy, 28,* 153–158.

39. Lyubomirsky, S., & Nolen-Hoeksema, S. (1993). Self-perpetuating properties of dysphoric rumination. *Journal of Personality and Social Psychology, 65,* 339–349.

40. Borkovec, T. D., & Hu, S. (1990). The effect of worry on cardiovascular response to phobic imagery. *Behaviour Research and Therapy, 28,* 69–73.

41. Borkovec, T. D. (1994). The nature, functions, and origins of worry. In G. Davey & F. Tallis (Eds.), *Worrying: Perspectives on theory, assessment, and treatment* (pp. 5–33). New York: Wiley.

42. Hayes, S. C., Strosahl, K. D., & Wilson, K. G. (2012). *Acceptance and commitment therapy: The process and practice of mindful change* (2nd ed.). New York: Guilford Press.

43. Mauss, I. B., Levenson, R. W., McCarter, L., Wilhelm, F. H., & Gross, J. J. (2005). The tie that binds?: Coherence among emotion experience, behavior, and physiology. *Emotion, 5,* 175–190.

44. Lemke, M. R., Fischer, C. J., Wendorff, T., Fritzer, G., Rupp, Z., & Tetzlaff, S. (2005). Modulation of involuntary and voluntary behavior following emotional stimuli in healthy subjects. *Progress in Neuropsychopharmacology and Biological Psychiatry, 29,* 69–76.

45. Dimberg, U., & Thunberg, M. (1998). Rapid facial reactions to emotional facial expressions. *Scandinavian Journal of Psychology, 39,* 39–45.

46. Ortony, A., & Turner, T. J. (1990). What's basic about basic emotions? *Psychological Review, 97,* 315–331.

47. Davidson, R. J., Jackson, D. C., & Kalin, N. H. (2000). Emotion, plasticity, context, and regulation: Perspectives from affective neuroscience. *Psychological Bulletin, 126,* 890–909.

48. Davidson, R. J. (2000). Affective style, psychopathology, and resilience: Brain mechanisms and plasticity. *American Psychologist, 55,* 1196–1214.

49. Linden, D. E. J. (2006). How psychotherapy changes the brain: The contribution of functional neuroimaging. *Molecular Psychiatry, 11,* 528–538.

50. Brody, A. L., Saxena, S., Stoessel, P., Gillies, L. A., Fairbanks, L. A., Alborzian, S., et al. (2001). Regional brain metabolic changes in patients with major depression treated with either paroxetine or interpersonal therapy: Preliminary findings. *Archives of General Psychiatry, 58,* 631–640.

51. Amini, F., Lewis, T., Lannon, R., Louie, A., Baumbacher, G., McGuinness, T., et al. (1996). Affect, attachment, memory: Contributions toward psychobiologic integration. *Psychiatry: Interpersonal and Biological Processes, 59,* 213–239.

52. Liggan, D. Y., & Kay, J. (1999). Some neurobiological aspects of psychotherapy: A review. *Journal of Psychotherapy Practice and Research, 8,* 103–114.

53. Post, R. M., & Weiss, S. R. B. (1997). Emergent properties of neural systems: How focal molecular neurobiological alterations can affect behavior. *Development and Psychopathology, 9,* 907–929.

54. Shin, L. M., & Liberzon, I. (2010). The neurocircuitry of fear, stress, and anxiety disorders. *Neuropsychopharmacology, 35,* 169–191.

55. Schober, J. M., & Pfaff, D. (2007). The neurophysiology of sexual arousal. *Best Practice and Research: Clinical Endocrinology and Metabolism, 21,* 445–461.

56. Panksepp, J. (2000). Emotion as a natural kind within the brain. In M. Lewis & J. M. Haviland-Jones (Eds.), *Handbook of emotions* (2nd ed., pp. 137–155). New York: Guilford Press.

57. Davidson, R. J., Kalin, N. H., & Shelton, S. E. (1993). Lateralized response to diazepam predicts temperamental style in rhesus monkeys. *Behavioral Neuroscience, 107,* 1106–1110.

58. Davidson, R. J. (1998). Anterior electrophysiological asymmetries, emotion, and depression: Concep-

tual and methodological conundrums. *Psychophysiology, 35,* 607–614.

59. Davidson, R. J., Putnam, K. M., & Larson, C. L. (2000). Dysfunction in the neural circuitry of emotion regulation: A possible prelude to violence. *Science, 289,* 591–594.

60. Davidson, R. J. (2000). Affective style, psychopathology, and resilience: Brain mechanisms and plasticity. *American Psychologist, 55,* 1196–1214.

61. Henriques, J. B., & Davidson, R. J. (1991). Left frontal hypoactivation in depression. *Journal of Abnormal Psychology, 100,* 535–545.

62. Tucker, D. M., & Williamson, P. A. (1984). Asymmetric neural control systems in human self-regulation. *Psychological Review, 91*(2), 185–215.

63. Oatley, K. J. J. M. (1992). Human emotions: Function and dysfunction. *Annual Review of Psychology, 43,* 55–85.

64. Ekman, P. (1993). Facial expression and emotion. *American Psychologist, 48,* 384–392.

65. Ekman, P. (1994). All emotions are basic. In P. Ekman & R. J. Davidson (Eds.), *The nature of emotion* (pp. 15–19). New York: Oxford University Press.

66. Diamond, R., & Carey, S. (1977). Developmental changes in representation of faces. *Journal of Experimental Child Psychology, 23,* 1–22.

67. Nelson, C. A. (1987). The recognition of facial expressions in the first 2 years of life: Mechanisms of development. *Child Development, 58,* 889–909.

68. Montague, D. P. F., & Walker-Andrews, A. S. (2001). Peekaboo: A new look at infants' perception of emotion expressions. *Developmental Psychology, 37,* 826–838.

69. Cohn, J. F., & Tronick, E. Z. (1983). Three-month-old infants' reaction to simulated maternal depression. *Child Development, 54,* 185–193.

70. Lamb, M. E., Morrison, D. C., & Malkin, C. M. (2007). The development of infant social expectations in face-to-face interaction: A longitudinal study. *Merrill-Palmer Quarterly, 33,* 241–254.

71. Fogel, A. (1993). *Developing through relationships: Origins of communication, self, and culture.* Chicago: University of Chicago Press.

72. Matsumoto, D. (2008). Mapping expressive differences around the world: The relationship between emotional display rules and individualism versus collectivism. *Journal of Cross-Cultural Psychology, 39,* 55–74.

73. Lively, K. J., & Powell, B. (2006). Emotional expression at work and at home: Domain, status, or individual characteristics? *Social Psychology Quarterly, 69,* 17–38.

74. Buck, R. (1980). Nonverbal behavior and the theory of emotion: The facial feedback hypothesis. *Journal of Personality and Social Psychology, 38,* 811–824.

75. Soussignan, R. (2002). Duchenne smile, emotional experience, and autonomic reactivity: A test of the facial feedback hypothesis. *Emotion, 2,* 52–74.

76. Lieberman, M. D., Eisenberger, N. I., Crockett, M. J., Tom, S. M., Pfeifer, J. H., & Way, B. M. (2007). Putting feelings into words: Affect labeling disrupts amygdala activity in response to affective stimuli. *Psychological Science, 18,* 421–428.

77. Ackerman, B. P., & Izard, C. E. (2004). Emotion cognition in children and adolescents: Introduction to the special issue. *Journal of Experimental Child Psychology, 89,* 271–275.

78. Borkovec, T. D., Ray, W. J., & Stober, J. (1998). Worry: A cognitive phenomenon intimately linked to affective, physiological, and interpersonal behavioral processes. *Cognitive Therapy and Research, 22,* 561–576.

79. Williams, J. B. W., Stiles, W. B., & Shapiro, D. A. (2007). Cognitive mechanisms in the avoidance of painful and dangerous thoughts: Elaborating the assimilation model. *Cognitive Therapy and Research, 23,* 285–306.

80. Philippot, P., Baeyens, C., Douilliez, C., & Francart, B. (2004). Cognitive regulation of emotion: Application to clinical disorders. In P. Philippot & R. S. Feldman (Eds.), *The regulation of emotion* (pp. 71–100). Mahwah, NJ: Erlbaum.

81. Roseman, I. J. (2001). A model of appraisal in the emotion system: Integrating theory, research, and applications. In K. R. Scherer, A. Schorr, & T. Johnstone (Eds.), *Appraisal processes in emotion: Theory, methods, research* (pp. 68–91). New York: Oxford University Press.

82. Gross, J. J. (2001). Emotion regulation in adulthood: Timing is everything. *Current Directions in Psychological Science, 10,* 214–219.

83. Siemer, M., Mauss, I., & Gross, J. J. (2007). Same situation—different emotions: How appraisals shape our emotions. *Emotion, 7,* 592–600.

84. Hunter, P. G., Schellenberg, E. G., & Griffith, A. T. (2012). Misery loves company: Mood-congruent emotional responding to music. *Emotion, 11,* 1068–1072.

85. White, L. K., Suway, J. G., Pine, D. S., Bar-Haim, Y., & Fox, N. A. (2011). Cascading effects: The influence of attention bias to threat on the interpretation of ambiguous information. *Behaviour Research and Therapy, 49,* 244–251.

86. Forgas, J. P., & Vargas, P. T. (2000). The effects of moon on social judgment and reasoning. In M. Lewis & J. M. Haviland-Jones (Eds.), *Handbook of emotions* (2nd ed., pp. 350–368). New York: Guilford Press.

87. Barlow, D. H. (Ed.). (2014). *Clinical handbook of psychological disorders: A step-by-step treatment manual* (5th ed.). New York: Guilford Press.

88. Young, J. E., Klosko, J. S., & Weishaar, M. E. (2003). *Schema therapy: A practitioner's guide.* New York: Guilford Press.

89. Bateman, A., & Fonagy, P. (2004). *Psychotherapy for borderline personality disorder: Mentalization-based treatment.* New York: Oxford University Press.

90. Lackner, J. M., & Quigley, B. M. (2005). Pain catastrophizing mediates the relationship between worry and pain suffering in patients with irritable bowel syndrome. *Behaviour Research and Therapy, 43,* 943–957.

91. Riddle, D. L., Wade, J. B., Jiranek, W. A., & Kong, X. (2010). Preoperative pain catastrophizing predicts pain outcome after knee arthroplasty. *Clinical Orthopaedics and Related Research, 468,* 798–806.

92. Vlaeyen, J. W., Timmermans, C., Rodriguez, L. M., Crombez, G., van Horne, W., Ayers, G. M., et al. (2004). Catastrophic thinking about pain increases discomfort during internal atrial cardioversion. *Journal of Psychosomatic Research, 56,* 139–144.

93. Smith, R. H., & Kim, S. H. (2007). Comprehending envy. *Psychological Bulletin, 133,* 46–64.

94. Cuijpers, P., Van Straten, A., & Warmerdam, L. (2007). Behavioral activation treatments for depression: A meta-analysis. *Clinical Psychology Review, 27,* 318–326.

95. Antony, M. M., & Stein, M. B. (Eds.). (2009). *Oxford handbook of anxiety and related disorders* (Oxford library of psychology). New York: Oxford University Press.

96. Kassinove, H., & Tafrate, R. C. (2002). *Anger management: The complete treatment guidebook for practitioners.* Atascadero, CA: Impact.

97. American Psychiatric Association. (2013, May). *Social anxiety disorder fact sheet.* Washington, DC: Author. Available from *www.dsm5.org/Documents/Social Anxiety Disorder Fact Sheet.pdf.*

98. Gross, J. J., & Levenson, R. W. (1993). Emotional suppression: Physiology, self-report, and expressive behavior. *Journal of Personality and Social Psychology, 64,* 970–986.

99. Gross, J. J., & John, O. P. (2003). Individual differences in two emotion regulation processes: Implications for affect, relationships, and well-being. *Journal of Personality and Social Psychology, 85,* 348–362.

100. Moreland, R. L., & Beach, S. R. (1992). Exposure effects in the classroom: The development of affinity among students. *Journal of Experimental Social Psychology, 28,* 255–276.

101. Norton, M. I., Frost, J. H., & Ariely, D. (2007). Less is more: The lure of ambiguity, or why familiarity breeds contempt. *Journal of Personality and Social Psychology, 92,* 97–105.

102. D'Zurilla, T. J., & Nezu, A. M. (1999). *Problem-solving therapy: A social competence approach to clinical intervention* (2nd ed.). New York: Springer.

103. Paulus, P. B., & Brown, V. R. (2007). Toward more creative and innovative group idea generation: A cognitive–social–motivational perspective of brainstorming. *Social and Personality Psychology Compass, 1,* 248–265.

104. Porter, S., Spencer, L., & Birt, A. (2003). Blinded by emotions?: Effect of the emotionality of a scene on susceptibility to false memories. *Canadian Journal of Behavioural Science, 35,* 165–175.

105. Beck, J. S. (2011). *Cognitive behavior therapy: Basics and beyond* (2nd ed.). New York: Guilford Press.

106. Folkman, S., & Moskowitz, J. T. (2000). Positive affect and the other side of coping. *American Psychologist, 55,* 647–654.

107. Polivy, J. (1996). Psychological consequences of food restriction. *Journal of the American Dietetic Association, 96,* 589–592.

108. Fredrickson, B. L., & Joiner, T. (2002). Positive emotions trigger upward spirals toward emotional well-being. *Psychological Science, 13,* 172–175.

109. Williams, K. E., Chambless, D. L., & Ahrens, A. (1997). Are emotions frightening?: An extension of the fear of fear construct. *Behaviour Research and Therapy, 35,* 239–248.

110. Creswell, J. D., Welch, W. T., Taylor, S. E., Sherman, D. K., Gruenewald, T. L., & Mann, T. (2005). Affirmation of personal values buffers neuroendocrine and psychological stress responses. *Psychological Science, 16,* 846–851.

111. Davidov, E., Schmidt, P., & Schwartz, S. H. (2008). Bringing values back in: The adequacy of the European Social Survey to Measure Values in 20 countries. *Public Opinion Quarterly, 72,* 420–445.

112. Diener, E., & Seligman, M. E. P. (2002). Very happy people. *Psychological Science, 13,* 80–83.

113. Dobson, K. (1989). A meta-analysis of the efficacy of cognitive therapy for depression. *Journal of Consulting and Clinical Psychology, 57,* 414–419.

114. Bandura, A. (1977). Self-efficacy: Toward a unifying theory of behavioral change. *Psychological Review, 84,* 191–215.

115. Christensen, K., Stephens, M., & Townsend, A. (1998). Mastery in women's multiple roles and well-being: Adult daughters providing care to impaired parents. *Health Psychology, 17,* 163–171.

116. Atienza, F. L., Balaguer, I., & Garcia-Merita, M. L. (1998). Video modeling and imagining training on performance of tennis service of 9- to 12-year-old children. *Perceptual and Motor Skills, 87,* 519–529.

117. Kazdin, A. E., & Mascitelli, S. (1982). Covert and overt rehearsal and homework practice in developing assertiveness. *Journal of Consulting and Clinical Psychology, 50,* 250–258.

118. Jeannerod, M., & Frak, V. (1999). Mental imaging of motor activity in humans. *Current Opinion in Neurobiology, 9,* 735–739.

119. Hilbert, A., & Tuschen-Caffier, B. (2007). Maintenance of binge eating through negative mood: A naturalistic comparison of binge eating disorder and bulimia nervosa. *International Journal of Eating Disorders, 40,* 521–530.

120. Stritzke, W. G. K., Patrick, C. J., & Lang, A. R. (1995). Alcohol and human emotion: A multidimensional analysis incorporating startle-probe methodology. *Journal of Abnormal Psychology, 104,* 114–122.

121. Yoo, S. S., Gujar, N., Hu, P., Jolesz, F. A., & Walker, M. P. (2007). The human emotional brain without sleep: A prefrontal amygdala disconnect. *Current Biology, 17,* R877–R878.

122. Salmon, P. (2001). Effects of physical exercise on anxiety, depression, and sensitivity to stress: A unifying theory. *Clinical Psychology Review, 21,* 33–61.

123. Krakow, B., Hollifeld, M., Johnston, L., Kloss, M. S. R., Warner, T. D., Tandberg, D., et al. (2001). Imagery rehearsal therapy for chronic nightmares in sexual assault survivors with posttraumatic stress disorder. *Journal of the American Medical Association, 286,* 537–545.

124. Nappi, C. M., Drummond, S. P. A., Thorp, S. R., & McQuaid, J. R. (2010). Effectiveness of imagery rehearsal therapy for the treatment of combat-related nightmares in veterans. *Behavior Therapy, 41,* 237–244.

125. Moore, B. A., & Krakow, B. (2007). Imagery rehearsal therapy for acute posttraumatic nightmares among combat soldiers in Iraq. *American Journal of Psychiatry, 164,* 683–684.

126. Moore, P. J., Adler, N. E., Williams, D. R., & Jackson, J. S. (2002). Socioeconomic status and health: The role of sleep. *Psychosomatic Medicine, 64,* 337–344.

127. Hublin, C., Partinen, M., Koskenvuo, M., & Kaprio, J. (2007). Sleep and mortality: A population-based 22-year follow-up study. *Sleep, 30,* 1245–1253.

128. Harvey, A. G. (2011). Sleep and circadian functioning: Critical mechanisms in the mood disorders? *Annual Review of Clinical Psychology, 7,* 297–319.

129. Harvey, A. G., & Greenall, E. (2003). Catastrophic worry in primary insomnia. *Journal of Behavior Therapy and Experimental Psychiatry, 34,* 11–23.

130. Afaghi, A., O'Connor, H., & Chow, C. M. (2007). High-glycemic-index carbohydrate meals shorten sleep onset. *American Journal of Clinical Nutrition, 85,* 426–430.

131. Borkovec, T. D., & Boudewyns, P. A. (1992). The treatment of initial insomnia. In J. M. G. Williams (Ed.), *The psychological treatment of depression: A guide to the theory and practice of cognitive behaviour therapy* (2nd ed., pp. 138–142). London: Routledge.

132. Borkovec, T. D., & Ruscio, A. M. (2001). Psychotherapy for generalized anxiety disorder. *Journal of Clinical Psychiatry, 62,* 37–45.

133. Marlatt, G. A., Larimer, M. E., & Witkiewitz, K. (Eds.). (2012). *Harm reduction: Pragmatic strategies for managing high-risk behaviors* (2nd ed.). New York: Guilford Press.

134. Gross, J. J., & Levenson, R. W. (1997). Hiding feelings: The acute effects of inhibiting negative and positive emotion. *Journal of Abnormal Psychology, 106,* 95–103.

135. De Mello, A. (1984). *The song of the bird.* New York: Image Books.

Chapter 10

Distress Tolerance Skills

Goals of the Module

Most approaches to mental health treatment focus on changing distressing events and circumstances. They have paid little attention to accepting, finding meaning for, and tolerating distress. Although the distinction is not as clear-cut as I am making it seem, this task has more often been tackled by religious and spiritual communities and leaders. DBT emphasizes the benefits of learning to bear pain skillfully. The ability to tolerate and accept distress is an essential mental health goal for at least two reasons. First, pain and distress are part of life; they cannot be entirely avoided or removed. The inability to accept this immutable fact itself leads to increased pain and suffering. Second, distress tolerance, at least over the short run, is part and parcel of any attempt to change oneself; otherwise, efforts to escape pain and distress (e.g., through impulsive actions) will interfere with efforts to establish desired changes.

Distress tolerance skills constitute a natural progression from mindfulness skills. They have to do with the ability to accept, in a nonevaluative and nonjudgmental fashion, both oneself and the current situation. Essentially, distress tolerance is the ability to perceive one's environment without putting demands on it to be different; to experience one's current emotional state without attempting to change it; and to observe one's own thoughts and action patterns without attempting to stop or control them. Although the stance advocated here is nonjudgmental, this should not be understood to mean that it is one of approval. It is especially important that this distinction be made clear: Toler-

ance and/or acceptance of reality are not equivalent to approval of reality.

The distress tolerance behaviors targeted in DBT skills training are concerned with tolerating and surviving crises (including crises caused by addictive behaviors) and with accepting life as it is in the moment.

Crisis Survival Skills

The portion of the module devoted to crisis survival skills (Sections II–IX) begins by defining "crisis" and the types of situations in which these skills can be most useful. By definition, crisis survival skills are short-term solutions to painful situations. Their purpose is to make a painful situation more tolerable, so that it is possible to refrain from impulsive actions that can make the situation worse. These skills can be overused and must be balanced by problem solving (see Chapter 9, Section XI). There are six sets of crisis survival strategies.

The STOP Skill

The STOP skill helps individuals refrain from impulsive actions. STOP is a mnemonic for the following steps: Stop, Take a step back, Observe, and Proceed mindfully.

Pros and Cons

Evaluating pros and cons is a decision-making strategy. The focus here is on thinking through the positive and negative consequences of acting on impulsive urges in crisis situations and of not acting on them (i.e., tolerating distress).

TIP Skills

The TIP skills can be used to change body chemistry quickly, so as to counteract disabling emotional arousal. TIP is a mnemonic for Temperature, Intense exercise, Paced breathing, and Paired muscle relaxation. (Note that although there are two P skills, the mnemonic remains the word TIP.)

Distracting with Wise Mind ACCEPTS

Distracting methods work by reducing contact with emotional stimuli or, in some cases, with the most painful aspects of the stimuli. They may also work to change parts of an emotional response. There are seven sets of distraction skills. The word ACCEPTS is a mnemonic for these strategies: Activities (discordant to the negative emotion), Contributing, Comparisons, Emotions (opposite to the current negative emotion), Pushing away from the situation, Thoughts, and Sensations.

Self-Soothing

Self-soothing strategies focus on the five senses—vision, hearing, smell, taste, and touch. They consist of sensual activities that feel comforting, nurturing, and soothing. The body scan meditation also falls into this category.

Improving the Moment

The final set of crisis survival skills is an idiosyncratic collection of ways to improve the quality of the moment. The word IMPROVE is a mnemonic for each of these strategies: Imagery, Meaning, Prayer, Relaxing actions, One thing in the moment, Vacation, and Encouragement.

Reality Acceptance Skills

Whereas the goal of crisis survival is to get through the crisis without making it worse, the goal of reality acceptance skills (Sections X–XV) is to reduce suffering and increase freedom when painful facts cannot be changed immediately, if ever. There are five sets of reality acceptance skills.

Radical Acceptance

Radical acceptance is *complete and total* acceptance, from deep within, of the facts of reality. It involves acknowledging facts that are true and letting go of a fight with reality. Acceptance is often misunderstood as approval (it is not) or as being against change (it is not).

Turning the Mind

It usually takes multiple efforts over time to accept a reality that feels unacceptable. The skill of turning the mind toward acceptance is *choosing* to accept reality as it is. It is not itself acceptance, but it is the first step toward acceptance, and it must usually be taken over and over again.

Willingness

Willingness and its opposite, willfulness, are concepts derived from the work of Gerald May (1982).[1] May describes willingness as follows:

> Willingness implies a surrendering of one's self-separateness, an entering into, an immersion in the deepest processes of life itself. It is a realization that one already is a part of some ultimate cosmic process and it is a commitment to participation in that process. In contrast, willfulness is the setting of oneself apart from the fundamental essence of life in an attempt to master, direct, control, or otherwise manipulate existence. More simply, willingness is saying yes to the mystery of being alive in each moment. Willfulness is saying no, or perhaps more commonly, "yes, but . . . " (p. 6)

May continues:

> Willingness and willfulness do not apply to specific things or situations. They reflect instead the underlying attitude one has toward the wonder of life itself. Willingness notices this wonder and bows in some kind of reverence to it. Willfulness forgets it, ignores it, or at its worst, actively tries to destroy it. Thus willingness can sometimes seem very active and assertive, even aggressive. And willfulness can appear in the guise of passivity. (p. 6)

Half-Smiling and Willing Hands

The skills of half-smiling and willing hands are usually taught together and are ways to accept reality with the body. In half-smiling, facial muscles are relaxed, with lips slightly upturned at the corners. Because emotions are partially controlled by facial expressions,[2, 3] adopting this facial expression helps clients feel more accepting. In willing hands, the hands are unclenched, with palms up and fingers relaxed. Willing hands are the opposite of clenched hands, which are indicative of anger and of fighting to change reality.

Mindfulness of Current Thoughts

Mindfulness of current thoughts is observing thoughts as thoughts (i.e., as neural firing of the brain or as sensations of the brain), rather than as facts about the world. This skill teaches clients to differentiate thoughts from facts—to distance themselves from their thoughts and become less reactive to them, while allowing them to arise and fade away. The approach is different from that of cognitive therapy, which emphasizes analyzing thoughts and changing them when they are irrational or inaccurate.

Skills When the Crisis Is Addiction

The seven sets of skills included in the final portion of the module (Sections XVI–XXI) were developed in a series of studies treating individuals with drug dependence.[4–6] These skills are dialectical abstinence, clear mind, community reinforcement, burning bridges, building new ones, alternate rebellion, and adaptive denial. When most or all participants of a skills training group have serious addictions, these skills can be integrated into the core DBT skills (as outlined in Schedule 8 in this manual's Part I Appendices), or they can be taught as a separate skills module either in place of one of the standard modules or in addition to the standard skills modules. The skills can also be taught on an as-needed basis in group or individual therapy.

Dialectical Abstinence

Dialectical abstinence brings together an abstinence approach and a harm reduction approach. This synthesis of approaches has historical roots in the original cognitive-behavioral relapse prevention model proposed by Marlatt and Gordon;[7] the goal of this maintenance approach was to prevent lapses from occurring (i.e., lapse prevention) and to manage them when they did occur to prevent a full-blown relapse (i.e., relapse management). Many have critiqued relapse prevention for giving clients "permission" to engage in addictive behaviors, for helping clients plan how to cope with a lapse or relapse, or for describing the abstinence violation effect. However, a harm reduction approach suggests that when a person has relapsed and is ready to drop out or give up, helping the person cope with the lapse and its demoralizing consequences is very often the best course of action.[8]

Clear Mind

"Clear mind" is a synthesis or middle ground between the extremes of "addict mind," which is governed by the addiction, and "clean mind," which is abstinent but takes risks and forgets that relapse is possible. Clear mind is abstinent from addictive behaviors, but also knows that relapse is possible.

Community Reinforcement

Community reinforcement focuses on building reinforcers in the community that will reward abstinence instead of addiction.

Burning Bridges and Building New Ones

"Burning bridges" means actively eliminating potential triggers for the addiction. "Building new bridges" refers to finding physical sensations and creating mental images to compete with addiction urges.

Alternate Rebellion and Adaptive Denial

When addictive behavior functions as rebellion, "alternate rebellion" focuses on finding alternative ways to rebel that are expressive but safer. "Adaptive denial" refers to suspending logic and denying—shutting out—urges for addictive behaviors when they hit. Denial can also take the form of believing that the addictive behavior is not possible.

Selecting Material to Teach

As noted above, there is a great deal of material for each skill in the teaching notes that follow. You will not cover most of it the first several times you teach specific skills. The notes are provided to give you a deeper understanding of each skill, so that you can answer questions and add new teaching as you go. As in Chapters 6–9, I have put a checkmark (✓) next to material I almost never skip. If I am in a huge rush, I may skip everything not checked. Also as in the earlier Part II chapters, I have indicated information summarizing research in special "Research Point" features. The great value of research is that it can often be used to sell the skills you are teaching.

As always, it is important that you have a basic understanding of the specific skills you are teach-

ing. The first several times you teach, carefully study the notes, handouts, and worksheets for each skill you plan to teach. Highlight the points you want to make, and bring a copy of the relevant pages with you to teach from. Be sure to practice each skill yourself, to be sure you understand how to use it. Before long, you will solidify your knowledge of each skill. At that point you will find your own favorite teaching points, examples, and stories and can ignore many of mine.

· | **Teaching Notes** | ·

I. GOALS OF THIS MODULE (DISTRESS TOLERANCE HANDOUT 1)

> **Main Point:** Distress tolerance skills enable us to survive immediate crises without making things worse, and to accept reality when we can't change it and it's not what we want it to be.
>
> **Distress Tolerance Handout 1: Goals of Distress Tolerance.** This handout lists goals, not specific skills. Briefly review the three goals; provide enough information and discussion to orient participants to the module; link the module to participants' own goals; and generate some enthusiasm for learning the distress tolerance skills. An important point is that crisis survival skills are needed for getting through crisis situations, but they are not intended to become a way of life. Over the long term, reality acceptance and problem solving have to be practiced if a client is to have a life worth living.
>
> **Worksheet:** There is no worksheet for this handout.

Explain the goals of distress tolerance skills to clients as follows.

✓ A. Survive Crisis Situations without Making Them Worse

The skills in this module are ways of surviving and doing well in crisis situations without resorting to behaviors that will make the situation worse. They are needed when we can't immediately change a situation for the better, or when we can't sort out our feelings well enough to know what changes we want or how to make them.

> **Note to Leaders:** If you plan on teaching the skills for addiction (Distress Tolerance Handouts 16–21), it can be useful here to define "addiction" as "any behavior you are unable to stop, despite negative consequences and despite your best efforts to stop." Note that many repetitive behaviors qualify as addictions. Getting over addictions requires immense distress tolerance!

✓ B. Accept Reality As It Is in the Moment

Acceptance of reality—of life as it is in the moment—is the only way out of hell. It is the way to turn suffering that cannot be tolerated into pain that can be tolerated. We can think of it as follows:

- Pain + nonacceptance = Suffering and being stuck
- Pain + acceptance = Ordinary pain (sometimes extremely intense) and the possibility of moving forward

Emphasize to participants that **life is not all crisis.** Although some clients may live as if their lives are a constant crisis, life in its totality is not *all* crisis. Living life as if it is always a crisis perpetuates the experience of crises, because it interferes with problem solving that will resolve problems over the long term; thus it can actually backfire and create more crises. At some point, therefore, we all have to experience and accept the lives that we have in front of us (so to speak). This is ultimately the only way to build a life worth living.

✓ C. Become Free

We are truly free when we can be at peace and content with ourselves and our lives, no matter what circumstances we find ourselves in. In many ways, freedom is an outcome of mastering both crisis survival and radical acceptance. The crisis survival skills are the bulwark keeping us from giving in to cravings on the way to freedom. Radical acceptance skills produce the quieting of intense desire. When we are free, we can look in the face of our cravings and desires and say "I don't have to satisfy you." Our intense emotions become like a passing tempest at sea, instead of a demand for action we must give in to.

> **Note to Leaders:** The distress tolerance goal of becoming free is identical to the goal of freedom in practicing mindfulness from a spiritual perspective. The important point is that both mindfulness practice and reality acceptance practice lead inevitably to a greater sense of freedom. In a sense, mindfulness practice is a reality acceptance practice. If you have not covered this goal in teaching mindfulness, you can teach it now. If you have previously taught it, simply make the connection between the two sets of skills. (The teaching notes are very similar.)

✓ **Discussion Point:** Either before or after reviewing Distress Tolerance Handout 1, ask participants to check off each goal that is important to them in the boxes on the handout and then share choices.

II. OVERVIEW: CRISIS SURVIVAL SKILLS (DISTRESS TOLERANCE HANDOUT 2)

> **Main Point:** The goal of crisis survival is to get through a crisis without making things worse. Crisis situations are, by definition, short-term. Thus these are not skills to be used all the time or as a lifestyle.
>
> **Distress Tolerance Handout 2: Overview: Crisis Survival Skills.** This handout can be reviewed quickly. It is simply an overview to orient participants to what is coming next. It can also be skipped and the information written on the board. Do not use this handout to teach the skills.
>
> **Distress Tolerance Worksheets 1, 1a, 1b: Crisis Survival Skills.** These are three different versions of a worksheet that can be used with Handout 2. Each worksheet covers all of the crisis survival skills and can be employed here if you are using this handout as a review. These worksheets can also be given again and again for each of the crisis survival skills (Distress Tolerance Handouts 4–9a) if you do not want to use the worksheets specific to each skill. Worksheet 1 provides space for participants to practice crisis survival skills only two times between sessions. Thus this can be a good starter worksheet with individuals you are trying to shape into more frequent skills practice. Worksheet 1a provides for practicing each skill twice. Worksheet 1b provides for multiple opportunities to practice each skill. Choose the worksheet that best fits the participants you are teaching. Review the worksheet you assign with participants. Alternatively, you can allow participants to choose the handout they wish to use. Allowing choice gives participants a greater sense of control and may result in higher homework compliance.

A. Crisis Survival Skills

✓ **1. What Are Crisis Survival Skills?**

Crisis survival skills are skills for tolerating and surviving a crisis situation.

2. When Should These Skills Be Used?

These skills are for use when a crisis cannot be avoided. The basic idea is to get through crisis situations without making them worse.

✓ **3. Six Categories of Crisis Survival Strategies**

There are six groups of crisis survival skills. Each is a series of methods for short-circuiting or coping with overwhelming negative emotions and almost intolerable situations.

- The STOP skill, for stopping oneself from engaging in impulsive behavior.
- Pros and cons.
- TIP skills, for changing your body chemistry.

■ Distracting.
■ Self-soothing.
■ Improving the moment.

✓ **4. Effects and Limits of These Skills**

These skills are not a cure for all problems in life. Their beneficial effects may only be temporary (but achieving them is not a small feat, nonetheless). These skills are primarily ways to survive painful emotions. They are not designed to be emotion regulation strategies (i.e., ways to reduce or end painful emotions), although they may help to regulate emotions and to reduce stress. Their central goal is to enable us to survive a crisis without making things worse.

III. KNOWING A CRISIS WHEN YOU SEE ONE (DISTRESS TOLERANCE HANDOUT 3)

> **Main Point:** Crisis survival skills are for crisis situations, which are, by definition, short-term. Thus these are not skills to be used all the time. Overusing them can get in the way of problem solving and change, and thus of building a life worth living.
>
> **Distress Tolerance Handout 3: When to Use Crisis Survival Skills.** Do not spend much time on this handout, but the core information is important to review and clarify.
>
> **Worksheet:** There is no worksheet for this handout.

A. What Is a Crisis?

1. Crises Are Highly Stressful Situations with Potential for Very Negative Outcomes

Example: "Your rent money was stolen, and you have no other money and are facing eviction. You are overwhelmed and just want the problem to go away. You then run into your old drug dealer, who offers you free drugs. Taking drugs in such a situation is likely to make things worse."

2. Crises Are Short-Term

Crisis survival skills are designed to be used only in the short term. When they are overused (i.e., used in every painful situation or to avoid every unwanted emotion), problems will never be resolved.

When this happens, crisis survival skills can amount to avoidance of building a life worth living and can make things worse rather than better in the long term.

Example: "You may be able to get through a period of urges to use drugs or an urge to attack another person if you distract yourself from the urges by playing loud music, going to a movie, or the like. But if every time a difficult-to-solve problem comes along, you avoid it or distract from it, problems will remain unsolved and life is unlikely to improve."

💬 **Discussion Point:** Elicit from participants times when they have used coping strategies that work in the short term but are harmful when overused or used to excess (e.g., eating, ignoring problems, going to sleep, distracting from important work that needs to be done).

3. Crises Create Intense Pressure for Quick Resolution

Most crises fall into two broad categories. Explain these to participants:

■ "You have a strong desire to engage in a destructive behavior (such as to take drugs, commit suicide, strike out in anger, or quit a job). Acting on these strong urges is ineffective."

■ "You are facing a major demand that will have serious consequences if it goes unmet (such as to write a report before a deadline, submit taxes on time, or pay bills or credit card debt). You feel completely overwhelmed and unable to focus and get it done. Shutting down and avoiding such demands is not effective."

In both cases, crisis survival skills are needed.

✓ **B. When to Use Crisis Survival Skills**

1. *Having Intense Pain That Cannot Be Helped Quickly*

Tell participants: "Use short-term crisis survival strategies to reduce pain to manageable levels so that the crisis can be managed and destructive behavior can be avoided. Once the pain's intensity is lowered, use more long-term skills—such as emotion regulation skills, reality acceptance and/ or mindfulness skills, and/or interpersonal effectiveness skills."

Example: "You have had an operation and are in a lot of pain. You have taken your prescribed medications, but have a strong urge to take a lot more than prescribed or to get drunk to ease the pain. Using a crisis survival skill (such as distraction, self-soothing, improving the moment) can help you tolerate the pain in the moment."

💬 **Discussion Point:** Surviving crisis situations is part and parcel of being effective—"doing what works" (a core mindfulness skill). However, at times people are more interested in proving to others how bad a situation is than in surviving the situation. The problem with proving how bad things are is that it hardly ever works over the long term in meeting any constructive goals. That is, although it may result in short-term gains (e.g., being put in the hospital or getting a lover to return), it usually fails in the long run. Elicit situations where this has been the case with clients. If you can give personal examples here, so much the better.

2. *Wanting to Act in Emotion Mind When That Would Make Things Worse*

Continue: "Crisis survival skills are useful when you suddenly have an intense urge to do something that you know will make matters worse, and you want to stop yourself before you do it."

Example: "You are with your family at an outdoor concert, and a man near you pushes and shoves you to get a better seat ahead of you. You immediately have an urge to yell obscenities at this man, but realize it would be poor modeling for your children and might make matters worse if the man yells back at you. Using a crisis survival skill (e.g., STOP) can help you block such a reaction, so that you can enjoy the concert with you family."

💬 **Discussion Point:** At some point, all of us have made a crisis worse by our own behavior. Elicit such examples from participants, particularly examples where they would have liked new skills to handle the situation more effectively.

3. *Having Emotional Distress Threaten to Become Overwhelming*

At times it is more effective to reduce feelings immediately than to experience them fully.

Example: "You are at home alone and are craving a drink. You have an alcohol problem, but you have been clean and sober for 3 months. You don't have alcohol in the house, but you start thinking about going out and buying some. Crisis survival skills can help you get through the urges without acting on them. For example, you can use distraction by calling a friend and asking him to come over for a while and watch a movie on TV. To distract yourself until he gets there, you put on loud music, remind yourself of how lucky you are compared to others you know who have not gotten so far in sobriety, and start replying to e-mails and surfing the Internet."

4. *Feeling Overwhelmed but Needing to Meet Demands*

High stress can be so disorganizing that we lose our ability to solve problems and cope well with difficult situations. "Falling apart" emotionally under high stress can create a new crisis, which can then exacerbate the original emotional crisis or dramatically increase destructive urges.

Continuing with effective and functional behavior can be critical to divert an emerging crisis. Crisis survival skills can buy time to regulate distress, so that other DBT skills (e.g., problem solving—see Emotion Regulation Handout 12) can be used.

Example: "There was a fire in your apartment last night, caused by an electrical problem next door. The fire was contained to an outside porch, and you got out OK, but there was a lot of smoke in your apartment. You stayed at a friend's house overnight. When you come back the next day, everything above waist level is covered with smoke residue. You can see that you are going to have to do a lot of cleaning, sorting what to save and what to throw out, and so on. You are so overwhelmed that you can't think or organize what to do, so you sit down and read a magazine instead of getting to work on your apartment. Realizing that this is not effective, you use one of the crisis survival skills (such as a TIP skill) to calm yourself down enough to call your sister and ask her to come over and help you clean."

5. *Having Extreme Arousal and Problems That Can't Be Solved Immediately*

When emotional arousal is extreme and a situation feels like a crisis, it can sometimes be very difficult to distract and "put a problem on the shelf," so to speak. The urgency to solve a problem *right now* may make it very difficult to do anything that is not focused on the crisis. If the timing is not right for working on a particular problem, this sense of urgency can create its own problems. Crisis survival skills can be used to distract from the situation until it can be solved.

Example: "You are at home one evening when you get very upset after realizing that you made a big mistake earlier that day at work. However, there is nothing you can do to fix the problem until tomorrow morning, when the building opens again. So to get through until the next day, you play games with your daughter and read her a bedtime story. After she is in bed, you self-soothe by putting bubble bath into a nice hot tub, turning on your favorite music, getting in, and reading something that will take your mind off the day."

💭 **Discussion Point:** Elicit from participants examples of coping with crisis situations effectively.

C. How to Evaluate Whether Crisis Survival Skills Are Working

1. *Most Important*

Say to participants: "When time passes and you haven't done anything to make things worse, the skills are working. This is true even if you don't feel better."

2. *Next*

Continue: "Skills are working when you start feeling more able to tolerate the problem while using your other skills. To figure this out, rate your distress tolerance from 0 ('I can't tolerate it at all') to 100 ('Although this is painful, I can definitely tolerate it')."

3. *Last*

"Crisis survival skills *might* help you feel better (this is emotion regulation). If so, great, but if not, keep your focus on surviving the crisis!"

IV. STOP PROBLEMATIC BEHAVIOR IMMEDIATELY (DISTRESS TOLERANCE HANDOUT 4)

> **Main Point:** The STOP skill helps individuals refrain from acting impulsively on their emotions and making a difficult situation worse. The skill does that by helping an individual resist acting on the first impulse

to act (Stop); Take a step back and detach from the situation; Observe to gather information about what is going on; and then Proceed mindfully (by evaluating the most effective option to take, given the goals, and finally following that option).

Distress Tolerance Handout 4: The STOP Skill. This handout gives a brief description for each step of the STOP skill. Teach this handout by first describing each step on the handout and then illustrating with an example.

Distress Tolerance Worksheets 2, 2a: Practicing the STOP Skill. These are alternative worksheets to use with Handout 4. Worksheet 2 gives space for practicing the STOP skill two times, and Worksheet 2a gives space for daily practice. Choose the worksheet that best fits the participants you are teaching. Review the worksheet you assign. Alternatively, you can allow participants to choose the handout they wish to use. Again, allowing choice gives participants a greater sense of control and may result in higher homework compliance.

A. When to Use the STOP Skill

Say to participants: "When emotion mind takes over, you may find that you often act impulsively without thinking. When you react impulsively, you do not have time to use your skills and get to your wise mind. To be able to use your skills, you need first to stop yourself from reacting. To help you stay in control, use the STOP skill."

✓ B. What Is the STOP Skill?

The STOP skill consists of the following sequence of steps: Stop, Take a step back, Observe, and Proceed mindfully.

1. Stop

Tell participants: "When you feel your emotions are about to take control, stop! Don't react. Don't move a muscle! Just freeze. Freezing for a moment helps prevent you from doing what your emotion wants you to do—to act without thinking. Stay in control. Remember, you are the boss of your emotions."

Note to Leaders: For participants who have visual imagery, instruct them to visualize a STOP sign whenever they want to stop from reacting to a situation. If necessary, participants can be instructed to use paced breathing (see Distress Tolerance Handout 6) after stopping, to get their arousal down.

Example: "If someone says something that provokes your anger (like calling you names or cursing at you), you might have the urge to attack this person physically or verbally. That, however, might not be in your best interest. Doing that might result in getting hurt, being jailed, or being fined. So stop, freeze, and don't act on your impulse to attack."

Example: "Your partner, whom you still love, just broke up with you. You see her on the street, and your first impulse might be to go and give her a hug. However, that might not be wise. Given the situation, she is likely to reject you, and that would hurt. So stop. Don't act on the urge to hug her."

💬 **Discussion Point:** Elicit from participants times when they have had strong urges to act on emotions, but when doing that did or would have made the situation worse.

👥 **Practice Exercise:** Elicit an example of a difficult situation that usually results in an impulsive behavior (e.g., being called names and calling names back). Ask a participant to role-play the situation. First model freezing yourself, and then have the participant practice freezing. Next, challenge the participant by escalating the situation while encouraging him or her to be motionless.

2. Take a Step Back

Continue: "When you are faced with a difficult situation, it may be hard to think about how to deal with it on the spot. Give yourself some time to calm down and think. Take a step back (in your mind and/or physically) from the situation. Get unstuck from what is going on. Take a deep breath. Continue breathing deeply as long as you need to do this (to reduce extreme emotion mind quickly) until you are back in control. Do not let your emotion control what you do. Remember that you are not your emotion. Do not let it put you over the edge."

Example: "You're crossing the street and don't notice a car approaching. The driver stops the car, gets out, starts cursing at you, and physically pushes you. Your urge is to punch him in the face; however, you know that would escalate the situation and get you in trouble. So you first stop and then literally take a step back to avoid confrontation."

Practice Exercise: Practice taking a step back, using the same situation as in the example above of being pushed by a driver. Model freezing, and then physically take a step back and take a deep breath. Have a participant go through this sequence of steps. Challenge the participant by escalating the situation while encouraging continued deep breathing. Elicit from participants other situations that trigger strong emotional reactions and destructive urges. Role-play with participants some of these situations, and instruct them to practice stopping and taking a step back, both physically and in their minds.

3. Observe

Go on: "Observe what is happening around you and within you, who is involved, and what other people are doing or saying. To make effective choices, it is important not to jump to conclusions. Instead, gather the relevant facts so as to understand what is going on and what the available options are. Use your mindfulness skills of observing and nonjudgmentalness (as described in Mindfulness Handouts 4 and 5)."

4. Proceed Mindfully

Say: "Ask yourself, 'What do I want from this situation? What are my goals? What choice might make this situation better or worse?' Ask your wise mind how to deal with this problem. Being mindful is the opposite of being impulsive and acting without thinking. When you are calm, stay in control, and have some information about what is going on, you are better prepared to deal with the situation effectively, without making it worse."

Example: "You get home really late from work, due to a flat tire. Your partner starts yelling at you, accusing you of cheating on him, and calling you names. You get really angry, and your first impulse is to yell and call him names back. However, you want to deal with this skillfully. So you stop and then take a step back from your partner. You observe that your partner appears drunk, and that there are a lot of empty bottles of beer in the kitchen. You know that when he is drunk, there's no point arguing, and he's likely to apologize in the morning. So you proceed mindfully by explaining the flat tire, pacifying your partner, and going to bed. You postpone a discussion till the next morning."

Practice Exercise: Discuss effective ways of dealing with the situation you have already been practicing (i.e., the angry driver), and then role-play the situation by going through all four steps of the STOP skill. Role-play with participants other difficult situations from the past when they wished they had not reacted impulsively, or situations that are likely to be difficult in the future. Instruct them to put together all four steps of the STOP skill.

Discussion Point: Discuss situations at home, work, school, or other activities where the STOP skill is needed.

💬 **Discussion Point:** Ask participants if they have difficulty with a specific step of the STOP skills. Instruct participants that they can learn these skills one step at a time (i.e., practicing first S̲top, then S̲top and T̲ake a step back, etc.) until they've mastered the entire sequence.

V. PROS AND CONS AS A WAY TO MAKE BEHAVIORAL DECISIONS (DISTRESS TOLERANCE HANDOUT 5)

> **Main Point:** The eventual goal of using pros and cons is for the person to see that accepting reality and tolerating distress lead to better outcomes than do rejecting reality and refusing to tolerate distress. This skill consists of thinking about the positive and negative aspects of both acting and not acting on crisis behavior urges.
>
> **Distress Tolerance Handout 5: Pros and Cons.** Teach this skill by first describing what is meant by pros and cons, and then putting the basic 2 × 2 grid up on the board and working through several examples of pros and cons with participants. In a group whose members have drug addictions, for example, list the pros and cons of using drugs, and then list the pros and cons of resisting the urge to use drugs.
>
> **Distress Tolerance Worksheets 3, 3a: Pros and Cons of Acting on Crisis Urges.** These two worksheets ask for exactly the same work on pros and cons, but are set up differently. Some people find Worksheet 3 much easier to understand and work with, and others find Worksheet 3a much easier. Review both worksheets with participants, and let participants pick the one they like best. Stress that it is important to fill out each of the four quadrants. Instruct participants to keep a copy of the completed worksheet, since it can be *very* hard to remember why not to engage in crisis behaviors when they are in emotion mind.

✓ A. When to Use Pros and Cons

1. To Compare the Advantages and Disadvantages of Different Options

Say to participants: "When you have to make a decision between two or more options, and want to examine their advantages and disadvantages, pros and cons can be very important in helping you make a wise choice. All of us use pros and cons some of the time, even if only implicitly, to make decisions."

Example: My alarm goes off at 6:00 A.M. on a workday. I am tired and want to stay in bed. I say to myself, "Oh, it would feel so good to keep staying in bed," and then I might say, "Oh! If I stay in bed I will be late for work and then my boss will be really angry with me." I get up.

Example: A friend keeps me waiting at a restaurant before showing up an hour late. While waiting, I am reviewing in my mind all the pros for just leaving and standing him up, and all the pros for yelling at him when he finally does arrive. In fact, I rehearse in my mind all the reasons I should tell him I am never going to a restaurant with him again. However, I then remember that this is a good friend and that if I get really mad or refuse to eat out with him again, it will be a big loss for me. I start reviewing the pros of tolerating the distress and not yelling at him, even if he is late without much of a reason.

💬 **Discussion Point:** Elicit from participants times when they automatically (i.e., without deciding to do it) think of consequences, positive and or negative, of doing things.

💬 **Discussion Point:** Elicit from participants times when they have difficult choices to make and need to evaluate the pros and cons of various choices.

2. To Help Resist Impulsive or Destructive Urges

Continue: "Pros and cons can also help you resist urges to act impulsively or do things that are destructive, particularly when you are in emotion mind. Pros and cons can help us all resist urges to quit and give up on life. It can help us resist actions such as using drugs, bingeing and purging, or having angry outbursts at others."

Example: Many individuals react to uncontrollable stress and crises by doing things that in the short run, the long run, or both are damaging to their self-interest and well-being. These might be things such as using drugs or alcohol excessively to escape difficult emotions or situations; overeating when distressed; throwing tantrums or saying things when angry that they later regret; or threatening or attempting suicide when upset or experiencing intensely painful emotions.

Example: "When you are in the middle of a very important task at work that has to be done *now*, you might be tempted to interrupt it to deal with problems in your personal life, such as a friend's calling you to say she is really angry at you. However, it might be most effective for you to tolerate the distress of knowing your friend is upset without solving that issue right away, and instead to keep working on your urgent task at work. You would resolve the problem with your friend later."

The eventual goal is for participants to conclude that accepting reality and tolerating distress lead to better outcomes than do rejecting reality and refusing to tolerate distress. It is important to note here that all of us use pros and cons many times during each day, at least implicitly.

✓ B. How to Do Pros and Cons

Doing pros and cons involves writing down the positive and negative consequences of tolerating distress by resisting impulsive behaviors, as well as the positive and negative consequences of not tolerating distress by engaging in impulsive behaviors.

1. Describe the Crisis Behavior

Explain: "Start by describing the crisis behavior you are trying to stop. A crisis behavior is any behavior that in the short run, long run, or both is damaging to your self-interest and well-being."

2. Examine the Advantages and Disadvantages of the Behavior

Go on: "Next, examine the advantages and disadvantages (pros and cons) of the crisis behavior—of acting on your crisis urges."

3. Consider Both Short-Term and Long-Term Consequences

"When you are doing pros and cons, don't forget to consider both the short-term and long-term consequences of the behavior you are examining."

Example: Relief and feeling better immediately (pros) may be short-term consequences of drinking excessively, using drugs, or yelling at someone, but having a hangover that interferes with work or ruining a relationship due to using substances or yelling in anger (cons) may be the long-term consequences of the same behaviors.

4. Consider Pros and Cons for Each Different Crisis Urge

"Make up separate lists of pros and cons for each different crisis urge you are working on."

Example: "If you are deciding among using illegal drugs, filing for a divorce, quitting a job, or another impulsive action, it is important to consider the pros and cons of each action (using drugs, filing for a divorce, quitting a job) separately. It is also important to write separate lists for the pros and cons of *not* engaging in these actions."

> **Note to Leaders:** Participants often find it strange that they are asked to write out separate lists of pros and cons for acting on crisis urges and for resisting crisis urges. They usually believe that the pros of resist-

ing crisis urges and the cons of not resisting crisis urges will be the same. This is often not the case, but the only way to see it is to have participants actually practice working out pros and cons in the session. A good way to do this is with a practice exercise on a class whiteboard (see below). A strategy to help distinguish the lists is to focus on what *does* happen that is a positive or negative consequence of either choice, as opposed to what *does not* happen.

 Practice Exercise: Draw a pros-and-cons grid on the board. You can use Figure 10.1 as a model (this type of grid is also seen in Distress Tolerance Handout 5 and Worksheet 3), or you can use the type of grid seen in Distress Tolerance Worksheet 3a and in the pros-and-cons worksheets for other modules. Get participants to generate pros and cons of tolerating a crisis without doing something harmful and/or impulsive. Then have them generate pros and cons for *not* tolerating the crisis (i.e., for engaging in self-injury, substance abuse, impulsively quitting a job, attacking a friend, or other examples of nontolerating behaviors the participants want to analyze). Be sure to focus on both short-term and long-term pros and cons. Compare the two sets.

Note to Leaders: It is helpful to avoid working on suicidal urges as an example, as this can get bogged down in a discussion of what we definitely know or don't know about what occurs once one dies (i.e., we know nothing).

However, if participants have a firm grasp of how to do pros and cons, writing out pros and cons for suicide can be very helpful for some individuals. You will probably need to tolerate a situation where the pros and cons of acting on suicidal urges come out more or less equal in weight and where an individual is undecided. If a person seems to have clearly decided on committing suicide or is leaning toward suicide, it is important to move to suicide risk assessment and crisis management strategies. It is equally important to remember that working through the pros and cons of suicide with a participant in a validating, noncontrolling, and nondemanding manner

	Pros	Cons
Acting on crisis urges	Advantages	Disadvantages
Resisting crisis urges	Advantages	Disadvantages

FIGURE 10.1. Pros and cons for acting versus not acting on urges.

may be your most effective way for the participant to end up choosing life. See Chapter 15 of the main DBT text for crisis strategies and suicidal behavior strategies.

5. Rehearse Pros and Cons Multiple Times

Encourage participants: "Rehearse the pros of resisting urges and the cons of giving in to urges multiple times before overwhelming urges hit. Such rehearsal makes it more likely that the pros of avoiding destructive behavior and cons of engaging in destructive behavior will pop into your mind when needed. The idea here is to get thinking about the long-term benefits of avoiding destructive behavior to become stronger, and thinking about immediate benefits of destructive behavior to become weaker."

6. Review Earlier Pros and Cons When a Crisis Urge Strikes

Continue: "Review the pros and cons you have written earlier when an overwhelming emotion or urge hits. If these are not available, then this is the time to write up such pros and cons. However, it can be very difficult to do this in emotion mind, so it is advisable to solicit support from someone else for doing pros and cons while you are in a crisis."

7. Say No to Crisis Urges

"It can be very helpful to say out loud or yell 'No!' when an overwhelming emotion or urge hits. Once this is done, it is important to distract yourself from the urge and from tempting events. Say to yourself, 'No, that's it; there is no going back,' or something similar."

> **Note to Leaders:** The problem with strong urges is that they are associated with a very strong desire to act on the urge. Subliminally, an individual also knows that if he or she actually practices pros and cons, then the desired activity is much less likely. Thus, at this level, the individual realizes that thinking of pros and cons will get in the way of engaging in a reinforcing activity, even if the activity only provides short-term reinforcement and is destructive in the long term. Thus it is very common for clients to resist doing pros and cons, because it gets in the way of desired activities. This might be a good time to discuss with participants the fact that immediate reinforcement is always much more powerful than delayed reinforcement. Engaging in pros and cons strengthens the power of delayed reinforcement (reinforcement for resisting the urge) and weakens the power of immediate reinforcement (reinforcement for giving in to the urge).

> **Discussion Point:** Elicit from participants times when the idea of thinking of pros and cons does not come into their minds, or when even if it does, they resist thinking of pros and cons. Discuss strategies to bring pros and cons to mind when needed, as well as strategies to break down resistance.

> **Practice Exercise:** Ask each person to complete a pros-and-cons exercise for one targeted problem behavior they would like to stop. Use plain paper, or use one of the worksheets (3 or 3a). After each person has completed the exercise, discuss a few examples. Elicit from participants ideas about where to keep the exercise or worksheet for use in a crisis.

> **Note to Leaders:** Pros and cons can be very effective for helping individual participants make difficult decisions about their lives. It is very important at these points that you not communicate a preference for one side or the other of the pros and cons. The task here is to help the person develop a reasonably comprehensive list of all the pros and cons for each side of the decision. It is important, then, to trust the wise mind of the participant in making a decision. A good guide to using pros and cons in these situations is the principle related to a "decisional balance." This principle comes from Motivational Interviewing, which was developed for clients with substance use disorders, but is useful in other venues as well.[9]

> The one exception to relying exclusively on "wise mind" is when the decision is to commit suicide or not. See the earlier Note to Leaders on using pros and cons with suicide.

VI. TIP SKILLS FOR MANAGING EXTREME AROUSAL (DISTRESS TOLERANCE HANDOUTS 6–6C)

Main Point: Very high emotional arousal can make it impossible to use most skills. TIP skills are rapid ways to reduce emotion arousal. These skills are Temperature (use of cold water on the face to elicit the dive response), Intense exercise, Paced breathing, and Paired muscle relaxation. (As noted in the introduction to this chapter, there are two P skills, although there is only one P in TIP.)

    Caution: Alert participants that the effect of cold water on the face is to reduce heart rate. Any participants with any heart risk or allergy to cold should not participate in the ice water exercise unless cleared to do so by their physicians.

Distress Tolerance Handout 6: TIP Skills: Changing Your Body Chemistry. This handout lists all the TIP skills and is useful for a review. See the other materials below for teaching individual skills. In particular, progressive relaxation is best taught by conducting a brief relaxation exercise such as described on Handout 6b.

Distress Tolerance Handout 6a: Using Cold Water, Step by Step. This handout recapitulates the steps for the use of cold water. If you do not teach this skill for some reason, this handout can be skipped.

Distress Tolerance Handout 6b: Paired Muscle Relaxation, Step by Step. Use this handout to provide training in how to relax muscles and how to pair relaxation with breathing out. The relaxation training is based on progressive relaxation practice, and the handout summarizes instructions for going from tensing and relaxing individual muscles to tensing and relaxing the whole body. Letting go of muscles is then paired with exhaling while saying internally the word "relax." If you do not practice relaxation of all the muscle groups in sessions, point out that the rest of the muscles are listed on the handout. This handout may also be useful for individual therapists.

Distress Tolerance Handout 6c: Effective Rethinking and Paired Relaxation, Step by Step. This optional handout integrates cognitive restructuring with paired breathing. It can be very useful when teaching this skill to work with participants in filling out Steps 1–3 on Distress Tolerance Worksheet 4b, described below.

Distress Tolerance Worksheet 4: Changing Body Chemistry with TIP Skills. Review this worksheet with participants. If necessary, teach participants to rate their level of emotional arousal (often called "subjective units of distress" or SUDS) on a 0–100 scale. Make 0 equal to no distress at all, and 100 equal to the most stress ever experienced in their entire lives. Remind participants that they can never go over 100 points. Notice that this worksheet is primarily a recording device, so that participants can describe what they did during homework review. There is room on the sheet for describing each skill only once. Therefore, you might want to have several copies of the worksheet for each person, particularly if you assign daily practice of one or more TIP skills.

Distress Tolerance Worksheet 4a: Paired Muscle Relaxation. Use this worksheet only if you ask participants to practice paired muscle relaxation between sessions. This worksheet can help participants remember how to tense and relax muscles, and also distinguishes between practicing to learn the skill and practicing when the skill is needed. If you assign this worksheet, review it with participants.

Distress Tolerance Worksheet 4b: Effective Rethinking and Paced Relaxation. Assign this worksheet if you have taught Handout 6c.

    Other Materials: To teach use of cold water, bring to the session zip-lock bags with a few ice cubes and

> water, gel cold packs, or pans of cold water and towels. To teach paced breathing, bring a large clock with a secondhand to the session.

✓ A. What Are TIP Skills?

Tell participants: "There are four TIP skills: tipping the Temperature of your face with cold water, Intense aerobic exercise, Paced breathing, and Paired muscle relaxation. (Note that there are two P skills, though there is only one P in TIP.) Each skill has the effect of rapidly changing your biological response patterns, and thereby causing a reduction in your emotional arousal."

B. Why Use TIP Skills?

Explain the reasons for using TIP skills as follows:

- ✓ ▪ "TIP skills change your body chemistry to reduce high emotional arousal and feelings of being overwhelmed."
- ✓ ▪ "TIP skills work very fast, within seconds to minutes, to bring down emotional arousal."
- ▪ "TIP skills are as effective as dysfunctional behaviors (drinking, using drugs, eating, self-harm) at reducing painful emotions, but without the short- and long-term negative results."
- ▪ "TIP skills work like fast-acting medications, but without the cost of medications or the side effects that some medications cause."
- ▪ "TIP skills are easy to use and don't require a lot of thinking."
- ▪ "Some TIP skills (paced breathing, some parts of paired muscle relaxation) can be used in public without others' knowing that you are using the skills."

✓ C. When TIP Skills Are Useful

Go on: "Here are some times when TIP skills are useful."

- ▪ "You are caught in emotion mind and can't get out."
- ▪ "You are in a crisis—that is, a high urge to engage in destructive behavior hits and you can't distract yourself."
- ▪ "An important demand needs to be met, and you are too overwhelmed to think of what to do."
- ▪ "You are not processing information effectively."
- ▪ "You are emotionally overwhelmed."
- ▪ "Other skills are not feasible to do, or are not helpful even if you are not in a crisis."
- ▪ "You are at your **skills breakdown point**."

> **Note to Leaders:** The concept of a skills breakdown point and how to determine it is discussed in Chapter 9, Section XX. See that section and Emotion Regulation Handout 23: Managing Extreme Emotions for instructions on how to teach this concept. Feel free to use that handout or its teaching notes at this point. If emotion regulation has already been taught, refer participants back to that skill.

✓ D. How the TIP Skills Work

The TIP skills are designed to activate the human body's physiological nervous system for decreasing arousal. The nervous system consists of two parts: a "sympathetic nervous system" and a "parasympathetic nervous system." These two systems work in opposite directions. The sympathetic system activates the fight-or-flight syndrome and increases arousal. The parasympathetic system increases emotion regulation, which is associated with decreases in emotional arousal. All of the TIP skills regulate emotions by increasing activity of the parasympathetic nervous system and decreasing activity of the sympathetic nervous system.

> **Note to Leaders:** Remind or point out to participants that (1) physiological arousal is an important component of emotions, and (2) changing any part of the emotion system affects the entire system. You can refer to the model of emotions taught in Chapter 9, Section V and in Emotion Regulation Handout 5: A Model for Describing Emotions.

✓ **E. Tipping Facial Temperature with Cold Water**

Tell participants: "The first TIP skill is tipping the Temperature of your face with cold water or cold packs on the face, while holding your breath. This induces the human dive reflex, which in turn sets off the parasympathetic system and reduces physiological and emotional arousal very quickly."[10, 11]

> **Research Point:** The dive reflex is the tendency in humans (and other mammals) for the heart to slow down to below resting heart rate when the person is immersed in very cold water without oxygen. This effect is due to increased activation of the parasympathetic nervous system, which is the body's physiological system for decreasing arousal (see the explanation of the sympathetic and parasympathetic systems, above). States of emotional overarousal occur when the sympathetic nervous system becomes overactive and the parasympathetic nervous system is underactive. (Milton Brown of the DBT Center of San Diego provides more information and a series of handouts on TIP skills at the Center's website, *www. dbtsandiego.com/current_clients.html*.)

1. Procedures

Explain the different ways in which the dive reflex can be induced with cold water.

a. Use a Bowl of Cold Water

Tell participants: "Bend over, hold your breath, and put your face (up to your temples) in a bowl of cold water for between 30 and 60 seconds, or until you start to become uncomfortable. This is usually sufficient to induce the dive reflex. The colder the water and the longer the immersion, the better it works. However, do not have the water too cold. Water below 50°F may cause facial pain during immersion."

b. Use an Ice Pack, a Zip-Lock Bag of Ice with Water, or a Cold Wet Compress

Say: "Sit in a chair, and hold the ice pack or zip-lock bag (wrapped in a cloth to keep from being too cold) or cold compress over the eyes and upper cheeks. Wet the side touching your face. Standing, bending over, and holding your breath at the same time appears to increase the effect."

c. Splash Cold Water on the Face

Add: "Splashing cold water on your eyes and cheeks may even be sufficient. To make it work even better, stand, bend over, and hold your breath."

2. When to Use Cold Water

In addition to times of high emotional arousal, my colleagues and I have found cold water or cold packs to be helpful in the following situations:

- Inability to sleep due to ruminating or "background" anxiety
- Dissociation, including dissociation during therapy or skills training sessions

3. Cautions

- *Heart problems.* Using cold water to induce the dive reflex can reduce heart rate very rapidly. Individuals with any heart disorder, a heart rate below their normal baseline due to medications, other medical problems, anorexia nervosa, or bulimia nervosa should only use this procedure with permission of their medical providers. In general, recommending that participants check with their medical providers before using the procedure is a good idea. Adolescents should seek parental permission as well.

■ *Short-lived effects.* The physical effects of the cold water are actually very short-lived. Thus it is easy for the out-of-control emotion to return if participants are not careful. Once extreme arousal is reduced, it can then be important to practice a different set of skills appropriate for the problem at hand.

Example: "You are very angry, and you use ice water or a cold pack to reduce the intensity of the emotion. If you then start thinking about all the things that set off the anger in the first place, anger is very likely to be set off again. The same is true of any other emotion."

Example: "You use cold water or a cold pack to interrupt anxiety ruminations that are keeping you awake. It is important to go back to bed and focus on something other than anxiety-inducing thoughts, such as paced breathing [see below] or thoughts of pleasant events."

Example: "A strong urge to engage in a problem behavior hits, and you use ice water or a cold pack to reduce the urge. Your arousal and urges come down. A little later, you go back to thinking about the problem behavior, and the urge resurfaces. It is thus important to engage in a different activity (problem solving or distracting) immediately after using the ice."

✓ 👥 **Practice Exercise:** If possible, demonstrate the dive reflex with participants. After screening participants for medical issues, try to get all those for whom the use of cold water is not ruled out to do the exercise once. This is a practice trial and increases the likelihood that they will use it when needed. Another variation is to do this as an experiment. In this case, the procedure is for participants to rate their arousal before and right after putting cold water (in zip-lock bags or cold gel bags) on their upper faces, covering their eyes and upper cheekbones. Alternatively, participants can take their pulses before and after practicing (a procedure used in high school science classes). Make it very clear that participation in the practice session is optional, and that the exercise is in no way an endurance contest.

Supplies needed for each participant are these:

1. One pint-sized plastic storage bag with water, or a gel pack that has been kept cold, and wet paper towels.

2. Alternatively, a cooler of cold water, large bowls or foil roaster pans, a place to dump water, and towels to dry faces.

The **procedure** is as follows:

1. Have each participant sit, put a wet paper towel around the bag or gel pack, and then place the bag or pack over eyes and cheeks for up to 30 seconds.

2. Alternatively, have each participant bend over a bowl or pan of water, hold breath, and put face in water for up to 30 seconds.

3. Once participants have finished either Step 1 or Step 2, have them discuss their experiences.

Another chance to practice the TIP cold water skill may arise if a participant is experiencing high arousal during a group session (even when you are not teaching the TIP skills). In such an instance, you could bring the supplies into the meeting room and ask the participant to try that skill. In our group sessions, when needed, we bring in a cold pack (which we wet on the face side) and a towel. (We keep several cold packs in the refrigerator at all times.)

✓ **F. Intense Exercise**

The second TIP skill is to engage in Intense aerobic exercise of any kind for at least 20 minutes.

1. Why Intense Exercise?

> **Research Point:** Intense exercise (of any kind) for 20–30 minutes or so can have a rapid effect on mood, decreasing negative mood and ruminative thoughts and increasing positive affect after exercising.[12]

- Tell participants: "State anxiety decreases significantly if you get your heart rate to 70% of the maximum for your age."
- "Increases in positive emotions are associated with getting your heart rate up to 55–70% of maximum heart rate for your age, but the increases are maintained for a significantly longer time following exercise when you get your heart rate to 70% intensity."[12]
- "Look up 'calculating heart rate training zones' on your search engine. Or go to *www. chabotcollege.edu/faculty/kgrace/FitnessCenter/TargetZones.htm* for how to estimate maximum recommended heart rate for your age."

A major characteristic of emotions is that they organize the body for action. Anger organizes the body to attack or defend, fear organizes the body to run, and so on. When the body is highly aroused, it can be difficult to inhibit emotional action even if the action is dysfunctional. Intense exercise, in these situations, can re-regulate the body to a less emotional state.

> **Note to Leaders:** Point out to participants that (1) emotions prepare them for action and that actions themselves are important components of emotions; and (2) inhibiting emotion-linked actions can therefore be very difficult. As noted earlier, you can refer to the model of emotions taught in Chapter 9, Section V, and in Emotion Regulation Handout 5.

2. When to Use Exercise

Say to participants: "Use exercise when you are agitated, when you are angry, when ruminating just won't stop, when you need to bring up your mood and willingness in the morning, and at any other time it has been useful for you in the past."

Example: "At the end of your work day, you find out that a report you thought was due in a week is actually due tomorrow. If you don't get the report done, you'll have big problems at work. You feel so overwhelmed by this unexpected demand that you don't know where to start to get things done. You can take a short break, go for a run to decrease the strong negative emotions, and then return and do what is needed to finish the report by its deadline."

G. <u>P</u>aced Breathing

The third TIP skill is <u>P</u>aced breathing. This refers to slowing down the pace of inhaling and exhaling (to an average of five to six breath cycles per minute) and breathing deeply from the abdomen. Breathing out should be slower than breathing in (e.g., 4 seconds in and 8 seconds out).

> **Research Point:** Generally, the heart beats faster during in-breaths and slows down during out-breaths. This change in heart rate is influenced by sympathetic nervous system activation upon breathing in and parasympathetic nervous system activation upon breathing out.
>
> Paced breathing can itself cause changes in sympathetic and parasympathetic activity. In a way similar to the dive reflex, slowing breathing to approximately five or six breaths per minute (i.e., to one complete breath cycle lasting 10–12 seconds) is effective at reducing emotional arousal by activating the parasympathetic nervous system.[13–16]

 Practice Exercise: Demonstrate paced breathing as an exercise with participants. The goal is to do the exercise once in a session, to increase the likelihood that the skill will be used again when needed. You can also do this as an experiment by asking participants to rate their arousal before and after practicing paced breathing.

You will need one large clock with a secondhand, to help participants to count breathing in and out.

The **procedure** is as follows:

1. Place the clock facing participants.

2. Instruct participants to watch the clock and count the seconds they inhale and the seconds they exhale. Encourage them to work while counting to get to a comfortable slow breathing rate, where the count is longer breathing out than breathing in. Give an example, such as 5 seconds in and 7 seconds out. They can choose to count the pause at the top of inhaling and at the bottom of exhaling or not. Give participants a few seconds to work on this.

3. Elicit from participants what numbers in and out they chose. Discuss.

> **Note to Leaders:** For a set of breathing pacers that will help you and your clients track breathing in and breathing out, you can again go to Milton Brown's website at the DBT Center of San Diego (*www.dbt-sandiego.com/current_clients.html*). This site also provides his handout "Regulating Emotions through Slow Abdominal Breathing." In addition, smartphone apps for paced breathing are available for both iPhones and Android phones, and breath pacers are available on YouTube.

✓ **H. Paired Muscle Relaxation**

Paired muscle relaxation, the fourth TIP skill, is the pairing of muscles relaxing with breathing out.

- Paired muscle relaxation is a variation on progressive muscle relaxation, which is widely used across many behavioral therapies for anxiety disorders.
- The strategy is to tense muscle groups, noticing the sensation of tension while breathing in, and then relax them by letting go of the tension, noticing the sensations as the muscle tension gradually goes down. The goal is to increase awareness of both tension and relaxation.
- The emphasis on noticing muscle sensations is similar to a mindfulness procedure focusing on body sensations (i.e., mindfulness of sensations).
- As a crisis survival skill, paired muscle relaxation teaches participants to notice tension and then relax muscles, and while doing so to pair relaxation with exhaling while saying the word "relax."

> **Note to Leaders:** How you teach paired muscle relaxation depends on how much time you have. If time is short, you can quickly demonstrate (with all participating) how to tense and relax muscles either one by one from the progressive relaxation list in Figure 10.2, or by putting muscle groups together and practicing them in groups. *If you have learned relaxation* through using a different order or grouping of muscles, feel free to use the method you use now. You can also use any of the numerous audio recordings available for muscle relaxation. It can be particularly helpful to have participants mentally rate their arousal before and after the practice and then share any changes. It is important to point out that relaxing is a skill that takes a lot of practice. Practicing on a daily basis can prepare clients for engaging in more functional behaviors during crises.

Orient participants to the procedure as follows:

- "Tensing and then relaxing muscle groups cause your muscles to become more relaxed than they were in the beginning, and more relaxed than you can ordinarily achieve by trying to relax without first tensing."
- "Pairing letting go of tension with saying the word 'Relax' in your mind while exhaling conditions your body to let go of tension and relax in the future when you say 'Relax' in your mind while exhaling."

Large
Medium
Small

Tense each muscle group for 5–10 seconds and then let go for 5–10 seconds.

1. Hands and wrists: Make fists with both hands and pull fists up on the wrists.

2. Lower and upper arms: Make fists and bend both arms up to touch your shoulders.

3. Shoulders: Pull both shoulders up to your ears.

4. Forehead: Pull eyebrows close together, wrinkling forehead.

5. Eyes: Shut eyes tightly.

6. Nose and upper cheeks: Scrunch up nose; bring upper lips and cheeks up toward eyes.

7. Lips and lower face: Press lips together; bring edges of lips back toward ears.

8. Tongue and mouth: Teeth together; tongue pushing on upper mouth.

9. Neck: Push head back into chair, floor, or bed, or push chin down to chest.

10. Chest: Take deep breath and hold it.

11. Back: Arch back, bringing shoulder blades together.

12. Stomach: Hold stomach in tightly.

13. Buttocks: Squeeze buttocks together.

14. Upper legs and thighs: Legs out; tense thighs.

15. Calves: Legs out; point toes down.

16. Ankles: Legs out; point toes together, heels out, toes curled under.

FIGURE 10.2. Progressive relaxation: Muscles and muscle groups. Adapted from Smith, R. E. (1980). Development of an integrated coping response through cognitive–affective stress management training. In I. G. Sarason & C. D. Spielberger (Eds.), *Stress and anxiety* (Vol. 7, pp. 265–280). Washington, DC: Hemisphere. Copyright 1980 by Hemisphere Publishing Corporation. Adapted by permission.

Note to Leaders: Some individuals experience a phenomenon of "relaxation-induced panic." That is, they may panic because of not meeting expectations to relax. To prevent this, it is very important to instruct participants that tensing and relaxing muscles may not result in relaxation, and that the important part of the exercise is to learn awareness of body tension. Individuals should also be instructed to feel free to stop at any time during practice. Allow those who are self-conscious when practicing simply to observe the demonstration and/or to face the wall during practice. In contrast to regular mindfulness practice, participants should be instructed to close their eyes during relaxation practice.

 Practice Exercise: Demonstrate and practice tensing and relaxing muscles.
The **procedure** is as follows:

1. Ask participants to rate their current arousal (subjective units of distress) on a scale of 0–100 (0 means no distress or tension at all; 100 means the very highest they could ever imagine).

2. Sit facing participants. Once everyone is in a comfortable position and can stretch out somewhat, ask participants to follow your instructions. Go through each of the muscle groups in Figure 10.2 (these are repeated in Distress Tolerance Handout 6b), tensing each, then letting go of each. Be sure participants see which muscles you are tensing and how to do it. In this demonstration, hold the tension for about 5–10 seconds, saying, "Notice the tension." Then say, "Let go," while rapidly letting go of the muscles, and add, "Notice the difference." Let relaxation go for about 5–10 seconds, and then go on to the next muscle group. Be sure to talk in a slow, steady cadence with an inviting voice tone. You might say something like this:

"Make fists with both of your hands, and pull your fists up toward your wrists; clench them just three-quarters of the way. . . . Pay attention to the tension. . . . Notice the tension in your hands . . . notice the tension . . . notice the tightness . . . just notice. . . . Now LET GO . . . just let go, let your hands drop down . . . let all the tension flow out. . . . Notice as your hands start to relax . . . notice the muscles letting go . . . just notice . . . paying attention to the sensations in your hands and wrists . . . letting all the tension just flow away. . . . " (Continue with the muscle groups in Figure 10.2.)

3. As a final instruction, tell participants to tense all their muscles quickly from head to toe, as if they are stiff robots, while breathing in deeply. Then, while breathing out slowly, they should let go like rag dolls, saying in their minds the word "Relax."

4. Have participants rate their arousal again.

5. Ask participants whether their arousal went down, stayed the same, or went up. Although we usually do this practice in group sessions for only 5–10 minutes, we have found that many participants have a noticeable reduction in arousal.

After the exercise, explain to participants: "Brief paired muscle relaxation can also be used in a crisis or when you have very, very little time. You can inhale while briefly tensing sets of muscles that can be tensed without being obvious to others—such as your stomach, buttocks, and chest—and then, when exhaling, relaxing them with the internal word 'Relax.' "

Practice Exercise: If you have the time, you can have participants practice paired muscle relaxation with a CD or other recording. It can be very useful to listen to a relaxation recording. In our clinic, we use one I developed that includes both a 5-minute relaxation and a 20-minute relaxation.[17] Many such recordings can also be found online. Since most participants like to hear their own therapists or skills trainers, you can make a recording, copy it to CDs or thumb drives, and give it out to participants.

Note to Leaders: If teaching relaxation is a major part of your intervention, or if you teach advanced classes, the practice assignments can be as follows:

1. "Practice tensing and relaxing each of the 16 muscle groups, paying attention to the tension for 5–10 seconds and attending to the sensations of relaxing the muscles for 5–10 seconds."

2. "Practice tensing and relaxing each of the nine larger muscle groups."

3. "Practice tensing and relaxing each of the four even larger muscle groups until you are proficient at reducing tension."

4. "Practice tensing the whole body while inhaling and then letting go of all the muscles on exhaling, while saying in your mind the word 'Relax.' Practice this paced relaxation throughout the day."

Note to Leaders: It is important to remind participants that getting relaxation paired with the word "relax" while exhaling can take a fair amount of practice. Once participants learn awareness of both physical tension and the difference between that and relaxation, they are ready to work on getting relaxation paired with the word relax while breathing out. I generally suggest practicing 5–10 times a day until their bodies and minds "get" the pairing; this usually happens in 5–6 weeks.

I. Effective Rethinking and Paired Relaxation

The combination of effective rethinking with paired relaxation is a method of using both cognitive restructuring and progressive muscle relaxation to bring down arousal rapidly in moments of high stress.

Practice Exercise: If you teach this combination, the procedure is as follows:

1. Say to participants: "Identify a situation (a prompting event) that is often related to distressing emotions, and in which you want to work on reducing your emotional reactions."

2. "Ask yourself, 'What must I be telling myself for this situation to be so upsetting?' For example, if taking difficult exams is a really stressful event for you, you might be telling yourself during the exam things like 'I am going to fail this,' 'If I fail, I might as well quit because I will never go anywhere in life,' 'If I fail, people will know it and think I am no good,' or 'If I fail, it will mean that I am either a lazy good-for-nothing or am stupid.'"

3. "Now rethink the situation in such a way as to counteract the thoughts and interpretations that cause you so much stress. As you rethink the situation, write down as many effective thoughts as you can to replace each of the stressful thoughts."

4. "Prepare yourself for the next time the stressful event or one like it occurs. To do this, combine rehearsal of your effective thoughts with paired relaxation. To do this, as you breathe in, imagine the stressful event is happening to you. Be sure to imagine you are in the stressful scene, not watching it as on television. Before breathing out, say to yourself (in a convincing tone) an effective self-statement followed by "SO RELAX," as you breathe out while intentionally relaxing all your muscles."

5. "Practice, practice, practice."

6. "When the stressful situation occurs, practice your effective rethinking and paired relaxing."

7. Discuss how similar this is to the cope ahead skill.

Note to Leaders: If you are working with just one person, this procedure can be strengthened by working with the client to practice incorporating imaginal exposure to the stressful situation before starting the effective self-statements and paired breathing. The idea here is to get stressful emotions up very high and then have the client practice saying the effective thoughts, followed by "Relax," while at the same time letting go of muscle tension. It is best not to try this before you are sure the individual has been able to use paired relaxation successfully. A forthcoming book will have further ideas on using paired relaxation.[18]

J. Review of TIP Skills

If you have time, review the TIP skills briefly to make sure everyone understands them.

VII. DISTRACTING WITH WISE MIND ACCEPTS

Main Point: Distracting methods work by reducing contact with whatever set off the distress or its most painful aspects. A secondary value is that they also may work to change parts of an emotional response.

Distress Tolerance Handout 7: Distracting. After explaining the value of distracting attention as a distress tolerance skill in a crisis situation, go through each of the ACCEPTS skills on this handout. Give participants an opportunity to offer their own distracting methods. It can be useful to ask participants to put checkmarks in the boxes for distracting activities they are willing to use or try out.

Distress Tolerance Worksheets 5, 5a, 5b: Distracting with Wise Mind ACCEPTS. These worksheets offer three different ways to record ACCEPTS skills practice. Distress Tolerance Worksheet 5 provides space for practice only two times between sessions. Thus it can be a good starter worksheet with individuals you are trying to shape into more frequent skills practice. Worksheet 5a instructs practicing every skill twice. Worksheet 5b instructs participants to practice and gives multiple opportunities for each skill.

✓ A. When Is Distracting Useful?

Say to participants: "When you are in a crisis, distraction can help you avoid dangerous behaviors, but distracting can easily be overused. Do not use it as a routine method to avoid painful emotions. Here are some effective uses of distraction."

1. When Emotional Pain Threatens to Become Overwhelming

Tell participants: "When your emotional pain or upset becomes so great that you are in danger of being overwhelmed by it at work, at school, or at meetings, it may be more effective to distract yourself from the feelings in the moment instead of fully experiencing them."

💬 **Discussion Point:** Elicit examples from participants of occasions when pain is intense but it is not an appropriate time to work on changing the source of the pain or figuring out and changing the painful emotions.

2. When Problems Can't Be Solved Immediately

Go on: "You can also use distraction when you have a problem that can't be solved immediately, and urgency to solve the problem *right now* is making it very difficult to focus on anything except the crisis."

💬 **Discussion Point:** Distraction can help a person tolerate a problem until the time is right for problem solving. Elicit from participants times when not tolerating distress and instead trying to solve an emotional problem *immediately* has led to even bigger problems.

💬 **Discussion Point:** Discuss factors that get in the way of putting problem solving off until a better moment.

💬 **Discussion Point:** Ask participants whether they have a tendency to distract themselves too much or too little.

👥 **Practice Exercise:** Ask participants to read through all the items on Handout 7 and check those they think might work for them. Ask people what they checked. (This exercise can be done at the beginning or at the end of reviewing the handout.)

✓ B. Seven Sets of Distracting Skills

Distracting from painful emotion or distress means turning one's attention to something else. There are seven sets of distracting skills. The sentence "Wise mind ACCEPTS" is a useful way to remember these skills.

1. Activities

Engaging in activities that are neutral or opposite to negative emotions and crisis behaviors can work to reduce impulsive urges and distress in a number of ways. They distract attention and fill short-term memory with non-crisis-oriented thoughts, images, and sensations. They affect physiological responses and emotional expressive behaviors directly. They can reduce the emotional pain that often drives the crisis behaviors. Treatments that focus on behavioral activation, for example, are very effective in reducing depression.

2. *Contributing*

Contributing to somebody else's well-being refocuses attention from oneself to others and what one can do for them. Participating fully in the experience of helping someone else can make people completely forget their own problems for a while. For some individuals, contributing also increases a sense of meaning in life, thereby improving the moment (see Distress Tolerance Handout 9). For others, it enhances self-respect.

3. *Comparisons*

Making comparisons also refocuses attention from oneself to others, but in a different way. In this case, the situations of others—those coping in the same way or less well, or the less fortunate in general—are used to recast one's own situation in a more positive light. Alternatively, one can focus on past problems that are no longer occurring, and compare the present moment to this past difficult time.

> *Example:* "Watch soap operas or other TV shows where people have problems worse than yours."

4. *Emotions*

Generating different emotions distracts from the current situation and negative emotion. This strategy interferes with the current mood state. This technique requires first figuring out the current emotion, so that activities for generating a different one can be sought.

> *Example:* "Read an emotional book (such as a thriller). Then, after you put the book down, think back to the story in the book and experience that emotion. However, don't read something that will make you feel worse than you already feel, or that will cue crisis behaviors."

> **Note to Leaders:** Remind participants that they cannot get a different emotion by simply demanding it or using willpower alone. What is needed is an activity that will reliably set off an emotion different from the one that is generating so much pain.

5. *Pushing Away*

Pushing away from a painful situation can be done by leaving it physically or by blocking it from one's mind. Leaving the situation decreases contact with its emotional cues. Blocking is a somewhat conscious effort to inhibit thoughts, images, and urges associated with negative emotions. One form of blocking is to repeatedly put off destructive behaviors for brief periods of time. Blocking is a bit like riding a bicycle; people only understand it when they do it. Most individuals seem able to do this and will usually know what you mean as soon as you mention the technique. It is perhaps related to the ability to dissociate or depersonalize. It should not be the first technique tried, but can be useful in an emergency. The secret is not to overuse it.

> *Example:* "Build up an imaginary wall between yourself and others."

> *Example:* "Put your emotions in a 'box,' and put the box on a shelf. This can be done through visualization, or you could make an actual worry box and drop pieces of paper in it with labels of the stressors."

> *Example:* "Put off smoking a cigarette every 5 minutes for 5 minutes."

6. _Thoughts_

Distracting with other thoughts fills short-term memory, so that thoughts activated by the negative emotion do not continue to reactivate the emotion.

Example: "Sing a song in your head."

Example: "You are at a funeral and no one is crying, and you feel that at any minute you are going to burst out sobbing, which you don't want to do. Distract yourself by counting something at the funeral—for instance, bricks on the wall, people in the pews, or words that are said by the speakers."

7. _Sensations_

Intense, different sensations can focus attention on something other than the emotional distress, its source, or its crisis urges. Holding ice cubes,[19] in particular, can be very helpful. In a skills training group run by a colleague of mine, a client brought everyone small refreezable ice packs. Several clients would then take them (frozen) to therapy sessions to hold onto when discussing very painful topics (e.g., sexual abuse, which one client had not previously been able to discuss at all). This technique, while at times useful, also needs to be closely monitored so that it does not interfere with exposure to important and relevant cues. Other ideas for eliciting sensations are tasting Tabasco sauce, lemon wedges, and intensely sour candy, or putting on headphones and listening to fast, upbeat music.

💬 **Discussion Point:** Elicit any objections participants have to using distraction, and discuss these. Cheerleading may be needed.

💬 **Discussion Point:** Some individuals spend so much time distracting themselves from their own issues and focusing on others' problems that they never get around to addressing their own. Elicit examples from participants.

VIII. SELF-SOOTHING (DISTRESS TOLERANCE HANDOUTS 8–8A)

Main Point: Self-soothing is doing things that feel pleasant, comforting, and provide relief from stress or pain. It makes it much easier to pass the time without making things worse.

Distress Tolerance Handout 8: Self-Soothing. After describing the value of self-soothing, go through self-soothing methods on this handout, focusing on each of the five senses. Give participants an opportunity to offer their own methods. It can be useful to ask participants to put checkmarks in the boxes for those self-soothing activities they are willing to try out.

Distress Tolerance Handout 8a: Body Scan Meditation, Step by Step (_Optional_). This handout contains a set of instructions for the body scan. If you do not have time to go through this procedure with participants, you might suggest that they get a recording leading them in a body scan[20] or listen to one on YouTube.

Distress Tolerance Worksheet 6, 6a, 6b: Self-Soothing. As with the worksheets for the distraction skills, each of these provides for an increase in the number of practices, from two practices between sessions (Worksheet 6) to practice of every skill twice (Worksheet 6a) to multiple daily practices (Worksheets 6b).

Distress Tolerance Worksheet 6c: Body Scan Meditation, Step by Step. If you assign the body scan meditation as homework, ask participants to use this worksheet to record practice.

　Other Materials: It can be useful to bring a few soothing items from one or more of the sense categories to share with participants. Examples for soothing smell are lavender, vanilla, cinnamon, baked cookies, flowers, or pleasant-smelling scratch-and-sniff stickers; for touch, small swatches of fabric with different soothing textures, teddy bears, or other plush toys; for vision, pictures of nature; for sound, soothing music (e.g., lullabies, sound machines); for taste, chocolate or butterscotch candy.

✓ **A. What Is Self-Soothing?**

Self-soothing is being comforting, nurturing, peacemaking, gentle, and mindfully kind to oneself.

✓ **B. When to Self-Soothe**

Self-soothing activities reduce vulnerability to emotion mind and to acting impulsively and they reduce the sense of deprivation that is often a precursor to feelings of vulnerability. They help people tolerate pain and distress without making things worse.

✓ **C. How to Self-Soothe**

1. Soothe the Five Senses

A way to remember the skills for self-soothing is to think of soothing the five senses:

- Vision
- Hearing
- Smell
- Taste
- Touch

✓ **Practice Exercise:** Ask participants to read through all the items on Handout 8 and check those they think might work for them. Then ask them what they checked. (This exercise can be done at the beginning or at the end of reviewing the handout.)

Note to Leaders: Go over the specific self-soothing activities on Handout 8, offering a few examples from any materials brought into the session. You need review only a few in each category during the session. Devote more time to the following discussion point.

Discussion Point: Some individuals have difficulties with self-soothing. Some believe that they do not deserve soothing, kindness, and gentleness; they may feel guilty or ashamed when they self-soothe. Others believe that they should get soothing from others; they don't self-soothe as a matter of principle, or feel angry at others when they attempt to self-soothe. For these participants, self-soothing requires opposite action (see Emotion Regulation Handout 10). Elicit examples from each participant.

Note to Leaders: It is important that each participant learn to self-soothe. Even if at first it elicits anger or guilt, self-soothing should be repeatedly attempted. In time, it will become easier. Some clients may be quite resistant to practicing self-soothing. Keep a watchful eye on homework practice, to be sure that each participant is at least trying these skills. Assess and problem-solve difficulties.

Discussion Point: In contrast, other individuals overuse self-soothing or use it in self-destructive ways. Each of the items on Handout 8 can create problems if used to excess. Elicit examples from each participant.

2. Balance Soothing the Senses with Problem Solving

It is important to balance self-soothing with focusing and working on a task. This is especially important during crises, when sudden demands feel overwhelming and keep one from doing what is required. In such a scenario, self-soothing can be an effective first step to bring down the negative emotions. However, self-soothing is not sufficient for resolving crises. It needs to be followed by working on the task and getting it done. Alternatively, you might suggest one of the TIP skills as a way to reduce feeling overwhelmed, followed by problem solving, and then followed by self-soothing as a reward.

D. Self-Soothing with a Body Scan Meditation

Another option for self-soothing is a more focused attention to body sensations, the body scan (as described in the optional Distress Tolerance Handout 8a). This is a practice commonly used in meditation. Tell participants: "The idea here is to settle the mind by letting go of thoughts about the past or about the future, and instead focus the mind on the present and on your present experiences of your breath and of your body. It is a way of approaching the sensations of your body with the curiosity of a child. Through this process, you will discover a lot about how your body feels, its sensations, and your mental reactions to paying attention to various parts of your body."

Encourage practice with a CD or web-based recording. Body scan meditation, like paired muscle relaxation, can be very soothing when it is done while listening to a soothing voice's step-by-step instructions. As noted earlier in regard to paired relaxation, since most participants like to hear their own therapists or skills trainers, you can make a recording, copy it to a CD or thumb drive, and give it out to participants.

> **Note to Leaders:** The body scan is an important part of various insight meditation practices,[20, 21] and of the mindfulness-based treatments that evolved from these practices.[22–28] As with paired muscle relaxation and sensory self-soothing, how you teach this depends on how much time you have. The full body scan procedure takes up to 30 minutes. If time is short, you can quickly demonstrate the body scan (with all participating) by instructing participants to focus on just two or three body areas (5–10 minutes). If you do not have an audio recording of a body scan, review and give participants Distress Tolerance Handout 8a to use as a guide for how to move systematically through the body. As noted above, before and after the practice, ask participants mentally to rate their ability to tolerate distress (0–100) without making things worse. Ask them to share any changes.

The steps for teaching body scan meditation are as follows:

1. Orient Participants to the Procedure

Say to participants: "Focusing your mind on your breath and on specific body sensations can be a very soothing experience if it is done slowly, with curiosity and with gentleness. It does not require a lot of effort or use of imagination. Bringing your mind back to the present and focusing on your body sensations can anchor the mind, calming emotions that feel out of control."

> **Note to Leaders:** As noted previously, some individuals experience "relaxation-induced panic" because of unmet expectations. To prevent this, instruct participants that the body scan may not result in relaxation, and that the important part of the exercise is to learn awareness of their body. Individuals should be instructed to feel free to stop at any time during practice. Allow those who are self-conscious about practicing to simply observe the demonstration and/or face the wall during practice.

2. Demonstrate Scanning Body Sensations

Ask participants to rate their level of distress (0–100) before starting the practice; you can ask them to write it down in case they forget. Then ask them to get in a comfortable position with their eyes partially open. In a slow and easy voice tone, give instructions on which part of the body to focus on, pausing for a minute or so between each instruction. For example, you can say something like this, speaking slowly and giving participants time to focus on each part of the body:

"*Focus your awareness, as if it were a spotlight, on:*
- *Where your body is touching the chair, (or the floor, or the bed).*
- *Down the left leg, into the left foot all the way to the toes.*
- *On each toe in turn.*
- *Expand attention into the rest of the foot, to:*
    - *The ankle.*
    - *The top of the foot.*
    - *The bones and joints.*
    - *The lower left leg.*
    - *The calf, shin, knee, and so forth in turn.*
    - *The left thigh.*"

"*Move your focus to:*
- *The right toes, and on to*
    - *Foot and ankle.*
    - *The right lower leg.*
    - *The right knee.*
    - *The right thigh.*
- *Up to the pelvic area.*
    - *Groin, genitals, buttocks, and hips.*
- *The lower back and the abdomen.*
- *The upper back and the chest and shoulders.*
- *Then move to the hands.*
    - *The sensations in the fingers and thumbs.*
    - *The palms and the backs of both hands.*
    - *The wrists, the lower arms, and the elbows.*
    - *The upper arms, the shoulders, and the armpits.*
- *The neck, the face (jaw, mouth, lips, nose, cheeks, ears, eyes, forehead).*
- *And then the entirety of the head.*"

3. Ask Participants to Rate Distress

Following the end of the exercise, ask participants to rate their level of distress, again on the 0–100 scale.

4. Give Suggestions for a Brief Body Scan

Tell participants: "In a crisis or when you have very, very little time, you can do a brief body scan. Focus your attention completely on just one section of your body, moving to a second and then a third."

IX. IMPROVING THE MOMENT (DISTRESS TOLERANCE HANDOUTS 9–9A)

Main Point: Improving the moment is an idiosyncratic series of strategies that can be helpful in improving the quality of the present moment, making it easier to survive a crisis without making it worse.

Distress Tolerance Handout 9: Improving the Moment. Review each of the strategies on this handout, and give participants an opportunity to offer their own methods and to share other strategies that work well in a crisis. Ask participants to put checkmarks in the boxes for those activities they are willing to try.

Distress Tolerance Handout 9a: Sensory Awareness, Step by Step (Optional). This optional hand-out can be used as a participant guide for a relaxing action (the R in IMPROVE) or used as a script for recording an audio guided relaxation that is distributed to participants.

Distress Tolerance Worksheets 7, 7a, 7b: IMPROVE the Moment. Review worksheets with participants. As with the worksheets for the previous skills, each of these provides for an increase in the number of practices from two practices between sessions (Worksheet 7) to practice of every skill twice (Worksheet 7a) to multiple daily practices (Worksheet 7b).

✓ A. What Is Improving the Moment?

Improving the moment is replacing immediate negative events with more positive ones by making the moment more positive and easier to tolerate. Some strategies involve changing appraisals of oneself (encouragement) or the situation (creating meaning in the situation, imagining changes in the situation). Some involve changing body responses to events (relaxing). Prayer and focusing on one thing in the moment have to do with acceptance and letting go.

✓ B. When to Practice Improving the Moment

Explain to participants: "Improving the moment is particularly useful when you are feeling over-whelmed in a stressful situation that may be long-lasting, or when distracting activities and self-soothing are not working."

✓ C. How to Improve the Moment

Tell participants: "A way to remember these skills is the word IMPROVE: Imagery, Meaning, Prayer, Relaxing actions, One thing in the moment, Vacation, Encouragement."

✓ **Practice Exercise:** Ask participants to read through all the items on Handout 9 and check those they think might work for them. Ask people what they checked. (This exercise can be done at the beginning or at the end of reviewing the handout.)

1. Imagery

Mental visualization—imagery—can be used to distract, soothe, bolster courage and confidence, and make future rewards more salient.

Say to participants: "Using imagery, you can create a situation different from the actual one; in this sense, it is like leaving the current situation. With imagery, however, you can be sure that the place you go to is safe and secure. Going to an imaginary safe place or room within yourself can be very helpful during flashbacks. For this strategy to be useful, however, you have to practice it enough times when you are not in a crisis to get it firmly down as a skill."

Practice Exercise: Ask participants to breathe deeply and go within themselves to wise mind. Suggest that while there, they begin building a safe room inside themselves. Have them imagine the furniture in the room, the locks on the doors, the things they would put in the room to feel safe. Ask them also to imagine what they would put in the room to protect themselves from destructive urges. What would they keep out of the room? Ask participants to share how they built their room.

Imagery can also be used to cope more effectively with crises. Practicing effective coping in imagination can actually increase one's chances of coping effectively in real life. It can be helpful first to write out a script outlining how one would cope effectively with a crisis without making it worse, and then practice it in imagination. Used in this way, imagery is very similar to the emotion regulation skill of cope ahead (see Emotion Regulation Handout 19).

Example: "Imagine yourself tolerating a very painful emotion or powerful urge to do something destructive by visualizing yourself flying away into the clouds, looking down on the pain and intense urges."

2. *Meaning*

Finding or creating meaning helps many people in crises. Victor Frankl wrote *Man's Search for Meaning*, an important book about surviving Nazi concentration camps.[29] It is based on the premise that people need to find or create meaning in their lives to survive terrible suffering. Finding or creating meaning is similar to the dialectical strategy of making lemonade out of lemons. (See Chapter 7 of the main DBT text.)

Discussion Point: It is important to note that life is at times unfair for reasons that no one can understand. People do not have to assume that there is a purpose to their suffering, although those who are religious or spiritual may see it this way. Those who do not believe in a higher purpose can still create meaning or purpose, however. Get feedback about participants' views on the meaning or purpose of suffering.

3. *Prayer*

The essence of prayer is the complete opening of oneself to the moment. This practice is very similar to the notion of radical acceptance, discussed later in this module. Note that the suggested prayer is not one of begging to have the suffering or crisis taken away. Nor is it a "Why me?" prayer.

Practice Exercise: During the skills training session, have all participants close their eyes, imagine or "get in touch with" current pain or suffering, and then silently try different types of prayer. These might include an acceptance prayer (e.g., "Thy will be done"), a "Deliver me" prayer, or a "Why me?" prayer. Have participants refocus on current suffering (for only a moment) before each attempt at prayer. Discuss afterward. Or suggest that people who are comfortable with praying try each type of prayer during the next crisis, and keep track of which type actually helps.

4. *Relaxing Actions*

Relaxing actions as part of improving the moment are different from paired muscle relaxation as taught in the TIP skills. In paired relaxation, the emphasis is on directly modifying how the body is reacting to stress. In relaxing actions, the emphasis is on widening activities to include a wider variety of relaxing things to do. Explain to participants: "The key here is to select activities that ordinarily have the effect of calming you down. When you are relaxed, it is usually far easier to resist temptations to engage in crisis behaviors. Being relaxed gives you time to think and review your pros and cons."

Discussion Point: Many of the skills taught in this module or in the Mindfulness module can be very relaxing. It can be useful to have each participant make a list of activities that are especially relaxing. Elicit from participants types of activities they find relaxing. Discuss types of activities that are relaxing to some but that cause tension, anxiety, or irritation for other people.

Practice Exercise: It can be very relaxing to listen to mindfulness or relaxation exercises recordings. As noted earlier, a wide range of these is available from various sources; as also noted earlier, these are often most useful if a skills trainer or therapist provides the recording. A script that can be used for such a recording is provided in Distress Tolerance Handout 9a and described below.

5. *One Thing in the Moment*

"One thing in the moment" is another way of describing "one-mindfully," the second mindfulness "how" skill discussed in Chapter 7 of this manual. Although it can be very difficult to do, focusing on one thing in the moment can be very helpful in the middle of a crisis; it can provide time to settle down. The secret of this skill is to remember that the only pain one has to survive is "just this moment." We all often suffer much more than is required by calling to mind past suffering and ruminating about future suffering we may have to endure. But, in reality, there is only "just this moment." This skill is important in reality acceptance, and a number of specific exercises for improving focus and increasing awareness are taught in the next segment of this module.

Practice Exercise: During the session, have all participants close their eyes and imagine or "get in touch with" some current discomfort, irritation, or anxiety right now, at this moment in the session. Instruct participants to raise a hand slightly when they have the focus. Instruct them to notice their level of current discomfort. Now instruct them to start ruminating about all the past times when they have had to endure such feelings in sessions. Have them also bring to mind and ruminate about how much more these feelings have to be endured in this skills training session and all future sessions. Instruct them to notice now their level of discomfort. Then have them refocus the mind on "just this moment." Explain: "Say in your mind, 'Just this moment'; let go of thoughts of the future and the past." Now have them notice their level of discomfort after doing this. Discuss the exercise.

6. _Vacation_

Continue: "Taking a 'vacation from adulthood' is coping by retreating into yourself or allowing yourself to be taken care of for the moment. Everyone needs a vacation from adulthood once in a while. The trick is to take it in a way that does not harm you, and also to make sure the vacation is brief. It should only last from a few moments to no longer than a day. When you have responsibilities, taking a vacation depends on getting someone else to take over your duties for a while. The idea is similar to the notion of taking a time out to regroup."

Discussion Point: Some individuals are experts at taking vacations. The problem is that they are not in control of their vacations; that is, they take them at inappropriate times and stay on them too long. When vacation taking becomes a skill to be practiced, this gives them the potential for getting in control. Elicit from participants times when they have taken vacations in an out-of-control fashion. Discuss ways to get in control of vacations and use them effectively.

✓ 7. _Encouragement_

"Encouragement is cheerleading yourself and rethinking situations. The idea is to talk to yourself as you would talk to someone you care about who is in a crisis—or to talk to yourself as you would like someone else to talk to you. In couples, having a higher ratio of positive comments to negative comments predicts the partners' staying in the relationship.[30–32] You are in a relationship with yourself, so to increase well-being, you have to say more positive and encouraging things than negatives and put-downs. The idea here is to rethink situations when you start telling yourself they are hopeless, that they won't ever end, or that you cannot do what is needed."

Note to Leaders: You may at first need to do quite a bit of modeling of self-encouragement here, as well as cheerleading.

Discussion Point: Mention that it is important to balance improving the moment with staying in the present. Discuss with participants how when this balance is not achieved, the strategies for improving the moment can be overused, particularly in invalidating environments. However, point out that just because they can be overused, this does not mean they have no value at all. Elicit and problem-solve resistance to using these skills.

D. Improving the Moment with Sensory Awareness

Sensory awareness (as described in the optional Distress Tolerance Handout 9a) is aimed at centering oneself to enhance a sense of calmness and peace. It involves focusing attention on various sensations that one might have. Although the procedure is given in the form of questions, the goal is to direct participants' attention to the presence or absence of sensations asked about, and to encourage participants to focus on their experiences. Like body scan meditation, this skill is much easier for participants to learn if they can listen to a recording of the questions or a live reader. You can make a recording yourself and put it on a CD or thumb drive to give to participants, or you can have participants record (on smartphones if they have them) your reciting the questions in the session.

> **Note to Leaders:** How you teach this depends on how much time you have. If time is short, you can quickly demonstrate (with all participating) by asking just ten questions. If you do not have a recording of the questions, give participants Distress Tolerance Handout 9a to use as a guide for asking themselves questions. It can be particularly helpful to have participants mentally rate their distress before and after the practice, and then share any changes. It is important to point out that relaxing is a skill that takes lots of practice. Practiced on a daily basis, however, it can prepare clients for engaging in more functional behaviors during crises.

The steps for teaching sensory awareness are as follows:

✓ **1. Orient Participants to the Procedure**

Tell participants: "This procedure asks a series of questions about your body sensations. Focusing your mind on body sensations can bring you back into the present. This helps many people feel 'grounded' and more at peace, calming emotions that feel out of control."

The entire procedure, practiced at home or in an individual session, ordinarily takes about 10 minutes, but it can also be done quickly in 5 minutes (by skipping questions).

✓ **2. Demonstrate Noticing the Sensations**

Start with very simple instructions: "Find a comfortable position. . . . Now, in your mind, rate your current level of distress from 0 to 100. Staying in this position, listen to each question that I ask. Listen to each question, and notice what occurs before I ask the next question. There are no right or wrong responses. Just notice your reaction to each question." Then start asking each question in a modulated but warm voice tone, pausing for several seconds between each question. Questions take between 5 and 7 seconds to read, and pauses should last 10–13 seconds. With 20 seconds per question, all of the questions can be given in 10 minutes.

1. *"Can you feel your hair touching your head?"*
2. *"Can you feel your chest rising and falling as you breathe?"*
3. *"Can you feel the space between your eyes?"*
4. *"Can you feel the distance between your ears?"*
5. *"Can you feel your breath touching the back of your eyes while you inhale?"*
6. *"Can you picture something far away?"*
7. *"Can you notice your arms touching your body?"*
8. *"Can you feel the bottoms of your feet?"*
9. *"Can you imagine a beautiful day at the beach?"*
10. *"Can you notice the space within your mouth?"*
11. *"Can you notice the position of your tongue in your mouth?"*
12. *"Can you feel a breeze against your cheek?"*
13. *"Can you feel how one arm is heavier than the other?"*
14. *"Can you feel a tingling or numbness in one hand?"*
15. *"Can you feel how one arm is more relaxed than the other?"*

16. *"Can you feel a change in the temperature in the air around you?"*
17. *"Can you feel how your left arm is warmer than the right?"*
18. *"Can you imagine how it would feel to be a rag doll?"*
19. *"Can you notice any tightness in your left forearm?"*
20. *"Can you imagine something very pleasant?"*
21. *"Can you imagine what it would feel like to float on a cloud?"*
22. *"Can you imagine what it would feel like to be stuck in molasses?"*
23. *"Can you picture something far away?"*
24. *"Can you feel a heaviness in your legs?"*
25. *"Can you imagine floating in warm water?"*
26. *"Can you notice your body hanging on your bones?"*
27. *"Can you allow yourself to drift lazily?"*
28. *"Can you feel your face getting soft?"*
29. *"Can you imagine a beautiful flower?"*[33]*
30. *"Can you feel how one arm and leg are heavier than the other?"*[33]

3. Give Suggestions for Brief Sensory Awareness

Say to participants: "In a crisis or when you have very little time, ask yourself two or three of these questions."

💬 **Discussion Point:** Ask participants after the practice whether their arousal and distress tolerance went down, stayed the same, or went up. Although my colleagues and I often spend only 5 minutes on this exercise in session, we have found that many participants have a noticeable reduction in arousal, which often makes tolerating distress much easier.

E. Summarizing the Crisis Survival Skills

Summarize the crisis survival skills with participants before moving to the next portion of this module.

> **Note to Leaders:** In reviewing the crisis survival skills, note that whereas some of the skills involve distancing from the painful reality (e.g., pushing away and most of the other distraction skills), others allow for some continued contact with the painful circumstance (e.g., encouragement, one thing in the moment, finding meaning, comparisons). In this sense, the latter crisis survival skills involve some reality acceptance. This is a meaningful distinction, as sometimes it is important to interrupt a crisis response (e.g., when one is on the verge of self-harm), while in other situations it is ineffective to distract oneself completely (e.g., while completing a shift at work or while in a therapy session).

X. OVERVIEW: REALITY ACCEPTANCE SKILLS (DISTRESS TOLERANCE HANDOUT 10)

> **Main Point:** The goals of reality acceptance skills are to reduce suffering and increase a sense of freedom through coming to terms with the facts of one's life.
>
> **Distress Tolerance Handout 10: Overview: Reality Acceptance Skills: Review this handout quickly.** It can also be skipped and the information written on the board instead. Do not use this handout to teach the skills.
>
> **Distress Tolerance Worksheets 8, 8a, 8b: Reality Acceptance Skills.** Each of these three worksheets

---

*Both items marked with note number 33 are adapted from Goldfried, M., & Davison, G. (1976). *Clinical behavior therapy.* New York: Holt, Rinehart & Winston. Copyright 1976 by Marvin R. Goldfried and Gerald C. Davison. Adapted by permission of the authors.

covers all the reality acceptance skills and can be used here if you are reviewing skills already taught. The worksheets vary in the amount of practice they provide for starting with two practices on Worksheet 8. This worksheet can be a good starter worksheet with individuals you are trying to shape into more frequent skills practice. Worksheet 8a provides for practice of every skill twice, while Worksheet 8a provides for multiple daily practices. These worksheets can be given again and again for each of the reality acceptance skills if you do not want to use the worksheets specific to each skill.

A. Reality Acceptance Skills

1. What Are Reality Acceptance Skills?

Tell participants: "Reality acceptance skills are skills for accepting your life as it is in the moment. They are particularly useful when you are living a life that is not the life you want."

Note to Leaders: If you have not (or have not yet) taught crisis survival skills, review the goals of reality acceptance below as you start. If you have taught crisis survival skills and discussed the goals of distress tolerance before (Handout 1), then skip point 2 below and remind participants of the goals *very* briefly here. The value of reality acceptance as outlined below can also be reviewed when you are teaching radical acceptance (see Distress Tolerance Handout 10).

2. Goals of Reality Acceptance Skills

Say to participants: "The goals of reality acceptance skills are to reduce your suffering and increase your sense of freedom."

Discussion Point: Elicit from participants times when refusing to accept reality as it is has led to more pain and suffering instead of less pain and suffering.

Discussion Point: Elicit from participants times when letting go of having to have whatever they happen to want in a moment in time, and instead allowing reality to be what it is, have led to increased serenity and a sense of freedom.

✓ B. Six Basic Reality Acceptance Skills

There are six basic reality acceptance skills:

- Radical acceptance
- Turning the mind
- Willingness
- Half-smiling
- Willing hands
- Allowing the mind: Mindfulness of current thoughts

Note to Leaders: It is tempting to start teaching the skill of radical acceptance on this handout but *don't do it* unless you are *not* planning on using Distress Tolerance Handout 11: Radical Acceptance.

XI. RADICAL ACCEPTANCE (DISTRESS TOLERANCE HANDOUTS 11–11B)

Main Point: Radical acceptance is complete and total openness to the facts of reality as they are, without throwing a tantrum or responding with willful ineffectiveness.

Distress Tolerance Handout 11: Radical Acceptance. A good way to teach this skill is to review and discuss this handout first, but be sure to leave enough time for participants to work on the first one or two steps of Worksheet 9 during the session. (Do not, however, require sharing.) Most participants will see the relevance of the skill as they work on the worksheet. This also gives you a good chance to coach participants in working with the handout. A common misconception is that people must accept things in life that are not facts. Reviewing the list of what has to be accepted (and, by omission, what does not have to be accepted) can be very important. It can be useful also to have participants decide during the session what facts in their lives they still need to accept and what they will work on accepting during the week. The very concept of accepting the reality of facts that are not in dispute can be difficult for many participants. This is particularly true when participants have been victims of horrific abuse and believe that life has been very unfair to them. A common pattern here is believing that to accept something is to approve of it or to be passive and not change things that are destructive. A number of reasons for accepting reality are included on this handout. Orient participants, and advise them to remain aware that strong primary emotions like sadness may show up when they are practicing acceptance, either in group sessions or in other settings. Also explain to them that a sense of calmness often follows the practice.

Distress Tolerance Handout 11a: Radical Acceptance: Factors That Interfere (Optional). Factors that interfere with acceptance are outlined on this optional handout. Information on the handout can be discussed when you are teaching Handout 11.

Distress Tolerance Handout 11b: Practicing Radical Acceptance, Step by Step (Optional). It is useful to have this handout available, as it gives instructions for practicing radical acceptance. For some groups of participants, however, the handout may be overwhelming, and the list of practice exercises on Worksheet 9 will be sufficient.

Distress Tolerance Worksheet 9: Radical Acceptance. It can be very useful to have participants fill in the first several questions of this worksheet during the session. Be sure, however, to review the entire worksheet with participants before they leave. If participants have trouble figuring out what they need to accept in their lives, instruct them to do the best they can and to discuss this with their individual therapists or with persons who know them well. It is typical for individuals to decide they need to accept things that are not in reality facts (e.g., "I am a no-good, rotten person"). At times these judgmental thoughts may be hidden behind statements that sound like facts (e.g., "I am a street bum on drugs"). Discuss ratings of level of current acceptance. Point out that if a person writes something down to be worked on, this means that acceptance is already *above* 0. Notice that this worksheet is not only a worksheet, but a recording device to help participants remember what they did, so they can describe it during homework review. Once a person decides what to work on, the practice of radical acceptance is the homework, not the writing down of the practice. The exercises at the end are a summary of the exercises on Handout 11b. If a person is working on accepting more than one life fact, then you can either give out more than one copy of the worksheet or suggest using the back of the sheet.

Distress Tolerance Worksheet 9a: Practicing Radical Acceptance. Review the worksheet with participants. The instructions for how to use this worksheet are similar to those given for Worksheets 5a, 6a, and 7a.

A. Isn't Radical Acceptance Giving Up or Approving?

Pose these two questions to participants:

- "If the point of skills training is to change, why put in radical acceptance?"
- "If you accept evil and wrongdoing, isn't that approving of it?"

Note to Leaders: It is usually important to address these questions first and get them out of the way. Generally, I start with reasonably extreme stories where (1) no one will disagree that acceptance is needed; (2) the pain of the people in the story is severe enough that participants will not feel that you are trivializing their pain by suggesting they accept it; and (3) it is clear that acceptance does not mean approval.

✓ ⊗ **Story Point:** In reading books on how individuals survived in Nazi concentration camps during World War II, two things became apparent to me. First, a person had to have luck to survive. Second, if a person was lucky (i.e., was not killed for random reasons), then to stay alive the person had to radically accept that he or she was actually in the concentration camp and that the guards had all the power. What was right, wrong, or fair had no relevance. Those who gave up fell down and died or committed suicide. Those who openly rebelled, insisted guards stop breaking the law, or the like also died: The guards shot them or did something else equally brutal. Those who lived had luck, but they also radically accepted the rules imposed by the guards and people in power, and within those rules they did their very best to "work the system" and be effective in the environment they eventually survived.

✓ ⊗ **Story Point:** A man is in prison with a life sentence for a crime he did not commit. He has used up his appeals, has no money or resources to hire a lawyer, and cannot get the Innocence Project to take up his cause. Accepting that prison is his home for the time being is critical. Without such reality acceptance, the prisoner might not adapt to prison, learn the skills necessary to survive in prison, and get whatever good things he can have while in prison. Tantrums and fighting the system can interfere with problem solving within the system and can lead to more punishment. Lying down on his cot, and giving up and giving in, can be just as problematic for this man and can also lead to punishment and recriminations.

💬 **Discussion Point:** Ask participants for examples in their own lives where radical acceptance of the facts of their lives has been important, either because such acceptance made things a lot better or because failure to accept made things a lot worse.

✓ B. What Is the Difference between Acceptance and Radical Acceptance?

Tell participants that acceptance is:

- "Acknowledging or recognizing facts that are true; conceding the facts."
- "Letting go of fighting your reality (and also of throwing tantrums)."

And tell them that radical acceptance is:

- "Accepting all the way, with your mind, your heart, and your body."
- "Accepting something from the depths of your soul."
- "Opening yourself to fully experiencing reality as it is in this one moment."

The idea here is to acknowledge what exists without anger or grudge, without bitterness, without meanness. Despair (and passivity when action is needed), bitterness, resentment, and undue shame or guilt are all the results of failures in radical acceptance. They are also often results of accepting distorted facts—facts not in evidence. Thus the goal of radical acceptance is to *fully* accept just those facts that must be accepted. It is this full experience of the moment that ultimately will bring about peace and eventually, with repeated practice, some level of contentment with life.

> **Note to Leaders:** The point of radical acceptance is extremely difficult for some individuals (and some skills training leaders) to see. They have great difficulty seeing that they can accept something without approving of it. They believe that if they accept what is, they cannot change it. Trying to get them to accept the notion of acceptance can become a power struggle. As a shaping strategy, you might suggest the terms "acknowledge," "recognize," or "endure," and discuss these. You will probably have to discuss them over and over again. Great patience is needed, but don't give up on radical acceptance. Also, as noted above, be prepared to orient participants to the possibility that strong primary emotions like sadness and grief may show up when they are practicing radical acceptance. Again, these emotions are the results of the necessary emotional processing of acceptance and are often followed by a sense of calmness.

✓ C. What Has to Be Accepted?

✓ 1. Reality Is What It Is

We only have to accept actual facts about the present and the past, and reasonable probabilities about the future. Thus we have to be very careful not to accept distortions of the past (e.g., "My mother hated me from the very beginning of my life"), exaggerations (e.g., "I never get what I want," "I hate everything about where I live"), catastrophes (e.g., "My whole life was ruined when I got fired"), judgmental assertions (e.g., "My wife is a jerk, and my children are no good"), or other similar beliefs or assumptions that are not actual facts.

⊗ **Story Point:** Tell the story of the man who had to learn to love dandelions (see Chapter 9, Section XIX). As noted there, this story is adapted from one I was told by my Zen teacher, who read it in a book by another spiritual teacher, Anthony De Mello.[34] *406*

Examples: Accepting that a loved one has died is very hard, but also very necessary if one is to build a life without that person. If you are lucky to live long enough, at some point you will have to accept that your hair is turning gray.

⊗ **Story Point:** Marie had a job as a clerk typist for a big insurance company. But she really wanted to be a social worker. So she decided to find a job as a social worker. She went to an employment agency, asked them to help her get a new job, and told them she wanted a job in social work. They found her a job in social work. She gave notice at the job she had, which was a really good job in the sense that the people were fabulous and she got a good salary and benefits. But she really wanted a social work job, so she left.

She was so excited! "Ah! I've got a job in social work!" she thought. She went in to work the first day, and they asked her to type up reports and letters. She typed all day and was thinking, "Oh, well, it's not so terrible; I'm learning what type of work people do here, and I'm not going to have to keep typing." But the second day, the third day, and then for a whole week, what did they have her do? Typing! So she went to her supervisor and asked, "Well, when am I going to get to do the social work?" The supervisor said, "What do you mean?" Marie said, "Well, I mean when do I get to do something like social work?" The supervisor said, "Your job is typing. That's what we need. You don't have the social work degree required to work as a social worker."

The first thing that went through Marie's mind was "No, that is not true. I took a job with a social work agency. This can't be true."

She actually thought of staying. She thought of staying and trying to make it into a social work job. That would be denying reality. Because the fact of the matter was that this really was a typing job. So what were her options? Well, she could have stayed miserable. She could have gotten hysterical. She could have stayed, fought, and told them that they should make it into a social work job. She could have told them that they were mean for not doing that. She could have done a lot of things.

Marie's other option was just to radically accept that this was not a social work job. She had made a mistake. She needed to correct the mistake. And the way to correct that mistake was to get another job. So that's just what she did. When her next break came, she called the people at the employment agency; she told them she had made a mistake. She needed another job. They said that this was fine, and they would help her look for one. When they called her old job for a reference, her old boss said they had not found anyone yet for her old job and would like her to come back. So she went back to the old job and was a lot happier. She decided to start saving money so she could go to graduate school in social work. She also decided to look for a place to volunteer where she could do things like social work until she got into school.

✓ 2. Everyone's Future Has Limitations

A limitation on the future means that we may be less likely to achieve one or more desired outcomes. Limitations are like probabilities. Accepting these limitations (or probabilities) can be important in setting goals and in avoiding failures that may only decrease the quality of our lives. The key here is that only highly likely limitations have to be accepted.

Limitations on our futures are caused by factors that have occurred in our lives, in the lives of others, and in our environment. If we do not change the causes that limit our present and future, then we cannot change, and reality itself will not change.

✓ **a. We Can Be Limited by Our Biology and by Our Environment**

We can be limited by our genes, the biology we are born with, an absence of childhood education or effective parenting, a poor economic background, social status, country of birth, gender, race, sexual orientation, ethnicity, body shape, height, age, physical illness or disabilities, family members who need our care, or any number of other factors that we have little control over.

Examples: If you are born a boy, you cannot do some things girls can do (like get pregnant). If you are a woman, you may be limited by some social expectations that are not applied to men. If you have little artistic talent, it is less likely that you will be a successful artist. If you are born with one leg, it is less likely that you will win the New York Marathon.

✓ **b. We Can Be Limited by Our Own Past Behavior**

Examples: A person who skipped class a lot in high school, didn't study, and hung out with gang members is less likely to get accepted at a lot of colleges. A person who has been convicted and jailed for a felony is more limited in employment aspirations than one who has not. A person who left a job to stay home and take care of children may have more difficulty finding a high-paying job than one who has been working all along. Psychological disorders such as schizophrenia, bipolar disorders, repeated major depression, phobias, and crippling anxiety can make life more difficult for some than for others; if not effectively treated, these disorders may limit what one does in the future.

✓ **c. We Can Be Limited by Known Probabilities**

Examples: We all must accept that we will die (this is certain). Most of us have to accept paying taxes (this is almost certain) or having a shortened life if we continue to smoke, avoid exercise, and refuse to manage high blood pressure (these are high probabilities).

Refusing at times to accept that an undesired outcome is almost certainly going to occur if we don't change our behavior is denial of reality and a failure of radical acceptance.

Examples: "You are unlikely to do well on an exam if you refuse to accept that you have to study for it. You are unlikely to keep a job if you refuse to accept that continued hostile behavior at work is likely to get you fired. Facing and accepting the necessity of paying bills on time and saving money are necessary if you want to avoid financial instability."

✓ **d. Thoughts about the Future Do Not Have to Be Accepted as High Probabilities**

Fearful and hopeless thoughts about the future are not facts about the future. They do not have to be accepted as high probabilities unless the feared event is highly likely and the causes of the event cannot be changed.

Example: "You may have to accept that you will never get a job if you are on your deathbed or if you are unwilling to look for a job, but it does not need to be accepted if you can still work and are willing to apply for jobs."

Example: "No one will ever love me" is an extreme thought and is unlikely to be true for most of us. We may have to accept the fact that we have the thought "No one will ever love me," but this (the existence of the thought going through our minds) is all that must be accepted. The thought does not make it true. We don't have to accept that "I am a person who will never be loved."

> **Note to Leaders:** That thoughts about the future are not facts about the future is an extremely important point to make. Be sure that participants understand this point.

💬 **Discussion Point:** Elicit from participants times when they have tried to accept things about the future that they did not need to accept.

e. The Effects of Limitations on Our Lives Can Vary

We all have limitations, but the effects of specific limitations on our lives depend on our dreams and goals and on our willingness to accept not having everything we want in our lives. We cannot always control our own desires. We can wish we did not want something that is unattainable, but wishing does not always make things come true. Thus, when goals and possibilities conflict, it can cause much more pain than when they do not conflict.

Examples: Having limited athletic ability is not a limitation for a person who doesn't like athletics or doesn't care about winning; being tone-deaf is not such an important limitation for a person who doesn't play or sing music; being over 60 may not be a work limitation for a person who has a secure job and doesn't want to change.

✓ ### 3. Everything in the Universe Has a Cause

The point here is that everything that exists is an outcome of a cause. The point is not to identify specific causes or imply that we can always know the causes of events in reality. Nor is it to define what constitutes a cause. Thus causes can be physical, psychological, spiritual, or any other type of cause we may believe in.

✓ ### a. For Whatever Happens, We Can Assume a Cause and Effect

If a cause occurs, the effect should also occur. Acceptance from this point of view is saying, "Everything should be as it is." The point of this statement is that accepting what occurs in the universe is acknowledging that it is caused. What is caused should be, in other words. Or we can say, "Everything is as it is," or "Everything is," or "Everything is caused."

b. The Rules of the Universe Are What They Are

✓ Radical acceptance involves saying, "The rules of the universe are the rules of the universe." Then we can try to figure out what caused what. When we say that reality should be different, we are saying that somehow the rules of the universe should be different; not only that, but we are saying that we should get to say what the laws of the universe are. Of course, if we got to make up the rules of the universe, we might make a mistake. There might be some unintended negative consequences as a result. Refusing to accept reality as it is, in essence, is saying that causes (or at least some causes) should not have effects. This would be a remaking of the laws of the universe.

For the most part, we only say, "Things should not be the way they are," when we don't like the way things are. We rarely say that about things we like, we want, or we accept.

✓ ⚔ **Story Point:** Imagine that there's a little boy on a bicycle. The child is on a hill, and the child is racing down the hill really fast on his bicycle. He goes into an intersection. Coming from the other direction down a long, empty road is a car. The car is going way over the speed limit. The intersection is unmarked: There's not a stop sign, there's not a stoplight, and there's not a yield sign. The car's coming the other way. The driver sees the child too late to stop, and the car and the child on the bike meet up right in the middle of the intersection. The car hits the child, and the child dies.

Should this have happened? Yes, it should have. There wasn't a stop sign. There wasn't a stop light. There wasn't a yield sign. The car was speeding. The child was going fast. The car was going fast. The driver could not stop the car in time. The child was a child. Children go fast. People speed on long, empty roads. If we want to say that this should not have happened, we would have to create causes for it not to happen. We'd have to do something about all those causes.

That's an example of accepting reality as it is and accepting that reality has causes. We do not, of course, have to approve of this. But, until the causes are different, that event should happen. It was caused.

If we want children biking down a steep hill to stop being hit by cars coming across an intersection, we may need to put up warning and stop signs or lights. We may need more police patrols or speed bumps in the road. Parents may need to teach their children better bike-riding habits. Simply saying that cars should not speed, or drivers should not hit little children, or children should look right and left before crossing an intersection does not cut down on accidents.

🗩 **Discussion Point:** Elicit from participants situations in their lives where they have been saying, "Why me?" or "It shouldn't have happened."

Note to Leaders: Relate the emphasis on "what is caused should be" to nonjudgmentalness as taught in the Mindfulness module.

---

   c. Radical Acceptance Does Not Require Knowing the Causes of Things

In the story above of the car and the bicycle, we don't know if the cause was lack of a stop sign or if the accident could have been avoided if the driver was not speeding. But we can accept that there was a cause, even if we don't know it.

✓   **4. *Life Can Be Worth Living Even When It Contains Pain***

If life had to be pain-free to be worth living, no one would have a life worth living. Acceptance requires finding a way not to say that life is a catastrophe. Suppressing our desires for what we want is not an effective way out of this. When we do that, we are acting as if it would be terrible if we did not get what we want, as if we could not be happy and could not tolerate not having everything we want. These beliefs, of course, just make things worse.

⊗ **Story Point:** "Put yourself in a situation discussed earlier: You are a person in prison for life, for a crime you did not commit. The Supreme Court didn't overturn your conviction. What are your options?"

"You certainly cannot solve the problem. You're not going to get yourself out of jail. And it just doesn't seem possible that you're going to start being happy that you're an innocent person in jail. So we have to rule that one out. So what are your options?"

"You could be miserable, distraught, upset. You could cry every day for the rest of your life. Or you could accept it and figure out a way to build a life worth living inside a prison. To go from unendurable agony to endurable pain, you're going to have to accept that you can build a life. Because if you don't accept it, what will happen? You're not going to build a life. And building a life worth living actually takes a fair amount of work. Believing that you can't do it makes it almost impossible. Believing that you can do it makes it a lot easier—so the chances are a lot higher that if you'll actually accept that you are in prison for a crime you did not commit, you will build a life worth living."

🗩 **Discussion Point:** Elicit from participants times when they have overcome extremely difficult and painful situations or unfair treatment to build something they could bear. Discuss how they did it.

✓ 👥 **Practice Exercise:** Distribute copies of Distress Tolerance Worksheet 9, and ask participants to complete Item 1: "Make a list of two very important things in your life right now that you need to radically accept. Then put a number [0–5] indicating how much you accept this part of yourself or your life." It may seem early in the teaching to ask for this, but our experience is that almost all participants can do it. Most individuals have an intuitive understanding of what radical acceptance is and of the necessity of it in their lives. To ensure that group participants encounter what really needs to be accepted in their lives, it can be a good idea to tell them at the start that you will not require them to share what items they wrote down. Discuss participants' experiences with identifying and writing down what they must accept. Note that if a person writes down what they need to accept, that means they have already accepted it at least a little bit and should choose a number above 0.

D. Why Accept Reality?

✓ ### 1. Rejecting or Denying Reality Doesn't Change Reality

Rejecting reality usually involves avoiding seeing or experiencing reality, throwing a tantrum, and insisting (to the universe?) that reality change right this minute. It may simply be denying the facts that are right in front of our eyes. Although avoiding, tantrums, and denying might make us feel better in the moment, they do not change the facts that have occurred.

Example: Some parents have a difficult time accepting that their children have grown up and left for college or a job in a new city. This refusal can lead to unrealistic demands, unwanted advice, and oversolicitous interference in their children's lives, ultimately damaging their relationships with their children.

Examples: "Refusal to accept that drinking and driving is dangerous can lead to a DUI or a wreck that kills someone and lands you in jail for vehicular manslaughter. Refusal to accept some of your partner's habits that you dislike can lead to high conflict and ultimately a lost relationship."

💬 **Discussion Point:** A great myth is that "If you refuse to accept something—if you just put your foot down and refuse to put up with it—it will magically change." It is as if resistance and/or willpower alone will change it. Get examples of this. Discuss why participants might believe this. Elicit examples of when tantrums and verbal refusals to accept things have been reinforced.

✓ ### 2. Changing Reality Requires First Accepting Reality

Rejection of reality is like a cloud that surrounds pain, interfering with being able to see it clearly. Problems that are difficult to see clearly are difficult to solve.

Examples:
- "Refusing to accept an illness can lead you not to take care of yourself, which may cause even more illness or difficulties."
- "Staying in an abusive relationship for years because you simply cannot accept that your partner is unlikely to stop abusing you is likely to lead only to more abuse."
- "Insisting that if a person really cares for you, he or she will do what you want—when in so many ways the person already shows he or she does care for you—will probably lead only to disappointment, and perhaps to the end of the relationship too."
- "Refusing to accept that it could rain on your outdoor wedding, and therefore not making any contingency plans, may lead to a ruined wedding."

✓ ✂ **Story Point:** "Imagine that you have a car and the brakes have gone almost completely out. You take the car to a mechanic and tell him what your problem is, and he promises to fix your brakes. You come in the next week to get your car, and all seems fine. Two days later, however, you are driving your car and all of a sudden the same brakes go out again. You take it back to the mechanic again. Who do you think will get your brakes fixed faster—the mechanic who says, 'Oh, no, I fixed them, and they should run fine. You must have messed them up,' or the mechanic who says, 'Wow! The brakes went out again? There must be something wrong. Let me look at them again and see what I can do'?"

✓ ⚒ **Story Point:** "Imagine the following situation. You want to buy a new house, and you finally find the house of your dreams. There's only one problem with the house: It's purple, and you hate the color purple. So you make an agreement with the seller before you buy it. You say, 'All right, I'll pay you this much money, but you have to repaint the house before I move in so that it is not purple.' The person agrees, and you sign the papers sealing the deal. The big day comes to move into the house. It's so exciting! You pick up your new house keys and you go to the house. However, when you get there you find that not only is the house still purple, but the owners have moved to Europe and they are not coming back." (Pause.)

"All right, you have two options. You can throw a tantrum: 'Ah! I can't stand it! This is a disaster. Oh, God! Where are those people? I just can't believe this has happened to me. Ah! I'm so mad! Well, I'm not going to tolerate this! I'm going to sue and make them paint this house . . . ' And you can go on, and on, and on. You can storm out of the house, get in your car, leave, and say, 'We're not buying that house.' But you signed the papers, and now the house is yours. Now imagine another way. You go in and say, 'Ah, I'm so disappointed. I didn't want the house purple. I know I could sue them but it would take a really long time. Where's the nearest paint store?' "

"How do you think you will get the color of the house changed faster—if you accept that the house is purple, or if you throw a tantrum?"

💬 **Discussion Point:** Elicit from participants times when failure to accept the facts of a problem interfered with solving the problem.

✓ **3. Pain Cannot Be Avoided**

Pain cannot be avoided; it is nature's way of signaling that something is wrong. If we could avoid pain, we would do it. If we did avoid pain, however, we would be highly likely to die young, as we could easily inadvertently get ourselves in dangerous situations that could easily kill us (accidentally burn ourselves to death, go into freezing water that would put us in shock, etc.). Individuals who are born with no sense of pain have very difficult lives, as they must constantly be vigilant so as not to harm themselves inadvertently.[35]

As discussed in the Emotion Regulation module, emotions, including those that are very painful, also have functions that are critical to human survival.

Example: The pain of a hand on a hot stove causes a person to move the hand quickly. People without the sensation of pain are in deep trouble.

Example: The pain of grief causes people to reach out to find loved ones who are lost. Without it, there would probably be no societies or cultures. No one would look after those who are sick, search for loved ones who are lost, or stay with people who are difficult at times.

Example: Pain of experiencing fear makes people avoid what is dangerous.

💬 **Discussion Point:** What are the pros and cons of never having painful emotions? Would participants like people who never have painful emotions?

✓ **4. Rejecting Reality Turns Pain into Suffering**

Suffering is pain plus nonacceptance of the pain. Pain can be difficult or almost impossible to bear, but suffering is even more difficult. Refusal to accept reality and the suffering that goes along with it can interfere with reducing pain.

Suffering comes when:

- People are unable to or refuse to accept pain.
- People cling to getting what they want, refusing to accept what they have.
- People resist reality as it is in the moment.

Radical acceptance transforms unbearable suffering into bearable pain.

In sum, pain is pain. Suffering and agony are pain plus nonacceptance. If we take pain and add nonacceptance, we end up with suffering.

5. Accepting Reality Can Bring Freedom

Accepting reality can free us from happiness, bitterness, anger, sadness, shame, and other painful emotions. The drive to stop pain no matter the cost is the opposite of freedom. Much of life involves managing painful situations that cannot be solved immediately. Although it is easy to think that we can just get rid of pain by positive thinking or by ignoring or suppressing pain, the fact is that these strategies often do not work. Our use of these strategies is usually based on the delusion that we cannot stand the pain. We feel compelled to do something to stop the pain. We are slaves to our incessant urges to escape from the present moment.

Example: "You may have experienced the death of someone important to you. Most people, when someone dies, can't accept it at first. They keep thinking, 'That can't have happened,' and they keep expecting the person to be there. Then eventually they accept it and realize that that person really did die. When you accept it, you're still in pain, but you can move ahead with your life."

Discussion Point: When acceptance is used as a technique to create change—as a sort of "bargain with God" ("I'll accept it, and in return you promise to make it better")—it is not really acceptance, much less radical acceptance. Elicit examples of bargaining from participants.

Practice Exercise: Ask participants to think of a time when they were very disappointed in something (e.g., they were not accepted somewhere; someone died; they lost something very important; they didn't get something they wanted)—but they eventually went on with their lives anyway. Ask them first to recall when they first found out about the disappointment. How did it feel? What was their reaction? Then ask them to remember what it felt like once they finally did accept that the event had indeed happened. Discuss any differences in the experience before and after accepting the facts. Focus on whether participants felt better able to move on with their lives after accepting.

✓ ### 6. Acceptance May Lead to Sadness, but Deep Calm Usually Follows

Acceptance often comes with a lot of sadness, but even with the sadness, it feels as if a burden has been lifted. Usually once radical acceptance (i.e., acceptance all the way) has taken place, people feel ready to move on with their lives.

Fear of sadness is often at the core of difficulties with acceptance. There is no doubt that finally accepting the facts of a painful or traumatic past, or that one's present is excruciatingly painful and perhaps even not changeable, can indeed be extremely sad. For many, the fear of falling into the abyss of sadness is too overwhelming even to imagine. This may be why, when losses are severe and irreplaceable, complete acceptance usually unfolds over a very long period of time.

Examples: Acceptance of losing a child can take years. Acceptance of not being accepted to college for the third year in a row can take a long time to be fully integrated. Realizing, finally, that one does not have a childhood home to go home to for holidays can also take a long time to come to terms with.

When the past is tragic or the present is not what we would want, a sense of liberation and freedom followed by a sense of deep calmness often follows once we radically accept the facts of the situation—once we stop fighting it, suppressing it, and catastrophizing it.

💬 **Discussion Point:** Elicit from participants times when fear of sadness has interfered with acceptance. Has sadness when accepting something ever been followed by calmness or a sense of freedom? Discuss.

✓ **7.** *The Path Out of Hell Is through Misery*

Say to participants: "The bottom line is that if you are in hell, the only way out is to go through a period of sustained misery. Misery is, of course, much better than hell, but it is painful nonetheless. By refusing to accept the misery that it takes to climb out of hell, you end up falling back into hell repeatedly, only to have to start over and over again."

Examples: Exposure is a critical component of treatment for PTSD and other anxiety disorders, and it is undeniably painful. Behavioral activation and opposite action are necessary to overcome depression; each requires doing something that depressed people don't want to do at the time. It takes a lot of distress tolerance (i.e., misery tolerance) to stop self-injury, using drugs and alcohol, and anger outbursts as ways to escape emotional pain.

Research Point: PTSD is primarily a result of trying to avoid all contact with cues that cause discomfort. Pathological grieving—that is, grieving that never ends—is a result of the same avoidance. Avoiding all cues that are associated with pain ensures that the pain will continue. The more people attempt to avoid and shut emotional (as well as physical) pain off, the more it comes back to haunt them. Trying to suppress emotional pain or avoid contact with pain-related cues leads to ruminating about the painful events; paradoxically, trying to get rid of painful thoughts creates painful thoughts. For example, mindfulness is a core part of mindfulness-based stress reduction, an effective program for helping people with chronic physical pain, described in the book *Full Catastrophe Living* by Jon Kabat-Zinn.[36] (See also the section on exposure-based treatments in Chapter 11 of the main DBT text.) Experiencing, tolerating, and accepting emotional pain are the ways to reducing pain.

E. When to Use Reality Acceptance Skills

Say to participants: "There are three types of situations when reality acceptance skills are useful."

▪ "Life has dealt you major trauma, pain, or difficulty."

Examples: Many of us may have to accept not having had a loving family, things we have done in the past that we regret, opportunities that we have not had or that we passed up.

Examples: Many people have to accept that they have family members now who do not treat them well, or physical disabilities that cannot be helped.

▪ "You are in distress *but not in a crisis*. The situation is painful and cannot be changed right now. The absence of reality acceptance here can lead to irritation, grumpiness, and sometimes even tantrums that ruin your whole day. Acceptance soothes the pain."

Examples: "Reality acceptance skills can help if you are waiting in unmoving traffic and are about to be late for an important appointment; if it is raining on a holiday when you had outdoor plans; or if a person you are planning on going to a party with gets sick and can't go with you."

▪ "Problem solving isn't working. In this case, you may need to evaluate whether you are actually accepting all the facts of reality. To solve problems, you need reality acceptance skills to see and evaluate the situation clearly (or you might solve the wrong problem), to dream up effective and practical solutions, and to evaluate whether your solution is working."

Example: "You've been planning a vacation for going camping in the mountains for a long time, and you catch the flu 2 days before. You go to the doctor and dutifully follow the treatment, but your symptoms are not improving. This might be a good time to accept the reality that you are sick and should stay home in order to recover."

Example: "It's late at night. You're returning from work and are looking for your keys to enter your apartment. You look in your bag and in all your pockets, and you can't find the keys. You remember you had them when you left work, because you locked the building door on your way out. You look again in your bag and in all your pockets, and they're still not there. You keep looking, hoping that the keys will show up, although that's very improbable after the fourth thorough search. Not accepting that the keys are not in your pockets and not in your bag keeps you from walking the six blocks back to your car to see if you dropped them somewhere in your car."

Example: "You're in love with someone who tells you that he or she is in love with someone else and does not want to see you again. You believe in your heart that this is the person for you, and so for months on end you continue to try getting the person to come back to you. Failing at that, you sit in your room each night, pray to God to bring the person back, cry, and write love letters to the person (which you rip up). Not accepting that the person is not coming back keeps you from moving on and finding someone else to love and cherish you."

💬 **Discussion Point:** Elicit from participants facts of their lives that they must accept. Discuss difficulties accepting facts that are painful, unfair, or just not right.

✓ **F. What Radical Acceptance Is Not**

✓ **1. It Is Not Approval**

It is easy to accept things we like and approve of. It is very hard to accept things we don't like. This does not mean that we cannot accept things we do not like or approve of.

Example: "It is a lot easier to discover that the person you married has many more wonderful qualities than you thought than it is to discover the person has many more negative qualities than you thought. However, both are equally important to accept."

Examples: "People in jail for crimes they did not commit must accept that they are there, but they do not have to approve of the unfairness of this reality. Accepting the fact that you have been traumatized is critical to overcoming PTSD, but it does not mean that you approve of being traumatized. Accepting that you indeed have high blood pressure does not mean you approve of it."

💬 **Discussion Point:** Elicit from participants things they have had to accept in their lives that they do not approve of. Discuss.

✓ **2. It Is Not Compassion or Love**

Accepting what people do or say does not mean that we have to love them or even have compassion for them. Compassion is easier when we accept, but it is not a necessary condition of acceptance. We do not have to have loving feelings for people, animals, or things we radically accept.

Examples: "You can radically accept that there are rats in your attic, but you don't have to love them. You can radically accept that people abuse children, rape women and men, steal from the rich and poor, and start wars without liking or approving in any way. Compassion and love are easier if you radically accept the individuals and their behavior (without approving, of course), but acceptance does not require it."

✓ **3. It Is Not Passivity, Giving Up, or Giving In**

Many people are afraid to accept things, because they fear that they will then not try to change things—that they will become passive and helpless. This will happen only if, at the same time, they fail to accept (1) their feelings of dislike or disapproval, (2) the possibility that they can make changes if they put in enough effort, and (3) the possibility that it is worth their time to try to change what they don't like.

💬 **Discussion Point:** Fighting reality can interfere with problem-solving reality. Some people, however, are afraid that if they ever actually accept their painful situation or emotions, they will become passive and just give up (or give in). Elicit and discuss participants' fears that this might happen. Explain: "Imagine that you have ordered a pair of shoes online, and that when they come they are the wrong size. If you refuse to accept that the shoes are the wrong size, you will never send them back and get the size you want." Elicit examples of when accepting things as they are has helped to reduce suffering and resulted in a greater ability to reduce the source of pain. (This and the next point have been discussed above under "Why Accept Reality?" and are taken up again below in Section XIII.)

✓ ### 4. It Is Not against Change

Acceptance alone does not change a difficult situation, but it makes change possible or more likely. In fact, acceptance is essential to bringing about change.

The notion of acceptance is central to every major religion, East and West. Elicit participants' reactions to this and any experiences they have. The idea is also similar to the Alcoholics Anonymous notion of surrendering to a higher power and accepting things one cannot change. (Remember, one can change the future. What one cannot change are the facts of the past and this exact—and fleeting—present moment.)

G. Radical Acceptance: Factors That Interfere

✓ 👥 **Practice Exercise:** Ask participants to read through the items on Distress Tolerance Handout 11a, and to check those items on this optional handout that interfere with their own ability to radically accept really painful events and facts. (This exercise can be done at the beginning or at the end of reviewing the handout.) Discuss.

1. Lack of Skills for Acceptance

Say to participants: "As with other skills, you may have no idea how to do radical acceptance at first. Many individuals try to accept, but simply have no idea of how to go about it. Also, because radical acceptance is a skill, you get better at it with practice."

2. Beliefs That Accepting Reality Minimizes or Approves of It

Continue: "People often confuse acceptance with being passive or doing nothing to change or prevent future painful events. The two, however, are not the same. In fact, as we've noted throughout this discussion, you can't change something you don't accept. If you don't face the reality as it is—if you deny it—how are you going to change it? If you think that there is no cause, that it just happened magically through fate or luck, then how are you going to change it?"

"So if you want things to change, accept them, then change them. Because when we talk about accepting reality as it is, we're not saying, 'Accept reality as it is and believe it can never change.' Reality is always changing. If you want to have an influence on how it changes, your interest is to accept how it is right now."

3. Strong Emotions

"Strong emotions may interfere with acceptance, because you may feel that accepting will lead to experiencing unbearable, overwhelming emotions—such as sadness, anger at the person or group that caused the painful event, rage at the injustice of the world, overwhelming shame about who you are, or guilt about your own behavior."

H. Practicing Radical Acceptance, Step by Step

> **Note to Leaders:** Review the ways to practice radical acceptance by going over the optional Distress Tolerance Handout 11b or by reviewing Worksheet 9. If you are short on time, assign reading this handout as homework. If you review this handout, highlight the steps as checked below.

✓   *1. Observe That You Are Questioning or Fighting Reality*

Tell participants: "Describe in detail what you need to accept, without exaggerating or minimizing. Describe factually and without judgment. (See Mindfulness Handout 4b: Suggestions for Practicing Describing.) It is all too easy to fight reality without even realizing you are doing it. This is especially true when you consistently avoid contact with what you have to accept. Acknowledging that you are not accepting, therefore, is the first essential step to acceptance."

✓   *2. Remind Yourself That the Reality Is Just as It Is*

Say: "Often you can skip past nonacceptance by simply making an accepting statement to yourself. Useful statements might be 'Everything is as it should be,' 'The situation is,' 'Reality is,' or 'Every day is a good day.' This last one is a Zen saying meant to convey that everything simply is; it's neither good nor bad."

✓   *3. Consider Causes of the Reality You Need to Accept*

Go on: "Acceptance is a lot easier once you understand the causes of the situation you are trying to accept. Sometimes you may need to go far into the past to grasp all of them, but this can be very helpful. People often shy away from analyzing causes, because they equate understanding causes with making excuses. Making excuses is then equated with 'letting a person off' without a consequence for the behavior. However, you can ensure consequences for behavior and still understand the causes. In fact, without understanding the causes, it will be almost impossible ever to change the behavior you do not like."

💬 **Discussion Point:** Elicit from participants times when people have refused to understand the causes of their behavior. Elicit when participants have found it difficult even to try understanding the causes of others' behavior. Ask participants whether they have seen understanding causes as making excuses.

✓   *4. Practice Accepting with the Whole Self (Mind, Body, and Spirit)*

Continue: "The basic idea in radical acceptance is that you've got to accept all the way. To do this you need to practice 'letting go.' If you are not accepting, your body will tighten up and your muscles will tense. Letting go is letting go of the tension in your body."

Add: "If your mind screams 'No! I don't want to!' and you tighten back up, don't worry. That happens. Start over. Just start relaxing again and keep letting go. Practice saying yes to the universe. Practice mindfulness as a way to practice acceptance of the present moment."

> **Note to Leaders:** Note that the process of "letting go with your body" goes through the same muscles as progressive relaxation. (See Distress Tolerance Handout 6b.) The only difference is that participants do not tense the muscles before letting go.

All major religions and spiritual disciplines have as an important part of their contemplative and/or meditative practice a focus on breathing. The focus is intended to help the individuals accept and tolerate themselves, the world, and reality as it is. A focus on breathing is also an important part of relaxation training and the treatment of panic attacks.

✓   **5. Practice Opposite Action**

"Next, practice opposite action all the way, so that you can accept the present moment." (See Emotion Regulation Handout 10.)

- ▪ "Act as if you have already radically accepted something, and you will find in time that you have accepted it."
- ▪ "Say out loud in a convincing voice tone that you accept; say it over and over."
- ▪ "Do a half-smile and hold your hands in a willing-hands position to make acceptance easier. Do this while thinking or talking about what you are accepting."
- ▪ "Imagine yourself accepting."

✓   **6. Cope Ahead**

"Cope ahead with events that seem unacceptable." (See Emotion Regulation Handout 19.)

Often difficulties in accepting things are due to fears that the truth will be a catastrophe. In these situations, cope ahead replaces fear with a sense of mastery. Encourage participants:

✓
✓
✓
- ▪ "Imagine what you would do if you actually did accept what seems unacceptable."
- ▪ "Rehearse what you would do if you accepted."
- ▪ "Imagine solving or escaping problems that arise."

✓   **7. Attend to Body Sensations**

Say: "Attend to your body sensations while you are thinking of what you are trying to accept."

- ▪ "Notice sensations in your chest, your stomach, your shoulders."
- ▪ "Notice places in your body where you feel tight or tense."
- ▪ "Scan your body very slowly. Adopt a curious mind as you think of what you are trying to accept."
- ▪ "Practice mindfulness of current emotions when difficult emotions associated with acceptance arise—sadness, anger, fear, or shame." (See Emotion Regulation Handout 22.)

✓   **8. Allow Disappointment, Sadness, or Grief to Arise within You**

Acknowledge: "At times, acceptance leads to almost unbearable disappointment, sadness, and grief. It is very important to recognize that although you indeed may feel acute disappointment, sadness, or grief, you can survive it, and acceptance leads to finding peace at the end of the process."

✓
- ▪ "Notice sadness as it arises within you."

- ▪ "Do your best not to suppress it right away."
- ▪ "If anger follows immediately, notice how anger may be blocking or hiding sadness."
- ▪ "Do your best to let anger go and allow sadness to arise within you."

✓
✓
- ▪ "Breathe into the sadness, saying in your mind, 'Sadness is arising within me.'"
- ▪ "If it becomes unbearable or ineffective, use crisis survival skills and be kind to yourself."

- ▪ "Come back to sadness at a later point while practicing acceptance."

✓   **9. Acknowledge That Life Can Be Worth Living Even When There Is Pain**

- ▪ "Notice when you are refusing to accept painful events in your life."
- ▪ "Remind yourself that even with painful events, life can be worth living."
- ▪ "With compassion toward yourself, try to let go of resistance to accepting."
- ▪ "Let go of catastrophizing. Say in your mind, 'I can stand this. I can handle this.'"
- ▪ "Remind yourself that all lives have some margin of pain."

✓ **10. *Do Pros and Cons***

"Do pros and cons as a way to motivate yourself for acceptance."

- ■ "Fill out one of the pros-and-cons worksheets for accepting."
- ■ "Put this worksheet where you can read it when acceptance is hard."
- ■ "Review your pros and cons when resistance to acceptance arises within you."

XII. TURNING THE MIND (DISTRESS TOLERANCE HANDOUT 12)

Main Point: In order to accept a reality that feels unacceptable, we usually have to make an effort more than once. We sometimes have to keep choosing to accept reality over and over and over for a very long time.

Distress Tolerance Handout 12: Turning the Mind. A good way to teach this skill is first to discuss times when participants have tried to accept something, thought they did accept it, and then found later that they were not accepting it any more. This is a very simple handout and should not take more than a few minutes. Its goal is simply to make the main point described above.

Distress Tolerance Worksheet 10: Turning the Mind, Willingness, Willfulness. Review this worksheet with participants. When you are using this worksheet with Handout 12, review only the first section on turning the mind. You might also want to work with participants during the session in developing their plans for catching themselves when they drift out of acceptance. If so, have them write these plans down on the worksheet during the session.

Distress Tolerance Worksheets 8, 8a, 8b: Reality Acceptance Skills *(Optional)*. These worksheets cover all the reality acceptance skills. See the box at the start of Section X for instructions on use of these worksheets.

A. What Is Turning the Mind?

Turning the mind is choosing to accept. Acceptance seems to require some sort of choice. People have to turn their minds in that direction, so to speak. Acceptance sometimes only lasts a moment or two, so people have to keep turning the mind over and over and over. The more painful the event, the longer it can take to accept it fully. The choice has to be made every day—sometimes many, many times a day, or even multiple times in an hour or a minute.

Examples: "Accepting that no one wants to see the movie you want to see may be accepted rapidly. Accepting that you did not get into the school you wanted to attend, that you did not get the job offer you were hoping for, that you are disabled after a car accident, or that your child has died will each take progressively more effort and more times turning the mind to acceptance."

Turning the mind is sometimes like turning the head; it requires just a few degrees of movement. Sometimes, though, it is like turning the whole body; it requires a full turn back to the path.

Example: All of us ultimately have to accept that we are who we are, with all of our imperfections. Not doing so causes no end of suffering, grief, and sadness. For many, however, this takes repeated practice, accepting over and over and over.

Example: Often, especially when we are depressed or overly anxious, we must accept that depressive or anxiety-provoking thoughts are going through our minds. We may need to say, "A thought has arisen in my mind," and then refocus on another topic. We may need to say this many, many times before it sinks in.

💬 **Discussion Point:** Elicit reasons participants give themselves for not turning the mind to acceptance of reality as it is. What makes it so difficult to take that first step? Discuss.

✓ **B. Turning the Mind, Step by Step**

1. Observe That You Are No Longer Accepting

Explain to participants: "The first step in turning the mind is to notice that you're not accepting something. The tipoff is often anger, bitterness, annoyance, or falling into the sea of 'Why me?' Or you might find that you are always trying to escape reality; you're trying to block things out all the time; you're hiding behind other things. Or you're covering up how you're really feeling. You find yourself saying all the time, 'Why? Why is this happening? Why is this happening?'"

2. Make an Inner Commitment to Accept Reality As It Is

Continue: "The next step is to make an inner commitment to accept reality as it is. In other words, go inside yourself and turn your mind toward acceptance. The inner commitment isn't accepting. You don't have to accept right away. You just have to make the commitment."

3. Do It Again, Over and Over

Say: "Sometimes you may have to go through the first two steps again, over and over, many times in a minute. Sometimes you have to do it many times in a day."

Example: "A mundane but common example is losing your keys. You look in your pocket, and they are not there. You accept that and look elsewhere. But soon you lose your acceptance and look in your pocket again. It is still not there, you accept, and . . . you come back to the pocket again."

💬 **Discussion Point:** Elicit times participants have had to turn the mind over and over again to accept the facts of reality. Discuss.

4. Develop a Plan for Catching Yourself When You Drift Out of Acceptance

As in the skill of cope ahead (see Emotion Regulation Handout 19), planning for the future can be very helpful in behaving skillfully. Explain: "The idea here is to think through what you usually do when you are not accepting. What cues could you use to alert yourself that you are drifting away from acceptance? You might also decide to check in with yourself on some regular basis—for instance, every night before going to bed or each morning—to review whether you need to turn your mind to acceptance."

Example: "You have a job in a large store, managing returns. Customers often wait in long lines, and by the time they get to you, they are frequently hostile and angry. They insist you take back returns even when they have no receipts and the items are clearly used. You find yourself getting very judgmental and irritable, and find it very hard to accept that customers are not always nice. 'It is what it is' does not come into your mind. Thinking the problem through, you realize that the first clues that you are not accepting reality are a rising sense of irritability, and tense shoulders followed by judgmental thoughts. You then consider how you can turn your mind to acceptance when these customers come to your station. You decide, first, to try and replace judgmental thoughts with nonjudgmental thoughts. 'How could you act this way?' can be replaced with 'It is what it is' and other similar internal thoughts. 'I can't stand this' could be replaced with 'All right, this is a pain. But it's not a catastrophe.' You could say, 'I don't like it. I'm frustrated. I can stand it.' You could say, 'Everything has a cause. There's a reason these customers act this way. Maybe there are problems in their lives. Maybe they were never taught to treat people differently.' You could turn your mind all the way by relaxing your shoulders at the same time. You might remind yourself that whenever you are annoyed, frustrated, or thinking things should not be the way they are, this is an opportunity for turning the mind. The key idea here is that if you're trying to get from nonacceptance to radical acceptance, you first have to turn the mind. This will be a lot easier if you know how to identify when you need to turn your mind."

Add: "Next, practice 'cope ahead' by imagining interactions with various difficult customers. While imagining these scenes, notice your judgmentalness, tense shoulders, and irritability, and practice turning your mind by using some of the strategies you developed previously."

XIII. WILLINGNESS (DISTRESS TOLERANCE HANDOUT 13)

Main Point: Willingness is the readiness to respond to life's situations wisely, as needed, voluntarily, and without grudge.

Distress Tolerance Handout 13: Willingness. Review the handout with participants. Contrast willingness with willfulness. Most participants will know what willfulness is. Willingness is the complete opposite.

Distress Tolerance Worksheet 10: Turning the Mind, Willingness, Willfulness. When you are using this worksheet with Handout 13, review the second section on willingness. You might also want to work with participants during the session to help them better understand willfulness by filling out the part of the worksheet for willing behaviors they could engage in and willful behaviors they have done in the past. If you do this, then give participants a second copy of the worksheet to use as homework.

Note to Leaders: A good way to introduce the skill of willingness is to introduce willfulness first. You can do this by pantomiming a machine, with arms out, frantically trying to control an object. Then say, "Willfulness is also this," and sit on your hands. The point is that willfulness is trying to control the universe, as well as sitting on one's hands when something is needed. Explain that passivity is willfulness, not willingness. Willingness is complete openness to the moment and doing what is needed. Demonstrate this by standing with "willing hands," palms out.

As noted in the introduction to this chapter, the notion of willingness versus willfulness is taken from Gerald May's book[1] on the topic. If participants seem to grasp the concepts as defined below and want to hear more, you can use the two quotations from May's book in the introduction.

A. What Is Willfulness?

Define "willfulness" for participants as follows:

- ■ "Throwing yourself into trying to control events, those around you, and so on."
- ■ "Trying to control experience, avoid it or escape from it, and so on."
- ■ "Denying life or refusing to be a part of it. Giving up and sitting on your hands instead of doing what is needed in the moment."
- ■ "Holding back, saying no, or more commonly saying, 'Yes, but . . . ' "[1]
- ■ "Imposing your will on reality—trying to fix everything, or refusing to do what is needed. It is the opposite of doing what works."
- ■ "Focusing on ego, on self-centered wants, on 'me, me, me.' "
- ■ "Holding a grudge or bitterness."

Note to Leaders: Your best teaching examples here will be times when you yourself have been outrageously willful.

B. What Is Willingness?

Define "willingness" for participants as follows:

■ "Willingness is accepting what is and responding to what is in an effective or appropriate way. It is doing what works. It is doing just what is needed in the current situation or moment."
■ "Willingness is focusing on both individual and common needs."
■ "It is throwing yourself into life without reservation, wholeheartedly."
■ "It is saying yes to the mystery of being alive in each moment."
■ "It is responding from wise mind."
■ "It is committing yourself to participation in the cosmic process of the universe."

Analogy/example: Life is like hitting baseballs from a pitching machine. A person's job is just to do his or her best to hit each ball as it comes. Refusing to accept that a ball is coming does not make it stop coming. Willpower, defiance, crying, or whimpering does not make the machine stop pitching the balls; they keep coming, over and over and over. A person can stand in the way of a ball and get hit, stand there doing nothing and let the ball go by as a strike, or swing at the ball. Life is like that. People can get as upset as they want about life, but actually life just keeps coming—one moment right after the next.

Analogy/example: Life is like a game of cards. It makes no difference to a good card player what cards are dealt. The object is to play whatever hand one gets as well as possible. As soon as one hand is played, another hand is dealt. The last game is over, and the current game is on. The idea is to be mindful of the current hand, play it as skillfully as possible, and then let go and focus on the next hand of cards. Throwing a tantrum about losing the last game will interfere with winning the current game.

💬 **Discussion Point:** Elicit examples of willingness and willfulness. If you can point to recent examples of your and/or your participants' being willful or willing, so much the better. A light touch is needed. Again, if participants seem ready for a more sophisticated discussion, give May's definitions in full (see the introduction to this chapter); elicit agreements and disagreements.

👥 **Practice Exercise:** The best way to get the ideas of willingness and willfulness into active use is to start highlighting them during skills training sessions when you and/or the clients are behaving willfully and when willingly. Phrase it as a question: "Do you all think I am being willful here? Hmmm, let's examine this," or "You're not by chance being willful about this, are you?" (Clients will usually enjoy catching you in willfulness.) Or when a difficult situation or conflict emerges in a session, you can say, "OK. Let's all try to be completely willing for the next 5 minutes."

✓ **C. How to Go from Willful to Willing**

1. Observe the Willfulness

Explain to participants: "The first thing you want to do when willfulness shows up is to just notice it. You observe it. You identify it. You label it. You describe it. You experience it. You say, 'Willfulness has shown up.'"

💬 **Discussion Point:** Elicit examples of when it has been hard to notice willfulness. Discuss what gets in the way of observing it.

2. Radically Accept the Willfulness

Say: "The second step is to radically accept that at this moment you feel (and may be acting) willful. Denying willfulness is not helpful, and you cannot fight willfulness with willfulness. In essence, you have to love the willfulness."

💬 **Discussion Point:** Elicit examples of being judgmental of willfulness, either in oneself or in others. Discuss what happens when one is judgmental of willfulness. Does it reduce it or increase it?

3. Turn the Mind

Continue: "Next, turn your mind toward acceptance and willingness. Turn your mind toward participating in reality just as it is."

4. Try Half-Smiling and a Willing Posture

Go on: "If you're having trouble getting yourself to turn your mind—that is, you want to do it, but your mind isn't turning—try half-smiling and a willing posture. Relax your face, let your lips go up just slightly at the corners, and open your hands. It is hard to be willing with clenched fists. It is hard to be willing when you are grimacing and pursing your lips tightly. Half-smiling and a willing posture are opposite actions for willfulness if you have a willful facial expression (a grim tight mouth) and a willful posture. Your mind's going one way, and your body is going another."

> **Note to Leaders:** You will be teaching half-smiling and willing hands next. You can quickly teach these skills here, or just tell participants that you will be teaching these next.

5. Ask, "What's the Threat?"

Say: "When willfulness is intransigent, ask yourself, 'What's the threat?' Usually, immovable willfulness has to do with some sort of threat. We think that if we're willing, we will lose something big, or something terrible is going to happen to us. There's something dangerous out there. That may be true also."

> *Example:* "You and several friends are asked to go to the back of the line while trying to get into a concert. You get angry, because you know someone closer to the entrance and think you should be able to stand in line with them. You refuse to move, and now the people behind you are also angry. You try to let go of willfulness, but are just furious thinking that you 'should' be able to join your friends at the front of the line. Then the people nearby get angry at you, so you realize you need to calm down. You ask yourself, 'What's the threat?' and realize your fear is that if you have to go to the back of the line, you won't get good seats. But then you realize that it's not true; your friends will save you seats. Immediately your willfulness goes down, and you and your friends walk to the back of the line."

> *Example:* "You are part of a team at work, and a team member is asking you at the last minute to help out on a really important task that he or she fell behind on but that is due tomorrow. You notice willfulness coming up: 'Why me? I shouldn't have to do extra work!' You are about to say no, but you decide to ask yourself, 'What's the threat?' You realize you are willful because you want to get home and cook a special dinner you were planning for your family, and staying an hour late threatens that. When you notice this, you realize that you can call home and rearrange the special dinner for an hour later or even for tomorrow night, and no one will really mind. You can help your teammate and still have a special dinner. You decide to help out your team and be willing to do the extra task."

Really immovable willfulness usually also involves some sort of expected catastrophe. We start saying, 'Not only is there a threat, not only is it dangerous, but I won't be able to deal with it.' So we deny it. We push it away. We ignore it. Willfulness allows us to do that.

> *Example:* Mary hates her job, but is afraid to apply for a different job. She complains about it constantly at home, and her family is adamant that she should stop complaining or look for a new job. Mary is just furious at her family for putting pressure on her to do a job search. Finally she asks herself, "What's the threat?" and realizes her fear is that she will not be able to tolerate job rejections. Her family points out that her misery now is worse than any misery she will have looking for a job. She agrees, and begins looking for a new job.

Conclude: "Willingness is active participation in reality. Willingness is what you need to overcome a threat. Willingness isn't approval. And it's definitely not lying down and letting yourself get rolled over. Usually you will find that even if there is a realistic threat, it will not be a catastrophe. You will be able to use many other skills—check the facts, problem solve, cope ahead, build mastery, and so on—to avert a catastrophe."

💬 **Discussion Point:** Elicit examples of times when participants have found it really hard to let go of willfulness, due to fear of some threat. Discuss how hard it can be sometimes to actually figure out what the threat is.

XIV. HALF-SMILING AND WILLING HANDS (DISTRESS TOLERANCE HANDOUTS 14–14A)

Main Point: Half-smiling and willing hands are ways of accepting reality with the body.

Distress Tolerance Handout 14: Half-Smiling and Willing Hands. Demonstrate how to do half-smiling and willing hands before reviewing the handout. It is essential to practice both of them when you teach. The key to each is to relax the muscles of your face (in half-smiling) and of your shoulders, arms, and hands (in willing hands).

Distress Tolerance Handout 14a: Practicing Half-Smiling and Willing Hands. Review one or more of the exercises on this handout in the session.

Distress Tolerance Worksheet 11: Half-Smiling and Willing Hands. Review the worksheet with participants. Remind participants that when they practice these skills "while contemplating a source of anger," it is important that the anger not be overwhelming. See also the Note to Leaders at the end of this section.

Distress Tolerance Worksheet 11a: Practicing Half-Smiling and Willing Hands. This is an alternative worksheet to Worksheet 11. It is somewhat simpler conceptually than Worksheet 11, but also requires more writing.

✓ **A. Why Half-Smile?**

Tell participants: "Half-smiling is a way of accepting reality with your body."

Explain that emotions are partially controlled by facial expressions.[2,3] By adopting a half-smile—a serene, accepting face—people can control their emotions somewhat. For example, they can feel more accepting if their faces express acceptance. (See Chapter 9 of this manual and Chapter 11 of the main DBT text for further discussion.)

Example: "Half-smiling when thinking about someone you dislike helps you feel more accepting of them, more understanding."

✓ **B. How to Practice Half-Smiling**

Instruct participants: "To half-smile, relax your face, neck, and shoulder muscles, and then half-smile with your lips. Try to adopt a serene facial expression. Remember to *relax* the facial muscles."

Add: "It is not necessary that anyone else see the half-smile, but it is essential that you feel it. The half-smile is mainly a communication to yourself—that is, to your brain—and not to other people."

✓ 👥 **Practice Exercise:** Ask participants to imagine that they are at a party where they do not want to be. Ask them to put on a phony grin, as if they are trying to make everyone think they are enjoying themselves. Ask them to notice how their faces feel.

Then stop and instruct them to relax their faces, starting with their foreheads and going down their faces to the lower jaw. Then, with relaxed faces, they should turn their lips just slightly up at the corners—just until they feel it. Discuss the differences in the two smiles.

Note to Leaders: It is important that you do the exercise above with participants, as they may be too shy to do it. If necessary, tell participants they can face the wall when they first try half-smiling. The key to teaching this is to be sure they see that the "grinning" is phony smiling, but half-smiling is not.

It can take some individuals several practices of this skill before they experience the effect. It can be helpful for such individuals to hear feedback from others who have the experience of acceptance and lightness as they practice this. Then encourage them to continue practicing the skill with an open mind.

Practice Exercise: Have participants sit very still and try to make a very impassive face—one with no expression. Ask them to experience how that feels. Then have them relax the muscles of the face—from the forehead, to the eyes, to the cheeks, to the mouth and jaw—and experience how that feels. Finally, have them half-smile and experience how that feels. Discuss the differences.

In discussing both the "grinning" and "impassive" exercises, you can say to participants: "When your face is tense and you are grinning, you are sending your brain two conflicting messages: 'This is awful' and 'This is nice.' Another instance of sending conflicting messages is when you try to make your face into an impassive mask so that your actual emotions are not expressed. Masking, however, can have a boomerang effect. It leads to increased distress."[37, 38]

✓ **C. Why Willing Hands?**

Explain willing hands to participants as follows:

- "Willing hands is another way of accepting reality with your body."
- "The essence of willing hands is this physical position: hands unclenched, palms up, fingers relaxed."
- "Willing hands is part of opposite action all the way for anger. Clenched hands are indicative of anger. Anger is often the opposite of accepting reality. Anger says, 'What is should not be.' Anger is an emotion that motivates you to *change* reality, to fight it, to overcome it. Anger has its place. But here we are practicing reality acceptance."

Practice Exercise: Have participants sit very still with their eyes closed. First, have them imagine a conflict with someone that happened as recently as possible—one where they got really angry at the other person. Let them do this for a few moments. Then instruct them to put their hands on their thighs in a willing-hands position as they continue to imagine the conflict situation. Ask them to open their eyes and discuss the exercise. Anger is almost always a reflection of a belief or assumption that some current reality "should" be different than it is. As acceptance goes up, anger will go down, and a sense of understanding and sometimes peace will increase.

Note to Leaders: Almost always, it is difficult for people to stay as angry and nonaccepting as they were, once they move their hands to a willing-hands position. It is very helpful if you try this yourself before teaching it and then discuss how it went for you (assuming that it was helpful in reducing anger). See Emotion Regulation Handout 11: Figuring Out Opposite Actions.

D. Ways to Practice Half-Smiling and Willing Hands: Exercises

Suggest to participants these ways of practicing half-smiling or willing hands:

- "When you first awake in the morning."
- "During your free moments."
- "While you are listening to music."
- "When you are irritated."
- "In a lying-down position."
- "In a sitting position."
- "While you are contemplating a person you hate or despise."

> **Note to Leaders:** Before participants practice the final exercise listed above, it is essential that you discuss with each of them which hated or despised person they are planning to think about. Unfailingly, participants with severe problems will select the person they have had the most extreme experiences with, such as a person who has raped or abused them. They then frequently become overwhelmed while doing the exercise, and their ability to accept and tolerate goes down instead of up. Caution participants to start with "easy" people, and to move to more "extreme" people only as their skill develops. This should be presented as a shaping exercise. Compare using this skill with learning to drive a car: "You don't start learning to drive on the expressway."

XV. ALLOWING THE MIND: MINDFULNESS OF CURRENT THOUGHTS (DISTRESS TOLERANCE HANDOUT 15–15A)

> **Main Point:** When we "allow the mind," we simply let thoughts come and go—noticing them as they come and go, but not trying to control or change them. Mindfulness of current thoughts is observing thoughts as thoughts (i.e., as neural firing of the brain or sensations of the brain) rather than as facts about the world, so that observing thoughts becomes similar to observing any other behavior.
>
> **Distress Tolerance Handout 15: Mindfulness of Current Thoughts.** The key skill to teach here is the skill of differentiating thoughts about oneself and the world from facts about oneself and the world. You may need to do repeated exercises until participants can reliably notice or observe thoughts as they go through their minds. It is essential that you differentiate this skill from the emotion regulation skill of checking the facts, as well as from efforts at cognitive modification. When observing thoughts, one is in essence allowing the mind to be itself, a thought-generating, pattern-making machine as Pat Hawk, my Zen and contemplative prayer teacher used to say.
>
> **Distress Tolerance Handout 15a: Practicing Mindfulness of Thoughts** *(Optional)*. This is a list of examples of how one can practice mindfulness of current thoughts. This can be skipped or reviewed very briefly and then given out to read between sessions.
>
> **Distress Tolerance Worksheet 12: Mindfulness of Current Thoughts.** Review this worksheet with participants. If necessary, work with participants in identifying distressing thoughts. The thoughts identified can be accurate or inaccurate. Be sure participants see that the point of the worksheet is to describe thoughts running through their minds, rather than describing the events that set off the thoughts. Regardless of whether the thoughts fit the facts or not, the idea is to be more mindful of and less reactive to thoughts.
>
> **Distress Tolerance Worksheet 12a: Practicing Mindfulness of Thoughts.** This is an alternative worksheet to Worksheet 12. It is somewhat simpler conceptually than Worksheet 12, but also requires more writing.

> **Note to Leaders:** It can be helpful as you start this skill to relate mindfulness of current thoughts to Emotion Regulation Handout 22: Mindfulness of Current Emotions: Letting Go of Emotional Suffering, as well as Interpersonal Effectiveness Skills Handout 12: Mindfulness of Others.

✓ A. What Is Mindfulness of Current Thoughts?

1. It Is Noticing and Radically Accepting Thoughts

Explain to participants that mindfulness of current thoughts is noticing our thoughts and radically accepting them for what they are—sensations of the brain that come and go. The focus here is on thoughts that simply come into our minds. When these thoughts are negative or worry thoughts, we often either react to them immediately or grab hold of them and can't let go.

✓ **Practice Exercise:** Because some individuals may not know how to observe their thoughts, this is a good first exercise to be sure all can do it. Instruct participants to close their eyes and then notice thoughts that come into their minds immediately after you say a word out loud. Then, pausing between words, say five or six words (e.g., "salt," "high," "red," "circle," "up," "good"). Select some words that are likely to elicit a thought quickly (e.g., "salt" to elicit "pepper"). Ask participants what words came into their minds.

Practice Exercise: We can differentiate thoughts that come into our minds from those that we choose when we decide to think about something. Instruct participants to close their eyes and then review in their minds what they have done today. Give them a minute or so. Discuss what they thought about and how thinking about something on purpose is different from observing thoughts that come to mind.

2. It Is Changing Our Relationship to Thoughts

Observing thoughts is about changing our relationship to our own thoughts, rather than on changing the thoughts themselves. Painful and distressing thoughts, both accurate and inaccurate, go through everyone's mind at some point. The task is to find a new way of relating to negative or painful thoughts so that they do not induce so much suffering.

> **Note to Leaders:** Observing thoughts means observing not only thoughts, but also beliefs, assumptions, interpretations, internal descriptions/labels, and any other cognitive concepts. If you also have participants who are hearing voices, the same strategies can be used to be mindful of current voices: Participants can learn to react to them as simple firings of the brain, not beacons of truth.

3. The Goal Is Not a Mind Empty of Thoughts

Both secular and spiritual mindfulness practices have as an important part of their instructions simply noticing thoughts as they come and go while practicing mindfulness. Everyone, when learning to meditate or be mindful to the present moment, becomes distracted by thoughts at times. Many people erroneously believe that when practicing mindfulness they should suppress thoughts. They believe that the goal of mindfulness practice is to have an empty mind (i.e., a mind with no thoughts). Nothing could be further from the truth. Human brains generate thoughts, beliefs, assumptions, and concepts of all sorts. The idea in mindfulness is to notice thoughts—while neither becoming attached to them nor pushing them away.

💬 **Discussion Point:** Learning to let go of thoughts is extremely difficult. It takes a lot of practice. Letting go of thoughts is not the same as pushing them away. Trying to suppress painful thoughts usually makes them worse. Instead, it is allowing them to be as they are, coming and going. Discuss difficulties in letting go of thoughts.

B. Why Observe Thoughts?

✓ > **Research Point:** More and more research is showing that trying to block or suppress thoughts actually makes them worse.[39–41] One of the effective treatments for excessive worries and ruminations has individuals set aside a specific period each day to take time out and focus completely on worry thoughts.[42, 43] The treatment for obsessional thoughts involves consciously focusing on the obsessional thoughts, over and over and over.

1. Unnecessary Suffering and Reactive Problem Behaviors Are Often Caused by Thoughts

We react to thoughts instead of to the facts they are meant to represent.

> **Note to Leaders:** Relate this to the same point made in Emotion Regulation Handout 8: Checking the Facts. This idea is also the central idea underlying cognitive therapy, which focuses on the role of thoughts in eliciting negative emotions. The difference between cognitive therapy and mindfulness of current thoughts is that cognitive therapy emphasizes analyzing thoughts and, when they are irrational or inaccurate, changing the thoughts. Mindfulness of current thoughts observes but does not change thoughts.

2. Observing Thoughts Provides Distance from Them

Tell participants: "Observing your thoughts helps you separate yourself from your thoughts. It makes it easier for you to figure out what is a thought, what is a fact, and what is your emotional reaction to the thought."

Go on: "Distance also allows you to discover that you are *not* your thoughts. You are not defined by your thoughts (or by others' thoughts about you). Many people cannot separate themselves from their thoughts; they become their thoughts. Thoughts often masquerade as facts. We respond to our thoughts as if they are facts about ourselves, others, or the world. The problem here, inevitably, is that people have great difficulty accepting that a thought is just that, a thought. Most of us are attached to the belief that our thoughts represent facts about reality. Or we are attached to the idea that meaning and concepts are important—more important than the facts of 'what is.' "

✓ 3. Observing Thoughts Reveals Them for What They Are

Say: "Observing thoughts helps you see that thoughts are just thoughts. That is, they are sensations of the mind, coming and going. All thoughts are temporary, just as all sensations are temporary. A thought might come back to mind often, but it is still temporary; it comes and goes away."

✓ 4. Reacting to a Thought As If It Is a Fact Obscures Seeing "What Is"

✓ *Analogy/example:* "Asking why (an intellectual question) is usually not helpful. Life is often like mountain climbing. If you are climbing high on a mountain and you come across a crevasse, you need to know how to get across it, not why the crevasse is there."

> **Note to Leaders:** If you are including a spiritual perspective in your teaching, consider the following point that supports this rationale for mindfulness of thoughts: Experiencing reality ("what is") directly, without attending to thoughts or concepts, is the essential mystical experience. Indeed, it is the core spiritual experience across religions and spiritual traditions. If you want to expand this topic, put "mystical experience" into your search engine, and review the many sites that discuss mystical experiences.

✓ 5. Observing Thoughts Shows That They Are Not So Catastrophic

Continue: "Observing thoughts and maintaining your attention on them, instead of avoiding them or trying to get rid of them, can help you become less reactive to thoughts. Although events in life can be catastrophic, thoughts about these events are not themselves catastrophic."

6. Observing Thoughts Is the Path to Freedom

Reassure participants: "Over time and with practice, you will gradually feel more and more free, less controlled by your thoughts about the world. Letting go of trying to control thoughts or trying to get rid of them is a path to freedom. Many people believe that they should have control over their thoughts at all times. When you believe this, it is easy to become controlled by your thoughts. You lose your freedom to think as you do. Other people believe that they simply cannot bear painful thoughts; they think that they will fall into the abyss or they will die if they do not control their thoughts and what they believe. This is the road to losing freedom. Wisdom and freedom require the ability to allow the natural flow of thoughts, beliefs, and assumptions to come and go. They require experiencing thoughts but not being controlled by them. Always having to prevent or suppress thoughts is a form of being controlled by thoughts."

✓ C. **How to Be Mindful of Current Thoughts**

1. *Observe Your Thoughts*

Tell participants: "The first step is to observe your thoughts (beliefs, assumptions, interpretations, and internal descriptions or labels). Acknowledge their presence. Step back. Imagine you are on top of a mountain looking down on your thoughts below."

2. *Adopt a Curious Mind about Your Thoughts*

Say: "Next, try to observe your thoughts coming and going. Watch in your mind and ask: Where do the thoughts come from? Where do they go? Notice that every thought you have ever had has both come into your mind and also left your mind. Notice your thoughts, but do not evaluate your thoughts. Let go of judgments."

3. *Remember That You Are Not Your Thoughts*

Go on: "Do not necessarily act on a thought. Remind yourself that you have had thousands and thousands of thoughts in your life. All are gone. You are not gone. You are not your thoughts."

4. *Try Not to Block or Suppress Thoughts*

"Open yourself to the flow of the thoughts. Do not try to get rid of the emotions that go along with the thoughts. Don't push them away. Don't judge or reject them. Be willing to have your thoughts. Trying to build a wall to keep thoughts, particularly worry or other disturbing thoughts, out of your mind always has the effect of keeping thoughts coming back."

> **Note to Leaders:** These general instructions for mindfulness of current thoughts are often not useful at first. Remind participants that the point of mindfulness is to become free, so that even very distressing thoughts are not so disturbing. This takes a lot of practice. It is important to practice this skill with participants. Throughout skills training in this and other modules, often refer back to mindfulness of current thoughts, mindfulness of current emotions, mindfulness of others, and mindfulness of this one moment.

D. **Practicing Mindfulness of Current Thoughts**

> **Note to Leaders:** For each of the mindfulness exercises on Distress Tolerance Handout 15a, you can substitute other words for "thoughts" ("emotions," "sensations," "urges," etc.).

👥 **Practice Exercise:** Select one or two of the practice ideas for allowing thoughts "by observing them" from the optional Distress Tolerance Handout 15a. Instruct participants in how to do the exercise, using the instructions on the handout. Allow several minutes for each exercise. Discuss experiences.

👥 **Practice Exercise:** Go over one or several of the methods for practicing "by using words and voice tone." Practice as a group and then discuss experiences.

👥 **Practice Exercise:** Practice one or more of the methods for practicing "with opposite action." Discuss experiences.

XVI. OVERVIEW: WHEN THE CRISIS IS ADDICTION (DISTRESS TOLERANCE HANDOUTS 16–16A)

> **Main Point:** The skills in this portion of the module are specifically designed for dealing with various addictions. The skills can be taught to individual clients or added to a DBT skills program when the majority of participants in a group have serious addictions or repetitive dysfunctional behaviors they cannot stop.
>
> **Distress Tolerance Handout 16: Overview: When the Crisis Is Addiction.** This handout can be reviewed very quickly, or skipped and the information written on the board. Orient participants to what is coming next. Do not use this handout to teach the skills.
>
> **Distress Tolerance Handout 16a: Common Addictions** *(Optional)*. This handout can be used to help participants identify whether they have an addiction that might not be obvious (different from substance use disorders, etc.) and that they would like to work on.
>
> **Distress Tolerance Worksheet 13: Skills When the Crisis Is Addiction.** Review this worksheet with participants. This worksheet covers all of the skills for dealing with addictive behaviors. Use it for participants who are likely not to do a lot of homework. Bring extra copies when you teach new skills from the list.

✓ **A. Seven Basic Skills for Addiction-Related Behaviors**

List the seven basic skills for use when the crisis is addiction:

- Dialectical abstinence
- Clear mind
- Community reinforcement
- Burning bridges
- Building new ones
- Alternate rebellion
- Adaptive denial

✓ **B. Backing Down from Addiction**

Emphasize that these skills focus on "backing down from addiction." They can be remembered by starting at D and reciting the alphabet backward: D, C, B, A.

✓ **C. Common Addictions**

The definition of "addiction" is very broad and includes any repetitive behavior that an individual is unable to stop, despite the negative consequences of the behavior and the person's best efforts to stop. Individuals may have more than one addiction, but it is usually most helpful to focus on one addiction at a time.

> **Research Point:** Scientists have traditionally confined their use of the term "addiction" to substances that clearly foster physical dependence. That's changing, however. New knowledge suggests that as far as the brain is concerned, a reward is a reward, regardless of whether it comes from a chemical or an experience. And where there's a reward (as in gambling, eating, sex, or shopping, among others), there's the risk of getting trapped in a compulsion.[44] Once people get addicted, however, the pleasure of the addictive behavior may go down—but the urge to engage in the addictive behavior will not only increase, but will intensify. At that point, the addictive behavior may become reinforced not by pleasure, but by relief from the intense and unpleasant urges. Some people say that when they engage in addictive behaviors, they feel "normal" again. In these cases, a behavior that may have started with positive reinforcement (i.e., it gives pleasure) comes to be maintained by negative reinforcement (i.e., it stops unbearable distress).

Practice Exercise: Ask participants to read over the list of addictions on Handout 16a and check those that apply to them. Elicit from participants the number of addictions they checked. Asking participants to share what their addictions are can be risky, since several of the addictions may be very difficult to share publicly, and this can lead to shame, lying, or not participating. If all members of a group share the same addiction (e.g., drugs or gambling), you may want to skip this exercise until later in therapy.

> **Note to Leaders:** It is tempting to start teaching the skills from Handout 16 or 16a, but *don't do it* unless you are *not* planning on using the individual handouts for each skill.

XVII. DIALECTICAL ABSTINENCE (DISTRESS TOLERANCE HANDOUTS 17–17A)

> **Main Point:** Dialectical abstinence is a skill that synthesizes two approaches for dealing with addictive behaviors: abstinence (swearing off addictive behavior completely) and harm reduction (acknowledging that there will be slips and minimizing the damage). You and each client shift strategies between 100% absolute abstinence as long as the client stays off the addictive behavior, and relapse management should the client lapse.
>
> **Distress Tolerance Handout 17: Dialectical Abstinence.** The key idea here is that participants do not have to choose between abstinence and relapse prevention; a dialectical perspective suggests a synthesis of both. This synthesis can be difficult for some clients to accept, particularly those who are very active in Alcoholics Anonymous and other similar associations. Thus, it is important to teach the concepts clearly.
>
> **Distress Tolerance Handout 17a: Planning for Dialectical Abstinence.** The skills listed in the box "Plan for Abstinence" correspond to the skills covered in Handouts 18–21. If you do not have time to review each of these handouts in detail, you can teach the major content from this handout. A number of suggestions and DBT skills that might be helpful in putting together a harm reduction plan are also listed on this handout.
>
> **Distress Tolerance Worksheet 14: Planning for Dialectical Abstinence.** Review this worksheet with participants. Depending on how much time you have, instruct participants during the session to fill the worksheet with at least one entry for a number of the items. In session, discuss responses to the items so far. Assign worksheet as homework to be done more completely.

> **Note to Leaders:** Start by discussing the dilemma posed by alternating a commitment to abstinence with occasional or even frequent lapses.

The focus in treating addictions here follows a relapse prevention model: The intent is to foster abstinence from addictive behaviors, prevent relapse, and maximize harm reduction if there is a relapse. Relapse prevention[45–47] identifies high-risk situations and uses problem-solving skills to develop ways to both avoid and to cope skillfully with such situations and focuses on eliminating myths regarding the effects of addiction behaviors. Similar to building a life worth living as described in the Emotion Regulation module, relapse prevention focuses on building a life worth living without addictions.

✓ **A. What Is Dialectical Abstinence?**

Dialectical abstinence is a relapse prevention approach that incorporates a synthesis of focusing on absolute abstinence whenever one is abstinent even for a moment, and harm reduction following every slip even when it is very small.

1. *Abstinence*

Abstinence here means complete abstinence, which is never again engaging in the addictive behavior at any time for any reason.

2. *Harm Reduction*

Harm reduction, as the term is used here, has as its goal minimizing the harm done by a slip into the addictive behavior. It acknowledges that there may be slips, tries to minimize the damage, and is sympathetic to failures of complete abstinence. The basic goal is to manage lapses such that a lapse does not turn into a relapse.

3. *The Dialectical Tension*

Explain to participants: "The dialectical tension here is that on the one hand, you have agreed that you value living up to your potential and building a life worth living, and that your addictive behavior is incompatible with this goal. On the other hand, even with this commitment, you accept that you might have a lapse and once again engage in the addictive behavior. Thus you need a harm reduction plan."

4. *Dialectical Abstinence as a Synthesis*

In dialectical abstinence, the search is for a synthesis between abstinence and harm reduction that is more than the sum of the parts. The dialectical approach recognizes that both sides exist, and accepts both. It replaces the "either–or" relationship between abstinence and harm reduction with a "both–and" stance.

Example: Positive and negative poles on a battery are opposites, yet exist side by side.

Example: The yin and yang symbol is black and white, yet the synthesis of these is not the color gray. The synthesis transcends both.

5. *Pros and Cons*

The pro of abstinence is that people who commit to abstinence stay abstinent from their addictive behavior longer. The con of abstinence is that it usually takes people longer to recommit to abstinence once they've slipped. People who commit to harm reduction usually get back "on the wagon" faster after a slip, but also relapse quicker.

✓ 💬 **Discussion Point:** When it comes to addiction, people want to stop their addictive behaviors on the one hand, and on the other hand they very much want to engage in the addictive behaviors. When people are making a commitment to abstinence, there is usually a very intense desire to stay abstinent. After a lapse back to the addictive behavior, there is often an equally intense desire to continue with the addictive behavior. Discuss.

💬 **Discussion Point:** Ask participants whether they've tried either complete abstinence or harm reduction techniques in the past. Discuss the pros and cons of dialectical abstinence.

B. How to Do Dialectical Abstinence

Dialectical abstinence is a three-step process. First, participants must find a way to make a strong commitment to abstinence. Second, they need to plan for how to stay abstinent. And, third, they must plan for harm reduction if a lapse occurs. A shorthand version of how to do both abstinence and harm reduction is outlined on the optional Distress Tolerance Handout 17a. If you use this handout, ask participants to read through all the items and check those they think might work for them, both for staying abstinent and for harm reduction if there is a lapse. Ask people what they checked. (This exercise can be done at the beginning or at the end of reviewing the handout.)

✓ **1. Make a Strong Verbal Commitment to Abstinence in Wise Mind**

Tell participants: "Set a goal for yourself to stop your addictive behavior. Set a specific date to stop cold turkey. Make a verbal commitment to yourself, and share it publicly with other people. Because the urge to engage in addictive behavior is so strong, your commitment must be 100%. Anything short of that would set you up for failure. When faced with the urge to engage in your addictive behavior, you cannot have the idea that it is OK to give in for the moment, lapse just a little (for instance, have just one cigarette), and then plan to 'go right back on the wagon.' Such thinking undermines commitment and will make it more likely that you will decide to 'fall off the wagon' and slip back to addictive behavior."

This step can be viewed as "slamming the door shut" to addictive behaviors (see Distress Tolerance Handout 20: Burning Bridges and Building New Ones for more on this topic).

✓ Consider vegetarians. They never say "just this one time" and then eat meat or other prohibited food. Imagine you have become an "abstinitarian" who like vegetarians also never says "just this one time."

✓ ⊗ **Story Point:** "Stopping addictive behavior is like trying to win a major Olympic event. So imagine that you are like Olympic athletes and we, the skills trainers, are your coaches. For Olympic athletes, absolutely nothing is discussed before the race except winning or 'going for the gold.' If Olympic athletes thought or said that winning a bronze medal 'would be just fine,' then their training mentality, performance, and push would all be affected. Olympic athletes must also not think about falling down in a race or about what would occur if they should twist an ankle before the race. Those types of thoughts must stay out of their minds, even though these are possible outcomes. The athletes must only strive for the gold. In other words, think of yourselves as Olympic athletes in the Stop Addictive Behavior Event. The only thing you can possibly allow yourselves to think about and discuss is absolute and total abstinence."

✓ **2. Plan for Abstinence**

These points correspond to the points in the "Plan for Abstinence" sections of Distress Tolerance Handout 17a and Worksheet 14.

- ▪ "Enjoy your success, but with a clear mind; plan for temptations to relapse."
- ▪ "Spend time or touch base with people who will reinforce you for abstinence."
- ▪ "Plan reinforcing activities to do instead of addictive behaviors."
- ▪ "Burn bridges: Avoid cues and high-risk situations for addictive behaviors."
- ▪ "Build new bridges: Develop images, smells, and mental activities (such as urge surfing) to compete with information associated with craving." (Urge surfing is discussed in Section XX.)
- ▪ "Find alternative ways to rebel."
- ▪ "Publicly announce abstinence; deny any idea of lapsing to addiction" (as discussed above).

✓ **3. Prepare a Harm Reduction Plan, and Be Sure to Put It into Action Immediately after a Lapse**

Abstinence over the long run requires planning for abstinence and planning for lapses.

Example: A person practicing dialectical abstinence is like the quarterback in a football game. Quarterbacks are never fully content to obtain a few extra yards for a first down in each play; they are always striving in each play to obtain a touchdown. After the play is initiated, all efforts are oriented to run the full distance to the goal. The person practicing dialectical abstinence takes a similar approach—running like mad in the direction of the goal (abstinence), stopping only if he or she falls, and ready to resume full intent to obtain a touchdown in the next play.

Say to participants: "Adopt a dialectical view, and prepare for the possibility of failure. You must keep in your mind (way back in your mind in the very farthest part, so that it never interferes with your resolve) that if you do slip, you will deal with it effectively by accepting it nonjudgmentally and picking yourself back up. This means making a relapse prevention plan ahead of time for what you will actually do if you do slip. Who will you call? How will you remember to get right back to abstinence? What will you do to motivate yourself to get right back to abstinence? What skills will you use? Rehearse in your mind going through your crisis plan. Imagine success and a sense of mastery." Encourage participants to use the skill of cope ahead (see Emotion Regulation Handout 19).

Continue: "If you do slip, immediately fight with all your might the 'abstinence violation effect.' This can occur after a lapse when a person feels guilty, ashamed, and out of control, and wants to give up and give in. Common thoughts are 'I'm a loser,' or 'I might as well keep going now that I've started,' or 'A little more won't make a difference.' This kind of thinking can turn lapses into full-blown relapses."

Go over possible harm reduction skills for participants to rehearse and be ready to use. (These correspond to those listed in the "Plan for Harm Reduction" sections of Distress Tolerance Handout 17a and also Worksheet 14.)

- ▦ "Call your therapist, sponsor, or mentor for skills coaching."
- ▦ "Get in contact with other effective people who can help."
- ▦ "Get rid of temptations; surround yourself with cues for effective behaviors."
- ▦ "Review skills and handouts from DBT."
- ▦ "Practice opposite action (Emotion Regulation Handout 10) for shame. That is, make your lapse public among people who will not reject you once they know. If no other option works, go to an anonymous meeting of any sort and publicly report your lapse."
- ▦ "Build mastery and cope ahead (Emotion Regulation Handout 19), and checking the facts (Emotion Regulation Handout 8), can be used to fight feelings of being out of control."
- ▦ "Interpersonal skills (Interpersonal Effectiveness Handouts 5–7), such as asking for help from family, friends, sponsors, ministers, or counselors, can also be helpful. If you are isolated, help can often be found via online support groups."
- ▦ "You can conduct a chain analysis to analyze what prompted the lapse (General Handouts 7 and 7a)."
- ▦ "Problem solving right away (Emotion Regulation Handout 12) will suggest ways to 'get back on the wagon' and repair any damage you have done."
- ▦ "Distract yourself, self-soothe, and improve the moment (Distress Tolerance Handouts 7, 8, and 9) to let time pass without engaging in the addictive behavior again right away."
- ▦ "Cheerlead yourself."
- ▦ "Do pros and cons of stopping addictive behaviors."
- ▦ "Stay away from extreme thinking. Don't let one slip turn into a disaster."
- ▦ "Keep a list of all these harm reduction ideas with you all the time, ready if needed."

✓ ### 4. After a Lapse, Recommit to Total Abstinence

Emphasize: "After a lapse, recommit yourself to 100% total abstinence, knowing this was the last time that you will ever slip."

5. Cautions

Tell participants: "It is possible to do these two seemingly contradictory things—commit to absolute abstinence from addictive behavior, and accept a lapse should such behavior occur. This does not mean accepting a lapse before you have one. It will undermine your commitment to say to yourself, in the back of your mind, 'Oh, I guess it is really OK if I go ahead and engage in my addictive behavior, because if I do, I'll just do a chain analysis and recommit.' The possibility of a lapse must be buried somewhere outside of your awareness. You'll respond according to your plan, if it happens, but it will never happen."

XVIII. CLEAR MIND (DISTRESS TOLERANCE HANDOUTS 18–18A)

> **Main Point:** "Clear mind" is a middle ground between the extremes of "addict mind" (being governed by an addiction) and "clean mind" (thinking that the problems of addiction are over and there is no need to worry any more). Clear mind is the safest place to be, since it involves being clean and not engaging in the addiction, while remaining vigilant about the temptation to do so.
>
> **Distress Tolerance Handout 18: Clear Mind.** Review this handout, stressing the difference between clean mind and clear mind in particular.
>
> **Distress Tolerance Handout 18a: Behavior Patterns Characteristic of Addict Mind and of Clean Mind.** Review this handout with participants. Instruct participants to check the behaviors they engage in while in clean mind and while in addict mind.
>
> **Distress Tolerance Worksheet 15: From Clean Mind to Clear Mind.** Review this worksheet with participants. If time allows, practice with participants how they could replace one of the clean mind behaviors they marked on Handout 18a with a clear mind behavior. Assign the rest of the worksheet as homework.

✓ **A. Addict Mind, Clean Mind, and Clear Mind**

1. Addict Mind

Explain to participants: "Addict mind is your state of mind when you have given in to your addiction. You may have never tried to stop your addictive behavior, or you may have tried but relapsed. In addict mind, you are ruled by your addiction; urges to engage in the addictive behavior govern your thoughts, emotions, and behaviors. In addict mind, you are not even trying to resist your addictive behavior—or, when you are, the effort is half-hearted and ineffective."

Emphasize: "The danger of addict mind is that you are not engaging in any of the steps necessary to stop the addictive behavior. In addict mind, you are willing to do whatever is necessary to get the high that addictive behaviors bring. You may lie, steal, hide, break promises, and deny that you are in fact addicted."

💬 **Discussion Point:** Elicit examples from participants of behaviors or personal characteristics indicating that they are in the grip of addict mind.

2. Clean Mind

Continue: "Clean mind occurs when you are 'clean' and have not engaged in the problem behavior for a period of time, but you are oblivious to the dangers and temptation of relapsing. In clean mind, you may feel invincible in your fight against your addiction, and immune to the temptation to engage in the addictive behavior ever again. The distortion of clean mind is believing that you don't have an addiction problem any more."

Emphasize: "The danger of clean mind is that you may not avoid temptations and addiction cues, and may fail to use relapse prevention strategies you have developed at other times. In clean mind, you lower your guard and defenses against urges, and so you are not prepared when they hit."

3. Clear Mind

Go on: "Clear mind represents the synthesis between clean mind and addict mind. In clear mind, you are clean, while at the same time you stay aware of the dangers of relapse and actively engage in behaviors to prevent a lapse or relapse. It is the safest place to be. Clear mind is very similar to wise mind when addiction is involved."

✓ 🗩 **Discussion Point:** Elicit examples of times when participants have been in clean mind and were not vigilant to the dangers of relapsing. If you can point to examples of clean mind from your own life, do so.

> **Note to Leaders:** Be careful that the discussion stays at a general level as much as possible, so that it does not lead to an increase in participants' urges to engage in addictive behavior.

🗮 **Story Point:** "Overcoming addiction is like fighting a long war against urges to engage in the addictive behavior. The urges win a battle when you end up doing the addictive behavior, and you win when, despite the urges' attacks on you, you don't do the addictive behavior. Clean mind is forgetting the war once a few battles are over; it's thinking that because you've repelled the urges a few times, they will not come back, or that if they do come back they will be easy to repel. When you are in clean mind, you don't prepare for battle, and your defenses are down. Urges can catch you unprepared and win. Addict mind is like being under siege by the urges and believing that you can never repel them again. When you are in addict mind, you don't remember your victories; when you are defeated, you don't regroup and fight back. Clear mind is remembering both your victories and your defeats, fighting with all your might, and staying prepared for battle even when you are experiencing no urges."

✓ B. Behavior Patterns Characteristic of Addict Mind, Clean Mind, and Clear Mind

1. Addict Mind Behaviors

Say: "Behaviors characteristic of addict mind include engaging in the addictive behavior; glamorizing addiction; stealing to pay for addictive behaviors; lying, hiding, and isolating; stealing; not making eye contact with people; avoiding doctors, therapists, or people or groups who can help you; and so on."

✓ **Practice Exercise:** Ask participants to read through the list of addict mind behaviors on Distress Tolerance Handout 18a, and to check those behaviors they remember doing. (This exercise can be done at the beginning or at the end of reviewing the handout.)

2. Clean Mind Behaviors

Go on: "Behaviors characteristic of clean mind include thinking you have now learned your lesson and do not have to worry any more about the addiction; going into environments where others engage in addictive behaviors; seeing or living with people who have your addictions; acting as if all you need to get over addictions is willpower; isolating yourself; and so on."

a. Apparently Irrelevant Behaviors

Emphasize that **apparently irrelevant behaviors** are common in clean mind. Say: "These are actions that take you closer to engaging in the addictive behavior; they are steps toward addictive behaviors. On the surface, they look reasonable and unrelated to the addiction, but, collectively, they help set up a slip back into addictive behaviors. They are usually based on not thinking about your behavior and its consequences, on flat-out denial, or on delusion." Alan Marlatt[45] coined the term "apparently irrelevant decisions."

Example: "You are having a party for a close friend. Thinking that you really want to have her favorite foods, you buy her favorite cookies and ice cream for the party. You get a lot of each because you want to be sure you don't run out at the party. You have problems with bingeing and purging (and these are your usual binge foods)."

Example: "You are currently abstinent from alcohol. You have a craving for a hamburger, and you decide to go out to dinner at your corner bar, where they have really good hamburgers."

Continue: "Often the problem is not the first behavior, but rather a multiple set of behaviors in a sequence, all of which bring you closer to an overwhelming cue for addictive behavior."

Example: "Gambling is your addiction. You decide to go to visit a friend's country house north of your home. On the way, you decide to stop off at a shopping center. On the way out of the shopping center, you realize you are hungry for lunch. There is a really nice hotel next to the shopping center that serves good food in a relaxing environment. You go there and have a nice lunch. You have several hours before your friend is expecting you, so you decide you will just look in on the casino in the same hotel. As you look in, you decide you will just walk around but not gamble. Before you know it, you are gambling and never make it to your friend's house."

Practice Exercise: Ask participants to review the list of clean mind behaviors on Handout 18a. Ask them to add any behaviors that are indicative of clean mind for them.

Discussion Point: Elicit from participants examples of apparently irrelevant behaviors they engage in.

3. Clear Mind Behaviors

Conclude: "Clear mind behaviors are abstinent and vigilant for temptation. You are acutely aware that without skills, intense urges can return at any moment."

XIX. COMMUNITY REINFORCEMENT (DISTRESS TOLERANCE HANDOUT 19)

> **Main Point:** Community reinforcement focuses on restructuring the environment so that it will reinforce abstinence instead of addiction.
>
> **Distress Tolerance Handout 19: Community Reinforcement.** Review this handout, stressing the importance of reinforcement in changing and maintaining behavior.
>
> **Distress Tolerance Worksheet 16: Reinforcing Nonaddictive Behaviors.** Briefly review this worksheet with participants, and assign the worksheet as homework. Focus on replacing reinforcers for addiction with reinforcers for abstinence, and also on noticing the positive events that occur when participants are not engaging in addictive behaviors. Suggest (but do not assign) abstinence sampling.

✓ A. Reinforcement Maintains Addictive Behavior

> **Note to Leaders:** A very good description of the community reinforcement approach by William R. Miller and Robert J. Meyers, with Susanne Hiller-Sturmhofel, is available online (*http://pubs.niaaa.nih.gov/publications/arh23-2/116-121.pdf*).

1. Immediate Reinforcement Is Stronger Than Delayed Consequences

Unfortunately, the immediate reinforcement of an emotional high or emotional relief that an addictive behavior provides has a stronger effect than the delayed aversive consequences (such as remorse, guilt, and depression), which is why the addiction is maintained.

Discussion Point: Elicit from participants whether and how their addictive behavior leads to immediate pleasure or immediate relief from distress.

2. As Addictive Behavior Increases, Other Activities Decrease

As addictive behavior increases, other activities (e.g., sports, community involvement, social activities) decrease, and isolation increases. When this happens, the addictive behavior becomes more and more associated with the immediate reinforcing consequences, and thus becomes stronger and more entrenched.

Discussion Point: Elicit from participants both positive and negative consequences of their addictive behaviors.

B. Replace Addiction Reinforcers with Abstinence Reinforcers

Stopping addictive behaviors requires replacing addiction reinforcers with abstinence reinforcers. Why? It is because willpower is not sufficient to change behavior, or else we would all be perfect. In the long run, it requires making a lifestyle *without* the addictive behavior more rewarding than a lifestyle *with* that behavior. Go over the following action steps that can be helpful:

- "Search for people to spend time with who aren't addicted."
- "Increase the number of pleasant activities you engage in that do not involve your addiction." (See Emotion Regulation Handouts 16 and 17.)
- "If you cannot decide what addiction-free people or activities you like, sample a lot of different groups of people and a lot of different activities."

Practice Exercise: Ask participants to read through the "Replace Addiction Reinforcers . . . " section of Distress Tolerance Handout 19 (the list just above corresponds to this part of the handout) and check those they think might work for them. Ask people what they checked. (This exercise can be done at the beginning or at the end of reviewing the handout.)

✓ C. Get Reinforcement from Others for Not Engaging in Addictive Behaviors

1. Stay Away from Other Addicted People

Tell clients: "Stay away from other addicts who are uncomfortable with you if you are not also engaging in addictive behaviors."

2. Talk to People Who Really Love You

Say: "Teach your nonaddicted loved ones about reinforcement (if you have to). Then ask them to be vigilant for when you appear to be abstinent, and give you lots of reinforcing comments or other things they have available that could function as reinforcers."

3. Try a "Deprive, Then Reinforce" Strategy

The following strategy is designed for (1) people who do not have many potential reinforcers for abstinence in their lives; (2) people who already have most of the things that could be used as reinforcers (usually people with a fair amount of money); or (3) people who are so poor that they cannot add anything reinforcing to their lives. Say to such participants: "The basic idea is first to deprive yourself of something important that you would work hard to get back, and then give it back to yourself as a reward if you engage in the behavior you want to reinforce." Go over the steps with participants.

- "Decide on three things in your life that you really like, but that you could deprive yourself of for a week if you really had to."

Examples: Coffee; toothpaste; use of a car; carrying cash and/or credit cards; all jewelry; all but one pair of socks or underwear; texting or calling others on cell phones; sitting in chairs; watching TV; playing games.

- Week 1: "Deprive yourself of one item (Item 1) for the week." This is the equivalent of B. F.

Skinner's depriving rats of food before putting them in an experiment where food was the reinforcer. Note that the deprivation is not contingent on anything, and thus it is not being used as a punishment.

■ Week 2: "For each day you are abstinent, give yourself back Item 1 the day after. Deprive yourself of a second item (Item 2) for the week."

■ Week 3: "For each day you are abstinent, give yourself back Item 2 the day after. Give yourself back Item 1, but deprive yourself of a third item (Item 3) for the week."

■ Week 4: "For each day you are abstinent, give yourself back Item 3 the day after. Give yourself back Item 2, but deprive yourself of Item 1 again for the week."

■ "Continue to repeat the sequence."

> **Note to Leaders:** It is important to make it clear that this is not a punishment system, but a reinforcement system. For some people, this can only be done with a coach or another person to be accountable to. Suggest doing this with a counselor or therapist, a nonaddicted close friend, or a nonaddicted family member. Stress that the consequences have to be big enough that participants would actually work hard to get them.

4. Monitor Your Abstinence Motivation

"When your abstinence motivation starts to drop off, do these things."

■ "Review your plan for dialectical abstinence."

■ "Review your pros and cons for abstinence versus addictive behaviors."

D. Abstinence Sampling

Say to participants: "Abstinence sampling is deciding to try out abstinence to see what it is like and to see if there are any benefits to you of abstinence. This is like doing a personal experiment. You do not have to commit for the long term until you see how it goes. Although the short-term emotional high and relief of addiction will not be there, neither will the terrible consequences of addictive behavior."

■ "Commit to a specific number of days of abstinence, to *sample* what it would be like to live without addictive behavior."

■ "To get through abstinence sampling, implement your dialectical abstinence plan."

■ "Observe all the extra positive events occurring when you are not engaging in addictive behaviors."

XX. BURNING BRIDGES AND BUILDING NEW ONES (DISTRESS TOLERANCE HANDOUT 20)

> **Main Point:** "Burning bridges" means actively eliminating from one's life any and every connection to potential triggers for addictive behaviors. "Building new ones" refers to creating new mental images and smells to compete with the addiction urges.
>
> **Distress Tolerance Handout 20: Burning Bridges and Building New Ones.** First review the strategies for burning bridges and encourage participants to be completely honest about what bridges need to be burned to stop addiction behavior. Building new bridges here focuses on creating visual images and smells to compete with cravings. You can also discuss how building a community that will reinforce abstinence is another form of building bridges.
>
> **Distress Tolerance Worksheet 17: Burning Bridges and Building New Ones.** It can be very useful to have participants fill out at least one item in each section during the session and also have them write down the imagery they will use to help reduce cravings. The homework is then to fill out the rest of the items and also carry out the tasks of both burning bridges and building new ones.

✓ **A. What Is Burning Bridges?**

Say to participants: "Burning bridges is ultimately a skill of radical acceptance, commitment, and action, all directed toward never engaging in the addictive behavior again. The action component refers to actively cutting off, and removing from your life, all connections to potential triggers for the addictive behavior. You burn the bridge to addictive behavior so that this behavior is no longer an option."

✓ ✂ **Story Point:** "Imagine that you are in front of your house and a huge, angry elephant is closing in on you. You race into your garage and slam the door shut. The elephant is outside; you are inside. As long as you stay inside, the elephant can't harm you. But what if you've left the garage door slightly open at the bottom—just enough for the elephant to get its trunk in and lift up the door? What then? The elephant will get you. Or what if you are curious and hit the garage door opener just a little bit to see what's going on? In comes the elephant. Wham!" (Pause.)

"Burning your bridges is like going into the garage of abstinence and slamming that door shut in front of the elephant (urges to engage in the addictive behaviors). It is slamming that door down hard and not wavering or even considering opening it. It is shutting your mind to addictive behavior; it is putting up an iron wall between you and the addiction. What happens a lot of times is that you are still curious to see what the elephant is doing. So you don't close the garage door completely, or you decide after a while to open it just a little. As soon as the door is opened even a little, the elephant can get its trunk in and open the door."

✓ **B. Burning Bridges: How to Do It**

1. Make a Commitment to Getting Rid of Everything in Your Life That Makes Your Addiction Possible

Say: "First, make an absolute commitment to discarding all treats to abstinence. Walk into the garage of abstinence and slam the garage door shut."

2. List Everything in Your Life That Makes Addiction Possible

Go on: "Now make a list of all the things in your life that make your addiction possible." Now is the time for complete honesty; no holding back.

3. Get Rid of These Things

"Next, get rid of all these things. Consider getting rid of some things you might not have thought of before."

- "Phone numbers, e-mail addresses, and other contact information of people who will collude with your addiction."
- "People on social networking sites who might collude with you on your addiction."
- "Clothes and household items associated with or communicating addiction."
- "Cash that can be used to fuel addiction or secret credit cards."
- "Items in your house: food (e.g., Oreos, chocolate); drink (e.g., alcohol, coffee); magazines and catalogs; your computer, or at least your Internet connection; videos, CDs, and TV channels; smartphone apps; gym memberships; tobacco; and so on."
- Paraphernalia for your addictive behavior.
- Memberships in clubs, hotels, casinos, and so forth.

4. List and Do Things That Will Interfere with the Addiction

"Finally, list and do all the things you can do that will make it hard to continue your addiction."

- "Tell the truth about your behavior ruthlessly to others."
- "Tell your friends and family that you have quit your addictive behavior."

✓   👥 **Practice Exercise:** Ask participants to read through the "Burning Bridges" section of Distress Tolerance Handout 20 and check those they think might work for them. Ask people what they checked. (This exercise can be done at the beginning or at the end of reviewing the handout.)

💬 **Discussion Point:** Ask participants if they've had the experience of leaving a bridge intact toward addiction and having this end up contributing to a lapse or relapse. Discuss the difficulty of burning bridges and what gets in the way. Discuss pros and cons of burning bridges.

✓ C. What Is Building New Bridges?

Building new bridges is the strategy of actively imagining, as vividly as possible, visual images and smells that compete with those associated with the addictive behavior.

> **Research Point:** People who crave an addictive behavior start experiencing images and smells in their minds that are linked to the addiction. The more they focus on the addiction images, the more the craving increases, and the more difficult it gets to resist engaging in the addictive behavior. This means that the visual system and olfactory system are loaded with information when a craving occurs, so if new images and smells compete for "space" with that information, the craving can be reduced. Actively imagining images and smells that are very different from the addictive ones competes for attention with, and decreases the power of, the craved images.[48, 49]

✓ D. Building New Bridges: How to Do It

1. Create Nonaddictive Images and Smells

Say: "First, create new, nonaddictive images and smells to think about when you have an unwanted craving. These need to engage the visual and olfactory (smell) systems of your brain, and so 'steal' the space from the craving."

Example: "Whenever you crave a cigarette, imagine being on the beach. Keep the visual images and the smells of the beach in mind to reduce the craving for cigarettes."

2. Look at Moving Images; Surround Yourself with New Smells

"Also, when you have a craving, look at moving images or surround yourself with smells that are unrelated to the addiction. They will compete with information associated with your cravings."

Example: "When you crave chocolate, look at moving images or something that will engage the visual part of your brain. Or smell something that you find pleasant but that is not chocolate, such as perfume or pine needles."

3. Engage in Urge Surfing

The term "urge surfing" was coined by Alan Marlatt[50, 51] as a relapse prevention strategy for individuals addicted to alcohol and other drugs. It can be used to help with any addictive behaviors or destructive impulses.

a. Urge Surfing Is Like Surfing or Riding Out a Wave

Say: "The urge is the wave. Instead of trying to stop its movement, you surf on top of it."

b. Urge Surfing Is a Form of Mindfulness

Urge surfing involves using the mindfulness skills of observing and describing to "surf" over urges to engage in addictive behavior. Mindful urge surfing is a mindful, nonattached observing of these urges. With this skill, individuals learn over time to accept urges, cravings, and preoccupations without reacting to them, judging them, or acting on them.

c. **The Key to Urge Surfing Is Not Reacting**

Tell participants: "The key to urge surfing is stepping back and not reacting. Notice the urge moment by moment, particularly how, like a wave, it evolves and shifts over time."

d. **Urge Surfing Involves Retraining the Brain**

When people give in to their urges and engage in addictive behaviors, they reinforce the link between having an urge and acting on it. Urge surfing detaches the urge from the object of the urge (the food, drug, sex, casino, etc.). Over time, the brain learns that it is possible to experience an urge without acting on it.

e. **Urge Surfing Involves Imagery**

Say: "Imagine yourself on a surfboard riding the waves. Keep this image in your mind to help you remember that urges don't last forever—that this urge will go away, as others have done before it."

XXI. ALTERNATE REBELLION AND ADAPTIVE DENIAL (DISTRESS TOLERANCE HANDOUT 21)

> **Main Point:** Alternate rebellion and adaptive denial, as their names indicate, are adaptive alternatives to addictive behavior. If addictive behavior functions as a form of rebellion, some other type of rebellious behavior can be used as a more effective alternative to the addiction. In adaptive denial, persons with addictions convince themselves that they actually don't crave the addictive behavior (denial). For this to work, the individuals must be adamant in telling themselves that they don't have an urge for the addictive behavior.
>
> **Distress Tolerance Handout 21: Alternate Rebellion and Adaptive Denial.** The first half of this handout lists possible alternative options for rebellion. Have participants read and check off which of the examples they would be willing to try. The second half of the handout describes steps for adaptive denial.
>
> **Distress Tolerance Worksheet 17: Practicing Alternate Rebellion and Adaptive Denial.** Review this worksheet with participants. It can be very useful to have participants fill out the plans for alternate rebellion during the session, and also have them come up with something they could want or crave instead of their addictive behaviors. The homework is then to try these skills and record the outcomes.

A. Alternate Rebellion[52]

✓ **1. What Is Alternate Rebellion?**

Say to participants: "When addiction functions as rebellion, giving up addiction can be hard, because it implies that you need to give up rebelling. With alternate rebellion, you can satisfy the wish to rebel without destroying yourself or blocking your way to achieving important goals. 'Alternate rebellion' means finding another rebellious but nondestructive behavior to substitute for the addictive behavior."

✓ **2. Why Engage in Alternate Rebellion?**

Emphasize to clients: "Addiction as rebellion is ineffective. It does not help you toward your overall goal of a higher quality of life. Rebelling against a person, society, rules, boredom, or conventions, with addictive behavior is 'cutting off your nose to spite your face.' This is the opposite of the mindfulness 'how' skill of effectiveness." (See Mindfulness Handout 5.)

💬 **Discussion Point:** Elicit from participants reasons why addictive behavior is not an effective strategy for rebelling. Discuss how overall objectives for obtaining a higher quality of life are not kept in mind when addictive behavior is used to rebel.

Discussion Point: Ask participants whether addictive behavior functions in their lives partially or totally as a way to rebel. Prompt that this might be the case even if they did not intentionally choose the addiction for this purpose.

3. How to Do It

Again, alternate rebellion means rebelling *effectively*—finding a way to honor the desire to rebel in a creative way, instead of suppressing it, judging it, or mindlessly giving in to it through addiction. Make clear that there are many ways to employ this skill, and invite participants to use their imaginations.

Discussion Point: Ask participants to review the suggestions for alternate rebellion in Distress Tolerance Handout 21 and check ones they might like to try. Discuss the various alternatives.

Discussion Point: Ask participants for other effective ways to rebel.

Practice Exercise: Ask participants who don't buy into alternate rebellion (even if their addiction functions as rebellion) to do pros and cons for giving alternate rebellion a try. Point out that willfulness can get in the way of alternate rebellion.

> **Note to Leaders:** Since I originally developed this skill, a number of people have developed lists of options for alternate rebellion and put them on the Internet. Look up "alternative rebellion" or "alternate rebellion" on your search engine. Check these options out yourself before recommending any.

B. Adaptive Denial

✓ ### 1. What Is Adaptive Denial?

Explain to participants: "'Adaptive denial' refers to adamantly convincing yourself that you don't want to engage in the addictive behavior when an urge hits, or that the addictive behavior is not a possibility."

✓ ### 2. How to Do

- Begin: "Give logic a break when you are doing adaptive denial. Don't argue with yourself about believing that the urge is not there or that doing the addictive behavior is not possible."
- "Convince yourself that you want something else other than the addictive behavior."

  Example: "Fill a glass jar with dimes. Put the glass jar with dimes and another glass jar that is empty near you at all times. When you have a craving, say to yourself and out loud, 'Oh, I have to have a dime.' Then open the jar with dimes, take one out, and put it into the other jar."

- "Put off addictive behavior. Put it off for 5 minutes, then put it off for another 5 minutes, and so on. Each time, tell yourself that you only have to stand this for 5 minutes."
- "Do not replace craving for one addictive behavior with craving for another addictive behavior or for a behavior that is itself destructive."
- "Remember that replacing craving for one thing with craving for something else is to be used *only in a crisis*, when it appears clear that you are unable to tolerate intense cravings without giving in to it. Suppressing desire over the long run increases the level of desire rather than reduces it."

Discussion Point: Review the examples in Distress Tolerance Handout 21, and then ask participants to see if they can think up other examples.

References

1. May, G. G. (1982). *Will and spirit: A contemplative psychology.* San Francisco: Harper & Row.

2. Ekman, P., Friesen, W. V., O'Sullivan, M., Chan, A., Diacoyanni-Tarlatzis, I., Heider, K., et al. (1987). Personality processes and individual differences: Universals and cultural differences in the judgments of facial expressions of emotion. *Journal of Personality and Social Psychology, 53,* 712–717.

3. Ekman, P. (1993). Facial expression and emotion. *American Psychologist, 48,* 384–392.

4. Linehan, M. M., Schmidt, H., III, Dimeff, L. A., Craft, J. C., Kanter, J., & Comtois, K. A. (1999). Dialectical behavior therapy for patients with borderline personality disorder and drug-dependence. *American Journal on Addictions, 8,* 279–292.

5. Linehan, M. (2001). DBT versus comprehensive validation treatment + 12 step for multidiagnosed, opiate-dependent women with BPD: A randomized controlled trial. In A. Arntz (Chair), *Personality disorders II: Treatment research.* Symposium conducted at the World Congress of Behavioral and Cognitive Therapies, Vancouver, British Columbia, Canada.

6. Linehan, M. M, Lynch, T. R., Harned, M. S., Korslund, K. E., & Rosenthal, Z. M. (2009). *Preliminary outcomes of a randomized controlled trial of DBT vs. drug counseling for opiate-dependent BPD men and women.* Paper presented at the 43rd Annual Convention of the Association for Behavioral and Cognitive Therapies, New York.

7. Marlatt, G. A., & Gordon, J. R. (Eds.). (1985). *Relapse prevention: Maintenance strategies in the treatment of addictive behaviors.* New York: Guilford Press.

8. Supnick, J. A., & Colletti, G. (1984). Relapse coping and problem-solving training following treatment for smoking. *Addictive Behaviors, 9,* 401–404.

9. Miller, W. R., & Rollnick, S. (2013). *Motivational interviewing: Helping people change* (3rd ed.). New York: Guilford Press.

10. Jay, O., Christensen, J. P. H., & White, M. D. (2006). Human face-only immersion in cold water reduces maximal apnoeic times and stimulates ventilation. *Experimental Physiology, 92,* 197–206.

11. Foster, G. E., & Sheel, A. W. (2005). The human diving response, its function, and its control. *Scandinavian Journal of Medicine and Science in Sports, 15,* 3–12.

12. Tate, A. K., & Petruzzello, S. J. (1995). Varying the intensity of acute exercise: Implications for changes in affect. *Journal of Sports Medicine and Physical Fitness, 35,* 295–302.

13. Brown, M. Z. (n.d.). *Regulating emotions through slow abdominal breathing* (Handout). Available from *www.dbtsandiego.com/DBT2.pdf*

14. Clark, M., & Hirschman, R. (1990). Effects of paced respiration on anxiety reduction in a clinical population. *Biofeedback and Self-Regulation, 15,* 273–284.

15. McCaul, K., Solomon, S., & Holmes, D. (1979). Effects of paced respiration and expectations on physiological and psychological responses to threat. *Journal of Personality and Social Psychology, 37*(4), 564–571.

16. Stark, R., Schnienle, A., Walter, B., & Vatil, D. (2000). Effects of paced respiration on heart period and heart period variability. *Psychophysiology, 37.*

17. Linehan, M. M. (2005). *Putting your worries on a shelf: Progressive muscle and sensory awareness relaxation* [Audio recording]. Seattle, WA: Behavioral Tech.

18. Smith, R. E., & Ascough, J. C. (2015). *Engaging affect in cognitive-behavioral therapy.* Manuscript submitted for publication.

19. Hollon, S. (1989). Personal communication.

20. Goldstein, J. (1993). *Insight meditation: The practice of freedom.* Boston: Shambhala.

21. Goldstein, J., & Kornfield, J. (1987). *Seeking the heart of wisdom: The path of insight meditation.* Boston: Shambhala.

22. Kabat-Zinn, J., Massion, A. O., Kristeller, J., Peterson, L. G., Fletcher, K. E., Pbert, L., et al. (1992). Effectiveness of a meditation-based stress reduction program in the treatment of anxiety disorders. *American Journal of Psychiatry, 149,* 936–943.

23. Kabat-Zinn, J., Wheeler, E., Light, T., Skillings, A., Scharf, M. J., Cropley, T. G., et al. (1998). Influence of a mindfulness meditation-based stress reduction intervention on rates of skin clearing in patients with moderate to severe psoriasis undergoing phototherapy (UVB) and photochemotherapy (PUVA). *Psychosomatic Medicine, 60,* 625–632.

24. Kabat-Zinn, J., Lipworth, L., & Burney, R. (1985). The clinical use of mindfulness meditation for the self-regulation of chronic pain. *Journal of Behavioral Medicine, 8,* 163–190.

25. Bowen, S., Chawla, N., & Marlatt, G. A. (2011). *Mindfulness-based relapse prevention for addictive behaviors: A clinician's guide.* New York: Guilford Press.

26. Segal, Z. V., Williams, J. M. G., & Teasdale, J. D. (2013). *Mindfulness-based cognitive therapy for depression* (2nd ed.). New York: Guilford Press.

27. Zylowska, L., & Siegel, D. (2012). *The mindfulness prescription for adult ADHD: An 8-step program for strengthening attention, managing emotions, and achieving your goals.* Boston: Trumpeter Books.

28. Semple, R., & Lee, J. (2011). *Mindfulness-based cognitive therapy for anxious children: A manual for treating childhood anxiety.* Oakland, CA: New Harbinger.

29. Frankl, V. (2006). *Man's search for meaning*. Boston: Beacon Press. (Original work published 1959)

30. Gottman, J. (1994). *Why marriages succeed or fail: And how you can make yours last*. New York: Simon & Schuster.

31. Gottman, J. M., & Levenson, R. W. (1986). Assessing the role of emotion in marriage. *Behavioral Assessment, 8,* 31–48.

32. Gottman, J. M., & Levenson, R. W. (1992). Marital processes predictive of later dissolution: Behavior, physiology, and health. *Journal of Personality and Social Psychology, 63,* 221–233.

33. Goldfried, M. R., & Davison, G. C. (1976). *Clinical behavior therapy*. New York: Holt, Rinehart & Winston.

34. De Mello, A. (1984). *The song of the bird*. New York: Image Books.

35. Nagasako, E. M., Oaklander, A. L., & Dworkin, R. H. (2003). Congenital insensitivity to pain: An update. *Pain, 101*(3), 213–219.

36. Kabat-Zinn, J. (1990). *Full catastrophe living: Using the wisdom of your body and mind to face stress, pain, and illness*. New York: Delacorte Press.

37. Gross, J. J., & Levenson, R. W. (1997). Hiding feelings: The acute effects of inhibiting negative and positive emotion. *Journal of Abnormal Psychology, 106,* 95–103.

38. Gross, J. J., & John, O. P. (2003). Individual differences in two emotion regulation processes: Implications for affect, relationships, and well-being. *Journal of Personality and Social Psychology, 85,* 348–362.

39. Roemer, L., & Borkovec, T. D. (1994). Effects of suppressing thoughts about emotional material. *Journal of Abnormal Psychology, 103,* 467–474.

40. Wegner, D. M., Schneider, D. J., Carter, S. R., & White, T. L. (1987). Paradoxical effects of thought suppression. Journal of Personality and Social Psychology, 53, 5–13.

41. Wegner, D. M., & Erber, R. (1992). The hyperaccessibility of suppressed thoughts. *Journal of Personality and Social Psychology, 63,* 903–912.

42. Borkovec, T. D., & Inz, J. (1990). The nature of worry in generalized anxiety disorder: A predominance of thought activity. *Behaviour Research and Therapy, 28,* 153–158.

43. Borkovec, T. D., & Ruscio, A. M. (2001). Psychotherapy for generalized anxiety disorder. *Journal of Clinical Psychiatry, 62,* 37–45.

44. Holden, C. (2001). 'Behavioral' addictions: Do they exist? *Science, 294,* 980–982.

45. Marlatt, G. A. (1978). Craving for alcohol, loss of control and relapse: A behavioral analysis. In P. E. Nathan, G. A. Marlatt, & T. Lobe (Eds.), *Alcoholism: New directions in behavioral research and treatment*. New York: Plenum.

46. Marlatt, G. A., & Tapert, S. F. (1993). Harm reduction: Reducing the risks of addictive behaviors. In J. S. Baer, G. A. Marlatt, & R. J. McMahon (Eds). *Addictive behaviors across the life span: Prevention, treatment and policy issues* (pp. 243–273). Newbury Park, CA: Sage.

47. Marlatt, G. A., & Donovan, D. M. (Eds.). (2005). *Relapse prevention: Maintenance strategies in the treatment of addictive behaviors* (2nd ed.). New York: Guilford Press.

48. Kemps, E., Tiggermann, M., Woods, D., & Soekov, B. (2004). Reduction of food cravings through concurrent visuospatial processing. *International Journal of Eating Disorders, 36,* 31–40.

49. Kemps, E., & Tiggermann, M. (2007). Modality-specific imagery reduces cravings for food: An application of the elaborated intrusion theory of desire to food craving. *Journal of Experimental Psychology: Applied, 13,* 95–104.

50. Marlatt, G. A., Witkiewitz, K., Dillworth, T. M., Bowen, S., Parks, G. A., MacPherson, L. M., et al. (2004). Vipassana meditation as a treatment for alcohol and drug use disorders. In S. C. Hayes, V. M. Follette, & M. M. Linehan (Eds.), *Mindfulness and acceptance: Expanding the cognitive-behavioral tradition* (pp. 261–287). New York: Guilford Press.

51. Marlatt, G. A., Larimer, M. E., & Witkiewitz, K. (Eds.). (2012). *Harm reduction: Pragmatic strategies for managing high-risk behaviors* (2nd ed.). New York: Guilford Press.

52. Safer, D. J., Telch, C. F., & Chen, E. Y. (2009). *Dialectical behavior therapy for binge eating and bulimia*. New York: Guilford Press.

Index